CONGENITAL DISORDERS - LABORATORY AND CLINICAL RESEARCH SERIES

HIRSCHSPRUNG'S DISEASE: DIAGNOSIS AND TREATMENT

Congenital Disorders - Laboratory and Clinical Research Series

Hirschsprung's Disease: Diagnosis and Treatment
Ramón Núñez Núñez and Manuel López-Alonso
2009. ISBN 978-1-60741-349-3

CONGENITAL DISORDERS - LABORATORY AND CLINICAL RESEARCH SERIES

HIRSCHSPRUNG'S DISEASE: DIAGNOSIS AND TREATMENT

RAMON NÚÑEZ NÚÑEZ
AND
MANUEL LÓPEZ-ALONSO
EDITORS

Nova Biomedical Books
New York

Library of Congress Cataloging-in-Publication Data

Hirschsprung's disease: diagnosis and treatment / [edited by] Ramón Núñez Núñez and Manuel López-Alonso.
p. ; cm.
Includes bibliographical references and index.
ISBN 978-1-60741-349-3 (hardcover: alk. paper)
1. Hirschsprung's disease. I. Núñez, Ramón Núñez. II. López-Alonso, Manuel.
[DNLM: 1. Hirschsprung Disease--diagnosis. 2. Hirschsprung Disease--surgery. WI 528 H6693 2009]
RC862.M35H57 2009
616.3'4--dc22 2009008023

Published by Nova Science Publishers, Inc. ✦ New York

Contents

Foreword ix
Arnold Coran

Preface xi

List of Contributors xiii

Part I: **History, Development of the Enteric Nervous System, Physiology, Pathophysiology, Epidemiology, Classification, Genetics, and Histopathology of Hirschsprung's Disease** 1

Chapter I Hirschsprung's Disease: Historical Review 3
José Boix-Ochoa and Pilar Abad Calvo

Chapter II Biological Development of the Enteric Nervous System 15
Marie A. Breau and Sylvie Dufour

Chapter III Anorectal Physiology 45
Juan Ribas

Chapter IV Pathophysiology of Hirschsprung's Disease 55
Prem Puri and Anne-Marie O' Donnell

Chapter V Hirschsprung's Disease: Epidemiology, Classification and Associated Congenital Defects 73
Emilio Blesa, Enrique Galán and Juan J. Cardesa

Chapter VI Genetics and Hirschsprung's Disease 87
Enrique Galán, Emilio Blesa and Juan J. Cardesa

Chapter VII Histopathology of Hirschsprung Disease 107
William A. Meier-Ruge and Elizabeth Bruder

Part II:	**Hirschsprung's Disease: Clinical Features, Manometric Diagnosis, Radiological Diagnosis, Morphological Diagnosis, Differential Diagnosis, Medical Care, Enterostomies, And Bowel Preparation For Pull-Through**	**123**
Chapter VIII	Hirschsprung's Disease: Clinical Features *Ramón Núñez, Emilio Blesa and Rodolfo Cabrera*	**125**
Chapter IX	Manometric Diagnosis of Hirschsprung's Disease During the Neonatal Period *Manuel López-Alonso*	**137**
Chapter X	Radiological Diagnosis of Hirschsprung's Disease During the Neonatal Period *Manuel López-Alonso and J.Fernando Prieto*	**159**
Chapter XI	Morphological Diagnosis of Hirschsprung's Disease: Rectal Suction Biopsy *Dolores I. Segura and Manuel López-Alonso*	**169**
Chapter XII	Differential Diagnosis of Hirschsprung's Disease in the Neonatal Period *José Mª Gil-Vernet, Marta De Diego and Jesús Broto*	**183**
Chapter XIII	Hirschsprung's Disease: Preoperative Medical Care. Enterostomies. Bowel Preparation for Pull-Through *Ramón Núñez, Isabel Vargas and Mª José Estepa*	**197**
Part III:	**Hirschsprung's Disease: Classical Surgical Treatment (Swenson, Duhamel, Soave, and Rehbein), Laparoscopy in Hirschsprung's Disease, Exclusive Transanal Pull-Through, Total Colonic Aganglionosis, A Critical Review of the Different Operations for Hirschsprung's Disease**	**219**
Chapter XIV	Swenson's Technique *Luis Lassaletta*	**221**
Chapter XV	Duhamel's Technique *Piyawan Chiengkriwate*	**229**
Chapter XVI	Original Soave Procedure *Antonio Hernández-Orgaz A and Manuel López-Alonso*	**243**
Chapter XVII	Rehbein's Technique *José Mª Gil-Vernet, Jesús Broto and Marta De Diego*	**255**
Chapter XVIII	Laparoscopic-Assisted Transanal Pull-Through for Hirschsprung's Disease *Atsuyuki Yamataka and Akihiro Shimotakahara*	**261**

Chapter XIX	One-Stage Transanal Endorectal Colectomy and Pull-Through for Hirschsprung Disease in Neonates and Infants *Luis De la Torre-Mondragón and J. Arturo Ortega-Salgado*	**275**
Chapter XX	Total Colonic Hirschsprung Disease *Barbara E. Wildhaber, Daniel H. Teitelbaum and Arnold G. Coran*	**289**
Chapter XXI	A Critical Review of the Different Operations for Hirschsprung's Disease *Juan A. Tovar*	**305**
Part IV:	**Enterocolitis in Hirschsprung's Disease, Long-Term Results, Variant Hirschsprung's Disease, Intestinal Transplant, and Nutrition in Hirschsprung's Disease**	**317**
Chapter XXII	Enterocolitis in Hirschsprung's Disease *Ramón Núñez, Ana Torres and J.Ignacio Santamaría*	**319**
Chapter XXIII	Long-Term Results After Treatment of Hirschsprung's Disease *Scott A. Engum. and Jay L. Grosfeld*	**349**
Chapter XXIV	Variant Hirschsprung's Disease *Prem Puri*	**373**
Chapter XXV	Intestinal Transplant in Hirschsprung's Disease and Intestinal Pseudoobstruction *Manuel López Santamaría and Francisco Hernández Oliveros*	**385**
Chapter XXVI	Nutritional Status, Situations of Nutritional Risk, and Nutrition in Hirschsprung's Disease *Emilio Blesa and Luis Lassaletta*	**413**
Annex:	**Hirschsprung's Disease: The Parents' Experience and Informed Consent for Hirschsprung's Disease**	**429**
Chapter XXVII	Hirschsprung's Disease: The Parents' Experience *Sheyla Leal, Mª Carmen Vicente and Ángela Del Hoyo*	**430**
Chapter XXVIII	Informed Consent and Hirschsprung's Disease *Mª Ángeles López De La Torre*	**443**
Index		**463**

Foreword

Arnold Coran

It is a pleasure to write a Foreword for this new textbook devoted to Hirschsprung Disease. The editors have gathered together in this book a group of internationally known pediatric surgeons with major expertise in this disease. The spectrum of issue in the diagnosis and treatment of Hirschsprung Disease is very well covered in the 28 extensive chapters in the book. The text begins with physiology and genetics, two areas that have produced several new developments in this disease and continues on with the diagnosis, especially the histological diagnosis, an area that created great controversy in recent years. The second half of the book describes the various surgical techniques, including the laparoscopy approach for the management of this disease. A separate chapter is devoted to the very rare form of this disease, namely, total colonic aganglionosis. Finally, the last part of the book focuses on enterocolitis in Hirschsprung Disease, an entity that was poorly appreciated until recently, and the long term results of surgical treatment. The book completes its thorough coverage of all aspects of this disease with a chapter on atypical forms and other variants. Only a few books devoted to this entity have been published in the past. This new textbook adds additional information on this subject for all pediatric surgeons, especially those with a major interest in this disease.

Preface

Hirschsprung's disease is a common cause of neonatal intestinal obstruction, and represents one of the most important and fascinating pathologies for the pædiatric surgeon. Harald Hirschsprung would undoubtedly get a great surprise if he were to know how far the concept of the disease that he described in 1886 has evolved. In recent decades there have been great advances in knowledge of the genetics, pathophysiology, and treatment of this disease. Nonetheless, not everything has been resolved. Neonatal diagnosis is still difficult, and some patients may suffer grave postoperative complications such as enterocolitis, constipation, or fæcal incontinence. There is thus a need to continue working to minimize the morbidity of this disease.

Recently there was published the book: "Hirschsprung's Disease and Allied Disorders" by *Alexander M. Holschneider and Prem Puri* (Third Edition). It has extraordinary collaborators, and its content and presentation are excellent. Our sincerest congratulations.

For the editors, this new book about Hirschsprung's disease has meant a major personal challenge and great professional satisfaction. Its publication would not have been possible without the disinterested collaboration of such prestigious authors. We wish to acknowledge the great effort they have made and congratulate them on their work. Children with this disease and new generations of pædiatric surgeons will benefit from their contributions.

The aim of our book, "Hirschsprung's Disease: Diagnosis and Treatment", is to deal with the different aspects of this disease. It consists of 28 chapters covering a historical review, the biological development of the enteric nervous system, the physiology and physiopathology, genetics, histopathology, clinical features, diagnosis (with special reference to neonatal manometric diagnosis), differential diagnosis, surgical treatment (classical techniques and new methods by laparoscopy and exclusive transanal pull-through), total colonic aganglionosis, enterocolitis, the atypical forms of Hirschsprung's disease, and long-term postoperative results.

We have included some new chapters with respect to other treatises – intestinal transplant, nutrition in Hirschsprung's disease, a critical review of the different surgical techniques, Hirschsprung's disease:The parents' experience and informed consent for Hirschsprung's disease.

The book will be of great help to pediatric surgeons, pediatric gastroenterologists and pediatricians in general. But it may also be useful for parents of children with this disease.

In addition to the authors, we would like to express our gratitude for their collaboration in this book to Robert Chatwin, to Antonio Amador of the Service of Orientation and Teacher Training (SOFD) of the UEx, to the Faculty of Medicine of the UEx, to the *General Directorate of Knowledge Management and Quality Control* of the Extremadura Health Service (*SES*) and to the Foundation *Reina Mercedes* for Health Research (*Sevilla*). Also, we want to thank the authors of chapter 27 for their collaboration in this book. They are parents of children with Hirschsprung's disease who want to contribute with their experience in this book.

Finally we would like to thank the editorial Nova Publishers for their interest in publishing this book.

Ramón Núñez Núñez
Manuel López-Alonso

List of Contributors

Pilar Abad Calvo MD
Service of Paediatric Surgery,
Hospital Sabadell,
Corporació Sanitaria Parc Tauli,
Barcelona,Spain

Emilio Blesa MD PhD
Professor of Pediatrics
Service of Pediatric Surgery
Hospital Materno Infantil
Complejo Hospitalario Universitario
Calle la Violeta S/N
06010 Badajoz, Spain

José Boix-Ochoa MS PhD
Emeritus Professor
Paediatric Surgeon
Autonomous University
Barcelona, Spain

Marie A. Breau PhD
Division of Developmental Neurobiology,
National Institute for Medical Research,
Mill Hill, London NW7 1AA, United Kingdom.

Jesús Broto MD
Department of Pediatric Surgery
Hospital Universitario del Vall de Hebrón
Avda del Vall de Hebrón
Barcelona, Spain

Elizabeth Bruder MD
Department of Pathology
University of Basel
Schönbeinstrasse 40
4003 Basel
Switzerland

Rodolfo Cabrera MD PhD
Department of Pediatric Surgery
Hospital Universitario Infantil Virgen del Rocío
Avda Manuel Siurot s/n
41013 Sevilla, Spain

Juan José Cardesa MD PhD
Full Professor & Head
Department of Pediatrics
Hospital Materno Infantil
Complejo Hospitalario Universitario
Calle La Violeta S/N
06010 Badajoz, Spain

Piyawan Chiengkriwate MD
Pediatric Surgery Unit,
Department of Surgery, Faculty of Medicine,
Prince of Songkla University,
Hat Yai, Songkhla, 90110Thailand

Arnold G. Coran MD
University of Michigan Medical Center Head
Section of Pediatric Surgery
F3970 Mott Children's Hospital
Ann Arbor, MI 48109-0245 USA

Marta De Diego MD
Department of Pediatric Surgery
Hospital Germans Trias i Pujol.
Badalona Spain.

Luis De La Torre-Mondragón MD PhD
Full Professor of Pediatric Surgery
Universidad Nacional Autónoma de México
Hospital para el Niño Poblano and Hospital Ángeles Puebla
Av. Kepler No. 2143 Col. Unidad Territorial Atlixcayotl,
Puebla CP 72810
México

Sylvie Dufour PhD
UMR144, Centre National de la Recherche Scientifique
Institut Curie, 26 rue d'Ulm
75248 Paris Cedex 05
France

Scott A. Engum MD
James Whitcomb Riley Hospital for Children
Indiana University School of Medicine,
Department of Surgery
Indianapolis, Indiana, USA

Maria J. Estepa PhD
Service of Pharmacy
Hospital Perpetuo Socorro
Complejo Hospitalario Universitario
Avda: Damián Tellez Lafuentes S/N
06010 Badajoz, Spain

Enrique Galán MD PhD
Professor of Pediatrics. Genetics Unit
Department of Pediatrics
Hospital Materno Infantil
Complejo Hospitalario Universitario
Calle La Violeta S/N
06010 Badajoz, Spain

José Mª Gil-Vernet MD
Department of Pediatric Surgery
Hospital Universitario del Vall de Hebrón
Avda del Vall de Hebrón
Barcelona, Spain

Jay L. Grosfeld MD
Department of Pediatric Surgery
Riley Children's Hospital
702 Barnhill Drive-Suite 2500
Indiamapolis, IN 46202
USA

Francisco Hernández Oliveros MD
Department of Pediatric Surgery
Transplantation Unit
Hospital Universitario "La Paz"
P. de la Castellana 261
28046, Madrid, Spain

Antonio Hernández-Orgaz MD
Department of Pediatric Surgery
Staff Pediatric Surgeon
Hospital Universitario Infantil Virgen del Rocío
Avda Manuel Siurot s/n
41013 Sevilla, Spain

Luis Lassaletta MD PhD
Department of Pediatric Surgery
Hospital Universitario "La Paz"
P. de la Castellana 261
28046, Madrid, Spain

Manuel López-Alonso MD PhD
Department of Pediatric Surgery
Staff Pediatric Surgeon, Director Center for motility
and functional gastrointestinal disorders,
Hospital Universitario Virgen del Rocío.
Avda Manuel Siurot s/n
41013 Sevilla, Spain

Manuel López Santamaría MD PhD
Department of Pediatric Surgery
Transplantation Unit
Hospital Universitario "La Paz"
P. de la Castellana 261
28046, Madrid, Spain

Maria Ángeles López de la Torre
Graduate in Law
Laws Certificate in European and Comparative Law
Master in Labour and Social Security Law
Calle Bami 27 2A
41013 Sevilla, Spain

William A. Meier-Ruge MD PhD
Department of Pathology
University of Basel
Schönbeinstrasse 40
4003 Basel
Switzerland

Ramón Núñez Núñez MD PhD
Service of Paediatric Surgery
Hospital Materno Infantil
Complejo Hospitalario Universitario
Calle La Violeta S/N
06010 Badajoz, Spain

Anne-Marie O`Donnell
Children's Research Centre,
Our Lady's Children's Hospital,
Crumlin
Dublín 12, Ireland

J. Arturo Ortega Salgado MD
Professor of Pediatric Surgery
Centro Medico Nacional 20 de Noviembre – ISSSTE
Felix Cuevas 540 Mexico City
Mexico

J. Fernando Prieto MD
Staff Radiologist, Department of Radiology,
Hospital Universitario Virgen del Rocío.
Sevilla, Spain

Prem Puri MD FRCS FRCS(Ed) FACS
Professor & Director of Research
Children's Research Centre
Our Lady's Hospital for Sick Children
Crumlin
Dublin 12, Ireland

Juan Ribas MD PhD
Full Professor of Physiology
Facultad de Medicina
Universidad de Sevilla
Sevilla, Spain

J. Ignacio Santamaría MD PhD
Service of Paediatric Surgery,
Hospital Materno Infantil
Complejo Hospitalario Universitario
Calle La Violeta S/N
06010 Badajoz, Spain

Dolores I. Segura MD
Staff Pathologist, Section of Histochemistry,
Department of Pathology,
Hospital Universitario Virgen del Rocío.
Sevilla, Spain

Akihiro Shimotakahara, MD PhD
Assistant Professor
Department of Pediatric General and
Urogenital Surgery
Juntendo University School of Medicine
2-1-1 Hongo, Bunkyo-ku,
Tokyo 113-8421,
Japan

Daniel H. Teitelbaum MD
Section of Pediatric Surgery
University of Michigan Medical School
Ann Arbor, Michigan
C.S. Mott Children's Hospital
Ann Arbor, MI 48109
USA

Ana Torres MD
Service of Paediatric Surgery,
Hospital Materno Infantil
Complejo Hospitalario Universitario
Calle La Violeta S/N
06010 Badajoz, Spain

Juan A. Tovar MD PhD
Professor & Head
Department of Pediatric Surgery
Hospital Universitario "La Paz"
P. de la Castellana 261
28046, Madrid, Spain

Isabel Vargas ARNP
Service of Paediatric Surgery
Hospital Materno Infantil
Complejo Hospitalario Universitario
Calle La Violeta S/N
06010 Badajoz, Spain

Barbara E. Wildhaber MD
Section of Pediatric Surgery
Hôpital des Enfants
Rue Willi Donzé 6
1211 Genève 14
Switzerland

Atsuyuki Yamataka MD PhD
Professor & Head,
Department of Pediatric General and
Urogenital Surgery
Juntendo University School of Medicine
2-1-1 Hongo, Bunkyo-ku
Tokyo 113-8421
Japan

Part I: History, Development of the Enteric Nervous System, Physiology, Pathophysiology, Epidemiology, Classification, Genetics, and Histopathology of Hirschsprung's Disease

In: Hirschsprung's Disease: Diagnosis and Treatment
Ed: Ramón Núñez Núñez and Manuel López-Alonso
ISBN: 978-1-60741-349-3

Chapter I

Hirschsprung's Disease: Historical Review

José Boix-Ochoa and Pilar Abad Calvo

"Knowing the history will improve the future ..."
P.Abad 2009

In 1886, the great Danish pediatrician, Harald Hirschsprung, gave a lecture to the Berlin Paediatric Society describing the clinical and autopsy findings in two infants who had died of constipation associated with dilatation and hypertrophy of the colon.

Hirschsprung [1] was not the first to describe this condition; there had been previous over 20 case reports [2,3], but he was the first to recognize the fact that a congenital malformation might be the cause of the disease, which is named after him.

Hirschsprung's Disease and Harald Hirschsprung

The earliest description of a case of Hirschsprung's disease is an autopsy report on a five-year-old girl with "an enormous dilatation of the colon" by Frederick Ruysch in 1691 [4].

Harald Hirschsprung was born in Copenhagen in 1830. He was the eldest of three brothers and was expected to manage the father's tobacco company when his father retired. But Harald studied medicine and revealed an interest in research in pediatrics at the Royal Maternity Hospital. Hirschsprung studied congenital occlusion of the small intestine reviewing 31 patients (four Danish, and other from international literature). He subdivided the symptoms and pathologic signs into three groups: the congenital stricture, the valvular occlusion and the total break of the continuity. On 11 May 1861, defended his doctoral thesis "The Congenital Occlusion of the Esophagus, together with contribution to the knowledge of the congenital occlusion of the small intestine"[5].

In 1870 he was appointed chief paediatrician in the Children's Hospital in Rigensgade, Copenhagen, where worked from 1870 to 1879. This year was opened the new hospital "The

Queen Louise Hospital for Sick children after called Denmark's Queen Louise and during 25 years Hirschsprung was its chief. Every year would participate in pediatric conferences especially in Germany and Austria. In 1886 at the annual meeting in Berlin, Hirschsprung presented two cases observed in 1880 and 1885 respectively. "*As you will see, it is a colon, but a colon of such a size that it will no doubt surprise you to learn that it comes from a child only 11 months old when it died. ...When the abdominal cavity was opened, a couple of extremely dilated intestines emerged, that was the sigmoid and the other part of the intestine turned out to be somewhat dilated. Only rectum was no dilated, nor indeed subject to any obstruction.* "

Hirschsprung first saw this patient at eight months old and had a chronic propensity to constipation, with gross abdomen. Four years after, Hirschsprung observed another patient, a seven month old male and concluded ..."*the two cases must be caused by the same disease*". He was the first to explain the anatomic and clinical course of the disease. He observed the onset of symptoms in the first week of life and he assumed that it must be congenital [6]. Despite the fact that impacted stool was present in the colon on abdominal examination, digital examination of the rectum reveled an empty vault. He was not able to account for the pathogenesis of the disease, but his publication attracted the attention of the medical society to congenital megacolon and after 1888 the congenital megacolon has been known as Hirschsprung's disease. Harald died in 1916, at the age of 85 years. He was not a surgeon but he was a great contributor to pediatric surgery with descriptions about "constipation in newborns with colonic dilatation, cases of esophageal atresia with tracheoesophageal fistula and he was the first to described congenital hypertrophic pyloric stenosis E.H.P", all treatable surgical conditions. Today a bronze replica of Hirschsprung marble bust is in the garden of the Queen Louise Hospital for Children, Copenhagen, Denmark, remembering this great paediatrician [7].

The term "megacolon" was introduced by Mya in 1894, bringing attention to the current interpretation of the large colon as the source of the problem [8].

Incidentally, in 1897, Doctor Fredericks Treves performed resection of the involved narrow segment, he made a colo-anal anastomosis and the patient was cured." He said that *having made an elliptical incision around the evidently narrowed anus I proceeded to remove the anus and remaining portion of the rectum.* Treves resected the colon below the splenic flexure, including the narrow segment and the rectum, and he anastomosed the transverse colon to the anal skin [9] and the follow-up of this patient was reported by Johnson HD, et al. [10].

The aetiology of the condition remained in doubt and Hirschsprung's disease was often mistaken for acquired megacolon. This is surprising, because as early as 1901 Tittel [11] reported degeneration of the cells of Auerbach's and Meissner's plexus in the apparently normal colon distal to the dilated segment, in the rectum of a 15 month old infant who had been constipated since birth.

Similar observations were made by Hawkins [12] in 1907, Finney [13] in 1908, Dalla Valle in 1920 [14] and [15] in 1924 and Cameron [16] in 1928.

At the beginning of the 20th century,there were 3 different groups of authors and 3 concepts of pathogenesis of Hirschsprung' disease.The first group included those who promoted the theory of congenital megacolon: Hirschsprung, Mya, Genersich and Neugebauer.

The second group, which opposed the advocates of congenital causes of megacolon and instead proposed mechanical obstruction as an explanation, was represented by Fenwick, Wilms, Trevers, Fitz, and Chenisse. This faction saw megacolon as an analogy of hypertrophic pyloric stenosis.

The third group, represented mainly by Marfan, Griffith, Jacobi, Cooncetti, and Perthes, thought the mains cause of Hirschsprung disease was an unusually long sigmoid colon as well as vent mechanisms on the colon, which are caused by bending or folding of prolonged bowel [17].

Robertson and Kernohan [18] and Tiffin, Chandler and Farber [19] published papers prior to 1940, both of which expressed the belief that the cause of Hirschsprung's disease was the absence of peristaltic activity in the aganglionic segment of distal bowel.

Theodor Ehrenpreis: Megacolon in the Newborn

In 1940 Theodor Ehrenpreis of Sweden observed the motility disturbance present from birth in 10 infants with Hirschsprung's disease. In 1946 [20] doctoral thesis, an review of the etiology and pathogenesis of Hirschsprung's disease, pointed out that the diagnosis could be made in the neonate and published a detailed review of the disease in the neonatal period. The study contended that the megacolon developed after birth, and he attempted to prove this by performing barium enemas on newborns and monitoring them by repeated examinations. Some of the examinations films were reproduced in his monograph, and it's possible to suspect a narrow distal segment in some of the cases.

The Thesis [21]: "Megacolon in the newborn. A clinical and roentgenological study with special regard to the pathogenesis" was submitted to public discussion in the Great lecture Theatre of the Royal Caroline Institute on May 18th 1946, Stockholm. In the autumn of 1943 the author commenced a study of intestinal obstructions in newborns on the basis of a material from the Kronprinsessan Lovisas Children's Hospital covering ten years. *Some cases shows that the arisal of the megacolon disease is not necessarily due to a primary colon dilataion; the dilatation may occur secondary as a sequel to the chronic obstipation.* After the review of the literature he described the three principle theories:

I. *The malformation theory* is based on a number of cases described as megacolon, with colon dilatation in fetuses, newborns and infants verified roentgenologically or at autopsy.
II. *The obstruction theory.* It is an established fact that dilatation of the colon arises proximally to a manifest mechanical obstruction.
III. *The neurogenic theory.*The advances registered by neurosurgery in the treatment of megacolon have been accepted as proof of the accuracy of the neurogenic theory. The elimination of the sympathetic (inhibitory) influence on the motility of the colon ought naturally to yield improvement whether the disturbance in motility is entailed by a congenital colon dilatation, a relative obstruction, or a pathological innervation.

In the first chapter, T.Ehrenpreis, described the basis for the study of the size and length of colon thus consists of 100 normal cases in the ages of from 1-12 days. For study the megacolon in newborns the material consisted of 10 cases of megacolon, debuting at birth, subjected during the first 10 days of life to clinical and roentgenological examination and subsequently followed.

In chapter 2, described the technic. The basis for this study is roentgenograms, mainly obtained by means of contrast enema. The properties of the colon studied are the reaction to the contrast enema, the emptying power, the occurrence of haustral markings, the degree of redundancy, and the size of lumen.

Chapter 3 is titled roentgenological aspect of the colon in the healthy newborn infant, and concluded that the size of the colon shows great variations.

But it is in chapter 4, Megacolon in the newborn. Clinical and roentgenological onset and early development that described the onset of the disease is with great regularity distinguished by three cardinal symptoms, namely constipation, abdominal distension and vomiting. The obstipation was present from birth in seven of the cases in the form of absence of meconium discharge, scanty discharge or hard meconium discharge. Abdominal distension is diffuse and rounded and progressed rapidly after their initial appearance. The fairly good general condition of all of the cases is noteworthy. Roentgenological onset, scout films of the abdomen, and the administration of contrast in order to reveal or to exclude the presence of a mechanical obstruction. The reaction towards the contrast enema, the emptying, the haustrations, the degree of redundancy and the size of lumen have been studied and compared with the corresponding conditions in the normal material. Pictures taken after evacuation of the enema show practically no contractions of the colon, and a marked retention of the enema in comparison with the normal emptying films. Complete or nearly complete emptying did not occur in any case. The clinical development, improved after enemas and intestinal lavage, and the children temporarily became practically free of symptoms, but obstipation, abdominal distension and vomiting again set in after the lapse of one week. The symptoms were again relieved by enema and intestinal lavage but the effect was of short duration and the morbid picture gained an increasingly chronic character. The transition from a normal colon size in roentgenological development to the typical megacolon has thereby been gradual. Clinically the initial stage resembles the morbid picture of a low intestinal obstruction. *If a newborn infant does not normally pass the meconium during the first days of life, continues to be constipated, reveals vomiting and abdominal distension though a good general condition, the following reasons for the symptoms are to be taken into consideration: 1) atresia or marked stenosis within the distal portion of the bowel, 2) microcolon, 3) megacolon and, 4) meconium retention. An immediate X-ray examination is indicated. Contrast enema and films after evuation of the enema. When the occurrence of an organic obstruction can be ruled out the immediate object of the treatment in both cases will be limited to efforts to empty the bowel by conservative measures.*

At the end of the thesis, the discussion of the pathogenesis confirmed that the dysfunction of evacuation was manifest from the onset in all of the cases, and has thus no morphological nor mechanical explanation and should accordingly be denoted as primary in the pathogenesis of the megacolon disease. *The neurogenic theory, the assumption of a disturbance of innervation as the origin of the megacolon disease, the disfunction of evacuation has been demonstrated as primary to the dilatation of the colon and independent of the redundancy of the colon and other obstructive factors. It seems plausible and probable that the dysfunction of evacuation is the expression of a disturbance of innervation of the colon.*

Theordor Ehrenpreis stablished final conclusions: *The observations made in the present investigations seems to justify the conclusions that the dysfunction of evacuation is primary in the pathogenesis of the megacolon disease, that the dilatation of the colon develops secondarily, and that the redundancy of the colon is a phenomenon physiological for the infant age and without pathogen significance. The involvement of a disturvance of innervation in the pathogenesis of the megacolon disease is probable…and thus seems adequate to define the megacolon disease as a dysfunction of evacuation of the colon of as yet unknown origin, occurring in the absence of morphological and mechanical causations and giving rise secondarily to a characteristic dilatation of the colon.*

In 1943 Whitehouse et al. at the Mayo Clinic reviewed the various treatments in vogue they advocated resection of the dilated colon leaving the normal colon above and below [22].

Orvar Swenson

Orvar Swenson, after completing his training at the Peter Bent Brigham Hospital, worked as attending surgeon at the Boston Children's Hospital were a number of patients with congenital megacolon were cared for [23]. He spent time in a group of children with megacolon who were in very but condition despite some having had resection to remove the dilated portion of the colon and others having undergone sympatectomy.

The first child treated "JM" had rectosigmoid colostomy function. A recording balloon placed in the proximal limb of the colostomy recorded regular forceful contractions. In the distal limb there were no contractions. Instillation of barium showed a narrow irregular lumen. Injection of a thick paste also was done, and this failed to be expelled. Neuhauser's radiologic studies [24] demonstrated the narrow rectum and distal colon, the transition zone, and the proximal dilatation. They examined old barium enema films of patients with megacolon and in 20 instances they were suspicious that the rectosigmoid was considerably smaller than the massive proximal colon. This configuration of the distal colon in Hirschsprung's disease became the standard diagnostic test for this entity.These x-ray supported the belief that the etiology of the disease was a physiological defect in the narrow segment, wich served as a partial obstruction, and that removal of this segment of colon with reestablishment of intestinal continuity would be the treactment. These investigations, supported a new concept of the cause of this disease. And served as the basis for designing the operation [25].

In 1946 they tested this procedure in animals, removing the rectum down to the anus, and the animals remainded continent.

But the senior surgeons at Boston Children's Hospital did not accept this view, and when "JM" had recovered, his colostomy was closed. For several weeks worked well, after which his symptoms returned and a colostomy was performed again. After that, the symptoms disappeared. This confirmed that there must be partial physiological obstruction in the rectosigmoid. Two additional patients were observed whose clinical courses were identical. When their colostomy was closed, the constipation recurred and a new colostomy became necessary. Robert Gross, who succed Dr Ladd as Chief Surgeon at Boston Children's Hospital, permitted Swenson to embark on a radical treatment, which was the opposite of resection of the dilated colon. After these experiences, in June 1947, "JM" had resection in the manner planned at laboratory before. The patient did well, and 3 months later his colostomy was closed. Forty years after the operation, he was a normal, healthy married man with four children.

This was the fist evidence that the etiology of the disease was the defective narrow distal segment, and it explained why removal of the dilated segment did not cure the disease.

This work was presented at the January meeting of the Society of University Surgeons in 1948 [26].

During the same year Zuelzer and Wilson [27] and Whitehouse and Kernohan [28] published histological studies showing that the disease was due to congenital aganglionosis of the distal segment of the large intestine and these findings were confirmed by the subsequent observations of Bodian, Stephens and Ward [29], Swenson, Rheinhard and Diamond [30] and Hiatt [31].

Swenson conducted an investigation to define what the nature of the abnormality was in the defect segment. For five patients with megacolon who had transverse colostomies, they obtained recordings from two positions: the dilated colon and the narrow segment. They found that regular contractions were present in the dilated colon but that none existed in the narrow segment, except for small changes that were entirely different from those in the dilated colon. In addition, the intraluminal pressure was higher in the narrow segment than could be demonstrated in the normal colon. To be sure that these changes were not normal, two patients with a transverse colostomy and a normal left colon had recordings obtained in the same manner. Both had regular progressive contractions from all three recording positions. When distal resections were performed on the patients with megacolon, strips of tissue were removed from the specimens and ganglion cells were not present. Thus, it was established that it was aganglionic, and that its intraluminal pressure was higher than normal, indicating a failure of relaxation. [32].

In 1949 Swenson et al. published: "abstract of the original article, the clinical syndrome kown as Hirschsprung disease, or congenital megacolon, had been recognized for more than a century. The pathogenesis of the dilation/ hypertrophy of the colon without mechanical obstruction was puzzling, and the subject of great debate. Virtually all infants and children affected with this disorder died. The authors studied 26 patients with congenital megacolon admitted to Boston Children's Hospital during a 5 year period, from 1943 through 1947. Careful contrast radiografhic study of the distal colon in all 26 revealed a functional obstruction produced by a dyskinesia of the rectum. This was detected by running a small amount of barium slowly into the rectum with the patient in an oblique position. A portion of the rectum/ rectosignoid was consistently subnormal in calibre. Barium then was allowed to run through this narrowed area into the dilated colon. The authors interpreted the radiographic fidings as evidence of a physiologic partial obstruction of the rectum / rectosigmoid.

Colostomies were performed in the dilated portion of the colon in 3 early patients, and all symptoms / signs of HD disappeared in each instance. These returned, however, with closure of the colostomies and persisted until the ostomy in an additional 12 patients, and each was relieved os symptoms with restoration of a a normal calibre colon. The authors recognized that the distal obstructing segment would have to be removed before the colostomy could be closed. They divesed a special "pull-through" form of resection and tested it in the laboratory. The operation was performed subsequently on 23 patients, with no fatalities. Closure of the colostomy was possible in all but 2. The authors outlined the operation in detail in the article. Three infants, the youngest being 2 months old, tolerated a one-stage operation. The aurhtors indicated that all patients subsequently demonstrated the urge to defecate and had normal bowel control. Patients with HD have a physiologic obstruction in the nondilated segment of colon. Early colostomy relieves the symptoms/ signs of obstruction, and removal of the narrowed segment results in cure.[33]. They proposed in this 1948 article that a full thickness rectal biopsy shoud be performed to make the definitive diagnosis of HD [34].

Swenson published a follow up article in 1951 rewiewing his experience with 82 patients. He described a manometric study performed on 5 patients. Three small rubber tubes with ballons attached were inserted through a transverse colostomy and positioned so that one ballon was at the splenic flexure, one in the descending colon, and one in the rectosigmoid. The ballons were inflated with 10 mL of air and was attached to recording manometers. Two patients with transverse colostomies resulting from a right colectomy for gangrenous intussusception served as control subjects. The kymographic tracings revealed a progression of peristaltic waves from the transverse colon to the anus in the 2 control patients, and normal peristalsis in the dilated and hypertrophied colon in the patiens with congenital megacolon without progression of the waves into the rectosigmoid. The distal balloon recorde only slight contractions, a fraction of the amplitude of the normal peristaltic waves in the proximal colon. Swenson pointed out that the diagnosis of congenital megacolon may be difficult to establish in newborn and young ingfants, because dilatation of the colon was usually minimal and the abrupt change in calibre from the sigmoid to rectosigmoid was not present. Twelve of the 82 operated patients, suffered an acute illness characterized by vomiting, severe diarrhea, and abdominal distension with fever, enterocolitis. Swenson experienced a child who had a recurrence of obstructive symptoms, and at reoperation, an 8 cm aganglionic segment was found that had been missed at the mishap, "rapid sections" were made during surgery to identify the extent of the proximal aganglionic bowel.

In Gross's classic textbook, published in 1953, he described the various causes of intestinal obstruction. Atresia and stenosis of the large and small intestine were seen in 212 patients, malrotation in 156 patients, meconium ileus in 63 patients, and annular pancreas in 10 neonatal patients. A total of only 70 patients with Hirschsprung's disease were presented, and these represented infants and children as well as newborns. In contrast, in a series reported from the University of Michigan, Hirschsprung's disease was surpassed only by necrotizing enterocolitis (NEC) as a cause of neonatal intestinal obstruction.

In 1957 the Swenson follow up was 200 patients treated for HD. He realized that a number of operated patients developed one or more severe or fatal enterocolitis. Swenson made a technical revision in the pull-through procedure. The anastomosis of the properly innervated bowel was placed 1.5 cm from the anus in the initial operation. He proposed a partial internal sphinterectomy be performed.

Duhamel, Soave and Rehbein

The apparent morbidity of the Swenson pull-through operation led to the development of several other operative techniques.

Duhamel's operative procedure [35] and Soave's [36] application of the endorectal pull through procedure are outstanding contributions.

Duhamel looking for an easier and safer procedure, described a operation that avoided extensive pelvic resection and excluded the rectum [37]. In this operation, normally innervated proximal colon is anastomoses with the posterior rectal wall in a side-to-side manner. Stricture or a persistent septum often resulted in recurrent fecal impaction.

Soave proposed to remove the mucosa of the narrow rectal segment, leaving a seromuscular cylinder with normal blood and nerve supply. The normally innervated colon was brought though the aganglionic muscular cuff, allowing a redundant 10 cm portion to protrude through the anus. Twenty-one days later, when spontaneous healing was accomplished, the stump was resecte by cautery. Boley modified the operation by performing direct anastomosis of the anal verge during the initial anorectal pull-throug operation.

Professor Fritz Rehbein, developed a procedure for Hirschsprung's disease that bears his name in 1953. During his career he successfully used this operation on nearly 400 children. His procedure remains the operation of choice in many pediatric surgical centers world wide. Textbooks of pediatric surgery never mention Rehbein's procedure. But Swenson, Duhamel, Soave and Rehbein have published their present views on the surgical procedures they introduced in the book "Hirschsprung's disease" of which Professor Alexander Holschneider was the editor. The principle for treatment by Rehbein's procedure is to remove the aganglionic narrow segment including the dilated sigmoid colon by dissection of the upper rectum deep down into the pelvic cavity about 2 cm from peritoneal reflection and to elimination of the achalasia of internal anal sphincter by vigorous dilatation. Rehbein limited his operations to patients of approximately 3 months of age, removed the defective colon and made the anastomosis deep in the pelvis. [38].

Further, 46% of all patients with Hirschsprung's disease were diagnosed in the neonatal period. This increasing percentage of Hirschsprung's disease in newborns with intestinal obstruction is the result of the increased sophistication of clinical, radiologic, and pathologic diagnostic techniques. Data obtained by Kleinhaus et al. in their 1979 review of 1196 patients support this trend. Until 1955 the mean age of 6 months reported between 1971-1975. The percentage diagnosed by age 3 months increased from 20% before 1955 to 64% between 1971-75. The percentage diagnosed by 1 month of age simultaneously increased from 5% to 50% during the same periods. The importance of making the diagnosis in newborns is underscored by the increased mortality in newborns when this diagnosis is overlooked. Klein and Scarborough in 1954 reported a 70% mortality, Hoffman and Rehbein a 28% mortality, and Shimm and Swenson in 1966 reported a mortality of 33%. This was caused most often by the development of enterocolitis. Conversely, in those series where the diagnosis was made early and / or treatment of enterocolitis instituted more promptly, there was no mortality because of a greatly decreased incidence of enterocolitis or its complications [39].

Traditionally, surgical therapy for Hirschsprung's disease has consisted of a proximal defunctioning colostomy that is followed months later by a definitive reconstructive pull-through procedure in which the aganglionic colon is resected and the normally innervated bowel is brought down and sutured and to the area just above the anal sphinter.

So, Georgeson and De la Torre

In 1981. So et al. [40] were the first to report a one-stage pull-through operation in neonates with Hirschsprung's disease without a preliminary colostomy. The one-stage pull-through procedure became increasingly popular in the 1990s [41-43].

In 1995, Georgeson [44] described a minimal-access one stage laparoscopic approach consisting of transanal submucosal dissection combined with laparoscopic mobilization of the rectum.

De la Torre-Mondragon and Ortega-Salgado [45] in 1998 as well as Langer [46] in 1999, described a one-stage totally transanal approach that had the theoretical advantage of eliminating the need for intrabdominal rectal mobilization. Both the laparoscopic and transanal approaches have been associated with shorter hospital stays, less pain, shorter time to oral feeds, lower costs, and improved cosmesis.

Since then the transanal procedure has been used extensively [47-52]. Despite the fact that this technique has now been widely adopted by surgeons all over the world, there remain a number of controversies regarding the optimal approach.

Swenson said:

> The key to curing these patients is to remove the defective segment, and good results are achieved by all methods…but infortunately, some problems remain concerning the treatment of megacolon: 1. The management of children with total colonic aganglionosis is not uniformly satisfactory and 2. the enterocolitis.

Because Hirschprung's history is alive new papers arrive ours hands [53,54].

….Solid foundations, the last stone isn't yet in place.

References

[1] Hirschsprung H. Stuhlträgheit Neugeborener in Folge von Dilatation and Hypertrophie des Colons. *Jahrb Kinderheilkd*, 1888;27: 1-7.

[2] Joyle F. La dilatation congenital idiopathique du colon. *Presse Med*, 1909; 17: 803.

[3] Kleinschmidt H. Aetiologie des Megacolon. *Arch Dis Chir*, 1926;142: 91.

[4] Leenders E. Sieber W K. Congenital megacolon observation by Frederick Ruysch – 1691. *J Pediatr Surg*,1970;5: 1-3

[5] Hirschsprung H. *Den medfodt tillukning af spiseroret samt bidrag til kundskaber om den medfodte tyndtarms-tillukning* [Thesis]. Copenhagen: S. Trier, 1861.
[6] Roed Petersen K, Erichsen G. The Danish Pediatrician Harald Hirschsprung. The Surgeon's Library. *Surg, Gynecol Obstet* 1988;166: 181-5.
[7] Touloukian RJ. Pediatric Surgery between 1860 and 1900. *J Pediatr Surg* 1995; 30: 911-6.
[8] Mya G. Due osservazioni di dilatazione ed ipertrofia congenital del colon. *Sperimentale* 1894;48: 215.
[9] Treves F. Idiopathic dilatation of the colon. *Lancet* 1898;1: 267-79
[10] .Johnson HD, Dawis H, Ewans JH. Letters to editor. *Lancet* 1957;1: 1143-4.
[11] Tittel K. Über eine angeborene Missbildung des Dickdarms. *Wien Klin Wochenschr* 1901;14: 903-7.
[12] Hawkins, H P. Idiopathic Dilatation of the Colon. *Br Med J* 1907;1: 477.
[13] Finney J. Congenital idiopathic dilatation of colon. *Surg Gynecol Obstet* 1908;6:624.
[14] Dalla Valle A. Ricerche istologiche di un cas di megacolon congenital. *Pediatria*, 1920; 28: 740-52.
[15] Dalla Valle A. Contributo alla conoscenza della forma famigliare del megacolon congenito. *Pediatria*, 1924;32:568.
[16] Cameron J A M. On the Aetiology of Hirschsprung's Disease. *Arch Dis Child*, 1928; 3: 210.
[17] Skaba R. Brief historial review. Historic milestones of Hirschsprung's disease (commemorating the 90 th anniversary of Professor Harald Hirschsprung's death). *J Pediatr Surg* 2007, 42: 249-51.
[18] Robertson H E, Kernohan J W. The Myenteric Plexus in Congenital Megacolon. *Proc Staff Meet Mayo Clin* 1938;13:123.
[19] Tiffin, M E Chandler, L R, Farber H K Localised Absence of the ganglion Cells of the Myenteric Plexus in congenital Megacolon. *Am J Dis Child* 1940;59:1071.
[20] Eek S, Knutrud O. Megacolon congenitum Hirschsprung. *J Oslo Cy Hosp* 1962; 12: 245.
[21] Ehrenpreis T. Megacolon in the newborn. *Acta Chir Scand* 1946;94 Suppl 112, 1-111.
[22] Whitehouse F, Bargan JA, Dixon CF: Congenital megacolon: Favorable end results of treatment by resection. *Gastroenterology* 1943;1: 922-37.
[23] Swenson O. My early experience e with Hirschsprung's disease. *J Pediatr Surg* 1989; 24: 839-45.
[24] Swenson O, Neuhauser E B D, Pickett L K. New concepts of etiology, diagnosis and treatment of congenital megacolon (Hirschsprung's disease). *Pediatrics* 1949;4: 201-9.
[25] Swenson O. How the cause and cure of Hirschsprung disease were discovered. *J Pediatr Surg*, 1999; 34: 1580-7.
[26] Swenson O, Bill A H. Resection of Rectum and Rectosigmoid with Preservation of the Sphincter for Benign spastic lesions producing *Megacolon. Surg* 1948; 24: 212-220.
[27] Zuelzer W W, Wilson J C. Functional Intestinal Obstruction in a congenital Neurogenic Lesion in Infancy. *Am J Dis Child* 1948;75: 40.
[28] Whitehouse F R, Kernohan J W. Myenteric Plexus in Congenital Megacolon. *Arch intern Med* 1948;82: 75.

[29] Bodian M, Stephens F D, Ward B C. Hirschsprung's Disease and idiopathic megacolon. *Lancet* 1949;1: 6-11.

[30] Swenson O, Rheinhard H F, Diamond I. Hirschsprung's Disease. *New Engl J Med* 1949;241:903.

[31] Hiatt R B. The Pathological Physiology of Congenital Megacolon. *Ann Surg* 1951; 133: 313-320.

[32] Swenson O. Early of the therapy of Hirschsprung's disease: facts and personal observations over 50 years. *J Pediatr Surg* 1996; 31: 1003-8.

[33] Sieber WK. Hirschsprung's disease. In: Welch KJ, Randolph JG, Ravitch M M, O'Neill JA, Rowe MI (eds). *Pediatric Surgery*. Fourth Edition.Vol 2. Chicago: Year Book Medical Publishers INC.1986. p.995-1020.

[34] Fitzgerald J F. Commentary. *New Concepts of the etiology, diagnosis and treatment of congenital megacolon (Hirschsprung's disease)* by Osvar Swenson Pediatrics. 1998; 102; 205-7.

[35] Duhamel B: Retrorectal and transanal pull-through procedure for the treatment of Hirschsprung's disease. *Dis colon Rectum* 1964;7: 45-8.

[36] Soave F. Hirschsprung's disease: A new surgical technique. *Arch Dis Child* 1964;39:116-24.

[37] Duhamel B. Une nouvelle opération pour le megacolon congenital: L'abaissement retro-rectale et trans-anale du colon, et son application possible au traitement de quelques autres malformations. *Presse Med* 1956;64:2249-50.

[38] Rehbein F, Von S, Zimmermann H. Results with abdominal resection in Hirschsprung's disease. *Arch Dis Child* 1960;35: 29-37.

[39] *Essentials of Pediatric Surgery.* Rowe MI, J O'Neill JA, Jr, Grosfeld JL, Fonkalsrud EW, Coran AG. St Louis: Mosby; 1995.

[40] So HB, Schwartz DL, Berker JM, Daum F, Schneider KM. Endorectal "pull-through" without preliminary colostomy in neonates with Hirschsprung's disease. *J Pediatr Surg* 1980;1:470-1.

[41] Hackam DJ, Superina RA, Pearl RH. Single-stage repair of Hirschsprung's disease: a comparison of 109 patients over 5 years. *J Pediatr Surg* 1997;32:1028-31

[42] So HB, Becker JM, Schwartz DL, Kutin ND. Eighteen years' experience with neonatal Hirschsprung's disease treated by endorectal pull-through without colostomy. *J Pediatr Surg* 1998;33:673-5.

[43] Ramesh JC, Ramanujam TM, Yik YI, Go DW. Management of Hirschsprung's disease with reference to one-stage pull-through without colostomy. *J Pediatr Surg* 1999;34:1691-4

[44] Georgeson KE, Fuenfer MM, Hardin WD. Primary laparoscopic pull-through for Hirschsprung's disease in infants and children. *J Pediatr Surg* 1995:30:1017-21.

[45] De la Torre-Mondragon L, Ortega-Salgado JA. Transanal endorectal pull-through for Hirschsprung's disease. *J Pediatr Surg* 1998; 33: 1283-6.

[46] Langer JC, Minkes RK, Mazziotti MV. Transanal one-stage Soave procedure for infants with Hirschsprung disease. *J Pediatr Surg* 1999; 34: 148-52.

[47] Albanese CT, Jennings RW, Smith B, Bratton B, Harrison MR: Perineal one-stage pull-through for Hirschsprung's disease. *J Pediatr Surg* 1999 Mar;34:377-80.

[48] Teitelbaum DH, Cilley RE, Sherman NJ, Bliss D, Uitylugt ND, Ranaud EJ et al. A decade of experience with the primary pull-through for hirschsprung disease in the newborn period: a multicenter analysis of outcomes. *Ann Surg* 2000;232:372-80.

[49] Langer JC, Durrant AC, De La Torre L, Teitelbaum DH, Minkes RK, Caty MG, et al. One-stage transanal Soave pullthrough for Hirschsprung disease: a multicenter experience with 141 children. *Ann Surg*, 2003;238:569-83.

[50] Nasr A, Langer J C. Evolution of the technique in the transanal pull-through for Hirschsprung's disease: effect on outcome. *J Pediatr Surg* 2007:42:36-40.

[51] El-Sawaf MI, Drongowski RA, Chamberlain JN, Coran AG, Teitelbaum DH. Are the long-term results of the transanal pull-through equal to those of the transabdominal pull-through?. A comparison of the 2 approaches for Hirschsprung disease. *J Pediatr Surg* 2007: 42: 41-7.

[52] Pratap A, Gupta DK, Shakya VC, Adhikary S, Tiwari A, Sherestha P et al.: Analysis of problems, complications, avoidance and management with transanal pull-through for Hirschsprung disease. *J Pediatr Surg*, 2007;42:1869-76.

[53] Dasgupta R, Langer JC. Evaluation and management of persistent problems after surgery for Hirschsprung disease in a child. *J Pediatr Surg*, 2008;46:13-9.

[54] Yamataka A, Kaneyama K, Fujiwara N, Hayashi Y, Lane GJ, Kawashima K et al. Rectal mucosal dissection during transanal pull-through for Hirschsprung disease: the anorectal or the dentate line? *J Pediatr Surg*. 2009;44:266-9.

In: Hirschsprung's Disease: Diagnosis and Treatment
Ed: Ramón Núñez Núñez and Manuel López-Alonso
ISBN: 978-1-60741-349-3

Chapter II

Biological Development of the Enteric Nervous System

Marie A. Breau and Sylvie Dufour

The studies on the genetics of the most frequent human defect affecting the development of the enteric nervous system (ENS), the Hirschsprung's disease (HSCR), together with extensive analysis of various animal models of this disease, have allowed a growing understanding of both normal and pathological development of the ENS, at the tissue, cellular, and molecular scales. In this chapter, we aim at giving a picture of the current knowledge of the different steps of ENS development, mostly in the mouse model, as well as the cellular and molecular mechanisms involved.

Embryonic Origin of the ENS

The ENS comprises all the neurons and glial cells present in the wall of the intestine. It is composed of interconnected ganglia, which are organised in two concentric plexi: the myenteric plexus, located between the longitudinal and circular smooth muscles, and the more internal submucosal plexus. The entire ENS, excluding its extrinsic innervation and Cajal cells [1], develops from precursor cells formed in a particular embryonic structure, the neural crest. In vertebrates, neural crest cells (NCC) are formed following complex induction processes in a territory running along the antero-posterior axis of the embryo, at the boundary between the neural plate and the non-neural ectoderm [2, 3]. In mice, NCC detach from this zone just before closure of the neural tube on about day 8.5 of embryonic development (E8.5). They then migrate through embryonic tissues, following defined pathways and subsequently differentiating into various cell types, including melanocytes, Schwann cells, sensory, sympathetic and parasympathetic neurons, the neurons and glial cells of the ENS, and the neuroendocrine cells of adrenal medulla. In addition, it is also believed that connective structures (dermis, skeleton, cartilage and certain muscles) of the face and neck are also derived from NCC [4].

A panoply of molecular tools and techniques has made it possible to map NCC derivatives. It has been shown that the derivatives obtained from NCC depend on the location of their origin along the antero-posterior axis of the embryo. Cephalic, vagal (somites 1 to 7; VNCC), trunk (somites 8 to 28 in chick and 8 to 24 in mice) and sacral NCC (SNCC) have been identified, from the most anterior to the most posterior. Melanocytes arise from NCC distributed along the whole length of the antero-posterior axis, whereas the cells forming the different types of ganglia of the peripheral nervous system originate from well-delimited regions. In particular, the ganglia of the ENS arise from populations of NCC emanating from the vagal and sacral regions of the neural tube. The first demonstration of the embryonic origin of the ENS was obtained from experiments involving ablation of the dorsal neural primordium at the vagal level (somites 1 to 7), including the NCC and the dorsal part of the neural tube [5]; these ablations resulted in an absence of the ENS in the intestinal wall. More than 20 years later, the techniques for grafting between quail and chick developed by Nicole Le Douarin were used to confirm the contribution of VNCC to ENS development [6-8]. The use of these grafting techniques also led to the identification of a second source of precursors contributing to the ENS: the SNCC [6]. The existence and importance of this second source remained controversial for more than 25 years (see for example, [9-11]). It now appears that the SNCC are involved in the formation of only a small proportion of neurons and glial cells in the colon [11-13].

Modes of Intestinal Colonisation by NCC

The ENS originates from precursor cells forming in a particular region of the embryo, the neural crest, at some distance from the intestine. The development of the ENS must therefore necessarily involve the invasion of the growing intestine by the VNCC and SNCC. The VNCC enter the intestine via its anterior (rostral) extremity and then progress through the gut mesenchyme towards the posterior (caudal) end, in a rostrocaudal wave of colonisation [10]. The spatial and temporal details of the progression of these cells within the intestine were described using transgenic [14,15] and immunological [16-18] markers of VNCC. In mice, VNCC colonise the intestine between E9.5 and E14 (figure 1). The VNCC leave the dorsal zone of the neural tube on E8.5 and migrate to the anterior end of the intestine, which they reach by E9.5. By E10.5, the VNCC have penetrated the intestinal mesenchyme and colonised the future oesophagus, stomach and part of the future small intestine (midgut). They start to invade the caecum at E11.5. They arrive in the middle of the colon (hindgut) at E12.5 and reach the posterior end of the intestine at E14 [17]. In mice, the SNCC migrate from the dorsal neural tube to the pelvic plexus and invade the distal colon in a caudorostral manner after the arrival of the VNCC, with which they mix in the posterior-most part of the intestine [12,13]. In addition to determining the timetable of the gut invasion, some studies have revealed the existence of chains and sheets of cells at the migration front in mice ([16] and figure 2, A and B) and chick [18]. The colonisation of the intestine by VNCC has recently been analysed by videomicroscopy over several hours, in cultured intestines. The VNCC were visualised in the intestinal tissues of transgenic mice expressing green fluorescent protein (GFP) or yellow fluorescent protein (YFP, a variant of GFP) in NCC [13,19,20]

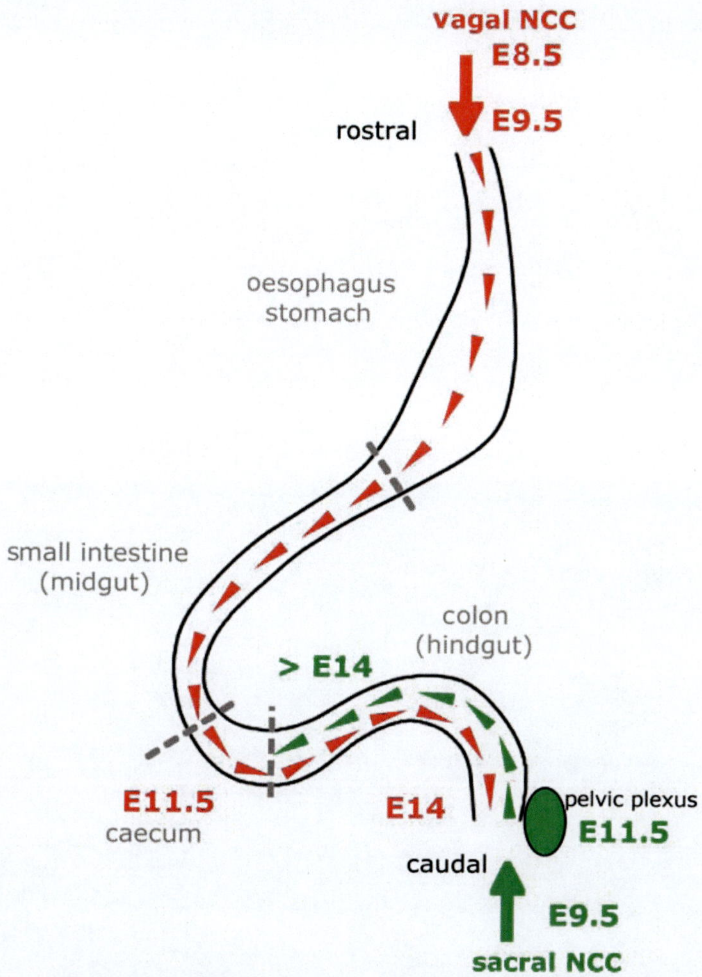

Figure 1. The colonisation of the developing gut by VNCC and SNCC (adapted from [174]).

These dynamic analyses confirmed that VNCC progress by forming chains of cells in the linear parts of the intestine — at E10.5 in the ileum and from E12.5 in the colon. Certain cells momentarily leave their chain and become isolated, later being reincorporated into the original chain or joining another chain. Two chains can also join up and then rapidly form new chains, moving in divergent directions, at the point of intersection (figure 2, C-F). The cells contributing to the formation and progress of these chains are located in a 300 μm-wide zone behind the migration front. In this zone, the VNCC seem to migrate caudally towards the front, along the chains established by the cells of the front. These dynamic studies have also shown that the migration front advances at 35 to 40 μm/h in the linear zones. In addition, many cell division events have been observed at the migration front, suggesting that proliferation is an important process in the colonisation of the intestine by the VNCC. The cells located more rostrally are more static than the VNCC of the migration front and migrate over only small distances. They form a network of nodes linked by branches. The positions of these nodes in any given region seem to correspond to the points of intersection between chains previously formed at the migration front in that region. Thus, the leading VNCC leave behind them a network structure that persists for several hours. This suggests that these VNCC constitute a sort of scaffold or frame over which the more rostral cells and neuronal projections advance [19].

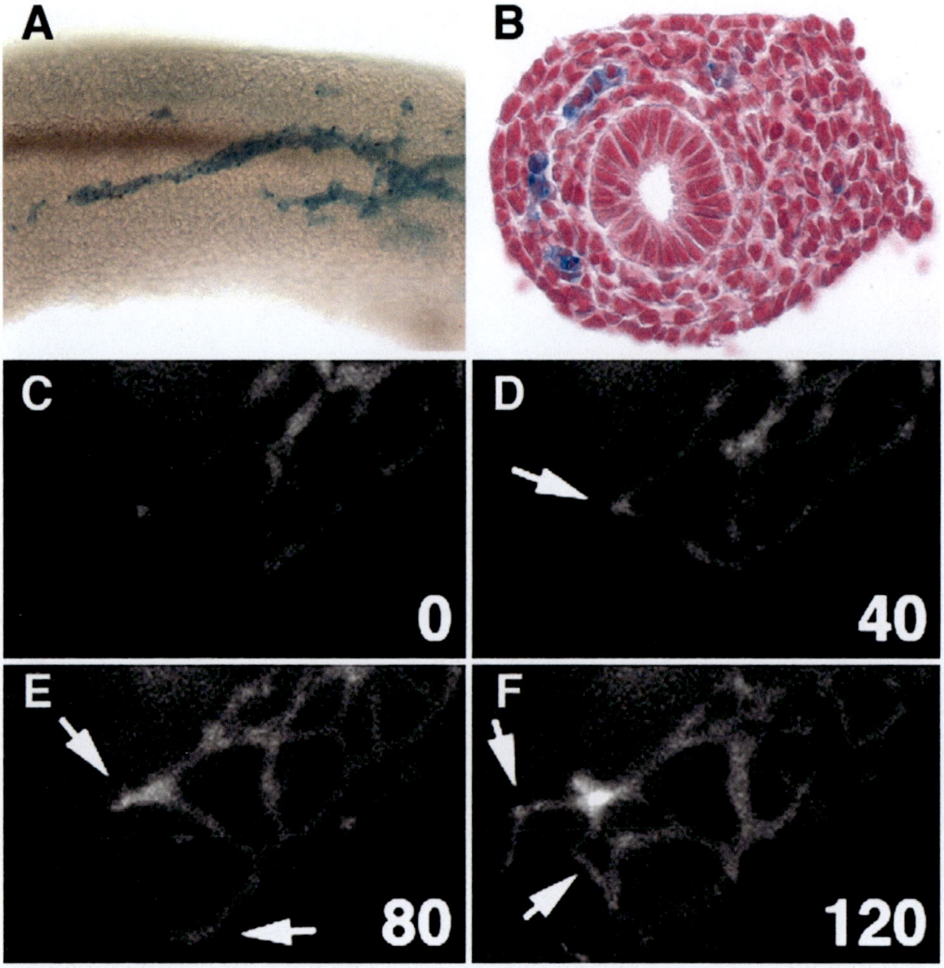

Figure 2. VNCC migrate as chains in the developing hindgut (E12.5). In A, VNCC are revealed by an Xgal whole-mount staining detecting beta-galactosidase activity in HtPA-Cre/R26R transgenic embryos [151]. Chains of cells, as well as isolated VNCC, can be observed at the migration front. VNCC interact with each other within the chains, but are also in close contact with neighbouring mesenchymal cells as shown in B, which represents a transverse section of the hindgut at the migration front. (C-F) The YFP fluorescence allows the visualisation of the VNCC within the living gut tissue dissected from transgenic HtPA-Cre/R26RYFP E12.5 embryos (Breau et al., unpublished results). The migratory chains progress in the gut wall in a highly dynamic manner (time scale in minutes). The arrows point out the developing chains and nodes that are formed at the intersection of two previous chains.

Studies of the invasion of the caecum region have shown that the behaviour of the VNCC in this zone differs from the chain-like migration pattern characteristic of the linear regions of the intestine [21,13]. Rather than forming chains, the furthest advanced cells detach from the population and migrate into the body of the caecum. There they join up to form small aggregates, projecting small chains towards other aggregates. The resulting interactions between small aggregates establish a network in the caecum and proximal colon [13]. The differences between VNCC behaviour in the caecum and in linear regions probably reflect differences in the cellular and molecular mechanisms controlling the progress of the VNCC population in successive regions of the intestine.

Importance of the Intestinal Growth and Differentiation Programme in the Establishment of the ENS

The intestine grows during the wave of rostrocaudal colonisation by the VNCC. However, this growth — involving elongation and, to a lesser extent, thickening — is not uniform in time and space. Midgut elongation in chick occurs after the arrival of the VNCC. By contrast, the most important episode of caecum and colon growth coincides with the arrival of these cells [22]. This also seems to be the case in mice, although the phases of growth of the different regions of the intestine in relation to VNCC colonisation have not been quantified.

The intestinal tube is formed by invagination of the endoderm, giving rise to the epithelium, which is then "enclosed" in the splanchnic mesoderm, which gives rise to the various cells types present in the wall. The intestine is thus specified and patterned along two axes: radial patterning controls the formation of the various concentric layers of the intestinal wall, whereas longitudinal patterning controls the specification of each region of the digestive tract — oesophagus, stomach, small intestine, caecum and colon [23]. Early in morphogenesis, signals exchanged between the epithelium and the surrounding mesenchyme induce changes in gene expression along the antero-posterior and radial axes, controlling and predetermining the longitudinal and radial patterning of the intestine [24]. Some of the molecular mechanisms involved in the radial patterning of the intestine have recently been identified. They involve a gene of the Hedgehog family, *Shh* (Sonic hedgehog), expressed by the intestinal endoderm. The Hox genes control the patterning of various embryonic organs and structures along the antero-posterior axis [25]. Some Hox genes display differential expression along the length of the antero-posterior axis of the intestine, suggesting that they also play a role in longitudinal patterning in this organ [23,26,27]. Interestingly, the anterior or posterior limits of the expression domains of different Hox genes correspond to morphological zones and specific subdivisions of the intestine, such as the stomach or the caecum. The regional expression of these genes and of genes encoding other transcription factors undoubtedly controls diverse aspects of intestinal development, and provides support for the notion that the intestinal environment is heterogeneous along its antero-posterior axis, even before or during the wave of colonisation by VNCC.

Thus, the signals responsible for the radial and longitudinal patterning of endodermic and mesodermic derivatives in the intestine wall may target VNCC during or after the colonisation, modifying their migration patterns, survival, proliferation or differentiation.

Formation of the Myenteric and Submucosal Plexi: Structural Aspects and Differentiation of Enteric NCC

Formation of the Myenteric Plexus

During the intestinal colonisation, VNCC migrate into the external mesenchyme of the gut wall, which itself later differentiates into smooth muscle cells. The zone occupied by migrating VNCC thus corresponds to the site of myenteric plexus formation. In adult mice, the ENS network has a reticulate organisation, in which the ganglia are elongated perpendicularly to the rostrocaudal axis of the intestine and linked by neuronal projections that are most of the time either perpendicular or parallel to this axis. This reticulate structure, which can be detected from the E16.5 stage (figure 3, B, D, E), contrasts strongly with the appearance of the initial network formed by the VNCC (figure 3, A, C). The steps by which this reticulated network is formed from the initial network and the mechanisms of this remodelling are unknown. The VNCC must proliferate actively and aggregate to form the ganglia. This second event must require a dynamic regulation of intercellular adhesion. The final reticulated appearance of the ENS strongly suggests that VNCC interact with smooth muscle cells of the circular and longitudinal layers. Some authors have suggested that the nodes of the initial network correspond to the future sites of ganglion formation in the myenteric plexus [19], but this remains to be confirmed.

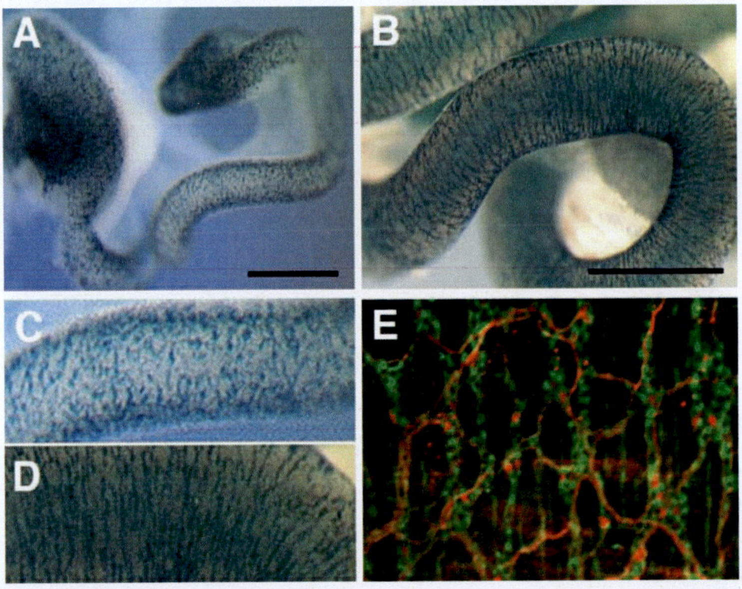

Figure 3. Shape of the network formed by VNCC at various stages of embryonic and postnatal development. A-D, VNCC are revealed after whole mount Xgal stainings of guts dissected from transgenic HtPA-Cre/R26R embryos at E12.5 (A,C) and E16.5 (B,D). C and D represent high magnifications of A and B, respectively [151,175]. E, whole mount immunostaining of a P14 gut (descending colon) labelled for neurofilament NF160 (red) and S100 (green). Scale bars in A and B represent 500 μm and 3 mm, respectively.

The neuronal projections of the myenteric plexus must also grow and find their targets among the diverse cell types within the intestinal wall. The axons of the first neurons detected in the intestine (those expressing the enzyme tyrosine hydroxylase (TH)) mostly project caudally, towards the migration front. They therefore appear to follow the pioneering VNCC. Elegant grafting experiments in which the VNCC in the colon migrated in the opposite direction to that usually observed have also shown that the neuronal projections are directed towards the rostral extremity in this case [28]. There is therefore a correlation between the direction of VNCC migration and the direction of the axonal projections of the first differentiated TH^+ neurons. The polarity of the intestine does not seem to affect the projection of the first neurons. However, a small proportion of differentiating neurons *in vivo* also have rostral projections. The reflex circuits of the ENS in adults involve neurons projecting rostrally, caudally or both. Thus, the direction of migration of the VNCC is not the only factor influencing the direction of neuronal projection during the formation of the myenteric plexus. Other mechanisms, such as the local secretion of attractive or repulsive molecules, must also be involved in these processes.

Formation of the Submucosal Plexus

In mice, the submucosal plexus begins to form in the duodenum on E14.5. It appears later in the colon, on E18.5, initially in the form of isolated neurons in the submucosal zone that aggregate into ganglia after birth [29]. The submucosal plexus is thus generated via an antero-posterior wave. Several studies have suggested that this structure is formed from myenteric plexus cells undergoing a secondary radial migration towards the epithelium. However, to our knowledge, this process has never been directly observed in mice. Secondary centripetal migration seems to be regulated by the netrin-DCC (for "deleted in colon cancer") guidance system in both mice and chick [30]. The netrins are a family of secreted, soluble proteins with sequences similar to that of laminins. They are involved in axonal navigation and cell migration. The family has four members in vertebrates, and two membrane receptors for netrins have been described: UNC-5 and DCC. The intestinal epithelium in mice expresses netrins 1 and 3 and that in chick expresses netrin 2, whereas the DCC receptor is present on the surface of VNCC [31]. *In vivo*, mice lacking DCC have no submucosal plexus. In addition, netrin-1 has a chemoattractant effect on VNCC in cultures of intestinal explants *in vitro*. Finally, neutralising antibodies directed against DCC inhibit the migration of VNCC towards the interior of explants [30]. These findings suggest that the formation of the submucosal plexus requires the attraction of a subpopulation of VNCC expressing DCC by the netrin-1 secreted by the intestinal mucosa.

The SHH protein is involved in another mechanism contributing to the correct positioning of the submucosal plexus in the intestinal wall. Mouse *Shh* double mutants display numerous ectopic neurons in the lamina propria [32]. Thus, in addition to the function of SHH in the patterning of mesodermic derivatives in the intestinal wall, it also acts as an inhibitor of neuronal differentiation or proliferation of at least some VNCC.

The Differentiation of Neurons and Glial Cells From Undifferentiated Progenitors

During the invasion of the gut by VNCC and later development, differentiated and undifferentiated VNCC coexist throughout the intestine. At the start of intestinal colonisation, most of the VNCC are undifferentiated. The undifferentiated progenitors are characterised by the expression of three main markers, SOX10, p75^{NTR} and RET (figure 4; [33]). They give rise to neurons and glial cells that are also characterised by a set of specific markers [33, 34].

Neuronal differentiation begins very early in the course of intestinal colonisation. Between stages E10.5 and E11.5, about 10 to 15% of VNCC begin to differentiate into neurons; they start to express TH and the pan-neuronal markers PGP9.5 and neurofilament (NF) [1,34], which are detected along the entire length of the colonised region and just behind the migration front. The TH$^+$ cells divide and their TH expression has been shown to be transient, subsequently replaced by nitric oxide synthase (NOS) production [28,35]. Consequently, these transiently catecholaminergic (TC) cells are considered to be progenitors in the process of differentiating into neurons, rather than fully differentiated neurons. This commitment to neuronal differentiation is accompanied by a rapid decrease in SOX10 levels and a slower decrease in p75^{NTR} expression. By contrast, PHOX2B expression is maintained in neurons (figure 4).

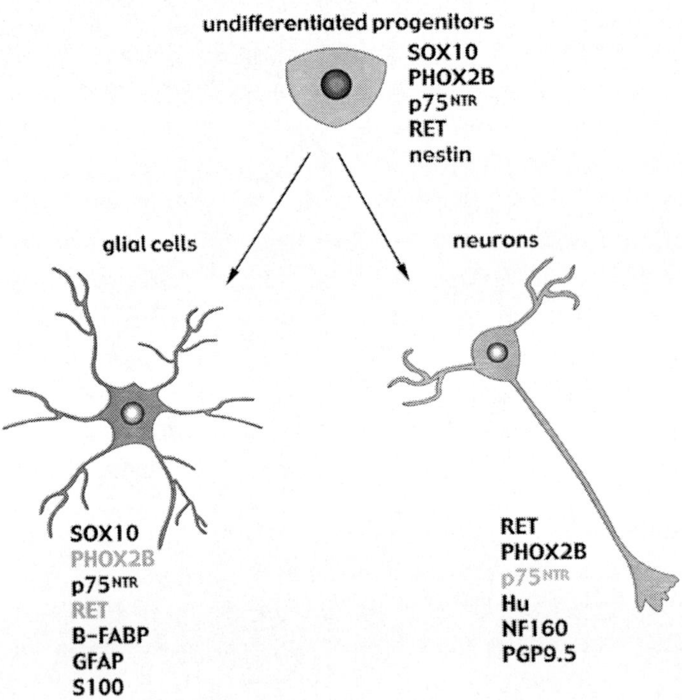

Figure 4. Expression markers of the ENS undifferentiated progenitor cells and their progeny along the neuronal and glial differentiation (adapted from [33]).

The first marker of glial differentiation, brain-fatty acid binding protein (B-FABP), is not detected in the small intestine until two days after the passage of the migration front, at stage E12.5 [34]. Unlike differentiating neurons, glial cells continue to produce the SOX10 transcription factor. They also continue to express PHOX2B but at lower levels, which thus appears to be specific to all VNCC in the embryonic mouse intestine, whether undifferentiated progenitors, or differentiating cells. During their differentiation, glial cells acquire other specific markers, including S100b (a calcium-binding protein), which is detected from E14.5, and glial fibrillary acidic protein (GFAP, an intermediate filament of the cytoskeleton) (figure 4). The mechanisms determining whether a given VNCC undergoes neuronal or glial differentiation are poorly known. SOX10 seems to play a key role in maintaining progenitors in an undifferentiated state [36], and then in differentiation of the glial lineage.

The Differentiation of Neurons into Neuronal Subtypes

Each enteric ganglion in adults contains multiple neuronal subtypes [37], differing in morphology, dendritic and axonal projections and/or neurotransmitter repertoire. Different subtypes of neurons seem to differentiate at different stages of development [38]. Some subtypes are present in such tiny quantities at birth that most of their differentiation is thought to be post-natal [39]. Transplantation experiments [40] and clonal analyses making use of the random inactivation of one of the two X chromosomes [17] have shown that not all the cells of a given ganglion originate from the same progenitor.

The mechanisms regulating the differentiation of neuronal subtypes are still poorly understood. However, it has been suggested that the neurturin (NTN)/GFRα2/RET pathway is involved in the differentiation of a subtype of enteric neurons. Mice mutant for GFRα2 or NTN have fewer cholinergic neurons than wild-type mice [41,42]. The transcription factor MASH-1 is involved in the production of certain types of neurons [43]. Also, mice lacking neurotrophin-3 (NT-3) and its receptor, TRKC, have fewer neurons than wild-type mice, and NT-3 stimulates the differentiation of certain types of neurons *in vitro*, suggesting that this pathway is required for the differentiation of certain neuronal subtypes [44]. HAND-2, a member of the twist family of basic helix-loop-helix (bHLH) transcription factors, is specifically expressed by NCC-derived cells in the gut and is involved in their terminal neuronal differentiation [45].

Despite the early commitment of some VNCC to the neuronal pathway, a pool of undifferentiated cells capable of generating neurons and glial cells persists throughout embryonic and post-natal development. These "stem cells" are attracting considerable interest for the development of cell therapies for diseases of the ENS and in particular for HSCR. Recent advances in this field have been recently nicely reviewed [33,46], and are beyond the scope of this chapter.

Mechanisms Guiding the Invasion of the Intestinal Tissue by VNCC at the Cell Population Scale: What is the Driving Force?

VNCC migration is a two-step process in the embryo: early migration from the neural tube to the rostral end of the intestine, followed by the invasion of intestinal tissues. The mechanisms controlling the first phase are not fully understood. Some studies have suggested that this step is regulated by chemotaxis: pre-enteric VNCC, which express RET before entering the intestine, would be attracted by a source of glial cell line-derived neurotrophic factor (GDNF), which is a ligand for RET, present in the anterior intestine [47].

Dynamic analyses of the behaviour of VNCC within the intestine have suggested that intestinal colonisation involves two major cellular processes: migration, at least over short distances, in the form of chains at the migration front, and proliferation, both at the migration front and in more rostral regions [13,19,20,48]. It also appears that only the VNCC close to the migration front are involved in the rostrocaudal progression of the population towards the uncolonised tissue. Neuronal differentiation begins just behind the migration front, so this zone contains a mixture of migrating undifferentiated and proliferative cells and differentiating, probably post-migratory and post-mitotic, neurons. However, the relative contributions of migration and proliferation to the invasive properties of the VNCC population remain unclear. Furthermore, we do not yet know whether migration and proliferation occur in a directional manner in response to particular factors distributed asymmetrically along the length of the rostrocaudal axis of the intestine. This would result in migration through chemotaxis and directed proliferation through chemokinesis. Finally, the exact nature of the "stop" signal instructing some VNCC to stop migrating or dividing is unknown.

The Link between Differentiation and Migration

Several studies have suggested that the migratory properties of VNCC decrease once they begin to differentiate into neurons [49-51]. However, neuronal differentiation cannot be the only stop signal, because post-migratory colonised zones also contain non-neural undifferentiated progenitors or glial cells. Transgenic mice producing fluorescent proteins have been used to address these questions. Indeed, it is straightforward to identify the mobile cells of the migration front, to fix the tissue rapidly and to carry out immunostaining to analyse the neuronal phenotype of cells identified as migratory in these samples. This approach was used by Young *and coll.* [19] at the E12.5 stage in the colon. They used three pan-neuronal markers, Hu (an mRNA-binding protein present in neuronal precursors and differentiated neurons), NF and PGP9.5, to detect the neurons, and SOX10 as a marker of undifferentiated VNCC. Less than 2% of the migratory VNCC expressed one or more of the neuronal markers studied, suggesting that migratory cells at the front are not neurons. However, this study only considered isolated cells, which could be identified unequivocally. It is therefore still possible that some neurons migrate within chains of cells. Recently, using

TH-GFP mice Hao *and coll.* [52] showed that GFP^+ immature enteric neurons migrate slowly but significantly in the developing gut. Their mode of migration is similar to what is described for neurons of the central nervous system with the extension of long process along which the cell body further translocates.

Chemotaxis

Chemotaxis may account for the progression of the VNCC along the intestine. In the chemotactic model, VNCC would migrate directionally in response to a gradient of a chemotactic factor in the intestinal tissue. The candidate molecule considered most likely to produce such an effect is GDNF, which has been shown to attract VNCC *in vitro* [17,47,53]. The source of GDNF may move over time, always lying slightly ahead of the migration front. Alternatively, the concentration of GDNF may be identical and limiting along the length of the intestine [17], with the VNCC creating a local gradient by sequestering GDNF, thereby stimulating migration towards non-colonised zones. Attempts to demonstrate GDNF synthesis by *in situ* hybridisation have given conflicting results, making it impossible to determine which of these hypotheses is correct. Some studies found no localised production of this factor in the intestine [17]. Others have reported that GDNF production is regulated spatially and temporally such that there is always a source of this molecule just ahead of the migration front, at least during colonisation of the small intestine and caecum [47]. However, VNCC are able to migrate caudorostrally in cultured explants of colon and ileum [28,54-56]. This suggests that the direction of VNCC migration is independent of a localised chemotactic factor, at least in these regions.

Cell Density and Population Pressure

Partial ablation of the VNCC population before migration from the neural tube decreases the distance covered by these cells in the intestine and leads to distal agangiogenesis in chick [54,57,58]. This suggests that the number of migrating VNCC in the intestine has a major effect on total tissue colonisation. In addition, high cell densities seem to promote the migration of trunk NCC *in vitro* [59-61]. These observations led to the concept of population pressure, according to which high cell densities, leading to frequent contact between cells stimulate migration away from these contacts. The number of VNCC in the intestine is essentially regulated by cell proliferation. Indeed, the wave of apoptosis observed elsewhere in the development of the peripheral nervous system is not detected during ENS development [62]. Instead, VNCC proliferate actively, during and after colonisation [48,55]. The effect of reducing the number of VNCC within the intestine during colonisation was investigated by isolating the most caudal VNCC from the rest of the population, by removing fragments of mesenchyme [19] or by cutting the intestine [13] at various distances behind the migration front. The results obtained suggested that the number of VNCC has an effect on the progression of these cells, at least in the distal colon. By contrast, in the caecum and proximal colon, decreasing the number of VNCC cells had no major effect on their invasive capacity.

These findings are consistent with the notion that the mechanisms controlling VNCC progression differ between regions of the intestine.

Cell Proliferation

A mathematical model checked by experimental verifications has recently suggested that proliferation is the critical mechanism underlying the directed invasion of VNCC at the migration front [55,63]. As VNCC density seems to be uniform in all the gut zones, the authors suggested that there is a maximum VNCC density in the intestine, beyond which cells cease to proliferate and migrate. This density threshold would correspond to a stop signal for the cells. This maximum density would be imposed by the intestine itself and might depend on the availability of a growth factor secreted in limited quantities by the intestine, such as GDNF. According to this hypothesis, the cells of the migration front are the only cells to migrate and multiply because only for them this maximum has not yet been reached. This idea is consistent with the findings of Druckenbrod and Epstein [20] indicating that only VNCC located in a 300 μm region immediately behind the migration front contributed to its progression. This hypothesis was tested experimentally with a graft system of the "kebab" type: the migration front or a colonised segment of the donor intestine was grafted into the host intestine at various points along the rostrocaudal axis — at the migration front, in a colonised region rostral to the migration front or in an uncolonised region caudal to the front. If the donor segment was transplanted into a colonised zone, the cells proliferated and migrated very little in the recipient tissue. By contrast, if the donor segment was transplanted in an uncolonised region, the donor VNCC invaded the tissue on either side of the graft, through a combination of migration and proliferation. Thus, the directional nature of VNCC progression seems to be due to the presence of an empty, non-colonised region being ahead of the migration front. The capacity of a given VNCC to migrate towards uncolonised tissue is not intrinsic to the cell; it depends on its position at the front, close to the region lacking VNCC.

Mechanisms Controlling the Invasion of the Intestinal Tissue by NCC and Later ENS Development: More about the Molecular Actors

HSCR is a congenital malformation (incidence 1/5000) characterised by the absence of myenteric and submucosal ganglia in a region of the distal intestine of variable length. This defect often results from the incomplete colonisation of the intestine by VNCC. In 12% of cases, it is associated with a chromosomal abnormality. In 18% of cases, it is associated with abnormalities affecting other NCC derivatives as part of syndromes such as Shah-Waardenburg syndrome, which also involves deafness and pigmentation defects [64]. HSCR as an isolated trait (non-syndromic form, 70% of patients) seems to have a complex multigenic origin. Mutations in at least eight genes have been identified in patients: genes encoding RET, GDNF, NTN, endothelin-3 (EDN3), endothelin B receptor (EDNRB), endothelin-converting enzyme-1 (ECE1), SOX10, PHOX2B and smad-interacting protein 1 (SIP1) or ZFHX1B. These mutations may be sporadic or inherited. Furthermore, the defect is highly variable, even if only a single mutation is considered (there is no strict correlation between genotype and phenotype), suggesting that genetic interactions and environmental factors affect phenotype. Mutations in the genes encoding the RET and ENDRB receptors are the most frequent causes of the disease, accounting for 50% and 5% of cases, respectively. Most of the gene products implicated in the disease modify the levels or activity of these two receptors, suggesting that the associated signalling pathways are essential for ENS development. The use of animal models with spontaneous or artificially induced gene mutations has made it possible to investigate the modes of action of these genes in ENS ontogeny.

The Biological Roles of the GDNF/RET Pathway during ENS Development

RET is a transmembrane tyrosine kinase receptor that can bind four different ligands: GDNF, NTN, artemin and persephin [65]. These ligands do not bind directly to the extracellular domain of RET. Instead, they bind to co-receptors inserted in the membrane via a glycosyl-phosphatidyl-inositol (GPI) group: GFRα1, GFRα2, GFRα3 and GFRα4, respectively.

RET is expressed on VNCC before and during intestinal colonisation [66-68] and on SNCC [69]. One of its ligands, GDNF, is produced in the intestinal mesenchyme during colonisation, but conflicting results have been obtained concerning its spatiotemporal pattern of expression [17,47]. Mice carrying homozygous null mutations of the *Ret*, *Gfrα-1* or *Gdnf* genes display complete agangliogenesis in the region downstream from the stomach, together with defects in renal morphogenesis [70-73]. This severe defect seems to result from apoptosis of VNCC very early in the colonisation of the anterior intestine [74]. The GDNF/RET pathway has been implicated in many processes, suggesting that GDNF has pleiotropic effects during ENS development. This pathway is particularly important for the survival and proliferation of VNCC *in vitro* [50,75] and *in vivo* [62,76], and thus for maintenance of VNCC population size. It is involved in VNCC migration *in vitro* [17,47] and *in vivo* [77], the retention of VNCC within the intestine [17], neuronal differentiation *in vitro* [50,51,74,78], but not *in vivo* [77] and neurite growth *in vitro* [50]. Some of these functions seem to be in opposition, such as the stimulation of proliferation and differentiation. GDNF may have different effects on the different VNCC subpopulations coexisting in the intestine: stem cells, commited progenitors, neuronal subtypes and glial cells. The signalling pathways activated by GDNF/RET in VNCC may be dependent on the amount of receptor at the surface and/or the amount of ligand locally available (threshold effect) or the signalling proteins produced by the target cells. Transplantation of wild-type ENCC into aganglionic RET mutant gut had previously revealed a cell-autonomous effect of RET within the gut [79]. Recently, it was shown that transplanted ENCC progenitors into vagal NCC pathway of wild-type embryos are able to colonize the entire intestin. In contrast, when grafted into RET-deficient embryos, ENCC progenitors are found restricted to the proximal foregut indicating a non-cell-autonomous effect of RET deletion in the early ontogeny of ENCC precursors [80].

The Biological Roles of the EDNRB/EDN3 Pathway during ENS Development

The endothelin family has three members: EDN1, EDN2 and EDN3. These molecules are 21-amino acid peptides that bind to seven-transmembrane domain G-protein-coupled receptors. Two types of receptor have been described in mammals: EDNRA, which binds preferentially to EDN1, and EDNRB, which binds all three peptides with the same affinity [81]. The EDN1/EDNDRA pathway is involved in the ontogeny of cranial and cardiac NCC, whereas the EDN3/EDNRB pathway is required for the development of melanocytes and the ENS.

EDNRB is expressed by VNCC before their entry into the intestine and throughout colonisation, and by certain mesenchymal cells in the proximal zone of the small intestine only [82]. EDN3 is expressed by gut mesenchymal cells. EDN3 mRNA production, unlike that of GDNF mRNA, is clearly closely associated with the VNCC migration front, at least until the caecum [83-84]. Surprisingly, EDN3 is still strongly expressed in the caecum after the passage of the VNCC, during colon colonisation. Various spontaneous mutations affecting the EDN3/EDNRB pathway have been identified in rodents. Lethal spotting (*ls*) mice lack EDN3. They have a point mutation in *edn3* resulting in a defectuous conversion of preproEDN3 into active EDN3 by ECE-1 [85]. Piebald lethal (s^l) mice and spotting lethal (*sl*) rats have a deletion of the *ednrb* gene [86-88]. Animals homozygous for these autosomal recessive mutations present agangliogenesis of the distal part of the intestine in addition to defects of skin and hair pigmentation, making them suitable models for HSCR. Mice with conditional deletion of the *ednrb* gene in NCC exhibit an aganglionic colon, defects of trunk pigmentation and die few weeks after birth due to the megacolon phenotype [89]. An elegant study tried to identify the embryonic stages at which EDN3/EDNRB signalling was required, using mice in which the endogenous *Ednrb* gene could be induced or repressed at various stages of development [90]. This pathway is necessary for ENS development between the E10.5 and E12.5 stages, its action coinciding with invasion of the caecum and proximal colon, and also probably with colonisation of the small intestine. The EDN3/EDNRB pathway inhibits neuronal differentiation and stimulates the differentiation of, and the production of laminin-α1 by, smooth muscle cells *in vitro* [50,51]. Furthermore, smooth muscle development is delayed in *ls/ls* mice [91], and laminin-1 accumulates in the colon [92,93]. These results suggest that EDN3 inhibits neuronal differentiation, acting directly against VNCC expressing EDNRB and indirectly, by stimulating the differentiation of smooth muscle cells and decreasing their production of laminin-α1, a component of the extracellular matrix that accelerates neuronal differentiation.

These observations suggested that, in the absence of this pathway *in vivo*, VNCC would differentiate early into neurons. This precocious differentiation would lead to exhaustion of the pool of undifferentiated progenitors and impaired colonisation [49-51]. This hypothesis has recently been refuted by various groups that have failed to detect precocious neuronal differentiation in the intestines of animals lacking EDN3 or EDNRB [94-96]. Depletion of the p75^{NTR+}/integrin $\alpha 4^+$ pool of progenitors is observed in the intestines of *sl/sl* rats before caecum invasion. Two defects may therefore be responsible for the observed agangliogenesis in the colon of these animals: depletion of the progenitor pool during small intestine colonisation and a migration defect at the time of caecum and proximal colon invasion [94]. These findings are consistent with a recent study implicating EDN3 in the maintenance of ENS progenitors [36], and it seems likely that these progenitors are the target population of EDN3 signalling.

Interactions between the GDNF/RET and EDN3/EDNRB Pathways

It has progressively become clear that the EDN3/EDNRB pathway acts principally by modifying various effects of the GDNF/RET on VNCC. This notion is supported by observations in humans and mice that genetic interactions between the *RET* and *ENDRB* loci seem to control the length of the aganglionic zone in the colon [82,97,98]. In addition, EDN3 can modify the effects of GDNF on VNCC proliferation, differentiation and migration *in vitro*. Indeed, it inhibits the neuronal differentiation triggered by GDNF [50,51), and increases the effect of GDNF on the proliferation of RET$^+$/TUJ$^-$ (TUJ being a pan-neuronal marker) progenitors [82]. Conflicting results have been obtained concerning the effect of EDN3 on VNCC migration in response to GDNF. VNCC lacking EDNRB display no apparent migration defect in response to GDNF in organotypic culture experiments *in vitro* [94]. However, EDN3 greatly decreases the migration of VNCC towards a source of GDNF *in vitro* [82,94,99]. Thus, the EDN3/EDNRB pathway seems to have a preferentially inhibitory effect on VNCC migration in response to GDNF that may maintain the migration front of the VNCC in the correct position in the intestine, preventing anarchic progression in response to GDNF [82], or allowing VNCC to progress beyond the caecum (where the GDNF concentration remains high as well) to colonise the colon. According to this model, the colonisation defect observed in mutants for this pathway would probably be primarily due to a combination of its effects on the proliferation and differentiation of VNCC. However, analyses of proliferation, apoptosis and neuronal differentiation in the intestines of *ls/ls* mice *in vivo* indicate that none of these cellular processes are affected, strongly suggesting that the defect concerns migration [95].

The GDNF/RET and EDN3/EDNRB pathways thus interact to control many cellular processes during ENS development and appear to mediate distinct effects in different VNCC subpopulations and at different stages of embryonic development. However, the conflicting results obtained, probably due to differences in the experimental systems used, make it difficult to draw firm conclusions about their respective functions.

Transcription Factors

The transcription factors SOX10, PHOX2B, PAX3, MASH-1, HOX11L1 and SIP1, are known to be involved in various aspects of ENS development [7,8].

SOX10 is a transcription factor belonging to the SRY family, which is characterised by the presence of a DNA-binding sequence known as the "HMG box" (high motility group). It is produced by VNCC before and during intestinal colonisation and by all migrating NCC destined to generate derivatives for the peripheral nervous system. Mutations in the *Sox10* gene have been found in some HSCR patients. Moreover, mutations of this gene cause Shah-Waardenburg type 4 syndrome (SW4). SW4 may also be caused by mutations in the genes encoding EDNRB and EDN3. Mice with spontaneous heterozygous *Dom* (dominant megacolon) mutations produce a truncated SOX10 protein and present distal agangliogenesis and pigmentation defects [100,101]. Mice with a homozygous null mutation for the *Sox10* locus have no ENS and have defects in the rest of the peripheral nervous system [102-104]. SOX10 is involved in the survival of VNCC before their arrival in the intestine and in maintaining stem cells in an undifferentiated state in the ENS [36]. Notch signaling is required for the maintenance of ENCC progenitors via the regulation of SOX10 and MASH-1 expression [105]. SOX10 also seems to control maintenance of the undifferentiated state in the rest of the peripheral nervous system [106,107]. It stimulates the expression of EDNRB [96,108,109] and RET [110,111] in VNCC and thus acts upstream from these two signalling pathways.

PHOX2B (paired-like homeobox 2B) is a paired-type homeodomain factor produced by the neuronal precursors of the autonomous nervous system, including VNCC. In humans, mutations in the Phox2B gene cause congenital central hypoventilation syndrome, in which HSCR is associated with tumours derived from the NCC, such as neuroblastomas and ganglioneuromas [112,113]. PHOX2B$^{-/-}$ mice have no ENS anywhere in the intestinal tract, including the stomach [114]; like SOX10, PHOX2B seems to be involved in the early survival of VNCC, before their entry into the intestine. In addition, the expression of RET, TH and dopamine-β-hydroxylase is regulated by PHOX2B, suggesting that this factor may also be involved in the neuronal differentiation of VNCC.

PAX3 is a paired-box-containing nuclear transcription factor expressed in the dorsal neural tube and in premigratory NCC [115]. Mutation in the *Pax3* gene is associated with the Waardenburg syndrome type I and II [116] in human and produce the *Sploch* phenotype [117] in mice. In *Sploch* mutant a severe loss of the NCC emerging from the neural tube [118] is observed leading to abnormal development of various NCC derivatives including the ENS [110]. PAX3 can interact with SOX10 to mediate the activation of the RET promoter [111] and the regulation of RET expression [110]. However, it is still unclear whether PAX3 can control the survival or proliferation of ENS precursors in a RET-dependent or independent manner.

MASH-1 belongs to the bHLH family of transcription factors. Null mutation of MASH-1 results in the loss enteric serotonergic neurons in the eosophagus (which are produced during the first wave of neuronal differentiation during gut colonization) [119]. The enteric neurons of the stomach and hindgut are less affected by the mutation indicating that there is a MASH-1-dependent and independent regulation of neuronal differentiation [43].

HOX11L1 is an orphan homeobox protein specifically expressed in several NCC-derivatives including enteric ganglia [120,121]. HOX11L1 was proposed as one of the PHOX2B effectors in the BMP signalling [122] and is thought to enhance the RET promoter activity in cell lines [123] and thus to contribute to the differentiation of the neuronal lineage during ENS development. HOXB5 is also expressed in vagal NCC. The perturbation of HOXB5 function reduces the RET expression and affect the ability of VNCC to migrate to the distal intestine [124].

SIP1, a two-handed zinc finger DNA binding protein, is a component of signal transduction pathways triggered by members of the TGF-b/BMP superfamily. Mutations in the gene encoding SIP1 are found in Mowat-Wilson syndrome, a complex dimorphic and mental retardation syndrome with occurrence of HSCR [125-127]. Generation of knock-out mice revealed that SIP1 is essential for the development of VNCC and the migratory behaviour of cranial NCC in the mouse [128,129]. The expression profile of this gene as well as the recent characterisation of BMP functions within the gut also suggest that SIP1 could play a role later during the development of the ENS [130,131].

Repulsive Cues

The expression of repulsive-attractive cues play crucial role in the regulation of cell migration and neural development [132-136]. Several studies have shown that pathfinding mechanisms of trunk, cardiac and cranial NCC are at least partially dependent on the spatiotemporal expression pattern of Ephrins/Eph receptors [137-139], Semaphorins/ Neuropilins [140-143] and Slit/Robo [144,145]. Considering the ENS development, Sema3A is expressed in the distal large intestine in chick [146]. In mice, Sema3A and Sema3F are strongly expressed in the caecum and the hindgut [56] and VNCC express neuropilin-1 [56]. Mice lacking Sema3A exhibit premature migration of some SNCC in the distal hindgut, suggesting that this protein has some inhibitory effect on SNCC and may contribute, in addition to other repulsive cues, to the delayed invasion of the distal gut by SNCC. In contrast, any noticeable defect was detected for VNCC indicating a different response of VNCC and SNCC to Sema3A. Additionally, Sema3A may also act as a repellent for VNCC in the inner mesenchyme contributing to the formation of the concentric VNCC layer in the outer mesenchyme [56]. DNA microarray analyses suggest that enteric NCC express Sema3E and mediators of the semaphorin signalling, Crmp1, Crmp2 (collapsin reponse mediator 1) and Dpysl3 (dihydropyrimidinase-like 3 protein) [147-148]. However, the biological significance of these proteins is currently not known during ENS development.

Adhesive Receptors

During their progression in the intestine and later in development, the VNCC interact physically both with each other and with their environment consisting of the extracellular matrix (ECM) and mesenchymal/smooth muscle cells (figure 2B). The VNCC and ganglion cells of the ENS express various intercellular adhesion proteins of the cadherin and CAM-Ig families (figure 5), such as N-cadherin [149-151], cadherin-6 and cadherin-11 [151], NCAM and its polysialated form PSA-NCAM, and L1CAM (L1) [151-155]. Some of these proteins are produced solely by VNCC in the intestine (L1), whereas others also seem to be expressed by the surrounding cells (NCAM and PSA-NCAM). NCAM and L1 are involved in diverse processes in nervous system development, including neuronal and glial migration, neurite growth and, in adults, synaptic plasticity and regeneration [156]. The soluble protein BMP4, which is secreted by intestinal mesenchymal cells, seems to control various aspects of ENS development by activating the polysialylation of NCAM [154,155]. BMP4 seems to act by inhibiting the migration of VNCC and triggering their aggregation into ganglia by stimulating the formation of PSA-NCAM just rostral to the migration front. This is quite unexpected, since PSA acts as an "anti-adhesion" component in the central nervous system, promoting cell migration. Here, PSA seems to act as a pro-adhesion component. In the embryonic intestine, L1 is expressed by VNCC from stage E10.5 [157]. In cultured intestines *ex vivo*, the migration of VNCC in the colon is affected by the inhibition of L1 function. Mice lacking L1 display a transient delay in VNCC colonisation. L1 seems to be involved in homotypic cell-cell contact between VNCC within invasive chains at the migration front. These results could be related to the possible role of the *L1* gene in certain patients with HSCR [158]. Ninjurin 2 (nerve injury induced protein 2) is a homophilic cell surface adhesion molecule expressed by enteric NCC when they differentiate into post-mitotic neurons. This molecule was proposed to play a role in the growth arrest of enteric NCC before they differentiate [159]. Differential screenings for genes specifically expressed in the VNCC have recently identified new intercellular adhesion molecules that may be involved in ENS development, including Syn-CAM and protocadherin α1, α4 and 15 [147,148].

Various components of the ECM are known to be present in the intestinal wall during VNCC colonisation. They include fibronectin, laminin-1, collagen IV, hyaluronic acid and chondroitin sulphate proteoglycans [160,161]. The α2 and α4 chains of laminin, which form different laminin isoforms, and tenascins C and W are also present in the intestine, but have been detected only from stage E14 onwards, after intestinal colonisation by the VNCC [162,163]. The laminin α5 chain is produced from stage E12 by cells of the intestinal mesenchyme [162,164]. Other characteristic components of basal laminae, such as entactin or nidogen, are detected in the intestine, during the later stages of gestation at least [165]. Integrins are the main receptors for ECM. 24 integrin heterodimers are described in Mammals, resulting from the combinatory association of 18 α subunits and 8 β subunits [166]. The α4, α6 and β1 subunits of integrins are expressed on the surface of at least some subpopulations of rat VNCC [53,94,167]. The β1, β3 and β5 subunits are expressed in mice VNCC [151], together with the 110 kDa laminin-binding protein (LBP110; [168-170]. Conditional deletion of the integrin β1 gene in NCC results in an absence of enteric ganglia in the descending colon, which leads to a megacolon phenotype similar to that observed in HSCR. This defect results from alteration of the capacity of the VNCC to migrate during the colonisation of the intestine, from the caecum onwards. Furthermore, the VNCC form abnormal aggregates in the intestinal wall in the colonised zones, resulting in the ENS being completely disorganised in the neonate. This suggests that β1 integrins may also be involved in the remodelling of the initial network after the gut colonisation [151]. The binding of LBP110 to laminin-α1 has been reported to stimulate the differentiation of VNCC into neurons *in vitro* [169-170], but the relevance of this mechanism *in vivo* remains to be determined. An increase in laminin-α1 and collagen IV levels was detected in the colon of *ls/ls* mice lacking EDN3, but not in mice lacking RET [93]. The absence of EDN3 may lead to the abnormal production of laminin-α1 by smooth muscle cells, favouring the precocious neuronal differentiation of VNCC and preventing their migration. Abnormalities in the composition of the ECM and the intestinal wall have also been observed in the aganglionic region of patients with HSCR. These abnormalities include the deposition of collagen IV and of several laminin chains [171-175]. Thus, defects in intestinal colonisation by VNCC may, in some cases, be associated with changes in the environment, rather than impairment of the invasive capacities of the VNCC.

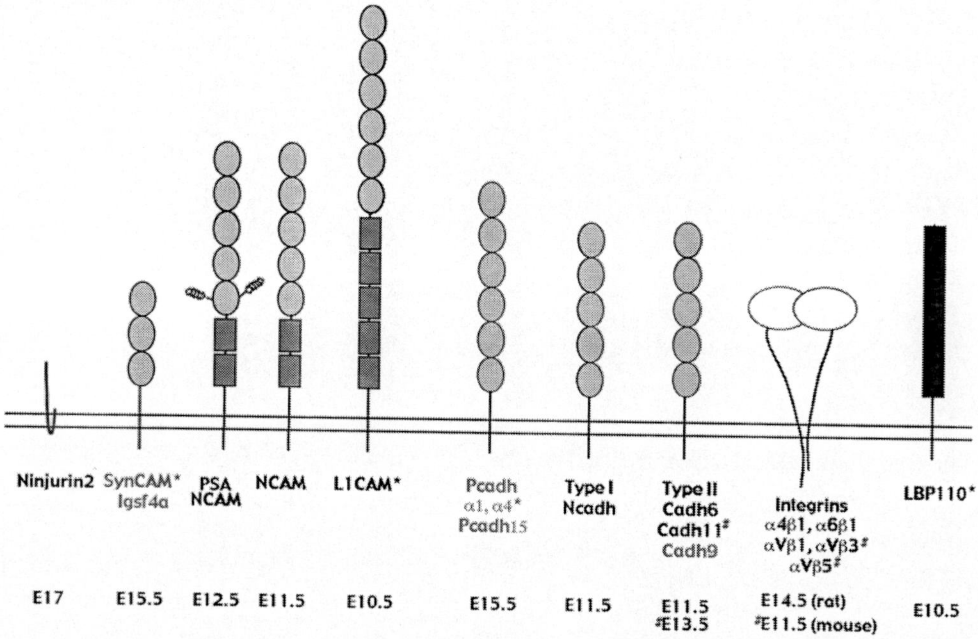

Figure 5. Adhesive receptors expressed by enteric NCC. These cells express various members of the three major adhesive receptor families, Ig-CAMS, cadherins and integrins. The grey color indicates molecules whose expression has been observed at the mRNA level only. Asterisks indicate molecules that are only expressed by NCC in the intestine. For each protein, we also indicate the stage of development from which the expression has been detected in the literature [147,151,155,157,159,170]. The protein domains represented by small rectangles and ovals correspond to FN-type III-like domain and Ig-like domain, respectively.

The numerous processes we described here are important to control the formation and function of the ENS. The functional study of the new ENS-specific genes recently identified in microarray analysis [147,148] will certainly help to identify new interesting players involved in normal ENS development and in HSCR etiology. One of the main challenges in the ENS field is to understand how transcriptional regulation, paracrine signalling through soluble molecules and dynamics of intercellular and cell/ECM adhesion are integrated together to control enteric NCC biology during the different steps of ENS development.

References

[1] Young HM. Embryological origin of interstitial cells of Cajal. *Microsc Res Tech* 1999; 47:303-8.

[2] Knecht AK, Bronner-Fraser M. Induction of the neural crest: a multigene process. *Nat Rev Genet* 2002; 3:453-61.

[3] Gammill LS, Bronner-Fraser M. Neural crest specification: migrating into genomics. *Nat Rev Neurosci* 2003; 4:795-805.

[4] Le Douarin NM, Kalcheim C. *The neural crest.* Second edition. Cambridge: University Press; 1999.

[5] Yntema CL, Hammond WS. The origin of intrinsic ganglia of trunk viscera from vagal neural crest in the chick embryo. *J Comp Neurol* 1954;101:515-41.

[6] Le Douarin NM, Teillet MA. The migration of neural crest cells to the wall of the digestive tract in avian embryo. *J Embryol Exp Morphol* 1973; 30:31-48.

[7] Newgreen D, Young HM. Enteric nervous system: development and developmental disturbances: part 1. *Pediatr Dev Pathol.* 2002; 5:224-47.

[8] Newgreen D, and Young MH. Enteric nervous system: development and developmental disturbances: part 2. *Pediatr Dev Pathol.* 2002; 5:329-49.

[9] Pomeranz HD, Gershon MD. Colonization of the avian hindgut by cells derived from the sacral neural crest. *Dev Biol* 1990; 137:378-94.

[10] Nishijima E, Meijers JH, Tibboel D, Luider TM, Peters-van der Sanden MM, van der Kamp AW et al. Formation and malformation of the enteric nervous system in mice: an organ culture study. *J Pediatr Surg* 1990; 25:627-31.

[11] Burns AJ, Le Douarin NM. The sacral neural crest contributes neurons and glia to the post-umbilical gut: spatiotemporal analysis of the development of the enteric nervous system. *Development* 1998; 125:4335-47.

[12] Kapur RP. Colonization of the murine hindgut by sacral crest-derived neural precursors: experimental support for an evolutionarily conserved model. *Dev. Biol* 2000; 227:146-55.

[13] Druckenbrod, N.R., Epstein ML. The pattern of neural crest advance in the cecum and colon. *Dev Biol* 2005; 287:125-33.

[14] Kapur RP, Yost C, Palmiter RD. A transgenic model for studying development of the enteric nervous system in normal and aganglionic mice. *Development* 1992; 116:167-175.

[15] Lay JM, Gillespie PJ, Samuelson LC. Murine prenatal expression of cholecystokinin in neural crest, enteric neurons, and enteroendocrine cells. *Dev Dyn* 1999; 216:190-200.

[16] Young HM, Hearn CJ, Ciampoli D, Southwell BR, Brunet JF, Newgreen DF. A single rostrocaudal colonization of the rodent intestine by enteric neuron precursors is revealed by the expression of Phox2b, Ret, and p75 and by explants grown under the kidney capsule or in organ culture. *Dev Biol* 1998; 202:67-84.

[17] Young HM, Newgreen DF. Enteric neural-crest derived cells: origin, identification, migration, and differentiation. *Anat Rec* 2001; 262:1-15.

[18] Conner PJ, Focke PJ, Noden MD, Epstein ML. Appearance of neurons and glia with respect to the wavefront during colonization of the avian gut by neural crest cells. *Dev Dyn*. 2003; 226:91-8.
[19] Young HM, Bergner AJ, Anderson RB, Enomoto H, Milbrandt J, Newgreen DF, Whitington PM. Dynamics of neural crest-derived cell migration in the embryonic mouse gut. *Dev Biol* 2004; 270:455-73.
[20] Druckenbrod NR, Epstein ML. Behavior of enteric neural crest-derived cells varies with respect to the migratory wavefront. *Dev Dyn* 2007; 236:84-92.
[21] Coventry S, Yost C, Palmiter RD, Kapur RP. Migration of ganglion cell precursors in the ileoceca of normal and lethal spotted embryos, a murine model for Hirschsprung disease. *Lab Invest* 1994; 71:82-93.
[22] Newgreen DF, Southwell B, Hartley L, Allan IJ. Migration of enteric neural crest cells in relation to growth of the gut in avian embryos. *Acta Anat (Basel)* 1996; 157:105-15.
[23] Roberts DJ. Molecular mechanisms of development of the gastrointestinal tract. *Dev Dyn* 2000; 219:109-20.
[24] Rubin DC. Intestinal morphogenesis. *Curr Opin Gastroenterol* 2007; 23:111-4.
[25] Krumlauf R. Hox genes in vertebrate development. *Cell*. 1994; 78:191-201.
[26] Sekimoto T, Yoshinobu K, Yoshida M, Kuratani S, Fujimoto S, Araki M et al. Region-specific expression of murine Hox genes implies the Hox code-mediated patterning of the digestive tract. *Genes Cells* 1998;3:51-64.
[27] Zacchetti G, Duboule D, Zakany J. Hox gene function in vertebrate gut morphogenesis: the case of the caecum. *Development* 2007;134:3967-73.
[28] Young HM, Jones BR, McKeown SJ. The projections of early enteric neurons are influenced by the direction of neural crest cell migration. *J Neurosci* 2002; 22:6005-18.
[29] McKeown SJ, Chow CW, Young HM. Development of the submucous plexus in the large intestine of the mouse. *Cell Tissue Res* 2001;303:301-5.
[30] Jiang Y, Liu MT, Gershon MD. Netrins and DCC in the guidance of migrating neural crest-derived cells in the developing bowel and pancreas. *Dev Biol* 2003;258:364-84.
[31] Seaman C, Anderson R, Emery B, Cooper HM. Localization of the netrin guidance receptor, DCC, in the developing peripheral and enteric nervous systems. *Mech Dev* 2001;103:173-5.
[32] Ramalho-Santos M, Melton DA, McMahon AP. Hedgehog signals regulate multiple aspects of gastrointestinal development. *Development* 2000; 127:2763-72.
[33] Heanue TA, Pachnis V. Enteric nervous system development and Hirschsprung's disease: advances in genetic and stem cell studies. *Nat Rev Neurosci* 2007; 8:466-79.
[34] Young HM, Bergner AJ, Muller T. Acquisition of neuronal and glial markers by neural crest-derived cells in the mouse intestine. *J Comp Neurol* 2003; 456:1-11.
[35] Baetge G, Pintar JE, Gershon MD. Transiently catecholaminergic (TC) cells in the bowel of the fetal rat: precursors of noncatecholaminergic enteric neurons. *Dev Biol* 1990; 141:353-80.
[36] Bondurand N, Natarajan D, Barlow A, Thapar N, Pachnis V. Maintenance of mammalian enteric nervous system progenitors by SOX10 and endothelin 3 signalling. *Development* 2006:133:2075-86.

[37] Brookes SJ. Classes of enteric nerve cells in the guinea-pig small intestine. *Anat Rec* 2001; 262:58-70.

[38] Pham TD, Gershon MD, Rothman TP. Time of origin of neurons in the murine enteric nervous system: sequence in relation to phenotype. *J Comp Neurol* 1991;314:789-98.

[39] Vannucchi MG, Faussone-Pellegrini MS. Differentiation of cholinergic cells in the rat gut during pre- and postnatal life. *Neurosci Lett* 1996; 206:105-8.

[40] Rothman TP, Le Douarin NM, Fontaine-Perus JC, Gershon MD. Colonization of the bowel by neural crest-derived cells re-migrating from foregut backtransplanted to vagal or sacral regions of host embryos. *Dev Dyn* 1993; 196:217-33.

[41] Heuckeroth RO, Enomoto H, Grider JR, Golden JP, Hanke JA, Jackman A et al. Gene targeting reveals a critical role for neurturin in the development and maintenance of enteric, sensory, and parasympathetic neurons. *Neuron* 1999; 22:253-63.

[42] Rossi J, Luukko K, Poteryaev D, Laurikainen A, Sun YF, Laakso T, et al. Retarded growth and deficits in the enteric and parasympathetic nervous system in mice lacking GFR alpha2, a functional neurturin receptor. *Neuron* 1999; 22:243-52.

[43] Blaugrund E, Pham TD, Tennyson VM, Lo L, Sommer L, Anderson DJ, Gershon MD. Distinct subpopulations of enteric neuronal progenitors defined by time of development, sympathoadrenal lineage markers and Mash-1-dependence. *Development* 1996; 122:309-20.

[44] Chalazonitis A, Pham TD, Rothman TP, DiStefano PS, Bothwell M, Blair-Flynn J et al. Neurotrophin-3 is required for the survival-differentiation of subsets of developing enteric neurons. *J Neurosci* 2001;21:5620-36.

[45] D'Autreaux F, Morikawa Y, Cserjesi P, Gershon MD. Hand2 is necessary for terminal differentiation of enteric neurons from crest-derived precursors but not for their migration into the gut or for formation of glia. *Development* 2007; 134:2237-49.

[46] Gershon MD. Transplanting the enteric nervous system: a step closer to treatment for aganglionosis. *Gut* 2007; 56:459-61.

[47] Natarajan D, Marcos-Gutierrez C, Pachnis V, de Graaff E. Requirement of signalling by receptor tyrosine kinase RET for the directed migration of enteric nervous system progenitor cells during mammalian embryogenesis. *Development* 2002; 129:5151-60.

[48] Young H.M, Turner KN, Bergner AJ. The location and phenotype of proliferating neural-crest-derived cells in the developing mouse gut. *Cell Tissue Res* 2005; 320:1-9.

[49] Gershon MD. Neural crest development. Do developing enteric neurons need endothelins?. *Curr Biol* 1995;5:601-4.

[50] Hearn CJ, Murphy M, Newgreen D. GDNF and ET-3 differentially modulate the numbers of avian enteric neural crest cells and enteric neurons in vitro. *Dev Biol.* 1998; 197:93-105.

[51] Wu JJ, Chen JX, Rothman TP, Gershon MD. Inhibition of in vitro enteric neuronal development by endothelin-3: mediation by endothelin B receptors. *Development* 1999;126:1161-73.

[52] Hao MM, Anderson RB, Kobayashi K, Whitington PM, and Young HM. The migratory behavior of immature enteric neurons. *Dev Neurobiol.* 2008. Epub Nov 4th.

[53] Iwashita T, Kruger GM, Pardal R, Kiel MJ, Morrison SJ. Hirschsprung disease is linked to defects in neural crest stem cell function. *Science* 2003;301:972-6.

[54] Burns AJ, Champeval D, Le Douarin NM. Sacral neural crest cells colonise aganglionic hindgut in vivo but fail to compensate for lack of enteric ganglia. *Dev Biol* 2000; 219:30-43.

[55] Simpson MJ, Landman KA, Hughes BD, Newgreen D. Looking inside an invasion wave of cells using continuum models: proliferation is the key. *J Theor Biol* 2006; 243:343-60.

[56] Anderson RB, Bergner AJ, Taniguchi M, Fujisawa H, Forrai A, Robb L et al. Effects of different regions of the developing gut on the migration of enteric neural crest-derived cells: a role for Sema3A, but not Sema3F. *Dev Biol* 2007; 305:287-99.

[57] Peters-van der Sanden MJ, Kirby ML, Gittenberger-de Groot A, Tibboel D, Mulder MP, Meijers C. Ablation of various regions within the avian vagal neural crest has differential effects on ganglion formation in the fore-, mid- and hindgut. *Dev Dyn* 1993; 196:183-94.

[58] Barlow AJ, Wallace AS, Thapar N, Burns AJ. Critical numbers of neural crest cells are required in the pathways from the neural tube to the foregut to ensure complete enteric nervous system formation. *Development* 2008; 135:1681-91.

[59] Newgreen DF, Ritterman M, Peters EA. Morphology and behaviour of neural crest cells of chick embryo in vitro. *Cell Tissue Res* 1979; 203:115-40.

[60] Rovasio RA, Delouvee A, Yamada KM, Timpl R, Thiery JP. Neural crest cell migration: requirements for exogenous fibronectin and high cell density. *J Cell Biol* 1983; 96:462-73.

[61] Thomas LA, Yamada KM. Contact stimulation of cell migration. *J Cell Sci* 1992; 103:1211-4.

[62] Gianino S, Grider JR, Cresswell J, Enomoto H, Heuckeroth RO. GDNF availability determines enteric neuron number by controlling precursor proliferation. *Development* 2003;130:2187-98.

[63] Simpson MJ, Zhang DC, Mariani M, Landman KA, Newgreen DF. Cell proliferation drives neural crest cell invasion of the intestine. *Dev Biol* 2007; 302:553-68.

[64] Amiel J, Lyonnet S. Hirschsprung disease, associated syndromes, and genetics: a review. *J Med Genet* 2001; 38:729-39.

[65] Sariola H, Saarma M. Novel functions and signalling pathways for GDNF. *J Cell Sci*.2003;116:3855-62.

[66] Pachnis V, Mankoo B, Costantini F. Expression of the c-ret proto-oncogene during mouse embryogenesis. *Development* 1993.119:1005-17.

[67] Robertson K, Mason I. Expression of ret in the chicken embryo suggests roles in regionalisation of the vagal neural tube and somites and in development of multiple neural crest and placodal lineages. *Mech Dev* 1995; 53:329-44.

[68] Durbec PL, Larsson-Blomberg LB, Schuchardt A, Costantini F, Pachnis V. Common origin and developmental dependence on c-ret of subsets of enteric and sympathetic neuroblasts. *Development* 1996;122:349-58.

[69] Delalande JM, Barlow AJ, Thomas AJ, Wallace AS, Thapar N, Erickson CA et al. The receptor tyrosine kinase RET regulates hindgut colonization by sacral neural crest cells. *Dev Biol* 2008;313:279-92.

[70] Schuchardt A, D'Agati V, Larsson-Blomberg L, Costantini F, Pachnis V. Defects in the kidney and enteric nervous system of mice lacking the tyrosine kinase receptor Ret. *Nature* 1994; 367:380-3.

[71] Moore MW, Klein RD, Farinas I, Sauer H, Armanini M, Phillips H et al. Renal and neuronal abnormalities in mice lacking GDNF. *Nature* 1996; 382:76-9.

[72] Sanchez, M.P., I. Silos-Santiago, J. Frisen, B. He, S.A. Lira, and M. Barbacid. Renal agenesis and the absence of enteric neurons in mice lacking GDNF. *Nature* 1996;382:70-3.

[73] Enomoto H, Araki T, Jackman A, Heuckeroth RO, Snider WD, Johnson EM Jr et al. GFR alpha1-deficient mice have deficits in the enteric nervous system and kidneys. *Neuron*. 1998;21:317-24.

[74] Taraviras S, Marcos-Gutierrez CV, Durbec P, Jani H, Grigoriou M, Sukumaran M et al. Signalling by the RET receptor tyrosine kinase and its role in the development of the mammalian enteric nervous system. *Development* 1999;126:2785-97.

[75] Heuckeroth RO, Lampe PA, Johnson EM, Milbrandt J. Neurturin and GDNF promote proliferation and survival of enteric neuron and glial progenitors in vitro. *Dev Biol* 1998; 200:116-29.

[76] Shen L, Pichel JG, Mayeli T, Sariola H, Lu B, Westphal H. Gdnf haploinsufficiency causes Hirschsprung-like intestinal obstruction and early-onset lethality in mice. *Am J Hum Genet* 2002; 70:435-47.

[77] Flynn B, Bergner AJ, Turner KN, Young HM, Anderson RB. Effect of Gdnf haploinsufficiency on rate of migration and number of enteric neural crest-derived cells. *Dev Dyn* 2007; 236:134-41.

[78] Chalazonitis A, Rothman TP, Chen J, Gershon MD. Age-dependent differences in the effects of GDNF and NT-3 on the development of neurons and glia from neural crest-derived precursors immunoselected from the fetal rat gut: expression of GFRalpha-1 in vitro and in vivo. *Dev Biol* 1998; 204:385-406.

[79] Natarajan D, Grigoriou M, Marcos-Gutierrez CV, Atkins C, and Pachnis V. Multipotential progenitors of the mammalian enteric nervous system capable of colonising aganglionic bowel in organ culture. *Development* 1999; 126:157-68.

[80] Bogni S, Trainor P, Natarajan D, Krumlauf R, and Pachnis V. Non-cell-autonomous effects of Ret deletion in early enteric neurogenesis. *Development* 2008; 135:3007-11.

[81] Sakurai T, Yanagisawa M, Masaki T. Molecular characterization of endothelin receptors. *Trends Pharmacol Sci* 1992; 13:103-8.

[82] Barlow A, de Graaff E, Pachnis V. Enteric nervous system progenitors are coordinately controlled by the G protein-coupled receptor EDNRB and the receptor tyrosine kinase RET. *Neuron* 2003;40:905-16.

[83] Leibl MA, Ota T, Woodward MN, Kenny SE, Lloyd DA, Vaillant CR et al. Expression of endothelin 3 by mesenchymal cells of embryonic mouse caecum. *Gut* 1999; 44:246-52.

[84] Woodward MN, Kenny SE, Vaillant C, Lloyd DA, Edgar DH. Time-dependent effects of endothelin-3 on enteric nervous system development in an organ culture model of Hirschsprung's disease. *J Pediatr Surg* 2000; 35:25-9.

[85] Baynash AG, Hosoda K, Giaid A, Richardson JA, Emoto N, Hammer RE et al. Interaction of endothelin-3 with endothelin-B receptor is essential for development of epidermal melanocytes and enteric neurons. *Cell* 1994;79:1277-85.
[86] Hosoda K, Hammer RE, Richardson JA, Baynash AG, Cheung JC, Giaid A et al. Targeted and natural (piebald-lethal) mutations of endothelin-B receptor gene produce megacolon associated with spotted coat color in mice. *Cell* 1994;79:1267-76.
[87] Ceccherini I, Zhang AL, Matera I, Yang G, Devoto M, Romeo G et al. Interstitial deletion of the endothelin-B receptor gene in the spotting lethal (sl) rat. *Hum Mol Genet* 1995; 4:2089-96.
[88] Gariepy CE, Cass DT, Yanagisawa M. Null mutation of endothelin receptor type B gene in spotting lethal rats causes aganglionic megacolon and white coat color. *Proc Natl Acad Sci U S A*. 1996;93:867-72.
[89] Druckenbrod NR, Powers PA, Bartley CR, Walker JW, and Epstein ML. Targeting of endothelin receptor-B to the neural crest. *Genesis* 2008; 46:396-400.
[90] Shin MK, Levorse JM, Ingram RS, Tilghman SM. The temporal requirement for endothelin receptor-B signalling during neural crest development. *Nature* 1999; 402:496-501.
[91] Tennyson VM, Pham TD, Rothman TP, Gershon MD. Abnormalities of smooth muscle, basal laminae, and nerves in the aganglionic segments of the bowel of lethal spotted mutant mice. *Anat Rec* 1986; 215:267-81.
[92] Payette RF, Tennyson VM, Pomeranz HD, Pham TD, Rothman TP, Gershon MD. Accumulation of components of basal laminae: association with the failure of neural crest cells to colonize the presumptive aganglionic bowel of ls/ls mutant mice. *Dev Biol* 1988;125:341-60.
[93] Rothman TP, Chen J, Howard MJ, Costantini F, Schuchardt A, Pachnis V et al. Increased expression of laminin-1 and collagen (IV) subunits in the aganglionic bowel of ls/ls, but not c-ret -/- mice. *Dev Biol* 1996; 178:498-513.
[94] Kruger GM, Mosher JT, Tsai YH, Yeager KJ, Iwashita T, Gariepy CE et al. Temporally distinct requirements for endothelin receptor B in the generation and migration of gut neural crest stem cells. *Neuron* 2003; 40:917-29.
[95] Woodward MN, Sidebotham EL, Connell MG, Kenny SE, Vaillant CR, Lloyd DA et al. Analysis of the effects of endothelin-3 on the development of neural crest cells in the embryonic mouse gut. *J Pediatr Surg* 2003; 38:1322-8.
[96] Lee HO, Levorse JM, Shin MK. The endothelin receptor-B is required for the migration of neural crest-derived melanocyte and enteric neuron precursors. *Dev Biol* 2003; 259:162-75.
[97] Carrasquillo MM, McCallion AS, Puffenberger EG, Kashuk CS, Nouri N, Chakravarti A. Genome-wide association study and mouse model identify interaction between RET and EDNRB pathways in Hirschsprung disease. *Nat Genet* 2002; 32:237-44.
[98] McCallion AS, Stames E, Conlon RA, Chakravarti A. Phenotype variation in two-locus mouse models of Hirschsprung disease: tissue-specific interaction between Ret and Ednrb. *Proc Natl Acad Sci U S A* 2003; 100:1826-31.
[99] Nagy N, Goldstein AM. Endothelin-3 regulates neural crest cell proliferation and differentiation in the hindgut enteric nervous system. *Dev Biol* 2006;293:203-17.

[100] Lane PW, Liu HM. Association of megacolon with a new dominant spotting gene (Dom) in the mouse. *J Hered* 1984;75:435-9.

[101] Herbarth B, Pingault V, Bondurand N, Kuhlbrodt K, Hermans-Borgmeyer I, Puliti A et al. Mutation of the Sry-related Sox10 gene in Dominant megacolon, a mouse model for human Hirschsprung disease. *Proc Natl Acad Sci U S A* 1998; 95:5161-5.

[102] Southard-Smith EM, Kos L, Pavan WJ. Sox10 mutation disrupts neural crest development in Dom Hirschsprung mouse model. *Nat Genet* 1998; 18:60-4.

[103] Kapur RP. Early death of neural crest cells is responsible for total enteric aganglionosis in Sox10(Dom)/Sox10(Dom) mouse embryos. *Pediatr Dev Pathol* 1999; 2:559-69.

[104] Britsch S, Goerich DE, Riethmacher D, Peirano RI, Rossner M, Nave KA et al. The transcription factor Sox10 is a key regulator of peripheral glial development. *Genes Dev* 2001; 15:66-78.

[105] Okamura Y, and Saga Y. Notch signaling is required for the maintenance of enteric neural crest progenitors. *Development* 2008; 135:3555-65.

[106] Kim J, Lo L, Dormand E, Anderson DJ. SOX10 maintains multipotency and inhibits neuronal differentiation of neural crest stem cells. *Neuron* 2003; 38:17-31.

[107] McKeown SJ, Lee VM, Bronner-Fraser M, Newgreen DF, Farlie PG. Sox10 overexpression induces neural crest-like cells from all dorsoventral levels of the neural tube but inhibits differentiation. *Dev Dyn* 2005;233:430-44.

[108] Zhu L, Lee HO, Jordan CS, Cantrell VA, Southard-Smith EM, Shin MK. Spatiotemporal regulation of endothelin receptor-B by SOX10 in neural crest-derived enteric neuron precursors. *Nat Genet* 2004;36:732-7.

[109] Stanchina L, Baral V, Robert F, Pingault V, Lemort N, Pachnis V et al. Interactions between Sox10, Edn3 and Ednrb during enteric nervous system and melanocyte development. *Dev Biol* 2006; 295:232-49.

[110] Lang D, Chen F, Milewski R, Li J, Lu MM, Epstein JA. Pax3 is required for enteric ganglia formation and functions with Sox10 to modulate expression of c-ret. *J Clin Invest* 2000;106:963-71.

[111] Lang D, Epstein JA. Sox10 and Pax3 physically interact to mediate activation of a conserved c-RET enhancer. *Hum Mol Genet* 2003; 12:937-45.

[112] Amiel J, Laudier B, Attie-Bitach T, Trang H, de Pontual L, Gener B et al. Polyalanine expansion and frameshift mutations of the paired-like homeobox gene PHOX2B in congenital central hypoventilation syndrome. *Nat Genet* 2003; 33:459-61.

[113] Trochet D, Hong SJ, Lim JK, Brunet JF, Munnich A, Kim KS et al. Molecular consequences of PHOX2B missense, frameshift and alanine expansion mutations leading to autonomic dysfunction. *Hum Mol Genet* 2005; 14:3697-708.

[114] Pattyn A, Morin X, Cremer H, Goridis C, Brunet JF. The homeobox gene Phox2b is essential for the development of autonomic neural crest derivatives. *Nature* 1999; 399:366-70.

[115] Goulding MD, Chalepakis G, Deutsch U, Erselius JR, Gruss P. Pax-3, a novel murine DNA binding protein expressed during early neurogenesis. *Embo J* 1991; 10:1135-47.

[116] Tassabehji M, Read AP, Newton VE, Patton M, Gruss P, Harris R et al. Mutations in the PAX3 gene causing Waardenburg syndrome type 1 and type 2. *Nat Genet* 1993; 3:26-30.

[117] Epstein DJ, Vekemans M, Gros P. Splotch (Sp2H), a mutation affecting development of the mouse neural tube, shows a deletion within the paired homeodomain of Pax-3. *Cell* 1991;67:767-74.

[118] Serbedzija GN, McMahon AP. Analysis of neural crest cell migration in Splotch mice using a neural crest-specific LacZ reporter. *Dev Biol* 1997;185:139-47.

[119] Lo L, Guillemot F, Joyner AL, Anderson DJ. MASH-1: a marker and a mutation for mammalian neural crest development. Perspect *Dev Neurobiol* 1994; 2:191-201.

[120] Hatano M, Iitsuka Y, Yamamoto H, Dezawa M, Yusa S, Cono Y et al. Ncx, a Hox11 related gene, is expressed in a variety of tissues derived from neural crest cells. *Anat Embryol (Berl)* 1997; 195:419-25.

[121] Shirasawa S, Yunker AM, Roth KA, Brown GA, Horning S, Korsmeyer SJ. Enx (Hox11L1)-deficient mice develop myenteric neuronal hyperplasia and megacolon. *Nat Med* 1997;3:646-50.

[122] Borghini S, Bachetti T, Fava M, Di Duca M, Cargnin F, Fornasari D et al. The TLX2 homeobox gene is a transcriptional target of PHOX2B in neural-crest-derived cells. *Biochem J* 2006;395:355-61.

[123] Bachetti T, Borghini S, Ravazzolo R, Ceccherini I. An in vitro approach to test the possible role of candidate factors in the transcriptional regulation of the RET proto-oncogene. *Gene Expr* 2005; 12:137-49.

[124] Lui VC, Cheng WW, Leon TY, Lau DK, Garcia-Barcelo MM, Miao XP, Kam MK et al. Perturbation of hoxb5 signaling in vagal neural crests down-regulates ret leading to intestinal hypoganglionosis in mice. *Gastroenterology* 2008; 134:1104-15.

[125] Cacheux V, Dastot-Le Moal F, Kaariainen H, Bondurand N, Rintala R, Boissier B et al. Loss-of-function mutations in SIP1 Smad interacting protein 1 result in a syndromic Hirschsprung disease. *Hum Mol Genet* 2001;10:1503-10.

[126] Dastot-Le Moal F, Wilson M, Mowat D, Collot N, Niel F, Goossens M. ZFHX1B mutations in patients with Mowat-Wilson syndrome. *Hum Mutat* 2007;28:313-21.

[127] Wakamatsu N, Yamada Y, Yamada K, Ono T, Nomura N, Taniguchi H et al. Mutations in SIP1, encoding Smad interacting protein-1, cause a form of Hirschsprung disease. *Nat Genet* 2001; 27:369-70.

[128] Higashi Y, Maruhashi M, Nelles L, Van de Putte T, Verschueren K, Miyoshi T et al. Generation of the floxed allele of the SIP1 (Smad-interacting protein 1) gene for Cre-mediated conditional knockout in the mouse. *Genesis* 2002; 32:82-4.

[129] Van de Putte T, Maruhashi M, Francis A, Nelles L, Kondoh H, Huylebroeck D et al. Mice lacking ZFHX1B, the gene that codes for Smad-interacting protein-1, reveal a role for multiple neural crest cell defects in the etiology of Hirschsprung disease-mental retardation syndrome. *Am J Hum Genet* 2003; 72:465-70.

[130] Chalazonitis A, D'Autreaux F, Guha U, Pham TD, Faure C, Chen JJ, Roman D, Kan L, Rothman TP, Kessler JA and Gershon MD. Bone morphogenetic protein-2 and -4 limit the number of enteric neurons but promote development of a TrkC-expressing neurotrophin-3-dependent subset. *J Neurosci* 2004; 24:4266-82.

[131] Van de Putte T, Francis A, Nelles L, van Grunsven LA and Huylebroeck D. Neural crest-specific removal of Zfhx1b in mouse leads to a wide range of neurocristopathies reminiscent of Mowat-Wilson syndrome. *Hum Mol Genet* 2007; 16:1423-36.

[132] Wilkinson DG. Multiple roles of EPH receptors and ephrins in neural development. *Nat Rev Neurosci* 2001; 2:155-64.

[133] Kullander K, Klein R. Mechanisms and functions of Eph and ephrin signalling. *Nat Rev Mol Cell Biol* 2002;3:475-86.

[134] Poliakov A, Cotrina M, Wilkinson DG. Diverse roles of eph receptors and ephrins in the regulation of cell migration and tissue assembly. *Dev Cell* 2004; 7:465-80.

[135] Casazza A, Fazzari P, Tamagnone L. Semaphorin signals in cell adhesion and cell migration: functional role and molecular mechanisms. *Adv Exp Med Biol* 2007; 600:90-108.

[136] Kuriyama S, Mayor R. Molecular analysis of neural crest migration. *Philos Trans R Soc Lond B Biol Sci* 2008; 363:1349-62.

[137] Krull CE, Lansford R, Gale NW, Collazo A, Marcelle C, Yancopoulos GD et al. Interactions of Eph-related receptors and ligands confer rostrocaudal pattern of trunk neural crest migration. *Curr. Biol.* 1997; 7:571-80.

[138] Wang HU, Anderson DJ. Eph family transmembrane ligands can mediate repulsive guidance of trunk neural crest migration and motor axon outgrowth. *Neuron* 1997; 18:383-96.

[139] Santiago A, Erickson CA. Ephrin-B ligands play a dual role in the control of neural crest cell migration. *Development* 2002; 129:3621-32.

[140] Gammill LS, Gonzalez C, Bronner-Fraser M. Neuropilin 2/semaphorin 3F signaling is essential for cranial neural crest migration and trigeminal ganglion condensation. *Dev Neurobiol* 2007;67:47-56.

[141] Sato M, Tsai HJ, Yost HJ. Semaphorin3D regulates invasion of cardiac neural crest cells into the primary heart field. *Dev Biol* 2006;298:12-21.

[142] Yu HH, Moens CB. Semaphorin signaling guides cranial neural crest cell migration in zebrafish. *Dev Biol* 2005;280:373-85.

[143] Osborne NJ, Begbie J, Chilton JK, Schmidt H, Eickholt BJ. Semaphorin/neuropilin signaling influences the positioning of migratory neural crest cells within the hindbrain region of the chick. *Dev Dyn* 2005; 232:939-49.

[144] De Bellard, M.E., Y. Rao, and M. Bronner-Fraser. Dual function of Slit2 in repulsion and enhanced migration of trunk, but not vagal, neural crest cells. *J Cell Biol.* 2003162:269-79.

[145] Jia L, Cheng L, Raper J. Slit/Robo signaling is necessary to confine early neural crest cells to the ventral migratory pathway in the trunk. *Dev Biol* 2005; 282:411-21.

[146] Shepherd IT, Raper JA. Collapsin-1/semaphorin D is a repellent for chick ganglion of Remak axons. *Dev Biol* 1999; 212:42-53.

[147] Heanue TA, Pachnis V. Expression profiling the developing mammalian enteric nervous system identifies marker and candidate Hirschsprung disease genes. *Proc Natl Acad Sci U S A* 2006;103:6919-24.

[148] Vohra BP, Tsuji K, Nagashimada M, Uesaka T, Wind D, Fu M et al. Differential gene expression and functional analysis implicate novel mechanisms in enteric nervous system precursor migration and neuritogenesis. *Dev Biol* 2006;298:259-71.

[149] Packer AI, Elwell VA, Parnass JD, Knudsen KA, Wolgemuth DJ. N-cadherin protein distribution in normal embryos and in embryos carrying mutations in the homeobox gene Hoxa-4. *Int J Dev Biol* 1997; 41:459-68.

[150] GaidarYA, Lepekhin EA, Sheichetova GA, Witt M. Distribution of N-cadherin and NCAM in neurons and endocrine cells of the human embryonic and fetal gastroenteropancreatic system. *Acta Histochem* 1998; 100:83-97.

[151] Breau MA, Pietri T, Eder O, Blanche M, Brakebusch C, Fassler R et al. Lack of β1 integrins in enteric neural crest cells leads to a Hirschsprung-like phenotype. *Development* 2006;133:1725-34.

[152] Mirsky R, Jessen KR, Schachner M, Goridis C. Distribution of the adhesion molecules N-CAM and L1 on peripheral neurons and glia in adult rats. *J Neurocytol* 1986; 15:799-815.

[153] Yoneda A, Wang Y, O'Briain DS, Puri P. Cell-adhesion molecules and fibroblast growth factor signalling in Hirschsprung's disease. *Pediatr Surg Int* 2001; 17:299-303.

[154] Faure C, Chalazonitis A, Rheaume C, Bouchard G, Sampathkumar SG, Yarema KJ et al. Gangliogenesis in the enteric nervous system: roles of the polysialylation of the neural cell adhesion molecule and its regulation by bone morphogenetic protein-4. *Dev Dyn* 2007;236:44-59.

[155] Fu M, Vohra BP, Wind D, Heuckeroth RO. BMP signaling regulates murine enteric nervous system precursor migration, neurite fasciculation, and patterning via altered Ncam1 polysialic acid addition. *Dev Biol* 2006; 299:137-50.

[156] Maness PF, Schachner M. Neural recognition molecules of the immunoglobulin superfamily: signaling transducers of axon guidance and neuronal migration. *Nat Neurosci* 2007; 10:19-26.

[157] Anderson RB, Turner KN, Nikonenko AG, Hemperly J, Schachner M, Young HM. The cell adhesion molecule L1 is required for chain migration of neural crest cells in the developing mouse gut. *Gastroenterology* 2006; 130:1221-32.

[158] Okamoto N, Wada Y, Goto M. Hydrocephalus and Hirschsprung's disease in a patient with a mutation of L1CAM. *J Med Genet* 1997; 34:670-1.

[159] Araki T, Milbrandt J. Ninjurin2, a novel homophilic adhesion molecule, is expressed in mature sensory and enteric neurons and promotes neurite outgrowth. *J Neurosci.* 2000;20:187-95.

[160] Fujimoto T, Hata J, Yokoyama S, Mitomi T. A study of the extracellular matrix protein as the migration pathway of neural crest cells in the gut: analysis in human embryos with special reference to the pathogenesis of Hirschsprung's disease. *J Pediatr Surg* 1989; 24:550-6.

[161] Newgreen DF, Hartley L. Extracellular matrix and adhesive molecules in the early development of the gut and its innervation in normal and spotting lethal rat embryos. *Acta Anat (Basel)* 1995;154:243-60.

[162] Lefebvre O, Sorokin L, Kedinger M, Simon-Assmann P. Developmental expression and cellular origin of the laminin alpha2, alpha4, and alpha5 chains in the intestine. *Dev Biol* 1999; 210:135-50.

[163] Scherberich A, Tucker RP, Samandari E, Brown-Luedi M, Martin D, Chiquet-Ehrismann R. Murine tenascin-W: a novel mammalian tenascin expressed in kidney and at sites of bone and smooth muscle development. *J Cell Sci* 2004; 117:571-81.

[164] Bolcato-Bellemin AL, Lefebvre O, Arnold C, Sorokin L, Miner JH, Kedinger M et al. Laminin alpha5 chain is required for intestinal smooth muscle development. *Dev Biol.* 2006;260:376-90.

[165] Simon-Assmann P, Kedinger M, De Arcangelis A, Rousseau V, Simo P. Extracellular matrix components in intestinal development. *Experientia.* 1995;51:883-900.

[166] Hynes RO. Integrins: bidirectional, allosteric signaling machines. *Cell* 2002; 110:673-87.

[167] Bixby S, Kruger GM, Mosher JT, Joseph NM, Morrison SJ. Cell-intrinsic differences between stem cells from different regions of the peripheral nervous system regulate the generation of neural diversity. *Neuron* 2002; 35:643-56.

[168] Pomeranz HD, Rothman TP, Chalazonitis A, Tennyson VM, Gershon MD. Neural crest-derived cells isolated from the gut by immunoselection develop neuronal and glial phenotypes when cultured on laminin. *Dev Biol* 1993; 156:341-61.

[169] Chalazonitis A, Tennyson VM, Kibbey MC, Rothman TP, Gershon MD. The alpha1 subunit of laminin-1 promotes the development of neurons by interacting with LBP110 expressed by neural crest-derived cells immunoselected from the fetal mouse gut. *J Neurobiol.* 1997;33:118-38.

[170] Howard MJ, Gershon MD. Development of LBP110 expression by neural crest-derived enteric precursors: migration and differentiation potential in ls/ls mutant mice. *J Neurobiol* 1998;35:341-54.

[171] Parikh DH, TamPK, Lloyd DA, Van Velzen D, Edgar DH. Quantitative and qualitative analysis of the extracellular matrix protein, laminin, in Hirschsprung's disease. *J Pediatr Surg* 1992;27:991-95.

[172] Parikh DH, Tam PK, Van Velzen D, Edgar D. Abnormalities in the distribution of laminin and collagen type IV in Hirschsprung's disease. *Gastroenterology* 1992; 102:1236-41.

[173] Alpy F, Ritie L, Jaubert F, Becmeur F, Mechine-Neuville A, Lefebvre O et al. The expression pattern of laminin isoforms in Hirschsprung disease reveals a distal peripheral nerve differentiation. *Hum Pathol* 2005;36:1055-65.

[174] Gariepy CE. Intestinal motility disorders and development of the enteric nervous system. *Pediatr Res* 2001; 49:605-13.

[175] Pietri T, Eder O, Blanche M, Thiery JP, Dufour S. The human tissue plasminogen activator-Cre mouse: a new tool for targeting specifically neural crest cells and their derivatives in vivo. *Dev Biol* 2003; 259:176-87.

In: Hirschsprung's Disease: Diagnosis and Treatment
Ed: Ramón Núñez and Manuel López-Alonso
ISBN: 978-1-60741-349-3

Chapter III

Anorectal Physiology

Juan Ribas

Introduction

Basically, the main function of the anorectal canal is to process the stool and to provide signals for discharging through the anus. Defecation is normally performed once at day in adults and 4-6 times at day in newborns, the rest of the day therefore faecal retention during long period is the physiological work of the anorectal canal. Doing so, this terminal part of the colon requires a powerful musculature and a reliable neural network including sensors, sensory-motor circuits and triggers for voluntary activation or inhibition in adults and involuntary activation in newborns.

The structure of the anorectal canal is different to that in the colon. The external longitudinal muscle layers increase in extension up to cover the whole circumference of the rectum. The slower velocity of propagation along longitudinal muscle layers than along circular muscle layers (characteristic of more aboral regions in the colon), is essential for the reservoir function of this region. At this level, the lumen of the rectum is occluded by several folders meanwhile the faeces are retained or defecation is not triggered. These folders act like selective valves that, under adequate sensing mechanisms, can allow the pass of gas, liquid or solid contents. Finally, the distal most region of the intestine, reaching the anus, consists on layers of both smooth and striated muscles. The latter normally devotes of voluntary control after the two or three years after born.

The internal sphincter consists on thick circular muscle layers and it is responsible of the 70-80 % of the anal tone in resting conditions. The external sphincter is formed by circular layers of striated muscles. However, this layer is able to keep up to the 20-30% of the muscular tone in the anal canal. Some other striated muscles belonging to the pelvic floor cooperate also with sphincter tone [1].

Local Neural Control of Ano-Rectal Motility

The intestinal motility is the result of wall musculature activation governed by the enteric nervous system. Signals from the mucosal epithelium and from the mechanical tension in the wall of the intestine are the stimuli for the enteric nervous system to be activated. The intramural blood flow is synchronously activated in order to feed both the muscles of the wall and the transport processes across the lining mucosa.

The enteric nervous system (ENS) owns three main types of neurons that resemble those in the Central Nervous System: Sensory neurons, interneurons and motor neurons. Sensory neurons have specialized regions to detect chemical, mechanical or painful stimuli which in turn are coded in neural signals such as action potentials. Interneurons are into the neural network connecting neurons by synapses. These neurons are thought to analyze and transmit information between sensor and motor neurons. Motor neurons are the final common pathway of the enteric nervous system transmitting information to the muscles in the wall of the gut (Figure 1).

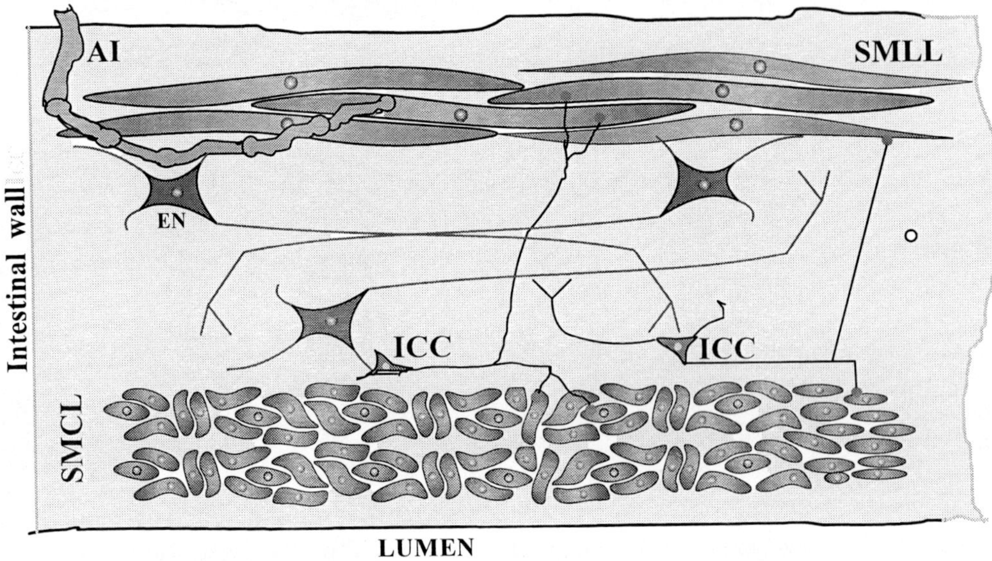

Figure 1. Schematic drawing of a section of gut wall. SMCL: smooth muscle circular layer; SMLL: smooth muscle longitudinal layer; EN: enteric neurons representing sensory, interneuron and motor neurons; ICC: interstitial cell of Cajal; AI: autonomic innervation. For the sake of clarity only ICCs close to circular muscle layer are represented. Notice the multiple connections of ICCs with both muscle layers and with enteric neurons.

Mechanoreceptors, in the specialized regions of sensory neurons, code the information on the mechanical state of the wall and mucosal epithelium of the intestine. Its role likes to be significant for the pathogenesis of some syndromes such as the irritable bowel or chronic constipation. Specially, sensory suppression in the recto-sigmoid area might account for by the inhibition or absence of ano-rectal reflexes or by the failure transmission of the recto-sigmoid conditions to the brain for the conscious perception of distension in this region[2,3].

The enteric nervous system exhibits activity pattern generators. This activity give rise to motor behaviour programs that, unlike reflex behaviour, do not require sensory input or feedback information from the sensory neurons to start the program. The whole sequence of a motor program may be triggered by the activation of a single cell named command neuron. Most of these behaviours are cyclic and the rate of repetitions is pre-programmed by the interneuronal circuitry interacting with the interstitial cells of Cajal (ICC), actual generators of electrical rhythm pattern in the digestive tract [4,5].

The pool of motor neurons of the enteric nervous system includes both excitatory and inhibitory neurons. The main neurotransmitters involved in excitation of wall muscle and mucosal secretion is acetylcholine and substance P, although other neurotransmitter like vasoactive intestinal peptide and serotonin are also involved. Inhibitory motor neurons release adenosine triphosphate, vasoactive intestinal peptide, pituitary adenylate cyclase activating peptide and nitric oxide which act as inhibitors at neuromuscular junctions. (For a more extensive review on digestive tract neurotransmission see [6])

The inhibitory motor neurons have a relevant role in the function of recto-sigmoid wall. Normally, these cells discharge in a tonic or continuous fashion so that contractions in the muscle of the gut occur only when these inhibitory neurons are turned off by input from interneurons in the enteric nervous system. The extension of the contracting segment of the circular muscle layer depends on the distance of spread of action potential in the geometry of the sincitium conformed by excitable cells in the intestinal wall. Gap junctions provide the bases for this tissue works like a functional sincitium. The order in which inhibitory motor neurons are switched off determines the direction and sense of the propagation of the contraction. The overall sense of the propagation is normally aboral, giving rise to the propulsive mechanical waves that facilitate the transit of the intestinal content. However, short length propagation of the wall contraction in adoral sense occurs also for mixture task during the digestive process. Overall abnormal sense (adoral) of the electrical and mechanical propagation occurs during vomit in thin intestine, stomach and oesophagus regions [4,7,8].

However, in the sphincter region, the inhibitory motor neurons are silent and tonic muscle contraction is the predominant state. In contrast to the colonic wall, inhibitory motor neurons in this region only are switched on for coordinate opening of sphincter and under adequate timing as respect functional events in proximal regions [9].

The Role of ICC

Santiago Ramon y Cajal was the first describing a type of cell that spread along the intestinal wall [10] (Figure 2). These cells had multiple branches and like to connect with neurons of the enteric nervous system and with smooth muscle cell in the wall. Formerly, Cajal thought these cells were primitive neurons connecting neurons to muscles. Later he realized that these cells originated from mesenchyme like fibroblasts and developed numerous mitochondrions and endoplasmic reticulum and were important to the normal function of the digestive tract. Therein these cells were labelled as non neural, despite they show auto-excitation in his electrical pacemaker activity [11].

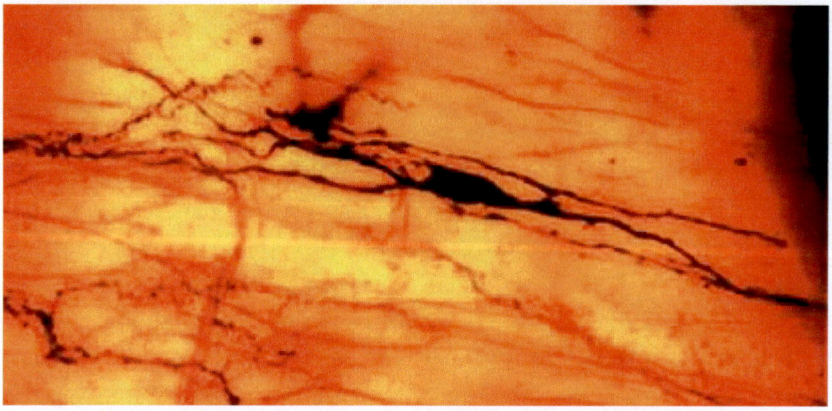

Figure 2. Cells of Cajal, stained and photographed by Cajal himself. *Courtesy of the Cajal Museum, Madrid*

Nowadays, ICCs are considered as the source of the intestinal pacemaker since it generates the electrical slow waves that characterize the basic electrical activity in the gut. On a hand, ICCs are synaptically contacted by neurons of the enteric nervous system. On the other hand, ICCs modulate their own electrical activity and pass through the output information to smooth muscle in the gut wall. ICCs express mechano-sensitive channels and mechanisms that can transduce length changes to mediate responses to stretch. Additionally, ICCs evidence sensitivity to carbon monoxide but its physiological role needs more research. The expression of a tyrosinkinase receptor called *Kit* allows the use of specific antibody to identify these types of cells and tumor derivatives from it [3,12,13](Figure 3).

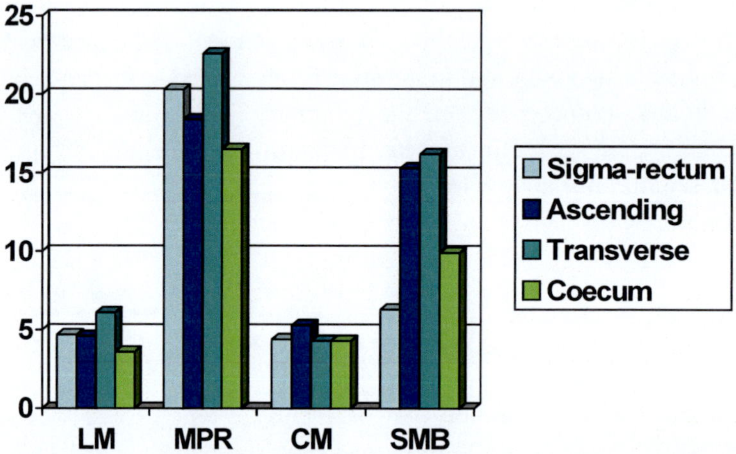

Figure 3. Distribution of interstitial cell of Cajal (ICC) in normal human colon. LM, longitudinal muscle layer; MPR, myenteric plexus region; CM, circular smooth muscle layer; SMB, submucosal border. (Adapted from 19).

The ICCs have been electrophysiologically and histochemically studied *in situ* and in culture as well as with genetic manipulation like knocked out animals for ICC expression. All data point out ICC as essential to generate slow electrical wave in its membrane potential which in combination with the trigger of action potentials determines the contractile activity of the smooth muscle. On the contrary, gut smooth muscle alone, without the concurrent activity of ICC are electrically quiescent [3,14,15].

Additionally, ICCs exhibit plastic properties which permit them to survive to stressing environmental condition. Some of these properties are a key to recover from transient mechanical obstruction or the side effect of intestinal surgery. In experimental animals, the mechanical clamping of an intestinal section provokes a hypertrophy of muscle layers ad oral to the obstruction without affecting ICCs. However, in aboral sense the ICCs become unresponsive to the enteric nervous stimulation and lost the ability to generate electrical slow waves. Nevertheless, ICCs do not die but change their phenotype and show features as fibroblasts as smooth cells. After release of the mechanical obstruction, this cells with intermediate phenotype diminishing and reappear cells with ICC histochemistry, eliciting slow waves and responding to electrical stimulation of enteric innervation [3,16].

ICCs are ubiquitous in the intestinal wall. ICC are localized in the submucosa, between the myoenteric plexus of Auerbach and the circular smooth muscle layer and in the outer longitudinal muscle layer. Attending to their location ICCs may be classified as ICC*my* with a reticular organization between intramural neurons and smooth muscle cells. Their main function like to be the pacemaker and triggering the slow waves; other class of ICC are named *intramuscular(im)* as they locate dispersal into the muscle layers, most of them are in the internal side of the circular muscle layer and are thought to serve for propagating the activation wave. Moreover, these ICC*im* express membrane receptors for neurotransmitters and hormones like CCK (cholecystokinine) suggesting an important role in neuromuscular and hormone-muscular transmission in the intestinal wall. There exist other subtypes of ICCs like ICC*dmp*, ICC*smp,* ICC*cm* and ICC*lm* corresponding to localizations in the deep muscular plexus, the sub-muscular plexus, in the bulk of the circular muscle layer and in the longitudinal muscle layer respectively. Whatever location of ICCs in the digestive track is functional significance is undoubted and its diminution or absence has been related to malfunction of the intestinal transit[5,16-19].

In the sphincteral region, the ICC*ims* receive synapses from enteric neurons and contact smooth muscle cells by gap junctions. The main neurotransmitter in this cell complex formed by neurons-ICC*ims*-smooth muscle cell is nitric oxide (NO).

Ano-Rectal Motility in Newborns

In addition to intrinsic activity in the enteric nervous system, reflexes may occur in response to stimulation of sensory neurons, normally undergoing a stereotypical behaviour. For example, a mechanical distension of the intestinal wall or a mucosal stress induces reflex contraction of the circular muscle of the wall above (ad oral) of the site of stimulation and reflex inhibition of the circular muscle below (ab oral) the stimulation [20]. This reflex behaviour is related to the morphological map of the neuronal circuit into the wall of the intestine. In fact, the distance at which occurs the muscle inhibition ab oral to the mechanical distension depends on the length of the axon terminals of the neuron underlying the reflex.

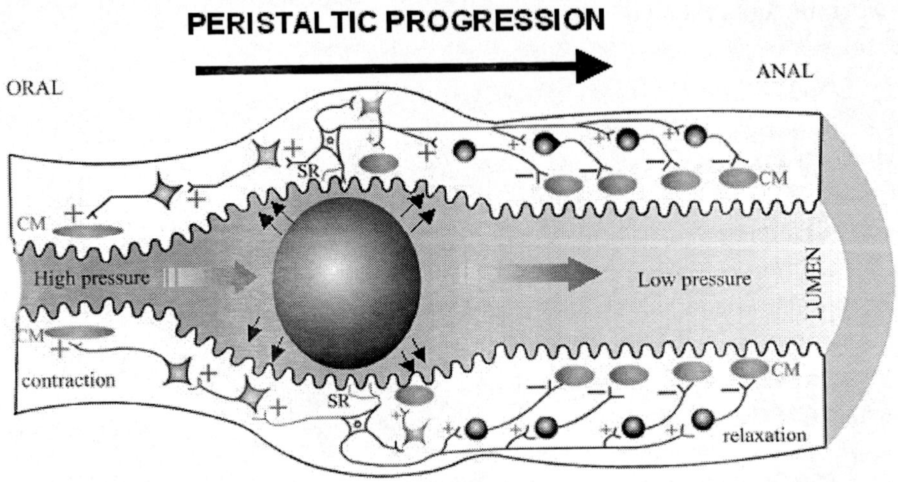

Figure 4. Schematic drawing of the gut component involved in peristaltic progression. The intestinal content, represented by the gray sphere, exert pressure on the intestinal wall which in turn reacts in different ways. At first, the stretched mucosa activates the mechano-sensitive terminals (stretch receptors) of sensory neurons in the submucosa plexus. Probably, mechanical and paracrine stimuli starts autoreflex response in the own segment stretched by the content, after a short lasting mechanical resistance, a multisegmentary reflex is triggered by means of interneurons and motor neurons which finally synapse ICC and smooth muscle cells. In the scheme, axonal projection in the anal direction is larger than that in the oral direction. In addition, final information to circular muscle layers in the aboral region is inhibitory, probably mediated by nitric oxide. On the contrary, circular muscle cells in the oral region are excited. As a consequence, contraction in the oral region generate a high pressure area whereas relaxation in the anal region provide a low pressure area, thus the pressure gradient so generated sure the adequate progression of the intestinal content through the gut lumen. CM, smooth muscle circular layer; SR, stretch receptors. Sensory neurons (hollow) interneurons and motor neurons excitatory (cian) and inhibitory (black) are representative of the whole neuronal network and interstitial cell of Cajal (ICC).

The motor behaviour of the intestinal wall in the ano-rectal region of the digestive tract follows the general pattern of other intestinal regions. However, because the especial organization of muscular layers in the aboral most part, where longitudinal muscular layers occupy larger extension on the gut circumference, the normal pressure profile is quite different, moreover in newborns. As shown in Figure 2 in Lopez Alonso's chapter, the intraluminal pressure in the ano-rectal canal rise up to 50 mmHg. In addition, spontaneous rhythmic oscillations at the beginning of the rectum decrease in amplitude as approach to the anus. Finally, the manometric recordings in prematures and newborns show a steady state plateau around the internal sphincter region, where the highest pressure is measured. This pressure profile accords to the main function of the final part of the rectum and the internal sphincter that is the retention of stools meanwhile reabsortive and compacting process are not ended.

Other interesting characteristics of the ano-rectal motility in newborns are the properties of the reflex responses induced by stretching stimulation of the intestinal wall. When a inflatable balloon is located in the rectum for stimulation purpose it is possible to obtain relaxation (inhibitory) responses few millimetres aborally. The insight into these reflex responses reveals features of the underlying nervous organization. As shown in the Lopez Alonso's chapter, increasing the volume of the stimulating balloon produce, with a short delay, a few mmHg pressure decays and then slowly increases up to the pre-stimulus condition. A typical time course response is shown in the figure 5. It is interesting to point out that when the stimulus is delivery at time the spontaneous wave is in the ascending way, the reflex response does not occur till the top value of the resting wave is reached. Contrariwise, when the mechanical stimulation coincides with top pressure on the spontaneous wave the relaxation response appear immediately with a minimal latency.

The recording of the reflex relaxation response in the region where the pressure is kept in almost steady state condition provides distinct features. The stimulus induced decay in pressure in the steady state region normally is larger in amplitude and duration than in more adoral rectum. Furthermore, during the relaxation response a new stimulus is unable to produce additional pressure decay. Even, when the stimulus is applied during the last 20% of the recovery phase it is unsuccessful in producing a new relaxation. In fact is necessary to wait the complete return to the pre-stimulus condition in order to get a new as schematically shown in Figure 5.

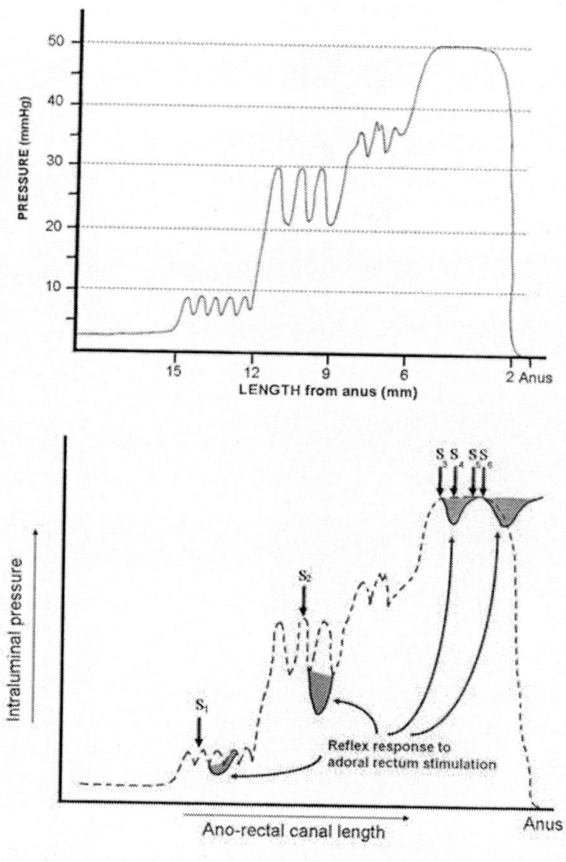

Figure 5. Schematic relaxation reflex responses (blue) superimposed on the manometric profile in the anorectal canal in newborns. Stimuli 1 was applied before of the top pressure in wave and the relaxation reflex response (blue) does not occur till the peak of the wave is over passed. Stimuli 2 in the top of the wave induced an instantaneous relaxation response. However, in the highest steady state pressure region, stimuli 4 and 5 are not producing any response because the refractoriness of the region during reflex relaxation. Finally, stimulus 6 after the complete recover of the pre-stimulus pressure level unchains a new relaxation response. (adapted from Lopez Alonso et al., 1991)

Since there exist a complex neuronal network underlying the motor reflex responses in the anorectal canal. Any change in cell excitability might explain the unresponsiveness of the wall gut during the reflex. This intra-reflex unresponsiveness is evidenced by the lack of effect after temporal summation of stimulation. Actually, any excitable (sensory neuron, interneuron, ICC, motor neuron or smooth muscle cell) in the network could enter refractory period accounting for unresponsiveness. However, smooth muscle cell and ICC seem to be the first choice candidate because their slow wave depolarization and the refractoriness of the muscular tissue to repetitive stimulation. One possibility set in the especial tissue structure in the final part of the anorectal canal, in the internal sphincter region. In this region the proportion of longitudinal and circular smooth muscles changes as do the intrinsic enteric nervous system connectivity. Particularly, the circular muscle layer is thicker than in the rest of the anorectal canal. Above can contribute altogether to explain the characteristic responses of the gut wall in this region. However, more electrophysiological research is needed to elucidate the fundamentals of these reflex responses.

References

[1] Barret KE. *Gastrointestinal physiology*. McGraw-Hill Ed. 2006. p. 304.

[2] Hagger R, Finlayson C, Kahn F, De Oliveira R, Chimelli L, Kumar D. A deficiency of interstitial cells of Cajal in chagasic megacolon. *J Auton Nerv Syst* 2000; 80:108-11.

[3] Sanders K, Ördög, T, Ward S. Physiology and pathophysiology of the interstitial cells of Cajal: From bench to bedside. IV. Genetic and animal models of GI motility disorders caused by loss of interstitial cells of Cajal. *Am J Physiol Gastrointest Liver Physiol* 2002; 282: G 747-56.

[4] Wood JD, Alpers DH, Andrews PLR. Fundamentals of neurogastroenterology. *Gut* 1999; 45: II6-II16.

[5] Costa M, Brookes SJH, Hennig GW. Anatomy and physiology of the enteric nervous system. *Gut* 2000; 47: iv15-iv19

[6] Kunze WAA, Furness JB. The enteric nervous system and regulation of intestinal motility. *Ann Rev Phsiol* 1999, 61:117-42.

[7] Ward S. Interstitial cells of Cajal in enteric neurotransmission. *Gut* 2000; 47: iv 40-3.

[8] Daniel E. Physiology and pathophysiology of the interstitial cell of Cajal: from bench to bedside III. Interaction of interstitial cells of Cajal with neuromediators: an interim assessment. *Am J Physiol Gastrointest Liver Physiol* 2001; 281: G 1329-32.

[9] Thomson L, Robinson TL, JCF, Farraway LA, Hughes MJG, David W. Andrews DW, Huizinga JD. Interstitial cells of Cajal generate a rhythmic pacemaker current. *Nature Medicine*, 1998: 4:848 –51.

[10] Cajal SR. *Histologie du système nerveux de l'homme et des vertèbrés*, vol. 2. Paris: Maloine; 1911, p. 891–942.

[11] Martínez A, Marín VG, Santiago Ramón y Cajal Junquera, Martínez-Murillo R, Freire M The contributions of Santiago Ramón y Cajal to cancer research — 100 years on. *Nature Reviews Cancer* 2005; 5: 904-9.

[12] Won K-J, Sanders KM, Ward SM. Interstitial cells of Cajal mediate mechanosensitive responses in the stomach. *PNAS*, 2005; 41: 14913-18.

[13] Blay J, Ray-Coquard I. *Gastrointestinal stromal tumors (GIST): a recently described entity with a specific treatment targeted on molecular causes.* Paris: Eurocancer, Jonn Libbey Eurotext, 2001.p. 171-2.

[14] Takayama I, Horiguchi K, Daigo Y, Mine T, Fujino MA, Ohno S. The interstitial cells of Cajal and a gastroenteric pacemaker system. *Arch Histol Cytol* 2002; 65: 1-26.

[15] Farrugia G, Kraichely RE. Deciphering the molecular basis for the pacemaker signal. *Gastroenterology*, 2005;129:1504-17.

[16] Sanders KM, Ward SM. Interstitial cells of Cajal: a new perspective on smooth muscle function. *J Physiol.* 2006 November 1; 576(Pt 3): 721–726.

[17] Yazigi R. Rincones olvidados de la gastroenterología: Las células intersticiales de Cajal. *Gastr Latinoam* 2006; 17: 35-42.

[18] Zárate N, Mearín F, Wang X, Hewlett B, Huizinga JD, Malagelada JR. Severe idiopathic gastroparesis due to neuronal and interstitial cells of Cajal degeneration: pathological findings and management. *Gut* 2003; 52: 966-70.

[19] Lyford G, He C, Soffer E,Hull TL, Strong SA, Senagore AJ et al. Pan-colonic decrease in interstitial cells of Cajal in patients with slow transit constipation. *Gut* 2002; 51:496–501.

[20] Bayliss WM, Starling EH. The movements and innervation of the small intestine. *J. Physiol.*1899; 24:99–143.

In: Hirschsprung's Disease: Diagnosis and Treatment
Ed: Ramón Núñez and Manuel López-Alonso
ISBN: 978-1-60741-349-3

Chapter IV

Pathophysiology of Hirschsprung's Disease

Prem Puri and Anne-Marie O' Donnell

Introduction

Hirschsprung's disease (HSCR) is a congenital disorder of the distal intestine, characterised by a narrowing and aganglionosis of the distal colon, resulting in functional obstruction and the prevention of normal peristalsis. HSCR is a relatively common cause of intestinal obstruction in the newborn, affecting one in every 5,000 live births. The disease is more common in boys, with a male to female ratio of 4:1 [1]. The functional characteristic of the disease is intestinal obstruction, or severe constipation, caused by the absence of ganglia in varying distances proximally from the rectum. The affected gut loses its ability to transmit a motile relaxation and contraction (peristaltic) wave; this section of the bowel is typically contracted and devoid of contents (Fig. 1). In contrast, the segment of intestine proximal to this becomes grossly distended by faecal accumulation and is termed a 'megacolon'. Despite extensive research in recent years, the pathophysiology of HSCR is still not fully understood.

The gastrointestinal tract is responsible for processing food into molecules that can be absorbed and utilised by the cells of the body. The cells lining the gastrointestinal tract perform digestion, secretion and absorption. They possess enzymes to digest sugars and peptides, and they transport specific substances present in the intestinal lumen. Food is broken down, bit by bit, until the molecules are small enough to be absorbed and the waste products eliminated. The neural network within the wall of the gut communicates with the adjacent smooth muscle layers to coordinate this digestion, absorption and excretion. Normal intestinal motility requires co-ordinated interaction of the enteric nervous system (ENS), smooth muscle cells and interstitial cells of Cajal (ICCs).

Neural Control of the Gastrointestinal Tract

The gastrointestinal tract is innervated both extrinsically and intrinsically, by the central nervous system (CNS) and ENS respectively. The gastrointestinal tract is connected to the CNS through the autonomic nervous system (ANS) (the brain-gut axis), via both motor and sensory pathways of the sympathetic and parasympathetic nervous systems (PNS).

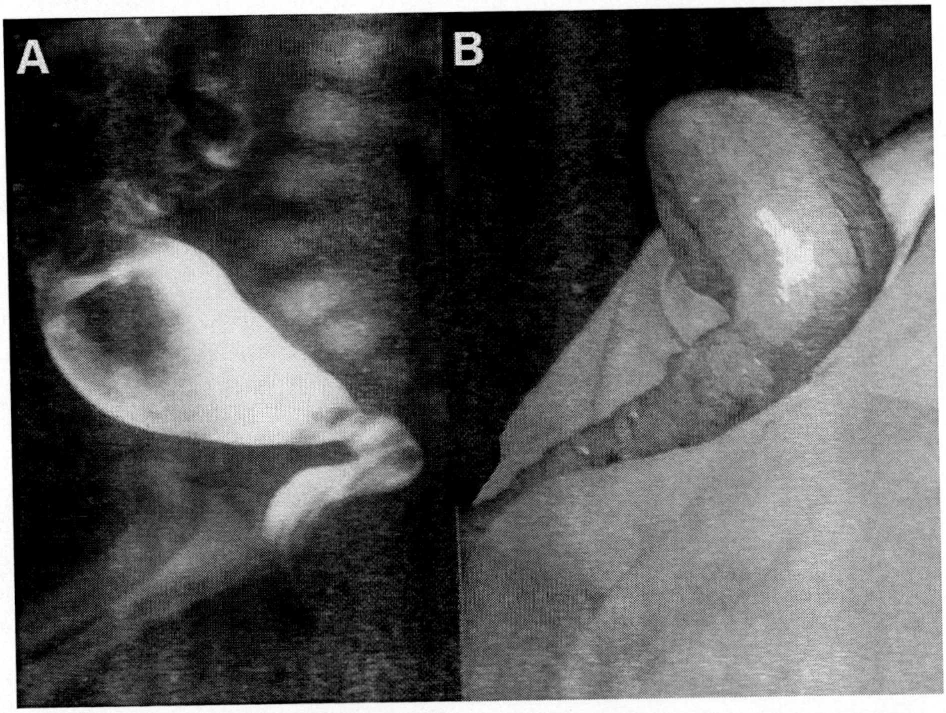

Figure 1: (A) Barium enema showing rectosigmoid Hirschsprung's disease with a classical contracted aganglionic segment. (B) Operative photograph of the same patient showing the aganglionic contracted segment and dilated ganglionic segment of bowel

Motor Input from the CNS

The parasympathetic motor pathways consist of the vagus nerves that control the motor and secretomotor functions of the upper gastrointestinal tract, and the sacral nerves that regulate the functions of the distal colon and rectum. The parasympathetic preganglionic neurons are all cholinergic and exert excitatory effects on enteric neurons through nicotinic and, in some regions, muscarinic receptors. These neurons provide rich connections to the myenteric neurons in the upper gastrointestinal tract as well as the distal colon and anorectum. In the small bowel, however, vagal preganglionic neurons innervate only small clusters of selected myenteric neurons, which may serve as command neurons [2]. The differences in the intensity of innervation by parasympathetic preganglionic fibres reflect the fact that the CNS exerts more direct control in the most proximal (ie. the oesophagus and stomach) and in the most distal (ie. the rectosigmoid) parts of the gastrointestinal tract and less direct control on the functions of the small intestine and proximal colon [3].

The sympathetic fibres entering the gut are adrenergic, postganglionic fibres with cell bodies in the prevertebral ganglia. They have at least four distinct targets in the gut: secretomotor neurons containing vasoactive intestinal polypeptide (VIP), presynaptic cholinergic nerve endings, submucosal blood vessels and gastrointestinal sphincters.

Sensory Output to the CNS

Neurons that carry sensory information out of the gut to the CNS are termed 'primary afferent neurons'. They are carried in the vagal and splanchnic nerves. Vagal primary afferent neurons have cell bodies in the nodose ganglia. It has been estimated that 80% of fibres in the vagal nerve trunk are afferent fibres [4]. The primary vagal afferent neurons in the smooth muscle layer are sensitive to mechanical distension of the gut; they have very low thresholds and convey information about physiologic motor activities in the gut [5]. Certain vagal primary afferent neurons in the mucosa are sensitive to luminal concentrations of glucose, amino acids, or long-chain fatty acids, whereas others respond to a wide variety of chemical and mechanical stimuli [6]. Chemical transmitters released by mucosal endocrine cells are involved in transducing the actions of some stimuli on the vagal afferent neurons.

The Enteric Nervous System

In addition to the CNS, the ENS provides the gastrointestinal tract with its own unique network of innervation within its walls. The ENS is the largest and most complex division of the PNS. The salient feature of the ENS, is that its neurons form highly complex local reflex circuits, which function largely independently of the CNS to control contractility of the smooth muscle layers of the bowel and secretions of the enteric glands [7]. The human ENS contains approximately 80-100 million neurons [7], even more than that contained within the spinal cord. For this reason, it is thought of by some researchers in the field as 'the second brain'. The structure of the ENS is actually more like that of brain than of peripheral nerve: collagen is absent, and enteric neurons are supported by glia rather than Schwann cells [8].

The neurons of the ENS, along with ICCs and muscle cells form a highly complex network within the gut wall, communicating with each other to regulate normal gut function. The ENS is composed of these neurons and glial cells organised into two ganglionated plexuses; the myenteric plexus and the submucosal plexus. These plexuses are arranged as two concentric rings within the gut wall extending throughout its entire length [7]. The myenteric plexus (Auerbach's plexus) is located between the outer longitudinal muscle layer and the inner circular muscle layer. The submucosal plexus can be divided into an outer plexus (Schabadasch's plexus), which is located in the submucosal layer adjacent to the circular muscle layer, and an inner submucous plexus (Meissner's plexus), located close to the muscularis mucosae [7]. The neurons of both these plexuses are organised as clusters of ganglion cells of various sizes.

Enteric Smooth Muscle

The muscular layers of the gastrointestinal tract are composed of smooth muscle cells that are continuous from the oesophagus to the anal canal. These cells can work partly against each other, or against a hydrostatic pressure within the lumen, and have a complex relation with each other. Smooth muscle cells are uninucleated and roughly spindle-shaped. Several structural specialisations are present at the cell surface, including cell-to-cell junctions and junctions between a cell and the surrounding connective tissue stroma. Smooth muscle cells are innervated by muscle motor neurons, and directly by the motor axons of ICCs, which are connected through electrically conducting gap junctions to the muscle [9]. Smooth muscle cells in the muscle coat are densely packed, with about 180,000 cell/mm^3. Smooth muscle cells possess a contractile apparatus, consisting of actin and myosin filaments and cytoskeleton [10]. The cytoskeletal system serves as a structural framework that surrounds and supports the contractile apparatus within the body of the cell and its primary function is to link or connect protein filaments to each other and to the anchoring sites.

Interstitial Cells of Cajal

The interstitial cells of Cajal (ICCs) are mesenchymal cells, spindle shaped or with several processes that form networks that are widely distributed within the submucosal, intramuscular and intermuscular layers of the gastrointestinal tract from the esophagus to the internal anal sphincter [10-12]. ICCs can be localised immunohistochemically by the expression of c-Kit, a trans-cell membrane tyrosine-kinase receptor. ICCs act as pacemakers in the gut wall, by developing spontaneous slow waves, which spread to the smooth muscle cells. Recent studies have demonstrated that ICCs also mediate enteric motor neurotransmission via synaptic-like contacts that exist between varicose nerve terminals and intramuscular ICCs [12]. However, the integrative role of the ICCs and the enteric nervous system in the control of gastrointestinal function is still unknown [13].

Classification of ENS Neurons

The functional complexity of the ENS is reflected in the number and phenotypic diversity of its neurons, which produce a large variety of neuropeptides and neurotransmitters [14,15]. The combinatorial expression of these molecules generates a chemical code that has been used to classify the neurons of the mammalian ENS into functionally distinct groups [16]. As well as functional classifications, ENS neurons can be classified according to their morphology and neurochemical properties.

Motor neurons are either excitatory or inhibitory. The excitatory motor neurons use acetylcholine and substance P as their main neurotransmitters, while the inhibitory motor neurons contain VIP and nitric oxide (NO). The primary afferent neurons are all cholinergic, thus use acetylcholine as their neurotransmitter, and may also contain substance P. Several subgroups of interneurons have been defined based on their neurotransmitter content [3].

According to their morphology, neurons are classified into Dogiel type I to type VII and giant neurons. Most neurons are Dogiel types I-III [17]. Dogiel type I neurons have flat cell bodies with many short, lamellar dendrites and a single long axon and they are implicated as enteric motor neurons. Dogiel type II neurons have relatively smooth cell bodies with short and long processes arising in a variety of configurations. The long processes may extend through interganglionic fibre tracts across several rows of ganglia. Shorter processes may project only within the home ganglion. Dogiel type III neurons are similar to the latter except there are more processes and more of the processes are shorter in length [18].

Neurons usually express a combination of different neurotransmitters, a phenomenon known as chemical coding [14]. The chemical code depends on the type of neuron and the intestinal segment. The general mechanism of chemically mediated synaptic transmission is the same in the enteric nervous system as elsewhere in the body, and seemingly as complex as in the central nervous system. More than 30 neurotransmitters have been identified in the ENS, which are usually co-localised according to their function [17,19] (Table 1). Enteric neurotransmitters are either small molecules (Norepinephrine, 5-HT), larger molecules (peptides) or gases (nitric oxide and carbon monoxide) [20].

Table 1. Main neurotransmitters involved in enteric nervous system neurotransmission

ENS	NEUROTRANSMITTERS
•Amines	**•Peptides**
-Acetylcholine	-Bombesin
-Histamine	-Calcitonin gene related peptide
-Norepinephrine	-Cholecystokinin
-Serotonin (5-hydroxytryptamine)	-Galanin
	-Gastrin-releasing peptide
•Amino acids	-Neurokinin A
-Glutamate	-Neuromidin U
-(-Amino)	-Neuropeptide Y
	-Neurotensin
•Purines	-Nociceptin (Orphanin)
-ATP	-Opoids
	-Dynorphin
•Gases	-Enkephalins
-Nitric oxide	-Endorphins
-Carbon monoxide	-Peptide YY
	-Peptide histidine isoleucine
	-Pituitary adenyl cyclase activating peptide
	-Secretin
	-Somatostatin
	-Substnace P
	-Thyrotropin releasing hormone
	-Vasoactive intestinal polypeptide
	-Vasoactive intestinal contractor (an endothelin)

Gut Motility

Two patterns of activity are recognized in the mammalian intestine, the activity of the interdigestive state and the fed pattern of activity [21]. During fasting, a specific motor activity- the migrating motor complexes- sweeps along the gut. The gut changes its motility from fasted to fed patterns through cephalic reflexes at the sight, smell or even anticipation of food [22]. After ingestion of food, the sensory input to the local and central control systems elicited by the food itself starts specific patterns of motility, such as swallowing, gastric emptying and peristalsis.

In the interdigestive state, complexes of contractions travelling in an anal direction have been recorded. These are known as migrating myoelectric complexes (MMC), which pass along the intestine every 80-110 min. in humans. The complex takes about 6-10 min to pass any point in the intestine, and as it passes, that region undergoes intense rhythmic contractions of the circular muscle [21]. These MMC probably act as housekeepers, to transport waste products in the interdigestive stage and they also control the bacterial flora, preventing overgrowth and returning bacteria to the large intestine [23,24]. Soon after a meal is consumed, MMCs disappear and are replaced by the fed pattern of activity, the peristaltic movements. Both the interdigestive pattern and the fed pattern are generated through the ENS but are modified by the extrinsic nerves. The continuity of the ENS is necessary for the orderly progress of the MMC; if the intestine is interrupted surgically and then rejoined, the MMC does not always pass the lesion and ectopic MMCs occur on the anal side [21].

The fed pattern of activity both mixes and propels the contents. In one human study, about 45% of individual contractions did not propagate and about 35% propagated for less than 9 cm [25]. These nonpropagating contractions correspond to the mixing activity. The propagated contractions are peristaltic waves, which consist of contraction of the circular muscle oral to a bolus in the lumen, the ascending excitatory reflex; and relaxation on the anal side, the descending inhibitory reflex. In addition, longitudinal muscle on the anal side may contract while the oral longitudinal muscle relaxes. Total extrinsic denervation of the bowel does not affect peristalsis [21], as all the neural elements for the peristaltic reflex are found intrinsically in the intestine.

Development of the ENS: The Neural Crest

The ENS is derived from the neural crest; a cell line exclusively produced by the neural tube of vertebrates in the early stages of embryonic development. It has fascinated embryologists for over a hundred years for two major reasons: it has the ability to differentiate into a vast number of cell types, and to migrate from its point of origin over considerable distances along defined routes to specific destinations [26]. Most of the PNS arises from the neural crest to include all the glia of the sensory ganglia, all neurons of the dorsal root ganglia and the majority of neurons of the cranial sensory ganglia. The ANS also derives entirely from the neural crest comprising all sympathetic and parasympathetic branches as well as the ENS [27].

It is now generally accepted that the enteric nerve cells are derived from neural crest cells that migrate primarily from the vagal neural tube [3,28]. Studies in the avian embryo provide strong evidence for the contribution of sacral neural crest cells to the hindgut ENS [29-31]. Whether the sacral neural crest contributes to the ENS in the human is less clear. Failure of the vagal derived neural crest cells to colonise the hindgut results in failure of ENS development in this region, suggesting an interaction between sacral and vagal enteric neural crest cells may be necessary for sacral neural crest cell contribution to the ENS [32].

Dynamics of Neural Crest Cell Migration in the Gut

The advance of neural crest cells along the gut is a result of a combination of both migration and proliferation. It is the co-ordination of these activities that leads to the colonisation of the gut and establishment of ganglia. Proliferation plays an important role and is required to maintain a population of migrating crest cells to offset the number that differentiate as colonisation progresses. This is underscored by the fact that the migratory path of enteric neural crest cells is longer than that of other crest-derived cells [33].

Migration is essential for the distribution of the cells throughout the gut. In fixed preparations of developing chick and mouse gut, enteric neural crest cells are arranged largely in strands or cords of cells [34,35]. The most caudal cells of the strand represent the 'migratory wavefront', while rostral to the wavefront, the neural crest cells show a pattern of branches and nodes.

Direct observation of neural crest cell migration in situ was first studied by Young et al. using mice in which cDNA encoding tau-EGFP-myc had been inserted into the first exon of the Ret gene [36]. These mice expressed green fluorescent protein in all enteric neural crest cells, and therefore permitted the study of their movement using time-lapse imaging. Their results revealed that in the ileum and distal colon, enteric neural crest cells migrate as chains and that the leading cells of strands follow complex and unpredictable pathways [36]. A similar study by Druckenbrod et al. using a different transgenic mouse examined the dynamics of neural crest cell movement within the caecum, proximal and distal colon [33]. Their results showed that the enteric neural crest cell wavefront regularly pauses at the caecum and then displays a very different pattern of migration from that found in other more proximal regions. Instead of advancing as a network of strands, neural crest cells initially migrate into the caecum and proximal colon as isolated single cells. These isolated cells then form groups, which over time extend strands towards other isolated groups of cells. This interaction re-establishes an unbroken network that is capable of advancing towards the terminal colon [33].

The Aganglionic Gut in Hirschsprung's Disease

The most striking finding in the distal intestine in HSCR is the absence of ganglion cells in the myenteric and submucous plexuses [37]. This aganglionosis is thought to be attributed to the early arrest of neural crest cell migration to the gut; the earlier the arrest of migration, the longer the aganglionic segment. Aganglionosis typically extends to the rectosigmoid region in approximately 80% of cases; the sigmoid, splenic flexure or transverse colon in 17% and total colon along with a short segment of terminal ileum in 8% of patients [38]. The aganglionosis is continuous and uninterrupted until the proximal transitional zone is reached. The length of this zone may vary and extend for several centimetres and is characterized by hypoganglionosis.

The characteristic gross pathologic feature of Hirschsprung's disease (HSCR) is a narrowed distal colon with a funnel shaped transition zone leading to a dilated and hypertrophied proximal colon. However, these features may vary with the duration of untreated disease. In the neonatal period, the intestine may appear normal; but as the child ages, the proximal intestine hypertrophies and becomes thicker and longer than normal. The taeniae disappear and the longitudinal muscle layer seems to completely surround the colon [39]. It has long been recognized that the obstructive symptoms in HSCR are secondary to the abnormal motility of the distal narrow segment, but there is still no clear explanation for the occurrence of contracted intestinal wall in the distal bowel in HSCR [40].

Impairment in Nitrergic Innervation in HSCR

Nitric oxide (NO) is the main inhibitory neurotransmitter used in the ENS and plays a key role in intestinal relaxation [41]. NO is produced in a reaction catalyzed by the enzyme nitric oxide synthase (NOS) using L-arginine and molecular oxygen as co-substrates to form L-citrulline and NO. When NO binds to cytosolic guanylate cyclase, it increases the production of 3′5′-cyclic guanosine monophosphate (cGMP) resulting in relaxation of the intestinal smooth muscle [42]. NOS has been shown to be colocalized with reduced nicotine adenine dinucleotide phosphate (NADPH) diaphorase, which has been demonstrated to have identical functions[43,44]. Several investigators have studied NOS distribution in the ganglionic and aganglionic bowel in patients with HSCR using nitric oxide synthase immunohistochemistry or NADPH diaphorase histochemistry [45-50]. Research in recent years has indicated that NO synthesis is somehow impaired in the aganglionic bowel in HSCR and that this deficiency in NO could prevent smooth muscle relaxation, thereby causing the lack of peristalsis in the aganglionic gut. In normal and ganglionic colon from patients with HSCR, Rolle et al have shown that there is strong NADPH diaphorase staining of ganglia and nerve fibres in the submucous and myenteric plexuses and a large number of positive nerve fibres in the circular and longitudinal muscle as well as in the muscularis mucosae [42]. However, in the aganglionic segment of HSCR patients, they observed no ganglia as well as an absence or marked reduction in NADPH diaphorase positive nerve fibres in both smooth muscle layers and in the muscularis mucosae. Hypertrophied nerve trunks typical of HSCR were seen to be weakly stained by NADPH diaphorase histochemistry [42]. Bealer et al. compared the effect of applying an exogenous source of NO, S-nitroso-Nacetylpenicillamine (SNAP) on the isometric tension of smooth muscle strips from aganglionic bowel and demonstrated a 70% reduction of resting tension [47]. Further evidence of nitrergic abnormalities were found by Kusafuka and Puri when they investigated the expression of neural NOS mRNA in the aganglionic segment from 7 patients who had

HSCR and found that NOS mRNA expression was decreased at least 1/50 to 1/100 times that compared to the level observed in ganglionic bowel [51]. The impairment of the nitrergic network within the aganglionic bowel is thought to contribute to the pathogenesis of HSCR.

Increased Cholinergic Activity in HSCR

One of the key histological findings, often used in the diagnosis of HSCR, is a marked increase in the amount of cholinergic nerve fibres in the intermuscular zone and submucosa in the aganglionic segment. These fibres appear as hypertrophied nerve trunks and they correspond to extrinsic preganglionic parasympathetic nerves [46,50-54]. These parasympathetic nerves continuously release acetylcholine which results in an excessive accumulation of the enzyme acetylcholinesterase in the lamina propria mucosae, muscularis mucosae and circular muscle and can be histochemically visualised with specific staining techniques [37]. Studies have shown that both the thick nerve trunks and the increased acetylcholinesterase activity are most pronounced in the most distal aganglionic rectum and progressively diminish proximally as the ganglionic region is approached [55]. However, it must be noted that the proximal extent of increased cholinergic activity does not necessarily correspond to the extent of the aganglionosis, and therefore cannot be used as a marker of aganglionosis, as it usually extends more proximally to a variable degree. Boston et al. have shown that the serum and erythrocytes from children with HSCR contain higher concentrations of acetylcholinesterase compared to normal age-matched children [56]. Considering the fact that acetylcholine is the major excitatory neurotransmitter in the ENS, it is thought that the tonic nature of the aganglionic segment in HSCR is partly attributed to the cholinergic nerve hyperplasia observed in this region. This theory has however been challenged by studies using animal models of HSCR, where chemically-induced animal models of aganglionosis were found not to display hypertrophic nerve bundles despite the characteristicly narrow appearance of the aganglionic region and typical obstructive symptoms exhibited [57,58].

Interstitial Cells of Cajal in HSCR

Several investigators have studied the distribution of ICCs in the ganglionic and aganglionic bowel in patients with HSCR using c-kit immunoreactivity, with a reduced number of c-kit immunoreactive ICCs in aganglionic bowel and also in the transitional zone of HSCR patients consistently reported [45,60-65]. Vanderwinden et al. described a reduced number of ICCs with a disrupted network in the aganglionic bowel [45]. These ICCs did not form a network and showed no clear relation to the hypertrophic nerve trunks. Yamataka et al. found few c-kit positive cells in the muscle layers of HSCR and a moderate number around the thick nerve bundles in the space between the two muscle layers in the aganglionic bowel [62,63]. Nevertheless, the latter study referred to the importance of regional differences in the distribution of c-kit positive cells in the normal colon since different expression of c-kit positive cells was shown in different regions of the bowel. This study did not differentiate between myenteric and muscular ICCs. Two more recent studies have shown that ICCs were either normal or only slightly reduced in the affected bowel in HSCR compared to normal bowel [66,67].

Advances in the management of Hirschsprung's disease afford most patients a satisfactory outcome after definitive surgery. However, some patients continue to have persistent bowel dysfunction despite adequate resection of the aganglionic bowel. Postoperative motility problems after proper resection of the aganglionic bowel have been attributed to intestinal neuronal dysplasia or altered distribution in ICCs. In a detailed study, Rolle et al. examined the three-dimensional morphology of c-kit immunoreactive ICCs in the aganglionic, ganglionic and transition zone of HSCR bowel [64]. All types of myenteric ICCs appeared to be markedly reduced in the aganglionic bowel and in the transition zone (Figure 2). Furthermore, ICCs were also diminished in the ganglionic part of the resected HSCR bowel. Whole-mount preparations of the ganglionic region of HSCR bowel displayed numerous myenteric ICCs forming sparse networks around the ganglia of the myenteric plexus, which were less developed than that seen in normal bowel [64]. The clear reduction of myenteric ICCs in the normoganglionic sigmoid colon in HSCR is assumed to be the cause of motility disturbances in some patients after pull-through operations [64].

A further study has confirmed that an abnormal distribution of c-kit positive cells in the normoganglionic segment can predict a poor clinical outcome in patients with HSCR [68], while a recently published study by Bettoli et al. introduced a new pathological protocol for the rapid assessment of enteric ICCs in order to improve the management of HSCR patients [69]. However, the provided data could not finally show if defective ICCs in aganglionic or ganglionic bowel of HSCR are the cause or the consequence of the neuropathy with subsequent chronic constipation.

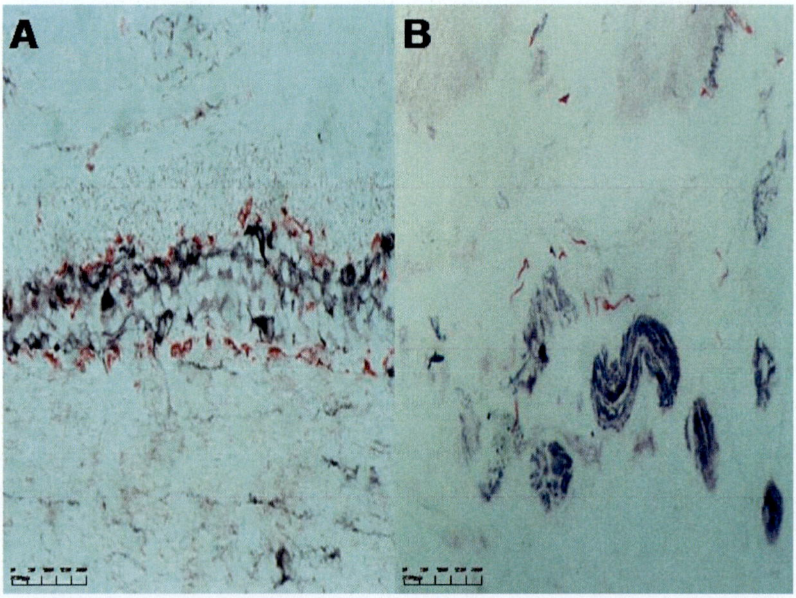

Figure 2. NADPH-diaphorase staining (blue) and C-kit immunohistochemistry (red) showing the overlap of ICCs and nitrergic neurons in ganglionic (A) and aganglionic (B) bowel of a Hirschsprung's patient.

Abnormalities of the Extracellular Matrix

Research over the years has suggested that extracellular matrix (EM) abnormalities could have an influence on the pathophysiology of HSCR. Parikh et al. have demonstrated that the concentration of laminin in the aganglionic bowel was twice as high as that in normoganglionic bowel of HSCR and three times higher than in age-matched controls [70]. The lethal spotted mouse, an animal model which develops aganglionosis in its distal bowel, displays an abnormal distribution of EM components including laminin, collagen type IV, glycosaminoglycans and proteoglycans in the smooth muscle layer [71,72]. In addition, they found an uneven distribution of laminin and collagen type IV in the muscularis propria of aganglionic bowel, with a more intense expression in the circular muscle layer compared to the longitudinal muscle layer [73]. Further work by the same authors showed that two EM components, tenascin and fibronectin, are more intensely expressed in aganglionic bowel from HSCR patients compared to the ganglionic segments [74].

Genetics of HSCR

During the past 15 years, there has been an explosion of information about the genes that control the development of the ENS. Molecular genetic analysis has identified several genes that control the migration, proliferation, differentiation and survival of neural crest derived cells (Figure 3) (Table 2). Formation of the mammalian ENS requires a co-ordinated and balanced interaction between signalling molecules and transcription factors which play a critical role in the formation of enteric ganglia. Failure of this integration leads to the absence of ganglion cells and therefore HSCR phenotype. Two signalling systems mediated by RET and EDNRB have been identified as the critical players in enteric neurogenesis. Another HSCR gene coding for protein members of an inter-related signalling pathways is Glial cell line derived neurotrophic factor (GDNF). The sex determining region Y-box (SOX10) gene has also been seen to be a key player in the pathogenesis of HSCR.

The tyrosine kinase receptor, RET, is vitally important for the migration and development of enteric ganglia derived from neural crest cells. Mutations in RET account for up to 50% of familial cases of HSCR and 15-20% of sporadic cases. This indicates that genetic mutations in other genes are also responsible for HSCR, and are yet to be discovered. GDNF stimulates the proliferation and survival of neural crest derived precursor cells in the embryonic gut. GDNF is the ligand of RET and GDNF mutations have been reported in HSCR [36,65]. The endothelins (EDN1, EDN2 and EDN3) are intracellular local messengers that act via cell surface receptors. EDN3 and endothelin receptor type B have been shown to be important for the normal migration and development of the ENS [75]. SOX10 is also essential for development of the ENS, with reports of mutations of this gene in patients with Waardenburg-Shah syndrome which includes ENS defects, pigmentation abnormalities as well as ANS abnormalities [76].

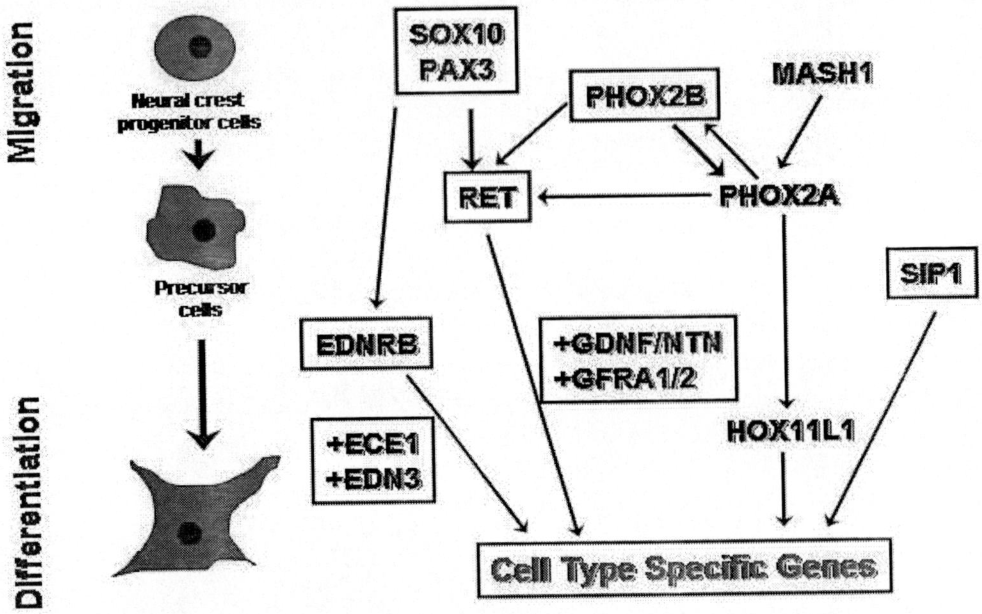

Figure 3. Schematic diagram outlining the major genes involved in the migration and differentiation of neural crest cells into neurons

Table 2. Major candidate genes involved in the pathogenesis of Hirschsprung's disease and their chromosomal alignments

Genes	Chromosomal assignment
RET	10q11.2
GDNF	5p12-13.1
GFRα	10q26
EDNRB	13q22
EDN-3	20q13.2
SOX10	22q13.1
NTN	19p13
ECE-1	1p36.1
PHOX2B	4p12
SIP1	2q22
PAX3	2q35
KIAA1279	10q21.3

Conclusion

Despite the fact that the most striking histological feature in Hirschsprung's disease is the absence of ganglion cells, it is unlikely that this is the only cause of the increased intestinal wall tone provoking a functional intestinal obstruction. As discussed throughout this chapter, there are a number of other histopathological findings both in the aganglionic segment and in the proximal ganglionic segment in Hirschsprung's disease which may account for the frequent discrepancy encountered between the length of the non-functional bowel and the degree of obstruction and also for the persistent obstructive symptoms after a pull-through operation for Hirschsprung's disease.

References

[1] Orr JD, Scobie W G. Presentation and incidence of Hirschsprung's disease. *Br J Med.*1983; 287: 1671.

[2] Kirchgessner AL, Gershon MD.Identification of vagal efferent fibers and putative target neurons in the enteric nervous system of the rat. *J Comp Neurol.* 1989; 285: 38-53

[3] Goyal RK, Hirano I.The enteric nervous system. *N Eng J Med.* 1996; 334: 1106-15

[4] Goyal RK, Hirano I. Mechanisms of disease: the enteric nervous system. *New Eng J Med.* 1996; 334: 1106-15.

[5] Sengupta JN, Gebhart G F.Gastrointestinal afferent fibres and sensation in *Physiology of the gastrointestinal tract.* J. LR, Ed. New York: Raven Press;1994. p. 483-520.

[6] Mei N. Intestinal chemosensitivity. Physiol Rev.1985; 65: 211-37.

[7] Furness J, Costa M. *The Enteric Nervous System.* New York: Churchill Livingstone, 1987.

[8] Gershon MD. Neural crest development. Do developing enteric neurons need endothelins? *Curr Biol.* 1995; 5: 601-4

[9] Sanders K. Interstitial cells of Cajal at the clinical and scientific interface. *J Physiol.*2006; 576: 683-7.

[10] Sanders KM, Ordog T. Ward S. Physiology and Pathophysiology of the Interstitial Cells of Cajal: From bench to bedside IV. Genetic and animal models of GI motility disorders caused by the loss of interstitial cells of Cajal. *Am J Physiol Gastrointest Liver Physiol.*2002; 282: 747-56.

[11] Takaki M. Gut pacemaker cells: the interstitial cells of Cajal (ICC). *J Smooth Muscle Res.* 2003; 39: 137-61.

[12] Ward SM, Sanders KM, Hirst G.Role of interstitial cells of cajal in neural control of gastrointestinal smooth muscles. *Neurogastroenterol Motil.* 2004; 16: 112-7.

[13] Albertí E, Mikkelsen HB, Larsen JO, Jimenenez M. Motility patterns and distribution of interstitial cells of cajal and nitrergic neurons in the proximal, mid- and distal-colon of the rat. *J Physiol Gastrointest Liver Physiol.* 2005; 17: 133-47.

[14] Costa M, Brookes S J, Steele P A, Gibbins I, Burcher E, Kondiach C J. Neurochemical classification of myenteric neurons in the guinea-pig ileum. *Neurosci*. 1996; 75: 949-67.

[15] Gershon MD, Kirchgessner A L, Wade PR. Functional anatomy of the enteric nervous system. In: *Physiology of the Gastrointestinal Tract*. New York: Raven Press; 1994 Vol 1: p. 381-442.

[16] Sang Q, Young HM. Chemical coding of neurons in myenteric plexus and external muscle of the small and large intestine of the mouse. *Cell Tissue Res*.1996; 284: 39-53.

[17] Furness J B. Types of neurons in the enteric nervous system. *J Auton Nerv Syst*. 2000; 81: 87-96.

[18] Brehmer A, Schrodl F, Neuhuber. W, Morphological classifications of enteric neurons-100 years after Dogiel. *Anat Embryol*. 1999; 200: 125-35.

[19] Hansen MB. Neurohumoral control of gastrointestinal motility. *Physiol Res*. 2003; 52: 1-30.

[20] Furness JB, Clerc N, Kunze WA. Memory in the enteric nervous system. *Gut*. 2000; 47: iv60-iv62.

[21] Kunze WA, Furness JB. The enteric nervous system and regulation of intestinal motility. *Annu Rev Physiol*. 1999; 61: 117-42.

[22] Olsson C, Holmgren S. The control of gut motility. *Comp Biochem Physio A Mol Integr Physiol*. 2001; 128: 481-503.

[23] Vantrappen G, Janssens J, Hellemans J, Ghoos Y. The interdigestive motor complex of normal subjects and patients with bacterial outgrowth of the small intestine. *J Clin Invest*. 1977; 59: 1158-66.

[24] Szurszewski JH. A migrating electric complex of canine small intestine. *Am J Physiol*. 1969; 217: 1757-63.

[25] Summers RW, Dusdieker NS. Patterns of spike burst spread and flow in the canine small intestine. *Gastroenterology*. 1981; 81: 742-50.

[26] Le Douarin NM, Creuzet S, Couly G, Dupin E. Neural crest cell plasticity and its limits. *Dev*. 2004; 131: 4637-50.

[27] Kalcheim C, Burstyn-Cohen T. Early stages of neural crest ontogeny: formation and regulation of cell delamination. *Int J Dev Biol*. 2005; 49: 105-16.

[28] Gershon M D, Chalazonitis A, Rothman TP. From neural crest to bowel: development of the enteric nervous system. *J Neurobiol*. 1993; 24: 199-214.

[29] Le Douarin NM, Teillet MA. The migration of neural crest cells to the wall of the digestive tract in the avian embryo. *J Embryol Exp Biol*. 1973; 30: 31-48.

[30] Pomeranz HD, Gershon MD. Colonization of the avian hindgut by cells derived from the sacral neural crest. *Dev Biol*. 1990; 137: 378-94.

[31] Burns AJ, Douarin NM. The sacral neural crest contributes neurons and glia to the post-umbilical gut: spatiotemporal analysis of the development of the enteric nervous system. *Dev*. 1998; 125: 4335-47.

[32] Gariepy CE. Intestinal motility disorders and development of the enteric nervous system. *Pediatr Res*. 2001; 49: 605-13

[33] Druckenbrod NR, Epstein ML. The pattern of neural crest advance in the cecum and colon. *Dev Biol*. 2005; 287: 125-33.

[34] Epstein ML, Poulsen KT, Thiboldeaux R. Formation of ganglia in the gut of the chick embryo. *J Comp Neurol*. 1991; 307: 189-99.

[35] Young HM, Hearn CJ, Ciampoli D, Southwell BR, Brunet JF, Newgreen DF. A single rostrocaudal colonization of the rodent intestine by enteric neuron precursors is revealed by the expression of Phox 2b, Ret, and p75 and by explants grown under the kidney capsule or in organ culture. *Dev Biol*. 1998; 202: 67-84.

[36] Young HM, Bergner AJ, Anderson RB, Enomoto H, Milbrandt J, Newgreen DF, et al. Dynamics of neural crest-derived cell migration in the embryonic mouse gut. *Dev Biol*. 2004; 270: 455-73.

[37] Meier-Ruge, W., ed. Histological diagnosis and differential diagnosis. *Hirschsprung's disease and allied disorders*, ed. A.M. Holschneider and P. Puri. Hardwood Academic Publishers. 2000; p. 252-265.

[38] Kleinhaus S, Boley SJ, SheranM, Sieber WK. Hirschsprung's disease: a survey of the surgical section of the American Academy of Pediatrics. *J Pediatr Surg*. 1979; 14: 588-97.

[39] Teitelbaum DH, Coran AG, Weitzman JJ, Ziegler MM, Kane T: Hirschsprung' disease and related neuromuscular disorders of the intestine. In O'Neill JA, Rowe MI, Grosfeld JL, Fonkairud EW, Coran AG. (Eds). *Pediatry Surgery*. Fifth Edition. St Louis: Mosby; 1998. p. 1381-1424.

[40] Dasgupta R, Langer JC. Hirshsprung disease. *Curr Probl Surg*. 2004; 41: 942-88.

[41] Bult H, Boeckxstaens GE, Pelckmans PA, Jordaens FH, Van Maercke YM, Herman AG. Nitric oxide as an inhibitory non-adrenergic non-cholinergic neurotransmitter. *Nature*. 1990; 345: 346-7.

[42] Rolle U, Nemeth L, Puri P. Nitrergic innervation of the normal gut and in motility disorders of childhood. *J Pediatr Surg*.2002; 37: 551-67.

[43] Dawson TM, Bredt DS, M. Fotuhi M, Hwang PM, Snyder SH. Nitric oxide synthase and neuronal NADPH diaphorase are identical in brain and peripheral tissues. *Proc Natl Acad Sci USA*. 1991; 88:7797-801.

[44] Hope BT, Michael GJ, Knigge KM, Vicent SR. Neuronal NADPH diaphorase is a nitric oxide synthase. *Proc Nat Acad Sci USA*. 1991; 88: 2811- 4.

[45] Vanderwinden J, Rumessem JJ, Liu H, Descamps D, De Laet MH, Vanderhaeghen JJ. Interstitial Cells of Cajal in human colon and in Hirschsprung's disease. *Gastroenterology*. 1996; 111: 901-10.

[46] Kobayashi H, O'Briain DS, Puri P. Lack of expression of NADPH-diaphorase and neural cell adhesion molecule (NCAM) in colonic muscle of patients with Hirschsprung's disease. *J Pediatr Surg*. 1994; 29: 301-4.

[47] Bealer J, Natuzzi ES, Buscher C, Ursell PC, Flake AW, Adzick NS et al. Nitric oxide synthase is deficient in the aganglionic colon of patients with Hirschsprung's disease. *Pediatrics*. 1994; 93: 647-51.

[48] Larsson LT.Hirschsprung's disease- immunohistochemical findings. *Histol Histopathol*, 1994; 9: 615-29.

[49] Guo R, Nada O, Suita S, Taguchi T, Masumoto K. The distribution and co-localization of nitric oxide synthase and vasoactive intestinal polypeptide in nerves of the colons with Hirschsprung's disease. *Virchows Arch*. 1997; 430:53-61.

[50] Watanabe Y, Ito T, Haraba T, Kobayashi S, Ozaki T, Nimura Y. Spatial distribution and pattern of extrinsic nerve strands in the aganglioic segment of congenital aganglionosis: stereoscopic analysis in spotting lethal rats. *J Pediatr Surg*. 1995; 30: 1471-6.

[51] Kusafuka T, Puri P. Altered mRNA expression of the neuronal nitric oxide synthase gene in Hirschsprung's disease. *J Pediatr Surg*. 1997; 32: 1054-8.

[52] Kakita Y, Oshiro K, O´Briain DS, Puri P. Selective demonstration of mural nerves in ganglionic and aganglionic colon by immunohistochemistry for glucose transporter-1: prominent extrinsic nerve pattern staining in Hirschsprung disease. *Arch Pathol Lab Med*. 2000; 124: 1314-9.

[53] Payette RF, Tennyson VM, Phan TD, Mawe GM, Pomeranz HD, Rothman TP et al. Origin and morphology of nerve fibers in the aganglionic colon of the lethal spotted (ls/ls) mutant mouse. *J Comp Neurol*. 1987; 25: 237-52.

[54] Tam PK, Boyd GP. Origin, course and endings of abnormal enteric nerve fibres in Hirschsprung's disease defined by whole-mount immunohistochemistry. *J Pediatr Surg*. 1990; 25: 457-61.

[55] Weinberg AG. Hirschsprung's disease- a pathologist's view. *Perspect Pediatr Pathol*. 1975; 2: 207-39.

[56] Boston VE, Cywes S, Davies MR. Serum and erythrocyte acetylcholinesterase activity in Hirschsprung's disease. *J Pediatr Surg*. 1978; 13: 407-10.

[57] Imamura K, Yamamoto M, Sato A, Kashiki Y, Kunieda T. Pathophysiology of aganglionic colon segment: an experimental study on aganglionosis produced by a new method in the rat. *J Pediatr Surg*. 1975; 10: 865-73.

[58] Sato A, Yamamoto M, Inamura K, Kashiki Y, Kunieda T, Sakata K. Pathophysiology of aganglionic colon and anorectum: an experimental study on aganglionosis produced by a new method in the rat. *J Pediatr Surg*. 1978; 13: 399-435.

[59] Piotrowska AP, Solari V, De Caluwe D, Puri P. Immunocolocalization of heme oxygenase-2 and interstitial cells of Cajal in normal and aganglionic colon. *J Pediatr Surg*. 2003; 38: 73-7.

[60] Nemeth L, Maddur S, Puri P. Immunolocalization of the Gap Junction Protein Connexin43 in the Interstitial Cells of Cajal in the Normal and Hirschsprung's Disease bowel. *J Pediatr Surg*. 2000; 35: 823-8.

[61] Nemeth L, Puri P. Three-dimensional morphology of c-Kit-positive cellular network and nitrergic innervation in the human gut. *Arch Pathol Lab Med*. 2001; 125: 899-904.

[62] Yamataka A, Kato Y, Tibboel D, Murata Y, Sueyoshi N, Fujimoto T et al. A lack of intestinal pacemaker (c-kit) in aganglionic bowel of patients with Hirschsprung's disease. *J Pediatr Surg*. 1995; 30: 441-4.

[63] Yamataka A, Oshiro K, Kobayashi H, Fujiwara T, Sunagawa M, Miyano T. Intestinal pacemaker c-kit+ cells and synapses in allied Hirschsprung's disorders. *J Pediatr Surg*. 1997; 32: 1069-74.

[64] Rolle U, Piotrowska A P, Nemeth L, Puri P. Altered distribution of interstitial cells of Cajal in Hirschsprung disease. *Arch Pathol Lab Med*. 2002; 126: 928-33.

[65] Newgreen D, Young HM. Enteric Nervous System: Development and developmental disturbances- Part 2. *Pediatr Dev Pathol*. 2002; 5: 329-49.

[66] Newman CJ, Laurini RN, Lesbros Y, Reinberg O, Meyrat BJ. Interstitial cells of Cajal are normally distributed in both ganglionated and aganglionic bowel in Hirschsprung's disease. *Pediatr Surg Int*. 2003; 19: 662-8.

[67] Taguchi, T, Suita S, Masumoto K, Nada O. Universal distribution of c-kit-positive cells in different types of Hirschsprung's disease. *Pediatr Surg Int*. 2003; 19: 273-9.

[68] Taguchi T, Suita S, Masumoto K, Nagasaki A. An abnormal distribution of C-kit positive cells in the normoganglionic segment can predict a poor clinical outcome in patients with Hirschsprung's disease. *Eur J Pediatr Surg*. 2005; 15: 153-8.

[69] Bettolli M, Rubin SZ, Staines W, Swinton E, Krantis A, Nizalik E. The use of rapid assessment of enteric ICC and neuronal morphology may improve patient management in pediatric surgery: a new clinical pathological protocol. *Pediatr Surg Int*. 2006; 22: 78-83.

[70] Parikh DH, Tam PK, Lloid DA, Van Velzen D, Edgar DH. Quantitative and qualitative analysis of the extracellular matrix protein, laminin, in Hirschsprung's disease. *J Pediatr Surg*. 1992; 27:991-5.

[71] Payette RF, Tennyson VM, Pomeranz HD, Pham TD, Rothman TP, Gershon MD. Accumulation of components of basal laminae: association with the failure of neural crest cells to colonize the presumptive aganglionic bowel of ls/ls mutant mice. *Dev Biol*. 1988; 125: 341-60.

[72] Tennyson VM, Payette RF, Rothman TP, Gershon MD. Distribution of hyaluronic acid and chondroitin sulfate proteglycans in the presumptive aganglionic terminal bowel of ls/ls fetal mice: an ultrastructural analysis. *J Comp Neurol*. 1990; 291: 345-362.

[73] Parikh DH, Tam PK, Van Velzen D, Edgar D. Abnormalities in the distribution of laminin and collagen type IV in Hirschsprung's disease. *Gastroenterology*. 1992; 102: 1236-41.

[74] Parikh DH, Tam PK, Van Velzen D, Edgar D. The extracellular matrix components, tenascin and fibronectin, in Hirschsprung's disease: an immunohistochemical study. *J Pediatr Surg*. 1994; 29: 1302-6.

[75] Parisi MA, Kapur RP. Genetics of Hirschsprung disease. *Curr Opin Pediatr*. 2000; 12: 610-7.

[76] Pingault V, Bondurand N, Kuhlbrodt K, Goerich DE, Préhu MO, Puliti A et al. Sox10 mutations in patients with Waardenburg-Hirschsprung disease. *Nat Genet*. 1998; 18: 171-3.

In: Hirschsprung's Disease: Diagnosis and Treatment
Ed: Ramón Núñez and Manuel López-Alonso
ISBN: 978-1-60741-349-3

Chapter V

Hirschsprung's Disease: Epidemiology, Classification and Associated Congenital Defects

Emilio Blesa, Enrique Galán and Juan J. Cardesa

Epidemiology

Hirschsprung's disease (HD) has very particular epidemiological characteristics. This has led to work on its overall incidence reporting different findings according to which variables were analyzed in the populations studied [1–3].

General Incidence

Nevertheless, it is currently accepted that the average incidence of HD is 1 in every 5000 live births [1–3]. The incidence varies, but not greatly, according to geographical area and race. It is also known to depend on sex, age, family antecedents, and the pathologies with which it can be associated. Other factors are suspected, but as yet not demonstrated, as being involved in its incidence. The underlying factors in part influence the clinical presentation and the morbidity/mortality of HD. Another very important factor is the length of the aganglionic segment.

Incidence by Geographic Area, Ethnicity and Time

In Western countries and Japan, the incidence of HD ranges essentially from 1 per 4500 to 5500 live births [1,4–7]. The extremes of the reported data are 1:12 000 for N Europe and

1:3000 for Oman [2,8]. There are geographical variations even within small countries, probably due to high levels of endogamy [8–9].

There are also differences in the reported incidence for various ethnic groups: 1 per 6666 live births for the 'white' population, 1 per 4754 for 'Afro-Americans', and 1 per 3571 for 'Asiatics' [10]. The ratio of the frequencies in 'non-whites' to 'whites' has been reported to be 1.67:1, and even greater if it is limited to males [1].

Longitudinal studies have shown no differences in incidence when comparing data for the different times at which the information was collected [1,2,10,11].

Sex

HD is commoner in men than in women. The accepted ratio between the sexes is 4:1, with only slight variation in this figure for different samples of patients [1,2,5,9,12–14], although some authors give the ratio as being closer to 3:1 than 4:1 [3,8,11]. In fact, it is considered to be a multifactorial disease modified by sex, with the expression of the genes involved being less restricted in men [3]. The greater incidence in men does not seem to have changed over long periods of time [7].

There is a clear decline in this predominance in men when only extensive and supra-sigmoidal aganglionosis is considered, and even more so for total colonic HD [2.3,5, 10–12].

Family Antecedents

The frequency of familial cases of HD is most commonly estimated at between 2.4% and 9%, with some authors coinciding in figures close to 7% [3,5,12,15–17]. A review of HD covering a long period of time reported a significant increase in familial incidence over recent years [7].

The risk of familial transmission of HD is considered to be 180 times greater than for the general population [15]. The distribution of the forms that occur in families is different from that of all HD patients when one considers sex, length of the affected segment, and the subset of the population studied.

Overall, in patients with familial forms of HD there disappears the increased incidence in men. This is especially so in patients with long segment disease, although the difference remains common in rectosigmoidal forms [12,15]. In patients with long segment aganglionosis, the reported incidence of familial forms (20–50%) is much higher than in short segment patients (3–5%) [2,3,15]. Among patients with familial forms of HD, the frequency of long segment aganglionosis is twice that of short segment disease, and in two families there has been documented a tendency to develop longer affected aganglionic segments in successive generations [15].

In populations with very high rates (>75%) of inbreeding, there is a greater incidence of familial forms of HD, with a clear tendency to concentrate in a few families with high rates of associated birth defects [8,9,16]. Authors who have described these 'peculiar' forms of aganglionosis consider the following to be special characteristics of their patients: similar or greater incidence in women, forms with more extensive involvement of the intestine, absence of hypertrophic nerve fibres in the affected segment, and increased morbidity and mortality, and suggested that these patients constitute a variant of HD [16].

Although the available data vary according to the experience of the different authors, HD is more frequent among the siblings than the parents or other relatives of the patients studied [3,5,8,14–16]. The incidence of more than one affected sibling is reported to be some 10 times greater than expected for patients with no familial history of HD [15].

Age at Diagnosis

In the pædiatric population, the age at which HD is diagnosed has improved dramatically, with diagnosis now being far earlier. While in series published more than thirty years ago, the patients diagnosed in the neonatal period were in the minority, even less than 10%, in recent publications they constitute about 90%. Diagnosis in children of more than one year in age, and even older than 5 years, has passed from being relatively frequent (>30%) to being exceptional [1,5,7,8,12,14]. The mean for diagnosis is now at 18 days of life, and is earliest in patients with family antecedents [17]. Early diagnosis includes the detection of HD in children with birth weights between 1500 g and 2500 g in 13.79% of patients, and between 2500 g and 3500 g in 72.4% of patients when associated with other anomalies and in 11.68% and 63.5%, respectively, when HD presents in isolation [14].

Other Variables

Although there have been many attempts to determine what other possible variables may influence the distribution of HD in the population, most show results that are difficult to interpret and of little value as epidemiological determinants of HD.

The socio-economic situation has been invoked as a factor conducive to HD in the least favoured social groups. Indeed, this seems to be suggested by the reported greater incidence (1.67:1) in 'non-whites' than in 'whites' in the USA [1]. Nonetheless, this finding needs to be confirmed with additional data before being accepted as valid.

Although a greater incidence has been reported when the mothers are white and older than 30 years, but not for non-white mothers, other studies either find no relationship between the mother's age and HD, or even a higher incidence when the mother is younger than 30. The case is similarly confusing with the first-born taken as parameter. Some studies have found the incidence to be higher, others have found it to be lower, and yet others find no difference from that of younger siblings (1,3,8).

The proportion of HD patients who were premature is between 4.66% and 8% [3,9,11], a percentage not very different from that of the general population. Birth weights below 2500 g corresponded to 5.5% of the patient sample of a certain population more than 25 years ago, with significant ($p<0.001$) increases 10 and 20 years later to 6.5% and 10.4%, respectively, in the same population [7].

Various complications have been described during the pregnancy of mothers of fœtuses with HD. They seem to be more frequent in recent periods, in cases of premature birth, and in mothers of patients with total colonic aganglionosis. One such complication is maternal hyperthermia, about which nothing is known concerning its significance or relationship with HD [8,11].

Studies of the possible influence of different seasons or toxic agents have not found any connection, and some of the authors consider the relationship unlikely, although they speculate on the possible link between HD and microenvironmental factors similar to those associated with neural tube defects [1,8]. Indeed, both are neurocristopathies, and both present greater incidence in certain populations.

Clinical Presentation

The diagnosis of HD is usually considered in patients who present delayed passage of meconium, or bowel obstruction or subobstruction as neonates or in early infancy, when they may also present diarrhœa [13]. In older patients, constipation is the usual presentation. It is therefore in patients with these characteristics where HD is suspected and almost all diagnoses of the disease are made.

The published incidence of HD in constipated patients varies between 9% and 43% [2,19]. Incidences have been reported of 17% of HD in a population of patients under one year in age with constipation, and of 14% in children of different ages [5,18]. But other workers have not detected any patients with HD in a limited population of constipated children, and hence advise diagnostic testing such as histochemistry and anorectal manometry only when the onset of the clinical pattern of constipation occurs early, before the age of three months [19]. The mean age (3.64 months) reported for the diagnosis of HD in children with constipation was much younger than the age (2.9 years) for constipated children in whom the diagnosis of HD was discarded [18]. Late diagnoses usually correspond to patients with constipation and encopresis who present an ultrashort aganglionic segment [5].

It is recommended to discard HD by rectal biopsy in constipated patients when there is a greater than 48-hour delay in the passage of meconium, lower bowel obstruction of unknown cause, severe constipation, chronic abdominal distension, or failure to thrive [18]. We believe that these indications may be made less stringent if the evaluation of patients with possible HD is by means of anorectal manometry.

Extent of the Affected Bowel

As we noted briefly above, and shall return to below in discussing the classification of HD, the length of the aganglionic segment from the ano-rectum is a factor of great interest in attempting to characterize the different forms of presentation, treatment, and prognosis in patients with aganglionosis.

Association with other Pathologies

HD is associated with many other pathologies. When they are present, HD is more likely to be detected than in the general population. Sometimes the association is so frequent that diagnosis of HD must be attempted in all these patients, and in general in any group of pathologies in which HD has a greater incidence than in the rest of the population.

Classification

We shall consider HD exclusively, excluding any other form of dysganglionosis (20).There are several criteria that can be used to construct different classifications of HD. Among them, as we noted briefly above, one can use the clinical presentation, familial antecedents, or association with various congenital defects. Whichever form of classification one tries to apply, many other variables will also have to be considered with the result that the borders between the types will be far from well defined. For practical purposes, the most widely used classification is based on the length of the aganglionic segment, from the anal sphincter to upper sections of the colon or small bowel. According to this criterion, the current trend is to classify aganglionoses into: (1) ultrashort, (2) short, (3) long, (4) total colonic, and (5) intestinal [21].

Some authors consider ultrashort segments of HD to be those which, from the internal anal sphincter, do not surpass the inferior third of the rectum or its peritoneal reflection [5,7]. Others, however, seem not to mean exactly the same thing when using this term [22]. For them, rather than a minimally extended form of typical HD, ultrashort aganglionosis is practically a variant of the disease. It is characterized clinically by constipation beginning at 6 to 12 months of age or at weaning, and histochemically by the absence of increased acetylcholinesterase activity in the nerve fibres of the lamina propria, although it is present in the muscularis mucosa and the corrugator cutis ani muscle. Some authors consider that up to 25% of all HD cases correspond to ultrashort segment involvement, although the incidence reported in most of the literature consulted is clearly less [7].

The most frequent form of HD is that which extends from the internal anal sphincter to variable portions of the upper two-thirds of the rectum or to the sigmoid colon. Also termed rectal or rectosigmoidal aganglionosis, it constitutes together with ultrashort aganglionosis the so-called short segment forms of HD. In the largest series of patients, these short segment forms represent between 75% and 80% of all HD cases [7,12,24]. Moreover, it is the most typical form in its clinical symptoms, and that which is treated surgically by applying the most widely used techniques.

Long segment aganglionosis is considered to include all those cases that extend to any part of the colon, proximal to the sigmoid colon, or up to the small bowel. Its various forms together account for between 20% and 25% of all HD cases [7,10]. The term 'long' in this context is generally used in reference to long colonic aganglionosis, its most frequent form [5,7,11,12].

Total colonic aganglionosis affects the entire colon, and usually a distal ileum segment of less than 30 cm proximal to the ileocæcal junction [7]. It accounts for between 3% and 12% of HD cases [2,3,7,10,11,23].

The most extensively affected forms of aganglionosis involve, in addition to the colon, major portions of the small bowel and even virtually the entire gut. Various published series do not refer to these forms, or they were not detected [2,11,12,24], but in the longest published series they account for 3.8% of all the cases [7].

This classification, summarized in Table I, involves differences in the epidemiological characteristics of the various categories of the disease, as were described above, as well as in the clinical manifestations, surgical treatment, and prognosis.

Table I. Classification of Hirschsprung's disease according to the length of the aganglionic segment.

FORM	AFFECTED SEGMENT	FREQUENCY	SIMPLIFIED FORM
ULTRASHORT	<1/3 distal of the rectum	Up to 25%	SHORT: 75% to 80%
SHORT	Rectal or rectosigmoidal	> 50%	
LONG	Supra-sigmoidal	< 15%	LONG: 20% to 25%
TOTAL COLONIC	Colon+/-30cm distal ileum	3% to 12%	
INTESTINAL	> 30 cm distal ileum	Up to 4%	

This simplification of the classification into short- and long-segment forms may in general be useful for the practical conceptualization of HD.

Associated Congenital Defects

The presentation of HD is in isolation in 70% of patients, in association with chromosomal abnormalities in 12%, and in association with other congenital defects in 18%, according to the incidences reported in a substantially general fashion by recent publications [10,21].

In the early extensive series of HD that reported associations with other congenital defects, these were not as frequent and diverse as in later publications [2–4,7,10,21,24,25]. There only appear to be very specific, one-off differences between racial groups or geographic areas in the incidence and variety of congenital defects described in the literature [7-9,14,25].

Because many of the congenital defects associated with HD form part of chromosomal anomalies and syndromes, it is difficult to estimate the incidence of each alone isolated from its context. Considered together, however, it has been possible to estimate the incidence, even though the different studies do not always follow the same criteria in their evaluation [7,14,25]. A review of 18 published series for congenital anomalies in HD found 21% of the 4328 patients with aganglionosis to have other associated congenital defects.

There is a tendency to classify the incidence of congenital defects associated with HD according to the affected organs [14,25], and one finds a major variability of their reported incidence between series. The usual classification is into affected structures of the gastrointestinal tract, central nervous system, genitourinary system, musculoskeletal system, cardiovascular system, craniofacial region, sense organs, skin, or association with tumours.

Gastrointestinal Tract

This is probably the system with most congenital defects associated with HD. The incidence has been estimated at 8.05% (25). The defects are malrotation, bowel atresias, and pathology of the omphalomesenteric duct.

There is general acceptance of the existence of a clinical association between HD and intestinal malrotation [7,25,26–30]. The same is the case for ano-rectal malformations, which are found to have an incidence of 2.5% in collectively reviewing more than 1200 HD patients [31–34]. In these patients, the diagnosis of HD is often delayed due to the frequent colostomy and to alterations in defæcation which are often attributed to the postoperative evolution of the ano-rectal defect.

Also in patients with small bowel and colon atresia, there has been a more frequent association with HD than expected for the general population [35–40]. A suggested explanation of these associations has been the secondary atresia and volvulus of the subobstructed bowel segment proximal to the transition zone, or some other cause of ischæmia, especially if it occurs during weeks 6 to 8 of gestation [35]. Association with HD must be suspected in both ano-rectal malformations and small bowel or colonic atresias, and when the patient who has undergone surgery for these problems has difficulty in defæcating normally [35].

Central Nervous System

Some authors report the incidence of congenital defects of the central nervous system in patients with HD to be greater than that of gastrointestinal tract defects [14], although others have estimated it to be 6.8% (25). The most frequently cited are congenital defects leading to psychomotor retardation, microcephaly, anencephaly, absence of the corpus callosum, and hydrocephaly [41–43]. Many of these defects may be considered as manifestations of neurocristopathies or other syndromes which will be discussed in the next chapter. The significance of the highly variable and low incidence of myelomeningocele in patients with HD is still an open issue of discussion (44).

Genitourinary System

The reported incidence of genitourinary system defects is also highly variable [10,14,15,45] but in general it is considered to be close to that of gastrointestinal tract and central nervous system defects in HD patients – 6.05% ([25]. The congenital defects in this category associated with aganglionosis include undescended testes, hypospadias, various kidney anomalies, hydronephrosis–hydroureter, intestinal duplications, and alteration of bladder function [14,25]. These congenital defects also often form part of syndromes associated with HD [46].

Skeleton, Muscles, and Limbs

This category of congenital defects are associated with 4.6% of HD patients according to the review that we are taking as the primary reference [25], although some workers report a higher incidence [14]. Among the most cited defects are muscular dystrophy, hernia of the diaphragm, polydactyly, syndactyly, limb hypoplasia, and spinal defects. Most of these congenital defects are associated with different, usually complex, syndromes which will be discussed in the next chapter.

Cardiovascular System

Several congenital cardiovascular defects are associated with HD, especially septation and conotruncal defects [10,47]. They are present in 5% of HD patients, above all in association with Down syndrome [15,25], but also with other syndromes, particularly those involving defects that are secondary to neurocristopathies [46–49].

Craniofacial Defects

Less frequent are craniofacial defects, with an estimated incidence of 2.9% [25]. They usually cause a peculiar aspect of the face. The commonest are the presence of narrow palpebral fissures, broad nasal root, cranial abnormalities, cleft palate, and micrognatia. Most of them usually form part of various syndromes, generally related to neural crest development pathologies [17,50–53].

Sensory Defects

There have also been described congenital defects that affect vision or hearing in HD patients. They include congenital deafness, microphthalmia, ptosis, iris coloboma, nystagmus, and anomalies of the papilla (14,25). Again, the defects detected in these cases often form part of various syndromes and are related to neurocristopathies [15,50,54–60].

Skin Defects

Skin defects described in association with HD include hypopigmentation, piebaldism, white forelock, keratitis, ichthyosis, and hair hypoplasia. Often these skin defects occur as part of syndromes that include, among other abnormalities, deafness [15,61–69].

Association with Tumours

Since HD is a neurocristopathy, and as a group these include various neural tumours, it seems unsurprising that there have been associations described between aganglionosis and different tumours of chromaffin cells – neuroblastoma, ganglioneuromas, retinoblastoma, pheochromocytoma, medullary thyroid carcinoma and other tumours typical of type-2 multiple endocrine neoplasia (MEN-2), and neurofibromatosis [25,70–72].

According to a major study [7] of cases recorded in periods separated by 10 years, there has been a clear increase in the proportion of diagnoses of congenital defects associated with HD from the first to the last records. Although in overall terms the defects reported in the three periods with greatest incidence did not vary greatly, there were marked differences for some specific defects [7].

We believe that the detection of symptoms suggestive of HD in patients with any of the isolated congenital defects described above means that the diagnosis of possible aganglionosis must be expected to be more likely than if these defects are absent. One must therefore attempt to exclude HD in these patients. This will be even more important if the congenital defects detected form part of a syndrome or of a group of genetic defects such as those to be analyzed in the next chapter, especially if their likely origin is a neurocristopathy [3].

References

[1] Goldberg EL. An epidemiological study of Hirschsprung`s disease. *Int J Epidemiol* 1984; 13: 479-85.

[2] Russell MB, Russell CA, Niebuhr E. An epidemiological study of Hirschsprung´s disease and additional anomalies. *Acta Pediatr* 1994; 83: 68-71.

[3] Ryan ET, Ecker JL, Chistakis NA, Folkman J. Hirschsprung´s disease: associated abnormalities and demography. *J Pediatr Surg* 1992; 27: 76-81.

[4] Spouge D, Baird PA. Hirschsprung´s disease in a large birth cohort. *Teratology* 1985; 32: 171-7.

[5] Orr JD, Scobie WG. Presentation and incidence of Hirschsprung´s disease. *BMJ* 1983; 287: 1671.

[6] Ikeda K, Goto S. Diagnosis and treatment of Hirschsprun´s disease in Japan. An analysis of 1628 patients. *Ann Surg* 1984; 199: 400-5.

[7] Suita S, Taguchi T, Ieiri S, Nakatsuji T. Hirschsprung′disease in Japan: analysis of 3852 patients based on a nationwide survey in 30 years. *J Pediatr Surg* 2005; 40: 197-201.

[8] Rajab A, Freeman NV, Patton MA. Hirschsprung′s disease in Oman. *J Pediatr Surg* 1997; 32: 724-7.

[9] Halevy H, Mares A, Cohen Z, Finaly R, Freud E, Pilpel D. Hirschsprung′s disease in the Negev. *Harefuah* 1994; 127: 148-54.

[10] Amiel J, Lyonnet S. Hirschsprung′s disease, associated syndromes, and genetics: a review. *J Med Genet* 2001; 38: 729-39.

[11] Klein MD, Philippart AI. Hirschsprung′s disease: three decades′ experience at a single institution. *J Pediatr Surg* 1993; 28: 1291-3.

[12] Kleinhaus S, Boley SJ, Sheran M, Sieber WK. Hirschsprung′s disease. A survey of the members of the Surgical Section of the American Academy of Pediatrics. *J Pediatr Surg* 1979; 14: 588-97.

[13] Singh SJ, Croaker GD, Manglick P, Wong CL, Athanasakos H, Elliott E, Cass D. Hirschsprung′s disease: the Australian Paediatric Surveillance Unit′s experience. *J Pediatr Surg* 2003; 19: 247-50.

[14] Sarioglu A, Tanyel FC, Buyukpamukcu N, Hicsonmez A. Hirschsprung-associated congenital anomalies. *Eur J Pediatr Surg* 1997; 7: 331-7.

[15] Moore SW, Millar AJ, AlbertynR, Cywes S. Familial aspests of Hirschsprung′s disease. *Eur J Pediatr Surg* 1991; 1: 97-101.

[16] Schiller M, Levy P, Shawa RA, Abu-Dalu K, Gorenstein A, Katz S. Familial Hirschsprung′s disease – A report of 22 affected siblings in four families. *J Pediatr Surg* 1990; 25: 322-5.

[17] Engum SA, Petrites M, Rescorla FJ, Grosfeld JL, Morrison AM, Engles D. Familial Hirschsprung ′s disease: 20 cases in 12 kindreds. *J Pediatr Surg* 1993; 28: 1286-90.

[18] Khan AR, Vujanic GM, Huddart S. The constipated child: how likely is Hirschsprung′s disease?. *Pediatr Surg Int* 2003; 19: 439-42.

[19] Wales JKH. Presentation and incidence of Hirschsprung′s disease. *BMJ* 1984; 288: 151.

[20] Martucciello G, Pini Prato A, Puri P, Holschneider AM, Meier-Ruge W, Jasonni V, Tovar JA, Grosfeld JL. Controversies concerning diagnostic guidelines for anomalies of the enteric nervous system: a report from the fourth International Symposium on Hirschsprung′s disease and related neurocristopathies. *J Pediatr Surg* 2005; 40: 1527-31.

[21] Godbole K. The many faces of Hirschsprung′s disease. *Indian Pediatr* 2004; 41: 1115-23.

[22] Meier-Rouge WA, Bruder E, Holschneider AM, Lochbuhler H, Piket G, Posslt HG, Tewes G. Diagnosis and Therapy of ultrashort Hirschsprung′s disease. *Eur J Pediatr Surg* 2004; 14: 392-7.

[23] Wildhaber BE, Teitelbaum DH, Coran AG. Total colonic Hirschsprung′s disease: a 28-year experience. *J Pediatr Surg* 2005; 40: 203-7.

[24] Swenson O, Sherman JO, Fisher J. Diagnosis of congenital megacolon: An analysis of 501 patients. *J Pediatr Surg* 1973; 8: 587-94.

[25] Moore SW. The contribution of associated congenital anomalies in understanding Hirschsprung´s disease. *Pediatr Surg Int* 2006; 22: 305-5.

[26] PoenaruD, Uroz-Tristan J, Leclerc S, Murphy S, Bensoussan AL. Imperforate anus, malrotation and Hirschsprung´s disease: a rare association. *Eur J Pediatr Surg* 1995; 5: 187-9.

[27] Corsois L, Boman F, Sfeir R, Mention K, Michaud L, Poddevin F, Mestdagh P, Gottrand F. Extensive Hirschsprung´s disease associated with intestinal malrotation. *Arch Pediatr* 2004; 11: 1205-08.

[28] Jain SK, Singla SK, Sharma M, Pathania OP, Taneja SB. Hirschsprung´s disease with intestinal malrotation and midgut volvulus: a rare association. *Indian J Gastroenterol* 1989; 8: 201.

[29] Brown RA, Cywes C. Disorders and congenital malformations associated with Hirschsprung´s disease. In Holschneider AM, Puri P (eds) *Hirschsprung´s disease*. Amsterdam: Harcourt; 1982. p.137-145.

[30] Sieber WK. Hirschsprung´s disease. In Welch KJ, Randolf JG, Ravitch MM, O´Neil JA, Rowe MI. *Peditric Surgery*. Chicago: Year Book Medical Publisher, Inc; 1986. 995-1019.

[31] Flageole H, Fecteau A, Laberge JM, Guttman FM. Hirschsprung´s disease, imperforate anus, and Down´s syndrome: a case report. *J Pediatr Surg* 1996; 31: 759-60.

[32] Meijers C, Mulder M. Anteroposterior diffences within caudal hindbrain neural crest cells population and the development of the enteric nervous system. Presented at the *Second International Meeting: Hirschsprung´s disease and related neurocristopathies*. Clevelan 1995.

[33] Watanatittan S, Suwatanaviroj A, Limprutithum T, Rattanasuwan T. Association of Hirschsprung´s disease and anorectal malformation. *J Pediatr Surg* 1991; 26: 192-5.

[34] Clarke SA, Van der Avoirt A. Imperforate anus, Hirschsprung´s disease and trisomy 21: a rare combination. *J Pediatr Surg* 1999; 34: 1874.

[35] Gupta M, Beeram MR, Pohl JF, Custer MD. Ileal atresia associated with Hirschsprung´s disease (total colonic aganglionosis). *J Pediatr Surg* 2005; 40: E5-E7.

[36] Gauderer M, Rothstein FC, Izant R. Ileal atresia and long segment Hirschsprung´s disease in a neonate. *J Pediatr Surg* 1984; 19: 15-7.

[37] Moore SW, Millar A, Rode H, Cywes S. Intestinal atresia and Hirschsprung´s disease. *Pediatr Surg Int* 1990; 5: 182-9.

[38] Currie ABM, Hemalatha AH, Doraiswamy NV, Cox SA. Colonic atresia in association with Hirschsprung´s disease. *J Roy Coll Surg Edinburgh* 1983; 28: 31-4.

[39] Siu KL, Kwok WK, Lee WY, Lee WH. A male newborn with colonic atresia and total colonic aganglionosis. *Pediatr Surg Int* 1999; 15: 141-2.

[40] Fishman SJ, Islam S, Buonomo C, Nurko S. Non fixation of an atretic colon predicts Hirschsprung´s disease. *J Pediatr Surg* 2001; 36: 202-4.

[41] Shahar E, Shinawi M. Neurocristopathies presenting with neurologic abnormalities associated with Hirschsprung´s disease. *Pediatr Neurol* 2003; 28: 385-91.

[42] Mathew A. Anencephaly-associated aganglionosis. *Am J Med Genet* 1998; 80: 518-20.

[43] Melaragno MI, Brunoni D, Patricio FR, Corbani M, Mutacchi Z, dos Santos R de et al. A patient with tetrasomy 9p, Dandy-Walker cyst and Hirschsprung´s disease. *Ann Genet* 1992; 35: 79-84.

[44] Merkler RG, Solish SB, Scherzer AL. Meningomyelocele and Hirschsprung´s disease: Theoretical and clinical significance. *Pediatrics* 1985; 76: 299-300.

[45] Festen C. Anomalies of the urinary tract in Hirschsprung´s disease. *Z Kinderchir* 1975; 17: 376-80.

[46] Hou JW. Bardet-Biedl syndrome initially presenting as McKusik-Kaufman syndrome. *J Formos Med Assoc* 2004; 103: 629-32.

[47] Nowaczyk MJ, James AG, Superina R, Siegel-Bartelt J. Hirschsprung´s disease, postaxial polydactyly, and atrial septal defect. *Am J Med Genet* 1997; 68: 74-5.

[48] Huang T, Elias ER, Mulliken JB, Kirse DJ, Holmes LB. A new syndrome: heart defect, laringeal anomalies, preaxial polydactyly, and colonic aganglionosis in sibs. *Genet Med* 1999; 1: 104-8.

[49] Lorda-Sánchez I, Ayuso C, Ibáñez A. Situs inversus and Hirschsprung´s disease: tow uncommon manifestation in Badet-Biedl syndrome. *Am J Med Genet* 2000; 90: 80-1.

[50] Yomo A, Taira T, Kondo I. Goldberg-shprintzen syndrome: Hirschsprung´s disease, hipotonía, and ptosis in sibs. *Am J Med Genet* 1991; 41: 188-1.

[51] Orrico A, Galli L, Cavaliere ML, Garavelli L, Fryns JP, Crushell E et al. Phenotypic and molecular characterisation of the Aarskog-Scott syndrome: a survey of the clinical variability in light of FGD1 mutation analysis in 46 patients. *Eur J Hum Genet* 2.004; 12: 16-23.

[52] Aurora P, Wallis CE. Jeune syndrome (asphisiating thoracic dystrophy) associated with Hirschsprung´s disease. *Clin Dysmorphol* 1999; 8: 259-63.

[53] Farlie PG, McKeown SJ, Newgreen DF. The neural crest: Basic biology and clinical relationships in the craneofacial and enteric nervous systems. *Birth Defects Res C Embryo Today* 2005; 72: 173-87.

[54] Edery P, Attie T, Amiel J, Pelet A, Eng C, Hofstra RM et al. Mutation of the endothelin.3 in the Waardenburg-Hirschsprung´s disease (Shah-Waardenburg syndrome). *Nat Genet* 1996; 12: 442-4.

[55] Guion-Almeida ML, Richieri-Costa A. Callosal agenesis, iris coloboma, and megacolon in a brazilian boy with Rubinstein-Taybi syndrome. *Am J Med Genet* 1992; 43: 929-31.

[56] Ohnuma K, Imaizumi K, Masuno M, Nakamura M, Kuroki Y. Magnetic resonance imaging abnormalities of the brain in Goldberg-Shpintzen syndrome (Hirschsprung´s disease, microcephaly, and iris coloboma). *Am J Med Genet* 1997; 73: 230-2.

[57] Fryer AE. Goldberg-Shprintzeng syndrome: report of a new family and review of the literature. *Clin Dysmorphol* 1998; 7; 97-101.

[58] Brook AS, Breuning MH, Osinga J, vd Smagt JJ, Catsman CE, Buys CH et al. A consanguineous family with Hirschsprung´s disease, microcephaly, and mental retardation (Goldberg-Shprintzen syndrome). *J Med Genet* 1999; 36: 485-9.

[59] Croaker GD, Shi E, Simpson E, Cartmill T, Cass DT. Congenital central hypoventilation syndrome and Hirschsprung´s disease. *Arch Dis Child* 1998; 78: 316-22.

[60] Lankosz-Lauterbach J, Sanak M. Oculoauriculovertebral syndrome (Goldenhar syndrome) Associated with Hirschsprung´s disease. *Pediatr Pol* 1987; 62: 249-52.

[61] Weinberg AG, Currarino G, Besserman M. Hirschsprung´s disease and congenital deafness. *Hum Genet* 1977; 38: 157-61.

[62] Toki F, Suzuki N, Inoue K, Suzuki M, Hirakata K, Nagai K et al. Intestinal aganglionosis associated with the Waardenburg syndrome: report of tow cases and review of the literature. *Pediatr Surg Int* 2003; 19: 725-8.

[63] Groos A, Kunze J, Maier RF, Stoltenburg-Didinger G, Grimmer I, Obladen M. Autosomal-recessive neural crest syndrome with albinism, black lock, cell migration disorder of the neurocytes of the gut, and deafness: ABCD syndrome. *Am J Med Genet* 1995; 56: 322-6.

[64] Verheij JB, Kunze J, Osinga J, van Essen AJ, Hofstra RM. ABCD syndrome is caused by a homozygous mutation in the EDNRB gene. *Am J Med Genet* 2002; 108: 223-5.

[65] Mahakrishnan A, Srinivasan MS. Piebaldness with Hirschsprung´s disease. *Arch Dermatol* 1980; 116: 1102.

[66] Makitie O, Kaitila I. Cartilage-hair hypoplasia—Clinical manifestation in 108 finnish patients. *Eur J Pediatr* 1993; 152: 211-7.

[67] Makitie O, Heikkinen M, Kaitila I, Rintala R. Hirschsprung´s disease in cartilage-hair hypoplasia has poor prognosis. *J Pediatr Surg* 2002; 37: 1585-8.

[68] Mallory SB, Hayni LS, Williams ML, Hall W. Ichthyosis, deafness, and Hirschsprung´s disease. *Pediatr Dermatol* 1989; 6: 24-7.

[69] Nadir E, Yerman S, Feldman M. A femal neonate with Hirschsprung´s disease and ichthyosis. *Isr Med Assoc J* 2005; 7: 342-3.

[70] Michna BA, McWilliams NB, Krummel TM, Hartenberg MA, Salzberg AM. Multifocal ganglioneuroblastoma coexisten with total colonic aganglionosis. *J Pediatr Surg* 1988; 23. 57-9.

[71] Hamel CJ, Sverijnen RS, De Van GA. Neurocristopathy in mother (ganglioneuroblastoma) and daughter (aganglionosis): incidental or causal?. *Genet Couns* 1994; 5: 303-5.

[72] Clausen N, Andersson P, Tommerup N. Famlial occurrence of neuroblastoma, von Recklinhausen´s neurofibromatosis, Hirschsprung´s agangliosis and jaw-winking syndrome. *Acta Pediatr Scand* 1989; 78: 736-41.

[73] Tovar JA. The neural crest in pediatric surgery. *J Pediatr Surg* 2007; 42: 915-26.

In: Hirschsprung's Disease: Diagnosis and Treatment
Ed: Ramón Núñez and Manuel López-Alonso
ISBN: 978-1-60741-349-3

Chapter VI

Genetics and Hirschsprung's Disease

Enrique Galán, Emilio Blesa and Juan J. Cardesa

Introduction

Harald Hirschsprung, a Danish pædiatrician, was the first to describe the disease that bears his name in two unrelated children. They both died from severe chronic constipation with abdominal swelling that led to a congenital megacolon [1]. In 1948, Swenson and Bill [2] developed the first surgical technique applicable to the treatment of this disease. Subsequent developments in surgery have enabled a great number of these patients to survive, and hence we have been able to observe the familial transmission of Hirschsprung's disease (HSCR) and determine its genetic nature. There also exist other factors demonstrating the genetic basis of HSCR. Firstly, there is a higher risk of recurrence for siblings of affected individuals relative to the risk for the general population. Secondly, the sex/incidence ratio is unbalanced. Thirdly, there is the association of HSCR with other genetic diseases (see the previous chapter of Blesa E *et al.*), including malformation syndromes and chromosomal anomalies. And finally, various animal models of aganglionic colon show specific patterns of Mendelian inheritance [3].

Advances in molecular genetics, especially in the last 10 years, have revealed the genetic basis of HSCR. The discovery of the locus of Multiple Endocrine Neoplasia (MEN) assigned to the chromosome 10q11.2 region, and where later was also found the locus of familial thyroid carcinoma, was the starting point to investigate the relationship with HSCR. Various lines of research led to the discovery that these entities as well as HSCR are related to the gene *RET* [4]. As we shall see later, today we know that *RET* is the major susceptibility gene, and that there are at least 10 genes related to HSCR. There probably exist additional modifier genes that influence the presentation and behaviour of HSCR.

It must not be forgotten that HSCR is due to an anomaly of the enteric nervous system whose origin is the neural crest, and therefore HSCR is presently regarded as a neurocristopathy [5].

Isolated HSCR appears to be complex. It has a non-Mendelian mode of inheritance with low sex-dependent penetrance and variable expressivity according to the length of the aganglionic segment, suggesting the involvement of one or more genes with low penetrance [6]. All these characteristics should be taken into account for the correct assessment of the risk of recurrence in the relatives of affected individuals. The relative risk of HSCR is as high as 200, and HSCR appears to be an excellent model for the common study of multifactorial diseases.

The presentation of HSCR, as we shall see in a previous chapter (Blesa E *et al.*), is in isolation in 70% of patients, associated with chromosomal anomalies in 12%, and associated with other birth defects in 18%. In this last group of patients, HSCR presents within a series of monogenic syndromes [7,8].

Definition and Classification

HSCR is a congenital malformation of the intestine which is characterized by the absence of cells of the parasympathomimetic intrinsic ganglia in the myenteric and submucous plexuses [9]. It is considered the consequence of a premature arrest of the craniocaudal migration of vagal neural crest cells in the intestine (forming the enteric nervous system) between 5 and 12 weeks of gestation.

Various criteria can be used to classify HSCR. Traditionally it was classified into two types: short-segment HSCR (80% of cases) when the aganglionic segment does not extend beyond the sigmoid colon, and long-segment HSCR (20% of cases) when the aganglionic segment extends proximally to the sigmoid colon [10]. From a practical point of view, the most used classification is that based on the extension of the aganglionic segment from the anal sphincter to the more proximal segments of the colon or small intestine. According to this criterion, aganglionoses are presently classified as: ultrashort, short, long, colonic, total, and intestinal (see previous chapter of Blesa E *et al.*) [11-14].

Summary of Genetic Epidemiology

The average incidence of HSCR is 1 per 5000 live births [15]. The incidence varies according to whether one considers such factors as population, race, geographic area, sex, age of presentation, family incidence, associated pathology, and length of the aganglionic segment.

One of the most comprehensive studies was that using data from the California Birth Defects Monitoring Program (1983–1997). This found an incidence of 1.5/10 000 newborn in Whites, 2.1/10 000 in Afro-Americans, 1/10 000 in Hispanics, and 2.8/10 000 in Asiatics [16].

HSCR is commoner in men than in women. The male/female ratio is 4/1, but this imbalance with respect to sex is particularly evident in the short forms, and declines as one considers more intense forms [17].

Associated Congenital Defects

As was mentioned above, HSCR presents in association with other congenital defects in 18% of cases and with chromosomal anomalies in 12% [7,8]. A recent review of 18 published series on congenital defects associated with HSCR which evaluated 4829 patients affected with HSCR found that 21% had some associated congenital defect. Although the incidence varies among the different studies, the trend is of higher percentages in the more recent studies, which tend to be more comprehensive and exhaustive.

Table 1 presents a summary of the congenital defects that are associated with HSCR. The topic is dealt with in detail in the previous chapter (Blesa *et al.*).

Table 1. Congenital defects associated with HSCR.

Organ/system with congenital defects	Percentage (%)
Gut	8.05 [18]
CNS	8.3–29 [19]
Genitourinary	6.05 [18,20]
Musculoskeletal and limbs	4.6–24 [18]
Craniofacial	4.99 [17,21]
Cardiovascular	2.86 [18]
Eye	2.2 [22]
Skin	Variable

Genetic Aspects of HSCR

Advances in molecular genetics in the last decade have led to progress in understanding the genetic basis of HSCR. Today we know that many of the genetic variations associated with HSCR are due to certain genes of susceptibility. There are mutations of these genes in 50% of familial cases, and in approximately 20–30% of sporadic cases [23].

The genetic influence seems to vary according to the length of the affected segment in HSCR patients. Long-segment HSCR is considered to have an autosomal dominant pattern of inheritance with incomplete penetrance (particularly with respect to the *RET* gene), while short-segment HSCR seems to have an autosomal recessive pattern or may be due to multiple genes [24]. Also, as we shall see below, there are known to be various syndromes with different Mendelian patterns which present HSCR.

The best classification of HSCR is to separate the cases into isolated or non-syndromic (which will include most cases with multifactorial inheritance) and syndromic (in which we shall also include the cases related with chromosomal anomalies).

1) Molecular Genetics in Isolated HSCR

Various genes have been described as involved in isolated HSCR. We currently know of 10 genes that are implicated (Table 2). The major ones are *RET* and *EDNRB*.

Table 2. Genes related to HSCR.

Gene	Locus	Inheritance	Phenotype	Penetrance
RET	10q11.2	AD	HSCR	70% males; 50% females
GDNF	5p13	AD	HSCR	5 published cases Weakly penetrant
NTN	19p13	AD	HSCR	1 published case
SOX10	22q13	AD	WS4	Around 80%
EDNRB	13q22	AR/AD	WS4/HSCR	Low
EDN3	20q13	AR/AD	WS4/HSCR	1 published case
ECE1	1p36	AD	HSCR, DC Craniofacial & cardiac	1 published case
ZFHX1B (SIP1)	2q22	AD	MCA-MR Facial gestalt	60%
PHOX2B	4p12	AD	CCHS	20%
TCF4	18q21	AD	Encephalopathy Epileptic	1 case

CCHS: congenital central hypoventilation syndrome
MCA: Multipe congenital anomalies
AD: autosomal dominant inheritance
AR: Autosomal recessive inheritance.

The RET Signaling Pathway

The first susceptibility locus was mapped to the 10q11.2 chromosome region in multigenerational families in which HSCR segregated with a pattern of autosomal dominant inheritance with incomplete penetrance [25,26]. This region was suspected of involvement in HSCR because of the observation that some patients with total colonic aganglionosis and mental retardation had a 10q11 interstitial deletion [27]. The *RET* proto-oncogene identified as responsible for MEN2 [28] and mapped to 10q11.2 was proposed as a candidate of HSCR because of two facts: (i) the joint presentation of MEN2A and HSCR in some families, and (ii) *RET* expression in neural-crest-derived cells. Subsequently, *RET* mutations were described in patients with HSCR [4, 29].

The *RET* gene is a 1114 amino acid membrane receptor that has an extracellular cadherin-like domain, a cysteine-rich region, and an intracellular tyrosine kinase domain. It is expressed in the developing peripheral and central nervous systems. The mutations in MEN2A appear in exons 10 and 11, in MEN2B they usually occur in exon 16, and in HSCR the mutations identified appear throughout the gene.

More than 100 mutations have been described in the *RET* gene. They are of various kinds, including large deletions, micro-deletions and insertions, and nonsense, missense, and splicing mutations [30-31]. It appears that the *RET* gene mutations in syndromes of predisposition to cancer are mutations that activate the gene causing constitutive dimerization and transformation of the receptor [33]. In contrast, mutations in HSCR are inactivating, and give rise to misfolding of the protein encoded by *RET* or a failure of the transport of the protein to the cell surface [34,35]. These mutations lead to a production of half the dose of the protein, a situation termed haploinsufficiency. Moreover, this haploinsufficiency has also been demonstrated in HSCR patients with *RET* deletions. This reduced amount of protein is insufficient for normal enteric development. Nonetheless, the case is more complex. A simple model of activation versus inactivation of the *RET* gene is not enough to explain the concurrence of HSCR and MEN2A in patients with MEN2A *RET* mutations.

With the development of screening for mutations in the *RET* gene, mutations are only found in 50% of familial cases of HSCR and 15–20% of sporadic cases [30,31,36,37]. However it has been shown that most families (with rare exceptions) are compatible with linkage at the *RET* locus. It is known that, in addition to mutations in the coding sequences, non-coding regions also play an important role in the development of HSCR. Collaborative studies of HSCR patients of different populations in Holland, Italy, France, Spain, USA, and Hong Kong have shown that HSCR is associated with the same haplotype of region 5' of *RET* (6–62% of patients) [38,39]. The same haplotype was also found in Asiatics in 85% of HSCR patients [40,41]. Moreover, different studies have characterized candidate polymorphisms for HSCR [40]. It has been postulated that there might exist a low-penetrance founder locus in linkage disequilibrium with the haplotype of two of the polymorphisms found [42].

Yet many individuals affected with HSCR have no *RET* mutations. In these patients, other factors of predisposition to the disease must be present in the form of rare non-coding mutations of the *RET* gene or mutations at other loci whether in their coding or non-coding sequences [43].

The *GDNF* gene is a member of the TGF family, and is a RET ligand. It is a major survival factor for many types of neurons. To activate *RET*, GDNF requires the presence of glycosyl-phosphatidylinositol coreceptors, of which four types have been described [44,45]. There have also been described other growth factors, ligands of *RET* (neurturin, artemin, and persephin). Combinations of these ligands are necessary for the development and maintenance of the neurons of the central and peripheral nervous systems. Mutations of *GDNF* have been identified in only 6 HSCR patients, and may therefore be regarded as a rare cause of HSCR (<5%) [46-48]. However, *GDNF* mutations may not be sufficient for the development of HSCR, since 4 of the 6 patients also presented other contributing factors such as *RET* mutations or trisomy 21 [46,47].

Another gene, *NTN*, may be related to HSCR. An *NTN* mutation has been described in a family that also presented a *RET* mutation [49].

The Endothelin Signaling Pathway

The other major signaling pathway in HSCR is that of *EDNRB*, the ligand of endothelin 3 (EDN3) and endothelin converting enzyme (ECE1). Approximately 5% of HSCR patients have (heterozygous) mutations in *EDNRB* or *EDN3* [25]. More recent studies showed how *RET* and *EDNRB* interact, *EDNRB* being the first modifier gene identified [26].

The endothelin pathway has a vasoconstrictive effect, and was therefore studied for its role in arterial hypertension. EDNRB and the A receptor, EDNRBA, are G-protein-coupled heptahelical receptors, which translate signals from endothelin. *EDNRB* has 443 amino acids, and is expressed mainly in the myenteric plexus, mucous layer, ganglia, and vessels of the colon submucosa [50,51].

The role of *EDNRB* in HSCR was described on the basis of different observations. First, there was the linkage at the 13q22 region in a population of Old Order Amish affected with HSCR [24,52]. Then there were reports of several HSCR patients with *de novo* interstitial deletions of 13q22 [53,54]. Subsequently, a comparative study of the piebald-lethal gene (a murine model of aganglionosis) showed its homology with *EDNRB* located at 13q22 [55]. The confirmation of the role of *EDNRB* came with the identification of the missense mutation W276C in the Amish population [56]. Like the case with *RET*, it appears that a haploinsufficiency mechanism could cause HSCR [57]. Nonetheless, the W276C mutation was neither necessary nor sufficient to cause HSCR, and penetrance was sex dependent (greater in males than in females) [57].

ECE1 is involved in the proteolytic processing of endothelins 1, 2, and 3. A case has been published of a patient with HSCR skip lesions, heart defects, craniofacial and hand anomalies, and autonomic dysfunction who had a mutation in one amino acid at position 742, very close to the active site of *ECE1* [58].

Other Genes: SOX10 and ZFHX1B (SIP1)

The recognition that *SOX10* could be related to HSCR came from the knowledge of a *de novo* mutation in the mouse. Murine dominant megacolon (*Dom*) is a model for Shah-Waardenburg syndrome (WS4) in heterozygotes; homozygous *Dom* mutations at embryonic level are lethal. *Dom* heterozygotes produce regional deficiencies of the neural-crest-derived enteric ganglia in the distal colon. *Dom* is homologous to human *SOX10* [59]. Truncation mutations have been observed in patients with heterozygous WS4 [60,61], Yemenite deaf-blind hypopigmentation syndrome and WS2 [62], and in other patients with neurological impairment. It seems unlikely that *SOX* is a major gene in isolated HSCR.

ZFHX1B (*SIP1*) is a transcription factor that has been reported to be mutated in HSCR patients with mental retardation and facial gestalt [64] in connection with a possible mechanism of haploinsufficiency [64].

As we have seen, altogether these genetic findings are complex, and many even have as yet no explanation. While *RET* and *EDNRB* once appeared to be independent, today they are known to be related. Considering everything together, one can make some general observations: (i) *RET* is the major gene involved in HSCR, (ii) the penetrance of *RET* mutations is incomplete and sex-related, (iii) the genotype-phenotype correlation is poor, (iv) HSCR is genetically heterogeneous, and is due to mutations that occur in different pathways, (v) there have been publications of patients who have mutations in more than one of the known susceptibility genes, and (vi) *RET* plays a role in the penetrance of some of the syndromic cases of HSCR [65].

Multigenic/Multifactorial Inheritance of Isolated HSCR Cases

The *RET* gene plays a key role in the genesis of HSCR, but multiple genes may be required to modulate its clinical expression. Genetic heterogeneity has also been demonstrated, where mutation in one of several genes is sufficient for the phenotypic expression of HSCR (*RET*, *EDNRB*, *EDN3*, *ECE1*). Segregation studies in HSCR have shown that the recurrence risk in siblings varies within the range 1.5–33% depending on the sex of the sibling, and on the sex and the length of the aganglionic segment in the proband [15]. Therefore, HSCR is assumed to be a sex-determined multifactorial disorder in which the effect of genes plays a greater role than that of environmental factors (relative risk of 200). Accordingly, and from the results of various segregation studies, one can consider an autosomal dominant model in long-segment HSCR and a multifactorial model in short-segment HSCR [65].

2) Molecular Genetics in Syndromic HSCR

As was noted above, HSCR is associated with chromosomal anomalies in 12% of cases, and on other occasions it is associated with monogenic syndromes especially in familial cases. Hence it is important that these patients be evaluated by an experienced clinical geneticist.

Chromosomal Anomalies

A large number of chromosomal anomalies have been described in HSCR patients. Table 3 lists the chromosomal anomalies that have been published as on some occasion associated with HSCR. Free trisomy 21 is the most frequent, affecting 2 to 10% of HSCR cases [8,15,66,67]. In these cases, there is an unbalanced sex ratio (5.5–10.5/1 male/female) and a predominance of short-segment HSCR greater than in isolated HSCR. Some authors have hypothesized gene overexpression on chromosome 21 predisposing to HSCR and a susceptibility gene mapping to the 21q22 region as observed in the Amish population [52].

As we have seen in describing the linkage of some genes related to HSCR, some chromosomal interstitial deletions found in HSCR patients have served to identify some predisposing genes. Among them are: the 10q11.2 deletion that led to the description of *RET*, the major susceptibility gene; the 13q22.1-32.1 deletion that led to the mapping of *EDNRB*; and the 2q22-23 deletion in patients with mental retardation and multiple congenital anomalies and with HSCR or severe chronic constipation that led to the description of the Mowat-Wilson syndrome [64,65] and the subsequent discovery of the *ZFHX1B* gene (previously known as *SIP1*) [63].

The Syndromes Observed

The recognition of known syndromes and the description of new entities associated with HSCR are very important for the prognosis of the disease and the appropriate genetic counseling, and in the search for new candidate HSCR genes [17]. The syndromes are many, with penetrance for HSCR ranging from 5 to > 80% [65]. Although there are various classifications, it seems that the most orderly divides these syndromes into five classes: (i) syndromes frequently associated with HSCR, (ii) other syndromes with HSCR as a common finding (mandatory), (iii) other syndromes with HSCR as an occasional associated finding, (iv) syndromes with rare association with HSCR, (v) miscellaneous associations [17,65].

There is a wide variety of syndromes that can include HSCR among their findings. They are all reflected in Table 5. In the following, we shall describe the most important.

Table 3. Chromosomal anomalies described in patients with HSCR

Anomaly	Clinical findings	Nº cases	Gene
Del 2q22-q23	RD, mental & growth retardation, microcephaly, epilepsy & HSCR	> 10 cases	*ZFHX1B*
Dup 2q		1 case	
Del 4p12	Dysmorphic features, mental & postnatal growth retardation, short HSCR	1 case	*PHOX2B*
Mos Tri 8			
Tetras 9p		1 case	
Del 10q11	Mental retardation, long HSCR	2 cases	*RET*
Del 13q22	Mental & growth retardation, RD & long HSCR		*EDNRB*
Del 17q21		> 1 case	
Dup 17q21-q23	Mental retardation,MCA	4 cases	
Del 18p		1 case	
Dup 18q		1 case	
Del 20p		1 case	
Tris 21	Down S., short HSCR	2–10% cases	?
Tri 22pter-q11	Cat's eye S.		
47,XXY			
Mos X/XX/XXX			

A) Syndromes that are often Associated with HSCR

Neurocristopathies: The neural crest is a transient and multipotent embryonic structure from which stem in part a range of tissues, organs, and systems, including neurons, the endocrine and paraendocrine system, craniofacial structures, conotruncal heart structures, and pigmentary tissues. The neurocristopathies can encompass tumours, malformations, and single or combined anomalies of the aforementioned organs and tissues. These anomalies include:

A1) Multiple Endocrine Neoplasia Type 2 and Familial Medullary Thyroid Carcinoma

Multiple endocrine neoplasia types 2A and 2B (MEN2A and 2B, respectively) and familial medullary thyroid carcinoma (FMTC) are syndromes of predisposition to cancer with an autosomal dominant pattern of inheritance. MEN2A is defined by an age-related predisposition to medullary thyroid cancer (MTC, risk of 70% by the age of 70 years), phæochromocytoma (50% of cases), and hyperplasia of the parathyroid glands (15% of cases). In addition to MTC and phæochromocytoma, patients with MEN2B present oral neuromas, Marfanoid habitus, and bowel hyperganglionosis [17]. Germline mutations of the *RET* gene have been identified in MEN2A, MEN2B, and FMTC patients, and some families with MEN2A and FMTC have shown association with HSCR [71-72]. These families present a germline *RET* mutation of the MEN2A or FMTC type. For this reason, individuals with HSCR, regardless of whether or not they have a family history of cancer, should be screened for *RET* exon 10 and 11 mutations to assess their predisposition for cancer.

A2) Neuroblastoma

Neuroblastoma is the commonest solid tumour in childhood (incidence of 1/10 000). The tumour may originate from anywhere within the sympathetic chains or the adrenal medulla (both derive from the neural crest). In some families, tumour predisposition segregates over generations with incomplete penetrance [73]. Neuroblastoma is associated with HSCR and CCHS in various combinations, and in each combination heterozygous mutations of *PHOX2B* (paired-like homeobox 2B) have been identified. However *PHOX2B* mutations in cases of isolated neuroblastoma are rare [74-76].

A3) Congenital Central Hypoventilation Syndrome (CCHS)

CCHS is characterized by abnormal ventilatory response to hypoxia and hypercapnia due to failure of autonomic respiratory control. Initially it was called Ondine's curse. CCHS is not in itself a neurocristopathy, but patients with this condition often present symptoms resulting from a dysfunction of the autonomic nervous system, and a predisposition to neural-crest-derived tumours (neuroblastoma, ganglioblastoma, and ganglioneuroma) [77,78]. The association of CCHS and HSCR is known as the Haddad syndrome, and occurs in 20% of CCHS patients. These cases correspond to long-segment HSCR (including total colonic aganglionosis). Mutations of *RET* and the endothelin signaling pathway have been found in patients with Haddad syndrome [79]. If the responsible gene is *PHOX2B*, the most frequent alteration in the affected patient is a *de novo* heterozygous mutation consisting of an in-frame duplication that gives rise to polyalanine expansion [80]. The parents of individuals with CCHS in whom the molecular alteration has been proven should also be evaluated, since 10% of them have a somatic mosaic mutation and some may develop late onset CCHS [81]. There may also be a genotype/phenotype correlation, because patients who have the molecular alteration that leads to polyalanine expansion are at a higher risk of developing tumours.

A4) Waardenburg Syndromes and Related Pigmentary Anomalies

The Waardenburg syndrome (WS) is an autosomal dominant process, and is the most frequent disorder associating pigmentary anomalies and sensorineural hearing loss due to the absence of skin melanocytes and the cochlear stria vascularis. WS is genetically heterogeneous with various loci that give rise to different types of WS. The association with HSCR defines type 4 (WS4), also known as Shah-Waardenburg syndrome, which is also a genetically heterogeneous process. Thus, homozygous mutations of the endothelin pathway, heterozygous *SOX10* mutations, and others have been described in WS4 patients.

Other syndromes that associate pigmentary anomalies and HSCR include: Yemenite deaf-blind hypopigmentation syndrome with a *SOX10* mutation found in some families [82], Black locks-Albinism-Deafness Syndrome (BADS) with HSCR/total colonic aganglionosis reported in one case [83], aganglionic megacolon associated with familial piebaldism [84], and HSCR with profound congenital deafness without other WS findings, *inter al.*

A5) Other Neurocristopathies

Other syndromic associations of HSCR have been reported: with familial dysautonomia syndrome (Riley-Day syndrome) (mapped to 9q31, where a susceptibility locus for HSCR has been described), cleft lip with or without cleft palate, myelomeningocele, and neurofibromatosis type 1. The significance of these associations is still not well established [65].

B) Other Syndromes With HSCR As A Frequent Finding (Mandatory)

B1) Mowat-Wilson Syndrome (MWS)

MWS is a syndrome of multiple congenital anomalies and mental retardation. It usually presents microcephaly, epilepsy, mental retardation, and facial gestalt. The malformations that can occur vary widely including, in descending order of frequency, hypospadias, kidney anomalies, congenital heart disease, and hypoplasia or agenesis of the corpus callosum and HSCR. Various kinds of mutations of *ZFHX1B* have been found, and it seems that the mechanism causing the syndrome is due to a loss of function of haploinsufficiency [85].

B2) Goldberg-Shprintzen Syndrome

This process is an autosomal recessive entity that combines multiple congenital anomalies, mental retardation, and HSCR. Among the findings that it presents are moderate mental retardation, microcephaly, polymicrogyria, facial dysmorphism, cleft palate, and iris coloboma. An inbred family has been identified with a KIAA1279 mutation. This syndrome must not be confused with the Shprintzen-Goldberg syndrome and craniosynostosis.

B3) HSCR with Limb Anomalies

A series of rare syndromes with HSCR and distal limb anomalies have been reported. They are listed in Table 4.

C) Other Syndromes with HSCR as an Occasional Finding

C1) Bardet-Biedl (BBS) and Mckusick-Kauffman (MKKS) Syndromes

BBS is characterized by pigmentary retinopathy, obesity, hypogenitalism, renal involvement (with kidney cysts), mental retardation, and postaxial polydactyly of the hands and feet. Previously described as a classic autosomal recessive hereditary pattern, this entity has been shown to have great heterogeneity of loci, and at least 12 loci have been found with 10 genes. Triallelic inheritance has been shown in BBS. HSCR has been found in several BBS cases [86].

MKKS is a rare disorder. It is allelic with BBS, and is characterized by hydrometrocolpos, postaxial polydactyly, and congenital heart disease. HSCR has been found in 10% of MKKS cases.

Table 4. Syndromes that are associated with HSCR.

Group	Syndrome	Clinical findings
Frequent association with HSCR	MEN2A	Medullary thyroid cancer
	Neuroblastoma	
	Haddad	Congenital central hypoventilation
	WS4	Pigmentation anomalies (white forelock, iris hypoplasia, hypopigmented patches)
	Yemenite deaf-blind hypopigmentation	Deafness, pigmentation and eye (microcornea, coloboma, nystagmus) anomalies
	BADS	Deafness, skin and retina hypopigmentation
	Piebaldism	Hypopigmented patches and white forelock
	Riley-Day	Anomalies of autonomic nervous system
Mandatory HSCR	Mowatt-Wilson	Microcephaly, epilepsy, facial gestalt, hypospadias
	Shprintzen-Goldberg	MR, polymicrogyria, microcephaly, CF, coloboma, dysmorphic features
	HSCR + limb anomalies	Polydactyly, renal agenesia, hypertelorism, deafness
		Postaxial polydactyly, VSD
		Dysmorphic features, nail and distal phalanx hypoplasia
Miscellaneous associations	HSAS/MASA	Hydrocephaly, aqueductal stenosis, adducted thumbs with spasticity, ACC, MR
	Jeune (asphyxiating thoracic dystrophy)	
	Pallister-Hall (CAVE)	
	Fryns	
	Aarskog	
	Frontonasal dysplasia	
	Osteopetrosis	
	Goldenhar	
	Lesch-Nyhan	
	Rubinstein-Taybi	
	Toriello-Carey	
	Spondylo-epi-metaphyseal dysplasia with joint laxity	
	Joubert	
	Persistent Mullerian duct S.	
	Asplenia with congenital cardiopathy	
		Preaxial polydactyly, congenital cardiopathy, larynx anomalies
		Brachydactyly type B

Table 4. Syndromes that are associated with HSCR. (Continued)

Group	Syndrome	Clinical findings
		BRESHEK (Brain abnormalities + Retardation + Ectodermal dysplasia + Skeletal malformation + Hirschsprung's disease + Ear/eye anomalies + Kidney dysplasia)
		Brachydactyly, macrocephaly, HSCR, spine anomalies
Occasional association with HSCR	Bardet-Biedl	Pigmentary retinosis, obesity, hypogenitalism, mild MR, postaxial polydactyly
	McKusick-Kauffman	Hydrometrocolpos, postaxial polydactyly, congenital cardiopathy
	Smith-Lemli-Opitz	Growth retardation, microcephaly, MR, hypospadias, syndactyly of toes 2-3, dysmorphic features
	Cartilage-hair hypoplasia	Short-limb dwarfism, metaphyseal dysplasia, immunodeficiency
Rarely associated with HSCR	Fukuyama's congenital muscular dystrophy	Muscular dystrophy, polymicrogyria, hydrocephaly, MR, seizures
	Clayton-Smith	Dysmorphic features, nail and toe hypoplasia, ichthyosis
	Kaplan	Agenesis of the corpus callosum (ACC), adducted thumbs, ptosis, muscular weakness
	Okamoto	Hydrocephaly, cleft palate, corpus callosum agenesis
	Werner's mesomelic dysplasia	
	Pitt-Hopkins	Epileptic encephalopathy, dysmorphic facial features, episodes of hypoventilation, autonomic dysfunction

C2) Smith-Lemli-Opitz Syndrome (SLO)

SLO is an autosomal recessive disease that is due to a mutation of the 7-dehydrocholesterol reductase gene (*DHCR7*) that results in impairment of cholesterol metabolism. It is characterized by pre- and post-natal growth retardation, microcephaly, severe mental retardation, facial dysmorphic features, hypospadias, and classic "Y" syndactyly of toes 2 and 3. HSCR has been found in a significant number of patients [87,8].

C3) Cartilage-Hair Hypoplasia Syndrome (CHH)

CHH is characterized by short limb dwarfism caused by metaphyseal dysplasia, sparse fine blond hair, transient microcytic anæmia, and immunodeficiency. It is due to mutations of *RMRP* mapped to chromosome region 9p13 [89]. HSCR is found in 10% of CHH cases [91].

D) Syndromes Rarely Associated with HSCR

There are various syndromes in which HSCR has been found on rare occasions (see Table 4).

E) Miscellaneous

There are diverse other entities and syndromes in which HSCR has been described. They include myopathies, syndromes with dermatological findings, and syndromes with central nervous system anomalies among which there stands out the MASA spectrum due to *L1CAM* mutations with X-linked recessive inheritance. Various mutations of this gene have been reported in patients with hydrocephaly and HSCR. It is as yet unknown whether *L1CAM* acts as a modifier gene in HSCR. There are a number of other rare associations of HSCR and certain syndromes which are listed in Table 4.

Genetic Counseling

HSCR is a multifactorial, sex-modified congenital malformation. The risk of recurrence in a proband's sibling is approximately 4% (relative risk of 200). This risk increases with increasing length of the affected segment. When HSCR presents within the spectrum of a disease, genetic counseling should refer to that disease rather than to HSCR itself. Due to the large number of syndromes with which HSCR may be associated, it is very important for patients who have HSCR and some associated congenital defect to be evaluated by a clinical geneticist with expertise in dysmorphology [93]. According to the Carter paradox, the greatest risk of recurrence in isolated HSCR cases is for a brother of a female proband with long-segment HSCR (Table 5).

Table 5. Epidemiology and risk of recurrence in isolated HSCR.

	L-HSCR	S-HSCR
Probands (%)	19	81
Sex ratio (M/F)	1.75	5.5
Inheritance pattern	Autosomal dominant	Multifactorial or recessive
Penetrance % (M / F)	52 / 40	17 / 4
Risk of recurrence (%)*		
Affected man	17 / 13	5 / 1
Affected woman	33 / 9	5 / 3

Relative risk = 200.
The risk of recurrence is presented according to the sex of the sibling (M / F).

Because HSCR is a very heterogeneous process, with the isolation of different susceptibility genes whose mutations have a low penetrance, systematic molecular study of the different genes in isolated HSCR patients is not indicated. Such studies are usually performed for purposes of research [91]. Moreover, the genotype-phenotype correlation is poor. It only seems to be useful to study exons 10 and 11 of *RET* for their predisposition to cancer in cases of MEN2A mutations. Indeed, if MEN2A mutations are identified, screening for these should be carried out in first degree family members, and, for carriers, prophylactic thyroidectomy should be considered before 5 years of age, together with long-term screening for phæochromocytoma and hyperparathyroidism.

Although prenatal diagnosis is possible if the mutation is known, it is of little utility because of the variable expression, the incomplete penetrance of the mutations of the genes predisposing to HSCR (especially *RET*), and the good prognosis after surgery in most patients suffering from HSCR.

References

[1] Hirschsprung H. Stuhlrägheit neugeborener infolge von dilatation und hypertrophic des colons. *Jb Inderheilk*, 1988;27:1.

[2] Stevenson O. Early history of the therapy of Hirschsprung's disease: fact and personal observation over 50 years [see comments]. *J Pediatr Surg*, 1996;31:1003-8.

[3] Tam PKH, García-Barcelo M. Molecular genetics of Hirschsprung's disease. *Sem Pediat Surg*, 2004; 13:236-48.

[4] Romeo G, Ronchetto P, Luo Y, Barone V, Seri M, Ceccherini I et al. Point mutations affecting the tyrosine kinase domain of the RET proto-oncogene in Hirschsprung's disease. *Nature*, 1994;367:377-8.

[5] Iwashita T, Kruger GM, Pardal R, Kiel MJ, Morrison SJ. Hirschsprung disease is linked to defects in neural crest stem function. *Science*, 2003; 301:972-6.

[6] Badner JA, Chakravarti A. Waardenburg syndrome and Hirschsprung disease: evidence for pleiotropic effects of a single dominant gene. *Am J Med Genet*, 1990; 35:100-4

[7] Passarge E. The genetics of Hirschsprung's disease. Evidence for heterogeneous etiology and a study of sixty-three families. *N Engl J Med*, 1967; 276:138-43.

[8] Goldberg EL. An epidemiological study of Hirschsprung's disease. *Int J Epidemiol*, 1984;13:479-85.

[9] Whitehouse F, Kernohan J. Myenteric plexuses in congenital megacolon: study of 11 cases. *Arch intern Med* 1948;82:75.

[10] Nihoul-Fekete C, Ricour G, Martelli H, Jacob SL, Pellerin D. Total colonic agangliosis (with or without ileal involvement): a review of 27 cases. *J Pediatr Surg*, 1986; 21:251-4

[11] Orr JD, Scobie WG. Presentation and incidence of Hirschsprung's disease. *BMJ*, 1983;287:1671.

[12] Suita S, Taguchi T, Ierie S, Nakatsuji T. Hirschsprung disease in Japan: analysis of 3852 patients based on a nationwide survey in 30 years. *J Pediatr Surg* 2005;40:197-201.

[13] Kleinhaus S, Boley SJ, Sheran Wk. Hirschsprung's disease. A survey of the members of the Surgical Section of the American Academy of Pediatrics. *J Pediatr Surg* 1979;14:588-97

[14] Swenson O, Sherman JO, Fisher J. Diagnosis of congenital megacolon: An analysis of 501 patients. *J Pediatr Surg* 1973; 8:587-94

[15] Bodian M, Carter C. A family study of Hirschsprung disease. *Ann Hum Genet* 1963;26:261

[16] Torfs C. An epidemiological study of Hirschsprung disease in a multiracial California population. The *Third International Meeting: Hirschsprung's Disease and Related Neurocristopathies*. Evian, France; 1988

[17] Amiel J, Lyonnet S. Hirschsprung's disease, associated syndromes, and genetics: a review. *J Med Genet* 2001;38:729-39.

[18] Moore SW. The contribution of associated congenital anomalies in understanding Hirschsprung's disease. *Pediatr Surg Int*; 22:305-15.

[19] Sarioglu A, Taniel FC, Buyukpamukcu N, Hicsonmez A. Hirschsprung-associated congenital anomalies. *Eur J Pediatr Surg* 1997;7:331-7.

[20] Festen C. Anomalies of the urinary tract in Hirschsprung's disease. *Z Kinderchir* 1975;17:376-80.

[21] Nowaczyk MJ, James AG, Superina R, Siegel-Bartelt J. Hirschsprung's disease, postaxial polydactyly, and atrial septal defect. *Am J Med Genet* 1997; 68:74-5.

[22] Moore SW, Rode H, Millar AJ, Albertin R, Cyves S. Familial aspects of Hirschsprung's disease. *Eur J Pediatr Surg* 1991;1:97-107

[23] Solari V, Ennis S, Yoneda A, Wong L, Messineo A, Hollwart ME, et al. Mutation analysis of the RET gene in total intestinal agangliosis by wave DNA fragment analysis system. *J Pediatr Surg* 2003; 38:497-501.

[24] Carrasquillo MM, McCallion AS, Puffenberger EG, Kaschuk CS, No N, Chakravarti A. Genome-wide association study as well as the study of mouse models help to identify the interaction between RET and EDNRB pathways in Hirschsprung disease. *Nat Genet* 2002; 3:237-44.

[25] Lyonnet S, Bolino A, Pelet A, Abel L, Nihoul-Fekete C, Briard ML, et al. A gene for Hirschsprung disease maps to the proximal long arm of chromosome 10 (see comments). *Nat Genet* 1993; 4:436-50

[26] Angrist M, Kauffman E, Slaugenhaupt SA, Matise TC, Puffenberger EG, Washington SS, et al. A gene for Hirschsprung disease (megacolon) in the pericentromeric region of human chromosome 10 (see comments). *Nat Genet* 1993; 4:351-6.

[27] Martiucciello G, Biocchini M, Dodero P, Cirillo M, Puliti A, Gimelli G. Total colonic aganglionsis associated with interstitial deletion of the long arm of chromosome 10. *Pediatr Surg Int* 1992,7:308.

[28] Mulligan ML, Kwok JB, Healey CS, Elsdon MJ, Eng C, Gardner E, et al. Germ-line mutations of the RET proto-oncogene in multiple endocrine neoplasia type 2A. *Nature* 1993; 363:458-60.

[29] Edery P, Lyonnet S, Mulligan LM, Pelet A, Dow E, Abel L, et al. Mutations of the RET proto-oncogene in Hirschsprung's disease. *Nature* 1994; 367:378-80.

[30] Angrist M, Bolk S, Thiel H, Puffenberger EG, Hofstra RM, Buys CH, et al. Mutation analysis of the RET receptor kinase in Hirschsprung disease. *Hum Mol Genet* 1995; 4:821-30.

[31] Attie T, Pelet A, Edery P, Eng C, Mulligan ML, Amiel J, et al. Diversity of RET proto-oncogene mutations in familial and sporadic Hirschsprung disease. *Hum Mol Genet* 1995; 4:1381-6

[32] Seri M, Yin L, Barone V, Bolino A, Celli I, Bocciardi R, et al. Frequency of the RET mutations in long and short segment Hirschsprung disease. *Hum Mutat* 1997; 9:243-9.

[33] Santoro M, Carlomagno F, Romano, Bottaro DP, Dathan NA, Grieco M et al. Activation of RET as a dominant transforming gene by germline mutations of MEN2A and MEN2B. *Science* 1995;267:381-3.

[34] Pasini B, Borrello MG, Greco A, Bongarzone I, Luo Y, Mondellini P et al. Loss of function effect of RET mutation causing Hirschsprung disease. *Nat Genet* 1995;10:35-40.

[35] Iwashita T, Murakami H, Asai N, Takahashi M. Mechanism of RET dysfunction by Hirschsprung mutations affecting its extracellular domain. *Hum Mol Genet* 1995; 5:1577-80.

[36] Sancandi M, Ceccherini I, Costa M, Fava M, Chen B, Wu Y, et al. Incidence of RET mutations in patients with Hirschsprung's disease. *J Pediatr Surg* 2000;35:139-42.

[37] García-Barcelo M, Sham MH, Lee WS, Lui VC, Chem BL, Wong KK, et al. Highly recurrent RET mutations and novel mutations in genes of the receptor tyrosine kinase and endothelin receptor B pathways in Chinese patients with sporadic Hirschsprung disease. *Clin Chem* 2004, 50: 93-100.

[38] Borrego S, Wright FA, Fernandez RM, Willians M, Lopez-Alonso M, Davuluri R, et al. A founding locus within the RET proto-oncogene may account for a large proportion of apparently sporadic Hirschsprung disease and subset of cases of sporadic medullary thyroid carcinoma. *Am J Hum Genet* 2003;72:88-100.

[39] García-Barcelo M, Ganster RW, Lui VC, Leon TY, So MT, Lau AM et al. TTF-1 and RET promoter SNPs: regulation of RET transcription in Hirschsprung's disease. *Hum Mol Genet* 2005;14:191-204.

[40] Emison ES, McCallion AS, Kashuk CS, Bush RT, Grice E, Lin S et al. A common sex-dependent mutation in a RET enhancer underlies Hirschsprung disease risk. *Nature* 2005; 434:857-863.

[41] Pelet A, de Puntual L, Clement-Ziza L, Salomon R, Mugnier C, Matsuda F et al. Monozygosity for a frequent and weakly penetrant predisposing allele at the RET locus in sporadic Hirschsprung disease. *J Med Genet* 2005;42:e18.

[42] Sancandi M, Griseri P, Pesce B, Patrone G, Pupp F, Lerone M, et al. Single nucleotide polymorphic alleles in the 5' region of the RET proto-oncogene define a risk haplotype in Hirschsprung's disease. *J Med Genet* 2003; 40:714-8.

[43] Plaza-Menacho I, Burzinski GM, De Goot JW, Eggen BJL and Hofstra RMW. Current concepts in RET-related genetics, signaling and therapeutics. *Trends Genet* 2006; 22:627-36.

[44] Jing S, Wen D, Yu Y, Holst PL, Luo Y, Fang M et al. GDNF-induced activation of the RET protein tyrosine kinase is mediated by GDNFR-alpha, a novel receptor for GDNF. *Cell* 1996;85:1113-24.

[45] Treanor JJ, Goodman L, de Savage F, Stone DM, Poulsen KT, Beck CD et al. Characterization of a multicomponent receptor for GDNF. *Nature* 1996; 382:80-3.

[46] Angrist M, Bolk S, Halunshka, Lapchak PA, Chakravarti A. Germline mutations in glial cell line-derived neurotrophic factor (GDNF) and RET in Hirschsprung disease patient. *Nat Genet* 1996; 14:341-4.

[47] Salomon R, Attie T, Pelet A, Bidaud C, Eng C, Amiel J et al. Germline mutations of the RET ligand GDNF are not sufficient to cause Hirschpung disease. *Nat Genet* 1996; 14:345-7.

[48] Ivanchuck SM, Myers SM, Eng C, Mulligan LM. De novo mutation of GDNF, ligand for the RET/GDNFR-alpha receptor complex, in Hirschsprung disease. *Hum Mol Genet* 1996;5:2023-6.

[49] Doray B, Salomon R, Amiel J, Pelet A, Touraine R, Billaud M, et al. Mutations of the ligand, neurturin, supports multigenic inheritance in Hirschsprung disease. *Hum Mol Genet* 1998; 7:1449-52.

[50] Inagaki H, Bishop AE, Escrig C, Wharton J, Allen-Mersh Tg, Polak JM. Localization of endothelin-like immunoreactivity and endothelin binding sites in human colon. *Gastroenterology* 1991;101:47-54.

[51] Sakamoto A, Yanagisawa M, Sakurai T, Takuwa Y, Yanagisawa H, Masaki T. Cloning and functional expression of human cDNA for the ETB endothelin receptor. *Biochem Biophys Res Commun* 1991; 178:656-63.

[52] Puffenberger EG, Kauffman ER, Bolk S, Matise TC, Washington SS, Angrist M et al. Identity-by-descent and association mapping of a recessive gene for Hirschsprung disease on human chromosome 13q12. *Hum Mol Genet* 1994; 1217-25.

[53] Lamont MA, Fitchett M, Dennis NR. Interstitial deletion of distal 13q associated with Hirschsprung's disease. *J Med Genet* 1989;26:100-4.

[54] Botani A, Xie YG, Binkert F, Schinzel A. A case of Hirschsprung disease with a chromosome 13 microdeletion, del(13)(q32.3q33.2): potential mapping of one disease locus. *Hum Genet* 1991;87:748-50.

[55] Hosoda K, Hammer RE, Richardson JA, Baynash AG, Cheung JC, Giaid A et al. Targeted and neural (piebald-lethal) mutations of endothelin-B-receptor gene produce megacolon associated with spotted coat color in mice. *Cell* 1994;79:1267-76.

[56] Puffenberger EG, Hosoda K, Washington SS, Nakao K, deWitt D, Yanagisawa M Chakravat A. A missense mutation of the endothelin-B-receptor gene in multigenic Hirchprung's disease. *Cell* 1994; 79:1257-66.

[57] Inoue K, Tanabe Y, Lupski JR. Myelin deficiencies in both the central and the peripheral nervous systems associated with a SOX10 mutation. *Ann Neurol* 1999;46:313-8.

[58] Hofstra RM, Valdenaire O, Arch E, Osinga J, Troes H, Loffler BM et al. A loss-of-function mutation in the endothelin-converting-enzyme 1 (ECE-1) associated with Hirschsprung disease, cardiac defects, and autonomic dysfunction. *Am J Hum Genet* 1999; 64:304-8

[59] Southard-Smith EM, Kos L, Pavan VJ. Sox mutation disrupts neural crest development in Dom Hirschsprung mouse model. *Nat Genet* 1998;18:60-4.

[60] Pingault V, Bondurand N, Kuhlbrodt K, Goerich DE, Prehu MO, Puliti A, et al. SOX10 mutations in patients with Waardenburg-Hirschsprung disease. *Nat Genet* 1998;18:171-3.

[61] Touraine RL, Attie-Bitach T, Manceau E, Korsch E, Sarda P, Pingault V, et al. Neurological phenotype in Waardenburg syndrome type 4 correlates with novel SOX10

truncating mutations and expression in developing brain. *Am J Med Genet* 2000; 66:1496-503

[62] Bondurand N, Kuhlbrondt K, Pingault V, Enderich J, Sajus M, Tommerup N, et al. A molecular analysis of the Yemenite deaf-blind hypopigmentation syndrome: SOX10 dysfunction causes different neurocristopathies. *Hum Mol Genet* 1999; 8:1785-9.

[63] Wakamatsu N, Yamada Y, Yamada K, Ono T, Nomura N, Taniguchi H et al. Mutations in SP1, encoding SMAD interacting protein-1, cause a form of Hirschsprung disease. *Nat Genet* 2001; 27:369-70.

[64] Mowat DR, Croaker GD, Cass DT, Kerr BA, Chaitw J, Ades et al. Hirschsprung disease, microcephaly, mental retardation, and characteristic facial features: delineation of a new syndrome an identification of a locus chromosome 2q22-q23. *J Med Genet* 1998;35:617-23.

[65] Amiel J, Sproat-Emison E, Garcia-Barcelo M, Lantieri F, Burzynski G, Borrego et al. Hirschsprung's disease, associated syndromes and genetics: a review. *J Med Genet* 2008;45:1-14.

[66] Spouge D, Baird PA. Hirschsprung disease in a large birth cohort. *Teratology* 1985:32-171.

[67] Garver KL. Law JC, Garver B. Hirschsprung disease: a genetic study. *Clin Genet* 1985; 28:503-8.

[68] Lurie IW, Supovitz KR, Rosenblum-Vos LS, Wulfsberg EA. Phenotypic variability of del(2)(q22-q23): report of a case with review of the literature. *Genet Couns*el 1994;5:11-4.

[69] Borst MJ, VanCamp JM, PeacocK ML, Decker RA. Mutational analysis of multiple endocrine neoplasia type 2A associated with Hirschsprung's disease. *Surgery* 1995;117:386-91.

[70] Caron P, Attie T, David D, Amiel J, Brousset F, Roger P et al. C618R mutation in exon 10 of the RET proto-oncogen in a kindred with multiple endocrine neoplasia type 2A and Hirschsprung's disease. *J Clin Endocrinol Metab* 1996;81:2731-3.

[71] Peretz H, Luboshitsky R, Baron E, Biton A, Gershoni R, Usher S et al. Cys 618 Arg mutation in the RET proto-oncogene associated with familial medullary thyroid carcinoma and maternally transmitted Hirschsprung's disease suggesting a role for imprinting. *Hum Mutat* 1997;10:155-9.

[72] Decker RA, Peacock ML, Watson P. Hirschsprung disease in MEN 2A: increased spectrum of RET exon 10 genotype-phenotype correlation. *Hum Mol Genet* 1998; 7:129-34.

[73] Chatten J, Voorhess ML. Familial neuroblastoma. Report of a kindred with multiple disorders, including neuroblastomas in four siblings. *N Engl J Med* 1967;277:1230-6.

[74] Rorher T, Trachsel D, Engelcke G, Hammer J. Congenital central hypoventilation syndrome associated Hirschprung's disease and neuroblastoma: case of multiple neurocristopathies. *Pediatr Pulmonol* 2002;33:71-6

[75] van Limpt V, Schramm A, van Lakeman A, Sluis P, Chan A, van Noesel M et al. The Phox2B homeobox gene is mutated in sporadic neuroblastomas. *Oncogene* 2004;23:9280-8.

[76] Perri P, Bachetti T, Longo L, Matera I, Seri M, Tonini GP et al. PHOX2B mutations and genetic predisposition to neuroblastoma. *Oncogene* 2005;24:3050-3.
[77] Roshkow JE, Haller JO, Berden WE, Sane SM. Hirschsprung's disease, Ondine's curse, and neuroblastoma. Manifestations of neurocristopathy [see comments]. *Pediatr Radiol* 1988;19:45-9.
[78] Levard G, Boige N, Vitroux C, Aigrain Y, Boureau M, Navarro J. Neurocristopathy. The association of Hirschsprung's disease-ganglioneuroma with autonomic nervous system dysfunction in 2 children. *Arch Fr Pediat* 1989;46:595-7
[79] Sakai T, Wakizaka A, Matsuda H, Nirasawa Y, Itok Y. Point mutation in exon 12 of the receptor tyrosine kinase proto-oncogene RET in Ondine-Hirschsprung syndrome. *Pediatrics* 1998;101:924-6.
[80] Weese-Mayer DE, Berry-Kravis EM, Zhou L, Maher BS, Silvestri JM, Curran ME et al. Idiopathic congenital hypoventilation syndrome: analysis of genes pertinent to early autonomic nervous system embryologic development and identification of mutations in PHOX2b. *Am J Med Genet* 2003;123:267-78.
[81] Weese-Mayer DE, Berry-Kravis EM, Zhou L. Adult identified with congenital central hypoventilation syndrome-mutation in PHOX2b gene and late-onset CCHS. *Am J Resp Crit Care Med* 2005;171:88.
[82] Gross A, Kunze J, Maier RF, Stoltenburg-Didinger G, Grimmer I, Obladen M. Autosomal-recessive neural crest syndrome with albinism, black lock, cell migration disorder of the neurocytes of the gut, and deafness: ABCD syndrome. *Am J Med Genet* 1995;56:322-6.
[83] Mahakrisnan A, Srinivasan JP. Piebaldness with Hirschsprung disease [letter]. *Arch Dermatol* 1980;116:1102.
[84] Zweir C, Thiel CT, Dufke A, Crow YJ, Meinecke P, Suri M et al. Clinical and mutational spectrum of Mowat-Wilson syndrome. *Eur J Med Genet* 2005;48:91-111.
[85] Radetti G, Frick R, Pasquino B, Mengarda G, Savage MO. Hypothalamic-pituitary dysfunction and Hirschsprung's disease in the Bardet-Bield syndrome. *Helv Paediatr Acta* 1988:43:249-52.
[86] Patterson K, Toomey KE, Chandra RS. Hirschsprung disease in 46,XY phenotypic infant girl with Smith-Lemli-Opitz syndrome. *J Pediatr* 1983;103:425-7.
[87] Stewart DR, von Allmen D. The genetics of Hirschsprung disease. *Gastroenterol Clin N Am* 2993;21:819-837.
[88] Godbole K. The many faces of Hirschsprung's disease. *Ind Pediatr* 2004;41:1115-23.
[89] Mäkitie O, Kaitila I. Cartilage-hair hypoplasia — clinical manifestations in 108 Finnish patients. *Eur J Pediatr* 1993;152:211-17.
[90] Gariepy CE. Genetic Basis of Hirschsprung disease: implications in clinical practice. *Mol Genet Metab* 2003;80:66-73.
[91] Brooks AS, Oostra BA and Hofstra RM. Studying the genetics of Hirschsprung's disease: unraveling an oligogenic disorder. *Clin Genet* 2004; 67:6-14.

In: Hirschsprung's Disease: Diagnosis and Treatment
Ed: Ramón Núñez and Manuel López-Alonso
ISBN: 978-1-60741-349-3

Chapter VII

Histopathology of Hirschsprung Disease

William A. Meier-Ruge and Elizabeth Bruder

Hirschsprung Disease and Total Aganglionosis of the Colon

Since 1957, Hirschsprung disease is routinely diagnosed in distal colon mucosa biopsies by an enzyme - histochemical acetylcholinesterase (AChE) reaction. These results were first published in 1967 [1-3]. Since these days, the AChE reaction, according to Karnovsky and Roots [4], is a standard procedure in the diagnosis of Hirschsprung Disease.

The characteristics of Hirschsprung disease are the increase of AChE activity in parasympathetic nerve fibres of lamina propria mucosae, muscularis mucosae and muscularis propria (Fig. 1). This typical picture of Hirschsprung disease is observed in the most distal 10 – 15 cm of the colon. An important precondition for a reliable diagnosis is a native frozen cryostat section of 15 μm. By thawing, spreading and drying of this section on a degreased microscopic slide, the section loses about 70% of its thickness. This results in a final thickness of 4 – 5 μm [5]. A cryostat section of 4 μm only allows a final thickness of 1.2 μm which is too thin to permit a reliable diagnosis (compare Fig. 11).

The fact that diagnosis of Hirschsprung disease can be reliably made in mucosal suction biopsies renders anaethesia of the patient unnecessary. A biopsy to exclude or diagnose Hirschsprung Disease, is recommended in neonates, which show a failure to pass meconium. Looking back on our 40 years experience, our diagnostic technique achieved a 100 % reliability. AChE examination of rectal suction biopsies is considered to be the gold standard in the diagnosis of Hirschsprung Disease [6-12]. The advantage of the AChE reaction is the fact that there is no need to look for nerve cells of the submucous plexus. Three mucosal biopsies, taken 1cm, 4cm and 8cm above the dentate line (rectal – anal transition line) allow a reliable diagnosis of Hirschsprung's Disease or its exclusion.

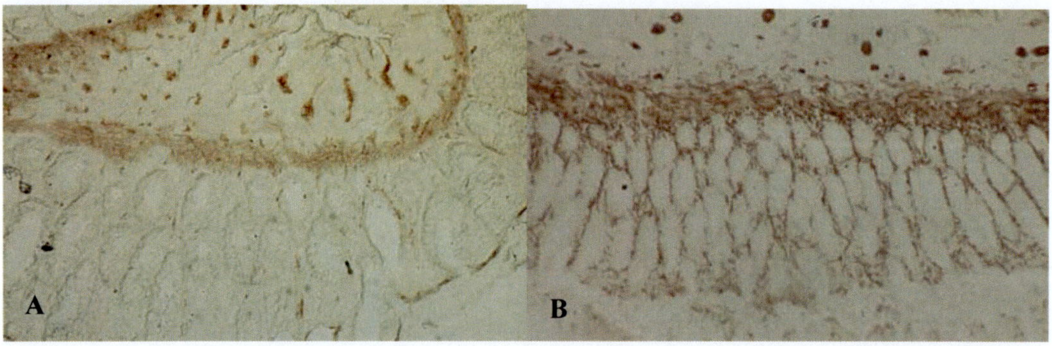

Figure 1. Rectal mucosa with acetylcholinesterase reaction without counterstaining. A: Normal innervated rectum mucosa (3 cm above the pectinate line). B: Aganglionic rectum mucosa with characteristic increase of Acetylcholinesterase (AChE) reaction in parasympathetic nerve fibres of lamina propria mucosae and muscularis mucosae (3 cm above the pectinate line; magnif. 90 x).

Despite the fact that staining of parasympathetic nerve fibres in lamina propria mucosae in neonates is less intense, the characteristics of Hirschsprung Disease are unambiguous [13-15] (Fig. 2). The AChE reaction overcomes the problems in identifying nerve cells in the submucosa. Some authors argue that an adequate diagnosis of submucous plexus in paraffin sections is possible not earlier than at an age of 3 years [16].

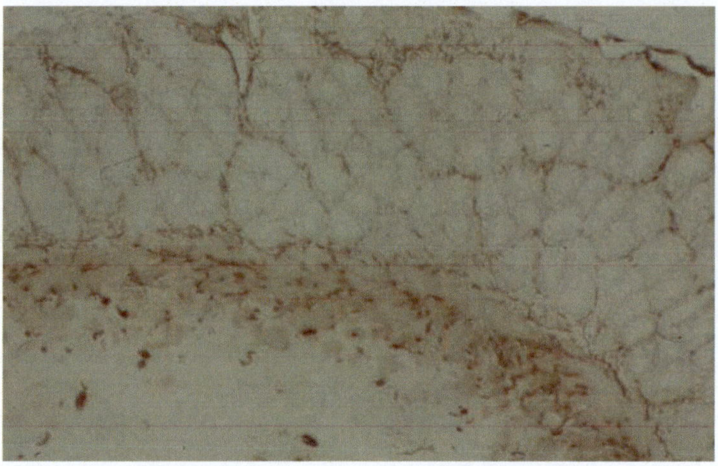

Figure 2. Low AChE reaction in aganglionic rectum mucosa of a neonate (magnif. 120 x).

It is important to be aware that due to embryological reasons the mucosal diagnosis of Hirschsprung disease is limited to the distal colon (Fig. 3). Morphometric measurements of nerve fibre density in circular muscles of total aganglionosis show an exponential decrease of nerve fibre density in a caudo – cranial direction [17] (Fig. 4). It is important to be aware that the extramural innervation of the distal colon arises from the sacral roots S 2 – S 5. These nerves invade circular muscles during the embryonic weeks 5 to 7. At this time, neuroblasts from the neck vagus have just arrived in stomach and jejunum. This becomes quite obvious in a coiled surgical specimen with total aganglionosis (Fig. 5 and 6). Therefore, a mucosal or a laparoscopically assisted [18] seromuscular biopsy of an aganglionic transversal or ascending colon show no characteristics of Hirschsprung disease as observed in rectal mucosa biopsies.

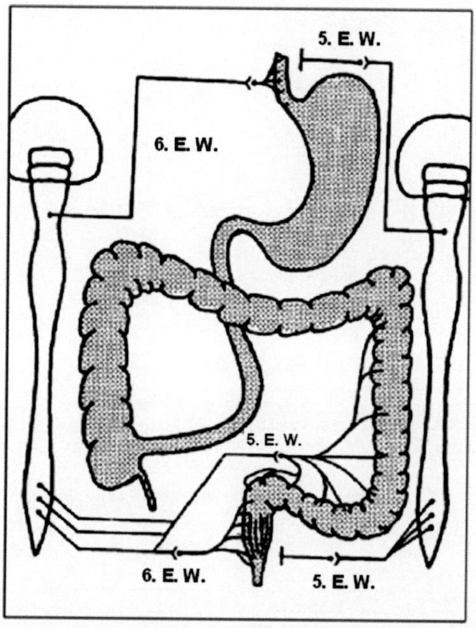

Figure 3. Development of the extramural innervation of the distal colon from the sacral roots S 2 – S 4 during the embryonic weeks 5 – 7. At the fifth embryonic week, the neuroblast colonisation of the stomach begins.

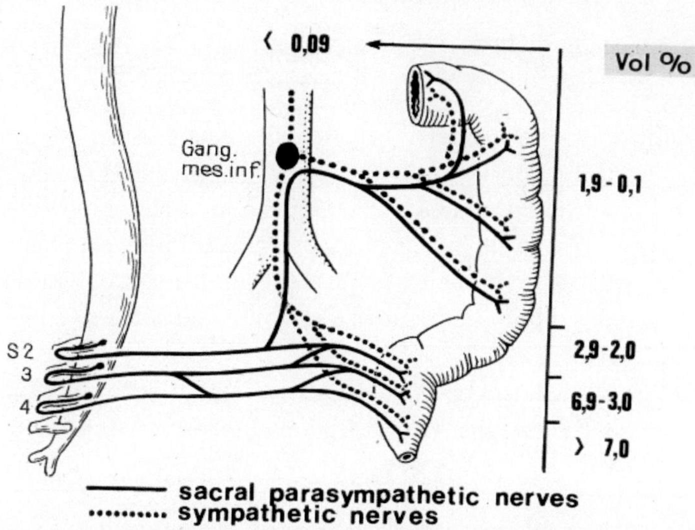

Figure 4. Exponential decline of nerve fibre density (morphometric measurements) in circular muscles of muscularis propria. This figure demonstrates that the increase of AChE activity in parasympathetic nerve fibres is limited to the distal colon [17].

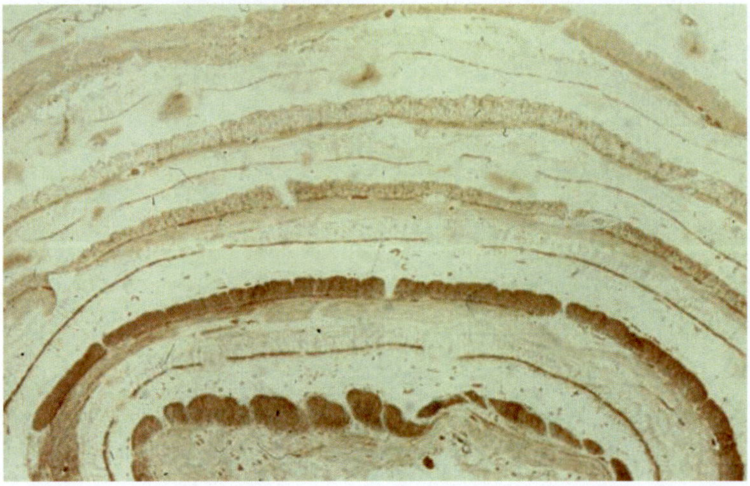

Figure 5. A coiled colon with total aganglionosis which shows the caudo – cranial decrease of AChE positive nerve fibres in circular muscles (magnif. 18 x).

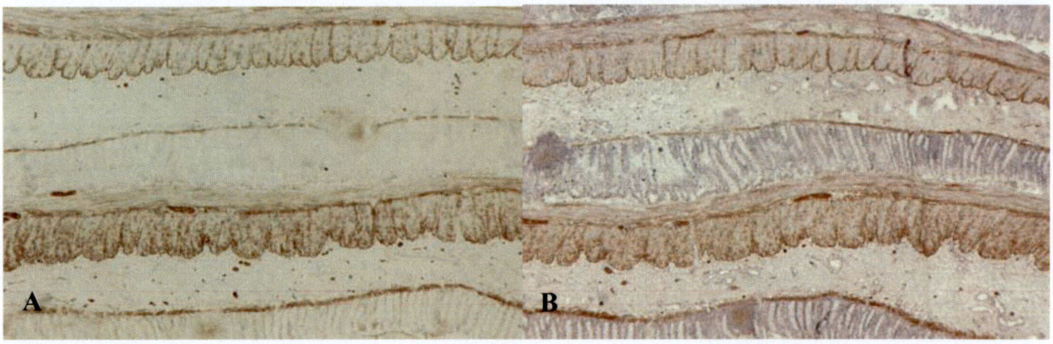

Figure 6. Higher magnification of two layers of the coiled aganglionic colon from Fig. 5. A: AChE reaction without counterstaining. B: AChE reaction with hemalum counterstaining (magnif. 60 x).

Laparoscopically taken seromuscular biopsies of sigma and / or descending colon are necessary to exclude innervation anomalies of myenteric plexus. This may be indicated if mucosal biopsies of the rectum have not shown HD. Seromuscular biopsies are necessary for the diagnosis of hypoganglionosis, hypogenesis or immaturity of myenteric plexus [19-21] (Fig. 7, 8 and 9) Also aplastic or atrophic desmosis of muscularis propria – a rare condition of the colon with aperistaltic syndrome – requires a seromuscular biopsy of the distal colon for a reliable diagnosis [22] (Fig. 10).

It is worthwhile to supplement an AChE reaction with a lactic, succinic dehydrogenase and NADPH diaphorase, because the AChE reaction does not stain electively nerve cells and ganglia.

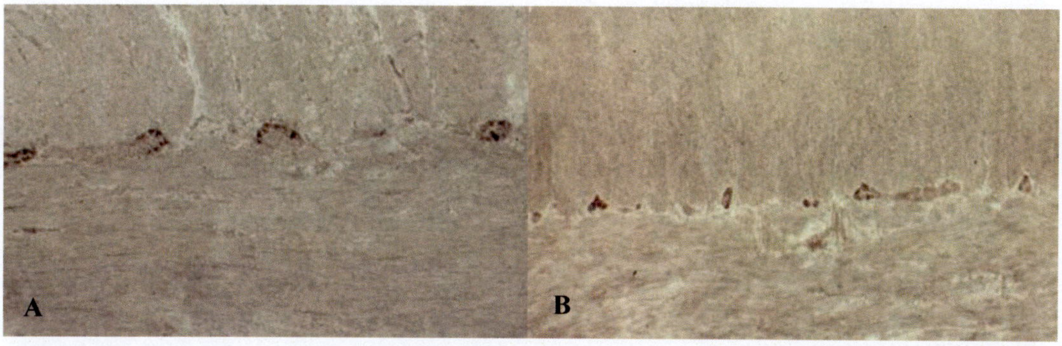

Figure 7. NADPH – Diaphorase (Nitroxid Synthetase) of a proximal resection margin. A: Normal innervated myenteric plexus (10cm proximal resection margin). B: Hypoplastic hypoganglionosis of myenteric plexus (3cm proximal resection margin; magnif. 180 x).

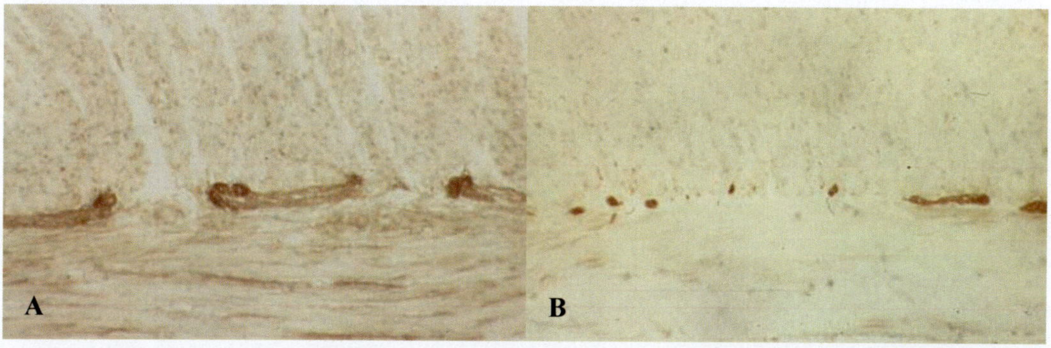

Figure 8. AChE reaction of a proximal resection line. A: Normal AChE activity of muscularis propria. B: Low parasympathetic tonus of muscularis propria in hypoganglionosis of myenteric plexus (magnif. 180 x).

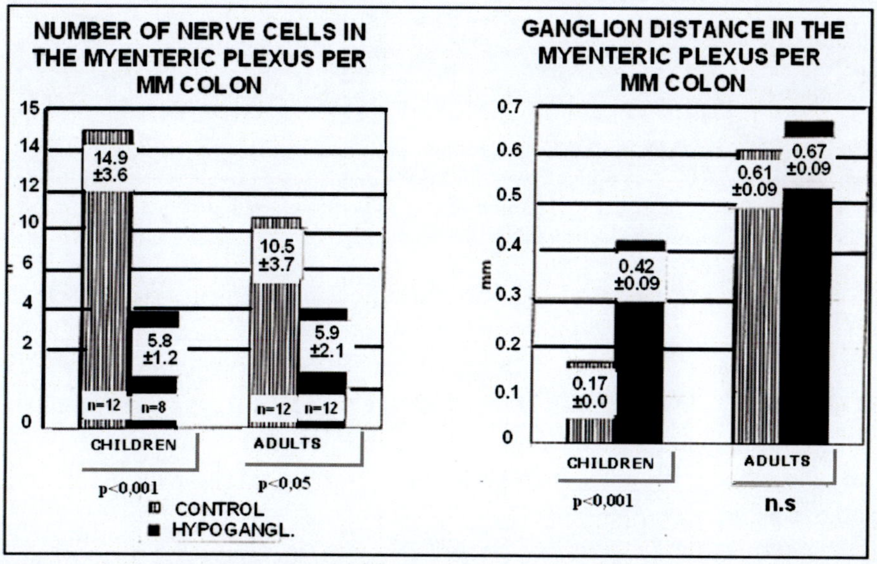

Figure 9 Morphometric values of nerve cell number and ganglion distances of myenteric plexus in hypoganglionosis of myenteric plexus in comparison to normal innervated colon.

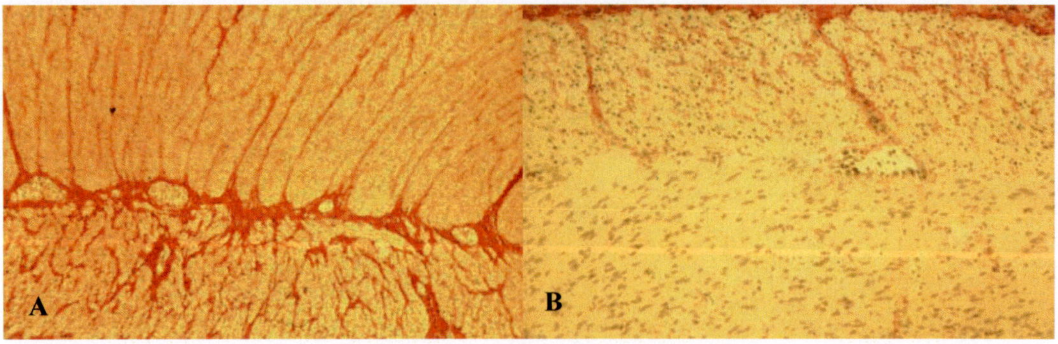

Figure 10. Picro-Siriusred staining of tendinous structures in muscularis propria. A: Normal developed tendinous net in circular and longitudinal muscles. Well developed tendinous myenteric plexus layer between circular and longitudinal muscles (cutting angle 45°). B: Atrophic desmosis of the colon with atrophy of tendinous structures in muscularis propria (magnif. 180 x).

In summary Hirschsprung disease is diagnosed by the following characteristics:

1. Increase of AChE activity in parasympathetic nerve fibres of lamina propria mucosae and muscularis mucosae (Fig. 1, 2 and 11).

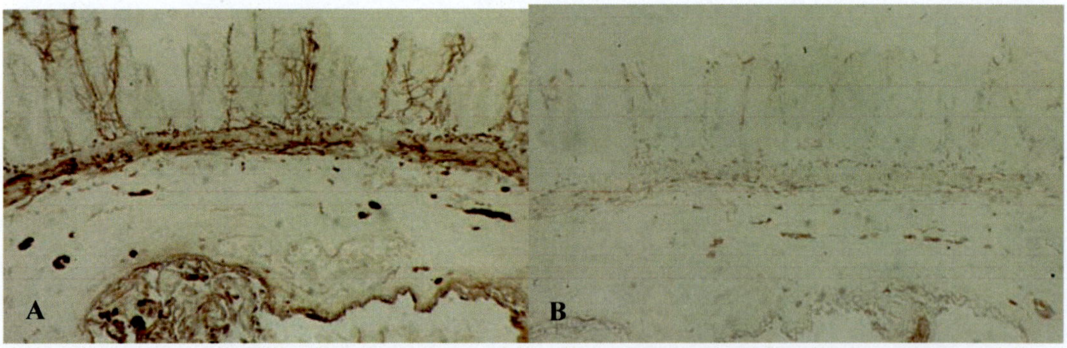

Figure 11. Comparison of a 4.5 μm thick cryostat section on a microscopic slide (A: cut as a 15 μm thick native cryostat section) with a 1.2 μm thick cryostat section (B: cut as a 4 μm native cryostat section) showing Hirschsprung's disease. A: AChE reaction of a 15 μm cryostat section with a final thickness of 4.5 μm. B: AChE reaction of a 4 μm thick cryostat section with a final thickness of 1.2 μm 60 x.

2. No nerve cells are observed in submucous and myenteric plexus in dehydrogenase reactions (Fig. 12).

For optimal evaluation of an AChE reaction, a section without counterstaining is mandatory (Fig. 1, 2, 6, 11 and 13). It is of advantage to stain always two sections for AChE: One section with hemalum counterstaining which allows an anatomical orientation (Fig. 6, 14 and 15) and the other section for the evaluation of the intensity of the AChE reaction in parasympathetic nerve fibres.

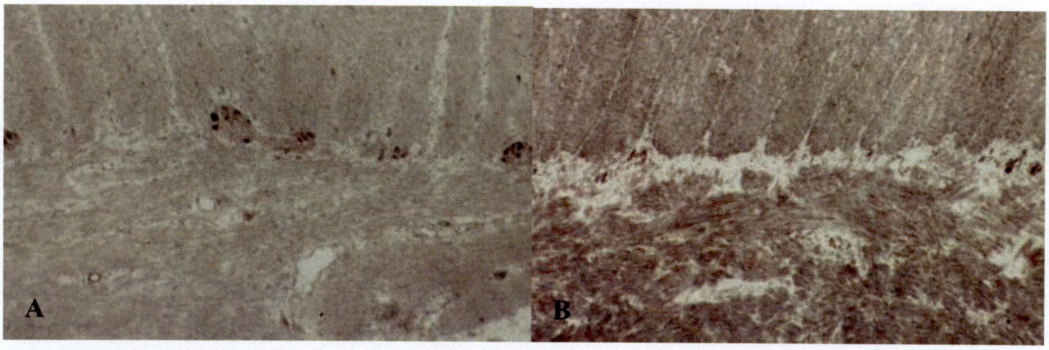

Figure 12. Dehydrogenase reaction to investigate myenteric plexus. A: Normal myenteric plexus. B: Aganglionosis of myenteric plexus (NADPH – Diaphorase, 8 min. Incubation; magnif. 180 x).

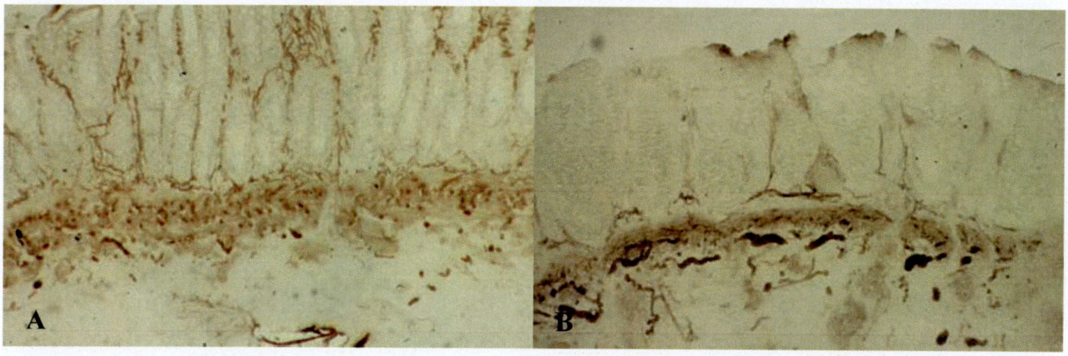

Figure 13. Ultrashort Hirschsprung's disease. A: Classical Hirschsprung's disease of a neonate (2 cm proximal dentate line). B: Ultrashort Hirschsprung's disease 2 cm proximal dentate line. Increase of AChE activity in muscularis mucosae and submucosa but not in nerve fibre nets in lamina propria mucosae (AChE reaction without counterstaining; magnif.120 x).

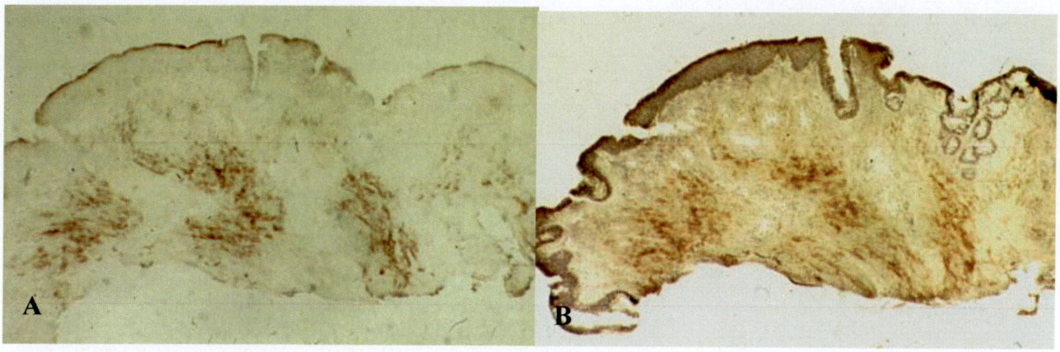

Figure 14. Aganglionosis of the anal ring. A: Musculus corrugator cutis ani with increased AChE activity in parasympathetic nerve fibres. B: Identical section with hemalum counterstaining (magnif. 120 x).

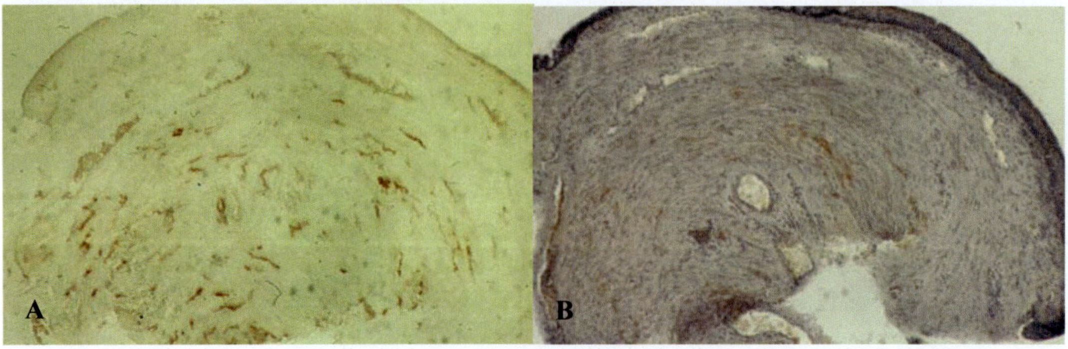

Figure 15. Normal musculus corrugator cutis ani in the dentate line A: AChE staining of musculus corrugator. B: Same section as left with hemalum counterstaining (magnif. 120 x).

Transitional Zone Examination of Pull Through Operations in Hirschsprung Disease

It is important to evaluate the quality of the myenteric plexus in seromuscular or full thickness biopsies of the proximal resection margin intraoperative in cryostat sections. To avoid a later revision of the one-stage pull-through operation, it is mandatory to identify a normal myenteric plexus [23,24] (compare Fig. 16). The intraoperative examination of the myenteric plexus with a NADPH-diaphorase reaction requires 5-7 minutes. This procedure is simple and reliable [25] (Fig. 7).

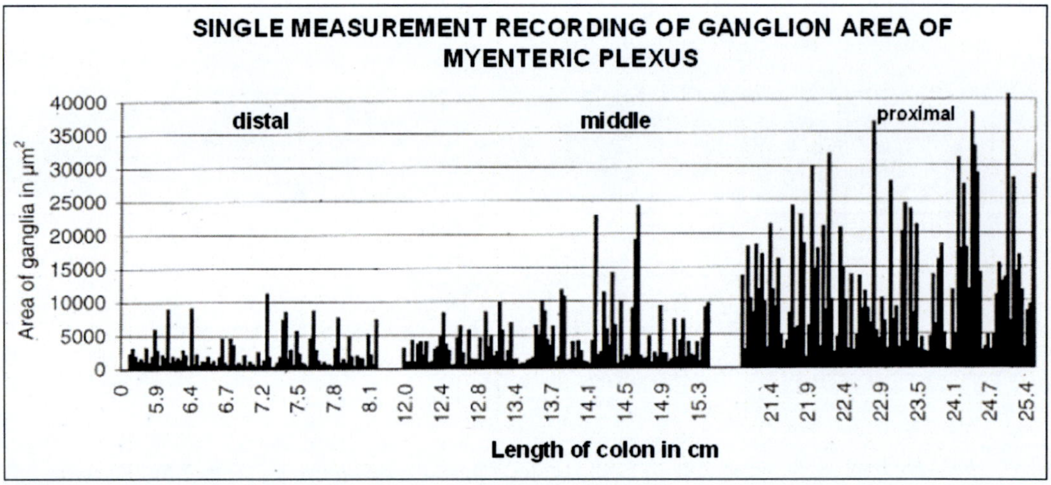

Figure 16. Morphometric data of ganglion area proximal an aganglionic segment (left) of Hirschsprung's disease. Data demonstrate a normal aspect of myenteric plexus 20 cm proximal to aganglionosis (Semiautomatic, computer operated measurement of a lactic dehydrogenasa reaction).

In this way it is possible to avoid an AChE reaction, which is caudo – cranial decreasing in the distal colon. An immaturity of the enteric nervous system is often accompanied by an increased AChE activity and may be misleading without an additional succinic dehydrogenase reaction and nitroxid synthase reaction [30].

The AChE reaction, however, provides further information to the experienced pathologist about the parasympathetic tonus of circular muscles (Fig. 8). Low AChE activity in nerve fibres of circular muscles, despite presence of nerve cells between circular and longitudinal muscles, is a clear indication that motility of this part of the colon is disturbed (Fig. 8B). Hypoplastic hypoganglionosis proximal of distal aganglionic colon shows nearly a 50% decrease of ganglion size and nerve cell number in the myenteric plexus. Ganglion distances have increased (about 30%) (Fig. 9).

The hypoganglionic part proximal of an aganglionosis can have a length of 3-5cm (Fig. 16) and in rare cases even 30 cm [21]. The pathologist needs some experience for a visual evaluation but this cannot be the reason to renunciate an intraoperative examination of the resection margin of a pull – through operation [24,26,27]. To overcome this problem, it is helpful to take laparoscopic assisted seromuscular biopsies from sigma, descending and transversal colon for an enzyme histochemical examination of the myenteric plexus before the resection.

The advantage to use an enzyme histochemical procedure is the possibility for a reliable evaluation of the function of the particular colon region. This is not possible in a hemalum eosin staining or an immunhistochemical reaction.

The enzyme histochemical staining of intraoperative biopsies gives the pathologist the possibility to inform the surgeon in 6 to 10 minutes about the innervation of the proximal resection margin of the colon. The use of a rapid AChE staining, introduced by Kobayashi et al. in 1994 [40,41] is not very helpful in examining the proximal resection line because of the caudo – cranial decline of parasympathetic nerve fibre density in circular muscles (Fig. 3, 4 and 5). In addition the increase in AChE in immaturity of the enteric nervous system is a risk for a false positive Hirschsprung diagnosis. A NADPH reaction which stains electively nerve cells and ganglia of the myenteric plexus is much more informative (Fig. 7 and 12).

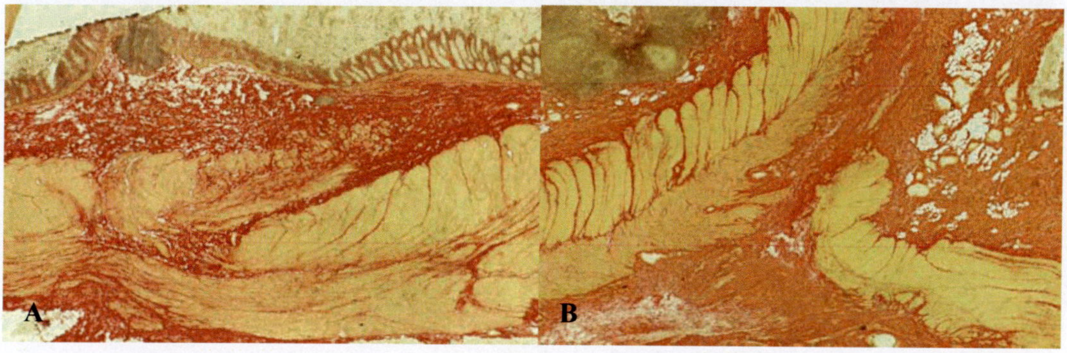

Figure 17. Anastomosis of distal and proximal colon after resecting an aganglionic segment. A: Regular end-to-end anastomosis. B: Stenosis of an atypical end–to–end anastomosis (Picro- Siriusred staining; magnif. 40 x).

We have examined in a series of more than 100 Hirschsprung patients [27] the postoperative course and observed that mainly hypoganglionosis in the proximal colon segment was the reason of a postoperative recurrence of chronic constipation. Independent from this study, we observed in patients with a scar stenosis an atypical anastomosis in which submucosa was not properly connected (Fig. 17B). The missing connection of submucous plexus disrupts peristalsis in the anastomosis which is preserved in a normal connection of proximal and distal submucous plexus (Fig. 17A).

We do not agree with Bax [37] that Hirschsprung disease is always incurable. The main reason of a postoperative obstruction in Hirschspung surgery is a missing orientation about the innervation of the proximal margin of the resection [27].

Ultrashort Hirschsprung Disease

Ultrashort Hirschsprung disease (UHD) is rare. Just 5-10% of Hirschsprung patients show an ultrashort aganglionic segment. UHD is defined to have an extension of 3 – 4 cm of the distal rectum [28]. In some cases UHD is limited to the anal ring or just the musculus corrugator cutis ani. UHD shows clinically an outlet obstruction.

In contrast to classical Hirschsprung disease (Fig. 14A) nets of parasympathetic nerve fibres with increased AChE in lamina propria mucosae are absent (fig 14 B). Nerve fibres with increased AChE are observed in muscularis mucosae and submucosa (Fig. 14A). This diagnosis can be difficult if the extramural parasympathetic innervation is hypoplastic (Fig. 18).

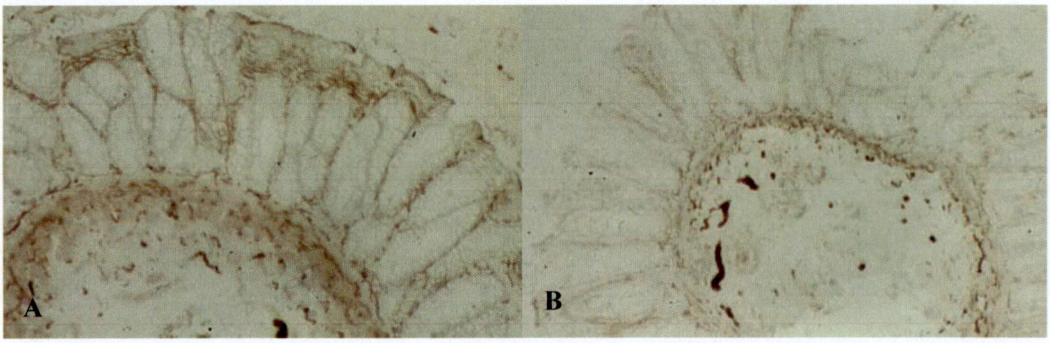

Figure 18. Ultrashort Hirschsprung's disease with hypoplastic parasympathetic innervation. A: Classical Hirschsprung (neonate, 3cm prox. dentate line; magnif. 120 x).B: Hypoplastic ultrashort Hirschsprung's disease (3cm prox. dentate line; magnify. 120 x).

If the aganglionosis is limited to the anal ring, the increase of AChE in nerve fibres is sometimes limited to the musculus corrugator cutis ani (Fig. 15). The diagnosis of UHD requires a biopsy of the recto – anal transitional zone with sufficient submucosa (Fig. 13).

UHD can exclusively be diagnosed in an AChE reaction, because nerve cells or ganglia are rare in the supra-anal rectum mucosa. With an AChE reaction the characteristic picture of UHD (Fig. 13) is quite obvious [29,30]. It is important to be aware that the diagnosis of UHD requires a sufficient amount of muscularis mucosae and submucosa. The biopsy may be taken with advantage by forceps and scissors.

The controversal opinions in literature about the existence of UHD are due to the fact that in paraffin sections with a hemalum - eosin staining a clear diagnosis is not possible

[31,33]. On the other hand the low nerve cell number in the supraanal rectum is not an appropriate parameter to reliably diagnose UHD.

It should be stressed that not only distal colon but also the internal sphincter contains nerve cells which can be simply identified in native frozen sections with a dehydrogenase reaction.

Zonal Aganglionosis

For embryonic reasons, zonal aganglionosis does not really exist. On the one hand nerve cells of myenteric plexus are resistant to hypoxia and inflammation. On the other, hypoganglionic segments are sometimes accompanied by wide intervals between ganglia of myenteric plexus (Fig. 9 and 12). This kind of anomaly requires serial sections with enzyme histochemical staining of ganglia or nerve cells.

In rare cases with total aganglionosis of the colon are sometimes small segments observed with normal innervation. In the recent 40 years we observed two such cases. A precondition is however, that the resected colon is coiled in its total length [30]. The term "Zonal aganglionosis" is in theses cases misleading. The expression "Focal ganglionic segment in aganglionosis" would be much more appropriate [34-36]. It is conceivable, that a few neuroblasts were transgressing into the aganglionic colon and develop a focal normal looking myenteric plexus. This anomaly is, however, without any functional consequence.

At this point, it may be mentioned that the progressive oligoneuronal hypoganglionosis develops time dependently an atrophy of ganglia which starts in the rectum and proceeds in cranial direction. These rare patients show a complete atrophy of the myenteric plexus at an age of 12 – 20 years. This disease is from a clinical point of view accompanied by an aperistaltic syndrome. It is hypothesized that the aetiology of this particular disease is caused by a lack of glia derived factors (GDF). GDF promotes the survival of the myenteric plexus.

Artefacts and Pitfalls in Enzyme Histochemical Hirschsprung Diagnosis

One of the most frequent reasons for unsatisfactory results in enzyme histochemistry is caused by cryostat sections which do not have the necessary thickness. It is important to be aware that a cryostat section loses 70% of its thickness by thawing, spreading and drying onto a microscopic slide. That means that a 15 μm thick native cryostat section has a final thickness of 4-5 μm on the microscopic slide [5]. A native cryostat section with thickness of 4 μm shows unsatisfactory results. The final thickness of this section will be just 1.2 μm (Fig. 11B).

In addition, a marked deviation from the enzyme histochemical techniques[38] e.g. more than 8-10 minutes incubation of dehydrogenases, missing iso OMPA (Sigma Ltd) for the inhibition of unspecific esterases, deviation from the recommended pH, incubation at room temperature etc. may cause unsatisfactory results. The diagnosis of HD is based on the brown staining of parasympathetic nerve fibres (Fig. 1, 13, 18 and 19).

A diffuse brown, cloudy staining in lamina propria mucosae is the result of a bleeding artefact from taking the biopsy (Fig. 19A). Even a diffuse brown coloration of muscularis mucosae and lymph nodes in the mucosa is unspecific. A lympho follicular hyperplasia may cover the characteristics of HD by a displacement of muscularis mucosae und lamina propria mucosae.

For embryological reasons, the enzyme histochemical characteristics of Hirschsprung disease are observed only in biopsies of the rectum or the distal colon (Fig. 3, 4 and 5). In total aganglionosis of the colon parasympathetic nerve fibres with increased AChE activity in mucosa and lamina propria are absent in transversal and ascending colon.

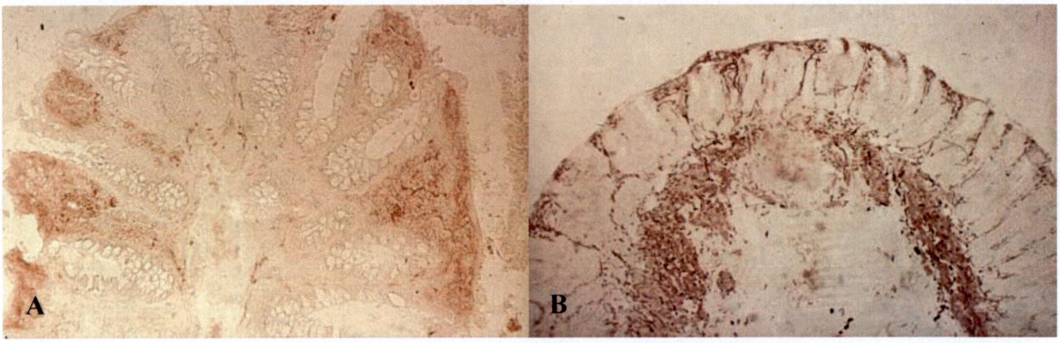

Figure 19. Bleeding artefact in lamina propria mucosae (A) of a normal innervated rectum mucosa. The artefact shows a diffuse amorphous brown staining of lamina propria mucosae. Compare rectum mucosa with classical Hirschsprung's disease (B) with an elective staining of parasympathetic nerve fibres in lamina propria mucosae and muscularis mucosae (AChE reaction without counterstaining; magnify. 70 x).

To exclude an UHD in the anal ring, it is recommended to take the first biopsy from the recto – anal ring and further biopsies 1cm, 2cm, 4cm and 8cm proximal the recto – anal ring. Full thickness biopsies from the rectal wall are not necessary for diagnosis of Hirschsprung disease. A primary laparoscopic assisted seromuscular biopsy from the sigma only has the risk that an aganglionosis in the distal rectum is missed [28,39]. A seromuscular biopsy from the sigma, however, has the advantage that a hypoganglionosis or hypoplasia of the myenteric plexus can be recognized (compare Fig. 7).

Summary

An acetylcholinesterase reaction on native cryostat sections is the gold standard for a reliable diagnosis of Hirschsprung disease. The advantage of this technique is the use of mucosa suction biopsies which can be performed without an anaesthesia of the neonate.

Ultrashort Hirschsprung disease has an extension of 1 – 4 cm above the pectinate line. To avoid overlooking a diagnosis of aganglionosis of the anal ring, the first biopsy may be taken from the recto – anal transitional zone. Ultrashort Hirschsprung disease shows parasympathetic nerve fibres only in muscularis mucosae and submucosa but – in contrast to classical Hirschsprung disease – no parasympathetic nerve fibres in lamina propria mucosae. Diagnosis can be made exclusively by an acetylcholinesterase reaction in native cryostat sections (15 μm). For a reliable diagnosis, a biopsy with muscularis mucosae and submucosa is necessary.

Total aganglionosis shows the characteristics of Hirschsprung disease in the mucosa of the distal colon, but no parasympathetic nerve structures can be observed in transversal and ascending colon. For embryological reasons the enzyme histochemical diagnosis of an aganglionosis is limited to the recto - sigmoid. One of the most frequent pitfalls in enzyme histochemistry is the use of 4 μm instead of 15 μm thick cryostat sections, because the cryostat sections loose 70% of its thickness by thawing, spreading and drying on a microscopic slide. Enzyme histochemistry allows insights into the pathophysiology of motility disorders of the intestinal tract.

References

[1] Meier-Ruge W: Zur Pathologie und bioptischen Diagnostik des Morbus Hirschsprung in Relation zum Megacolon acquisitum und funktionale. *Verh Dtsch Ges Pathol* 1967; 51: 323-8.

[2] Meier-Ruge W: Das Megacolon. Seine Diagnose und Pathophysiologie. *Virchows Arch* Abt A, Path Anat 1968; 344: 67-85.

[3] Meier-Ruge W, Lutterbeck PM, Herzog B, Morger R, Moser R, Schärli A: Acetylcholinesterase activity in suction biopsies of the rectum in the diagnosis of Hirschsprung's disease. *J Pediatr Surg* 1972; 7: 11-7.

[4] .Karnovsky MJ, Roots L: A "direct – colouring" thiocholine method for cholinesterase. *J Histochem Cytochem* 1964; 12: 219 –21.

[5] Meier-Ruge W, Bruder L: Preparation of cryostat sections from biopsies and colorectal specimen. *Pathobiology* 2005; 72: 93-4.

[6] Meier-Ruge W: Hirschsprung's disease: its aetiology, pathogenesis and differential diagnosis. *Curr Top Pathol* 1974; 59: 131 –79.

[7] Andrassy RJ, Isaacs H, Weitzman JJ: Rectal suction biopsy for the diagnosis of Hirschsprung's disease. *Ann Surg* 1981; 193: 419 –23.

[8] Nakao M, Suita S, Taguchi T, Hirose R, Shima Y: Fouteen-year experience of acetylcholinesterase staining for rectal mucosal biopsy in neonatal Hirschsprung's disease. *J Pediatr Surg* 2001; 36: 1357 – 63.

[9] Tomita R, Munakata K, Howard ER, Fujisaki S: Histological studies on Hirschsprung's disease and its allied disorders in childhood. *Hepatogastroenterology* 2004; 51: 1042 – 44

[10] De Lorijn F, Reitsma JB, Voskuijl WP, Aronson DC, Ten Kate FJ, Smets AM et al.: Diagnosis of Hirschsprung's disease: a prospective, comparative accuracy study of common tests. *J Pediatr* 2005; 146: 787-92.

[11] Meier-Ruge W, Bruder E: Characteristics of Hirschsprung's disease. *Pathobiology* 2005; 72: 10 –23.

[12] Pini-Prato A, Martucciello G, Jasonni V: Rectal suction biopsy in the diagnosis: 5 - year experience with Solo – RBT in 389 patients. *J Pediatr Surg* 2006; 41: 1043 –8.

[13] Goto S, Ikeda K, Toyohara T: Histochemical confirmation of the acetylcholinesterase – activity in rectal suction biopsy from neonates with Hirschsprung's disease. *Z Kinderchir* 1984; 39: 246-9.

[14] de Brito IA, Maksoud JG: Evolution with age of the acetylcholinesterase activity in rectal suction biopsy in Hirschsprung's disease. *J Pediatr Surg* 1987; 22: 425-30.

[15] Park WH, Choi SO, Kwon KY, Chang ES: Acetylcholinesterase histochemistry in rectal suction biopsies in the diagnosis of Hirschsprung's disease. *J Korean Med Sci* 1992; 7: 353-9.

[16] Croffie JM, Davis MM, Faught PR, Corkins MR, Gupta SK, Pfefferkorn MD et al: At what age is a suction rectal biopsy less likely to provide adequate tissue for identification of ganglion cells? *J Pediatr Gastroenterol Nutr* 2007; 44: 198 –202.

[17] Meier-Ruge W: The pathophysiology of aganglionosis of the entire colon (Zuelzer – Wilson Syndrome). Morphometric investigation of the extent of sacral parasympathetic innervation of circular muscles of the aganglionic colon. *Beitr Pathol* 1972; 147: 228 – 36.

[18] Munakata K, Okabe I, Morita K: Histologic studies of rectocolic aganglionosis and allied disorders. *J Pediatr Surg* 1978; 13: 67 –75.

[19] Keshtgar AS, Ward HC, Clayden GS, de Sousa NM: Investigations for incontinence and constipation after surgery for Hirschsprung's disease in children. *Pediatr Surg Int* 2003; 19: 4 – 8.

[20] Meier-Ruge W, Bruder E: Disturbed peristalsis of the gut.- Immaturity of the enteric nervous system. *Pathobiology* 2005; 72: 34-6.

[21] Meier-Ruge W, Bruder E: Aplastic neuronal dysganglionosis and hypoganglionic changes of the enteric nervous system. *Pathobiology* 2005; 72: 37-41.

[22] Meier-Ruge W, Bruder E: Aplastic desmosis of the gut (Aperistaltic Sydrome, Microcolon Megacystis Syndrome) and atrophic desmosis. *Pathobiology* 2005; 72: 42 – 7.

[23] Farrugia MK, Alexander N, Clarke S, Nash R, Nicholls EA, Holmes K: Does transitional zone pull-through in Hirschsprung's disease imply a poor prognosis? *J Pediatr Surg* 2003; 38: 1766 –69.

[24] Shayan K, Smith C, Langer JC: Reliability of intraoperative frozen sections in the management of Hirschsprung's disease. *J Pediatr Surg* 2004; 39: 1345 – 8.

[25] Kobayashi H, Hirakawa H, Puri P: NADPH – diaphorase histochemistry a reliable test for the intraoperative diagnosis of Hirschsprung's disease. *J Pediatr Surg* 1996; 31: 1552-3.

[26] Maia DM: The reliability of frozen – section diagnosis in the pathologic evaluation of Hirschsprung's disease. *Am J Surg Pathol* 2000; 24: 1675 –7.

[27] Schulten D, Holschneider AM, Meier-Ruge W: Proximal segment histology of resected bowel in Hirschsprung's disease predicts postoperative bowel function. *Eur J Pediatr Surg* 2000; 10: 378 – 81.

[28] Meier-Ruge W, Schärli AF: The epidemiology and enzyme histochemical characterization of ultrashort – segment Hirschsprung's disease. *Pediatr Surg Int* 1986; 1: 37 – 42.

[29] Meier-Ruge W: Histological diagnosis and differential diagnosis of Hirschsprung's disease. In: Holschneider AM, Puri P (eds.). *Hirschsprung's Disease and Allied Disorders.* Second Edition. Amsterdan: Overseas Publ Assoc, Harwood Academic Publishers; 2000.p.252-65.

[30] Meier-Ruge W, Bruder E: Pathology of chronic constipation in pediatric and adult coloproctology. *Pathobiology* 2005; 72: 1 –102.

[31] 31.Neilson IR, Yazbeck S: Ultrashort Hirschsprung's disease: myth or reality. *J Pediatr Surg* 1990; 25: 1135 –8.

[32] Ballard ET: Ultrashort segment of Hirschsprung's disease: a case report. *Pediatr Pathol Lab Med* 1996; 16: 319 –25

[33] Holschneider AM: Anal sphincter achalasia and ultrashort Hirschsprung's disease. In: Holschneider AM, Puri P (eds): *Hirschsprung's Disease and Allied Disorders*. Second Edition. Amsterdan: Overseas Publ Assoc, Harwood Academic Publishers; 2000.p.394-424.

[34] Yunis E,.Sieber WK, Akers DR: Does zonal aganglionosis really exist? Report of a rare variety of Hirschsprung's disease and review of the literature. *Pediatr Pathol* 1983; 1:33-49.

[35] Fu CG, Muto T, Masaki T, Nagawa H: Zonal adult Hirschsprung's disease. *Gut* 1996; 39: 765-7.

[36] Seldenrijk CA, van der Harten HJ, Klück P, Tibboel D, Moorman – Voestermans K, Meijer CJ: Zonal aganglionosis. An enzyme- and immuno – histochemical study of two cases. *Virchows Arch Abt A; Pathol Anat Histopathol* 1986; 410: 75 – 81.

[37] Bax KA: Duhamel lecture: The incurability of Hirschsprung's disease. *Eur J Pediatr Surg* 2006; 16: 380 –4.

[38] Meier-Ruge W, Bruder E: Preparation of incubation media for the daily routine of enzyme histochemical reaction. *Pathobiology* 2005; 72: 95 – 9.

[39] Moore BG, Sigaram C, Eckhoff DE, Gaumnitz EA, Starling JR: Immunohistochemical evaluation of ultrashort – segment Hirschsprung's disease. Report of three cases. *Dis colon Rectum* 1996; 39: 817 – 22.

[40] Kobayashi H, O'Briain DS, Hirakawa H, Wang Y, Puri P: A rapid technique of acetylcholinesterase staining. *Arch Path Lab Med* 1994; 118: 1127 – 9.

[41] Martucciello G, Favre A, Torre M, Pini Prato A, Jasonni V: A new acetylcholinesterase histochemical method for the intraoperative diagnosis of Hirschsprung's disease and intestinal neuronal dysplasia. *Eur J Pediatr Surg* 2001; 11: 300 –4.

Part II: Hirschsprung's Disease: Clinical Features, Manometric Diagnosis, Radiological Diagnosis, Morphological Diagnosis, Differential Diagnosis, Medical Care, Enterostomies, And Bowel Preparation For Pull-Through

In: Hirschsprung's Disease: Diagnosis and Treatment
Ed: Ramón Núñez and Manuel López-Alonso
ISBN: 978-1-60741-349-3

Chapter VIII

Hirschsprung's Disease: Clinical Features

Ramón Núñez, Emilio Blesa and Rodolfo Cabrera

Introduction

The clinical symptoms of Hirschsprung's disease (HD) – delayed passage of meconium, constipation, or intestinal obstruction – are secondary to the lack of peristaltic activity in the aganglionic segment and its state of contraction, and to the absence of internal anal sphincter relaxation during defæcation [1,2]. Typically, the severity of the clinical manifestations correlates with the length of the aganglionic segment, i.e., shorter extension of the disease, less clinical severity [3]. Nevertheless, in some patients there has been observed a discrepancy between the length of aganglionic segment and the degree of bowel obstruction [2]. Some authors [2,4,5] have attributed this lack of correlation to dysmotility of the bowel proximal to the aganglionic segment due to neuronal intestinal dysplasia (NID) associated with HD. Abnormal function of the proximal intestine would be one of the causes of the obstructive symptoms and episodes of enterocolitis that some patients present after the definitive surgery [2,6-9].

The clinical picture of HD depends on whether or not the disease manifests itself within the neonatal period [1,10]. Typically, a neonate with HD is born at term, and presents delayed meconium evacuation, abdominal distension, and vomiting. In most cases, medical care resolves the distal intestinal obstruction, but sometimes an intestinal derivation is required to relieve the compression [10-11]. Enterocolitis can be the first clinical manifestation of HD in the newborn [1,12]. This is the complication of greatest morbidity and mortality in HD [1,13]. To avoid it, early diagnosis is essential in the first days of life [14].

In some patients, HD presents no symptoms in the neonatal period, but is manifest later with severe constipation that resists treatment, with fæcaloma accumulation, abdominal distension, and failure to thrive [10].

Chromosomal abnormalities are associated with HD in 12% of cases, and other congenital malformations in 18% [15]. Therefore, in patients (newborn or other ages) with dysmorphic features or some other congenital malformation and a clinical pattern suggestive of HD, it is mandatory to exclude the possibility of this disease (see Chapters 5 and 6) [15]. Given the familial incidence of HD, especially of long segment aganglionosis, the family history of the disease must always be investigated [16]. Some authors [17,18] have mentioned the usefulness of prenatal ultrasound for the early suspicion of the disease, especially in extensive aganglionosis with intestinal distension. For others, however, this test is of limited value for the prenatal diagnosis or exclusion of HD [19].

Clinical Presentation in the Newborn

Some 80–90% of all patients with HD have symptoms typical of the disease in the first days of life [1,10,12]. Improved knowledge of the clinical manifestations of this disease in the newborn has led to most patients today being diagnosed in the neonatal period. Thus, in the survey of Singh et al. [12] of 114 cases of neonatal HD, 90.5% were diagnosed in the neonatal period, and their clinical presentation was characterized by abdominal distension (76% of patients), vomiting (69%), and delayed meconium (57%). Other authors [1,10], as also is our experience [20], have observed meconium delay of >24 hours in more than 90% of infants with HD. Indeed, according to Guo et al. [21], delay in passing meconium is a clinical sign of great sensitivity, specificity, and predictive value for the early suspicion of the disease (see Table 1). The statistics presented in Table 1 suggest that a history of delayed meconium passage in combination with any other clinical presentation should alert to the possibility of HD [21].

Table 1. Sensitivity, specificity, and predictive value of clinical features of Hirschsprung's disease in the neonatal period. Adapted from Guo et al. [21].

	Sensitivity %	Specificity %	Predictive value
Delayed meconium	83	88	0.77
Vomiting	77	38	0.30
Abdominal distension	83	33	0.26
Diarrhoea	86	13	0.11
Intestinal obstruction	80	18	0.14
Tight anus*	91	67	0.68

*Tight anus was considered as an impacted or resistant feeling when the little finger was inserted in the rectum.

Rectal examination of the newborn with HD (which must be done with the little finger) may show a tight anus [21], although this finding has also been described as unreliable [22]. Sometimes, when the examining finger is withdrawn, there is an explosive release of flatus and stools. This is typical of HD, and is accompanied by the decrease or disappearance of the abdominal distension.

The following paragraphs describe the most typical forms of clinical presentation of HD in the neonate.

Delay in Passing Meconium

In some 95% of healthy full-term infants, the first passage of meconium occurs within 24 hours of life, and in 99% within the first 48 hours [1,23,24]. In contrast, less than 10% of children with HD pass meconium within 24 hours [1,22].

Nevertheless, only 66% of the pre-term (<32 weeks gestation) or low birth weight (<2500 g) neonates pass meconium in the first 48 hours of life [1]. In pre-term neonates, maturation of intestinal motor function is delayed, with the consequent delay in evacuating meconium [1,23]. Kenny et al. [25] suggest that the particular cause may be a delay in the maturation of the interstitial cells of Cajal. Moreover, the chemical composition of the meconium (glycoprotein, saccharides, calcium, copper, iron, and phosphorus) in the pre-term neonate makes it more viscous, complicating its evacuation. In premature neonates, HD is rare. The frequency is about 7% of all newborn with HD [1,10]. In the first instance, a "wait and see" policy is often used in these infants. In those infants who do not develop a normal defæcation pattern in the following weeks, HD needs to be excluded [1].

Faced with a full-term neonate with a delay of >24 hours in passing meconium, one must suspect intestinal obstruction, with one of the possible causes being HD. This disease accounts for only 20-25% of cases of neonatal intestinal obstruction [26], so that, in addition to HD, one has to consider other causes of the delay in meconium passage, as reflected in Table 2.

Table 2. The conditions that may be associated with failure to pass meconium in the Newborn. Adapted from Lœning-Bauke et al [24].

The conditions	Prevalence (incidence per total births)	Abnormal findings
Meconium plug syndrome	1/500 to 1/1000 [27]	Meconium plugs
Small left colon syndrome	Rare	Transition zone * at splenic flexure
Anorectal malformation	1/2000 to 1/5000 [28]	Absent anus or anal fistula
Meconium ileus	1/2800 [29]	Abdominal distension at birth, cystic fibrosis
Hirschsprung's disease	1/5000 [1]	Tight anus, empty rectum, transition zone *
Hypoganglionosis	Rare	Transition zone*
Neuronal intestinal dysplasia	Rare	Megacolon, transition zone* abnormal ganglion cells
Megacysts-microcolon-intestinal Hypoperistalsis syndrome	Very rare	Microcolon, megacystis

*Transition zone (from small- to large-diameter bowel) refers to radiographic visualization on contrast study

In our experience [20] and that of other authors [21,30], anorectal manometry carried out on all infants who present delayed passage of meconium of more than 24 hours helps to select those lacking the recto-anal inhibitory reflex (RAIR), i.e., with suspected HD. Rectal suction biopsy confirms or excludes the aganglionosis [31]. The absence of RAIR in the newborn may also be due to NID [32] or to a transient functional obstruction of the colon (small left colon) [20]. In the latter case, an enema with gastrografin is of diagnostic and therapeutic value [20,24].

A meconium plug is the commonest and most benign cause (see table 2) of meconial delay [27]. Nonetheless, it has been reported that between 13% and 38% of cases of meconium plug are associated with HD (see table 3). In most neonates, rectal stimulation (with the finger or with a thermometer) or a saline enema will provoke passage of the meconium and normalize intestinal transit [24]. If subsequently in the newborn defæcation disorders persist, HD needs to be monitored and excluded [36].

Table 3. Association of meconium plug syndrome (MPS) with Hirschsprung's disease.

Series	No. of patients with MPS	Hirschsprung's disease (%)
Ellis et al. [33]	30	13.3
Van Leeuwen et al. [34]	8	25.0
Burge et al. [35]	21	38.1
Keckler et al [36]	77	13.0

Enterocolitis

Enterocolitis (diarrhœa, abdominal distension, vomiting, fever) is one of the forms of clinical presentation of HD in the newborn (see Chapter 22) [12,37]. It can be manifest exclusively as diarrhœa without prior vomiting or abdominal distension [1]. While the incidence of enterocolitis in infants with HD has fallen dramatically in recent decades [34], recent work [12,37] still reflects a frequency of 9%. Given the seriousness of this complication, the neonate with enterocolitis requires early treatment with IV antibiotics, correction of the electrolyte alterations, and the implementation of measures for intestinal decompression (colon irrigation with isotonic saline solution) [1,13,14,38]. Lack of improvement or worsening of the clinical parameters mandates an immediate laparotomy and the formation of a stoma (colostomy or ileostomy) proximal to the transition zone, and intestinal biopsies [39].

In a recent review, Haricharan et al. [40] report that children whose HD was diagnosed in the first days of life have a greater risk of postoperative enterocolitis than those in whom diagnosis of the aganglionosis was later.

Intestinal Obstruction

The severest form of HD (long segment HD, total colonic aganglionosis, (Fig. 1) is the commonest cause of low intestinal obstruction in the newborn [41,42]. The patient is usually a full-term neonate of normal birth weight, with delay in the passage of meconium, abdominal distension, and vomiting (alimentary or bile-stained). Rectal digital examination reveals a small, empty rectum which snugs itself around the examining finger. The frequent explosive passage of flatus and meconium or fæces when the examining finger is withdrawn from the rectum is a useful sign in pointing to the diagnosis [41].

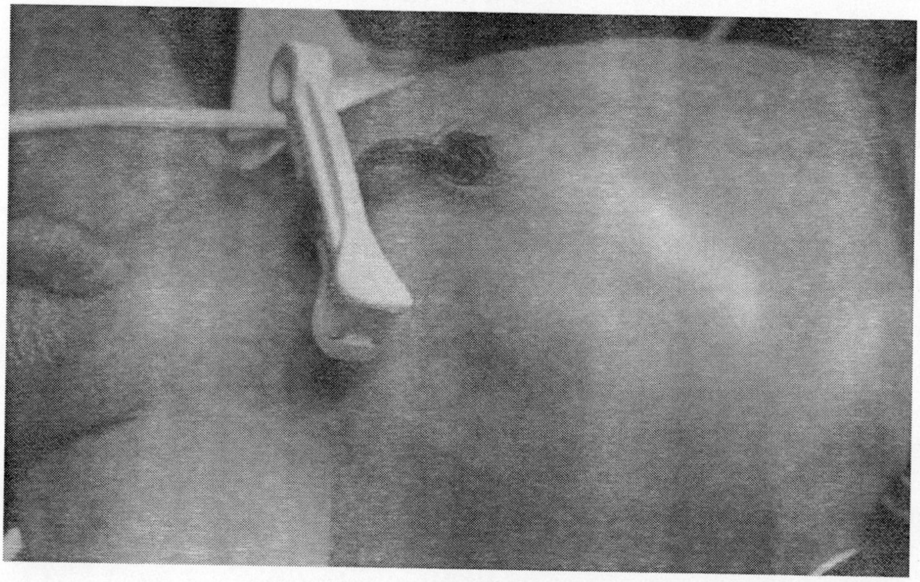

Figure 1. Newborn of 48 hours with total colonic aganglionosis and intestinal obstruction (visualization of bowel loops).

Rectal stimulation and rectal irrigation with normal saline empties the colon of meconium and can release the clinical pattern of distal intestinal obstruction [10]. If a first rectal irrigation does not relieve the patient of sufficient flatus and fæces it has to be repeated. If the rectal wash-out fails to relieve intestinal obstruction, a colostomy, or an ileostomy in the case of total colonic aganglionosis, must be done [11,12,43].

Differential diagnosis of HD includes meconium ileus, ileal atresia, colonic atresia, meconium plug syndrome, and small left colon syndrome (see Chapter 12). A properly performed contrast enema study can usually differentiate among these as HD shows the transition zone between dilated proximal normal bowel and the aganglionic spastic segment.

Patients with HD symptomatic enough to require hospitalization during the first three months of life exhibit more severe and non-specific symptoms of partial intestinal obstruction. This is an important element in prognosis, since almost all deaths from this disease occur during the first few months of life [43].

Pneumoperitoneum/Intestinal Perforation

Pneumoperitoneum / intestinal perforation is one of the clinical manifestations of HD in the neonate. The mechanism of perforation appears to be directly related to increased intraluminal pressure from distal obstruction. Rarely, patients with HD have a sufficiently high grade obstruction to perforate the bowel somewhere within the megacolon proximal to the transition zone. This catastrophic complication is likewise limited almost exclusively to the neonatal period of life [43]. In a literature survey of patients with HD presenting with perforation, in 47 patients (only one patient was older than 2 months at initial presentation) the site of perforation (see table 4) was in the proximal colon (68%), appendix (18%), or distal small bowel (6%), with 61% of patients having long segment or total colonic aganglionosis. Appendiceal and ileal perforation were particularly associated with long segment disease [42]. Aganglionosis is the commonest cause of large bowel obstruction in the young infant, and therefore colonic or appendiceal perforation in these patients should raise the suspicion of HD [42-48]. Once the diagnosis of pneumoperitoneum / intestinal perforation is made, surgical treatment is mandatory. To exteriorize the perforated bowel is the preferred treatment.

Most patients with total colonic aganglionosis have perforation in their colon rather than in the terminal ileum proximal to aganglionic bowel [41]. Perforation in these cases is in aganglionic bowel, and the appropriate treatment is an ileostomy. Differential diagnosis of distal small- or large-bowel perforation includes necrotizing enterocolitis and the other causes of distal bowel obstruction [43,45].

Table 4. Patients with Hirschsprung's disease presenting with bowel perforation [42]

Site of perforation	No. of patients	TCH	Proximal	Distal	Unknown
Colon					
Cæcum or AC	32 (68)	12	7	13	0
Splenic flexure	2 (4)	0	0	1	1
Sigmoid colon	2 (4)	0	0	2	0
Appendix	8 (18)	4	3	0	1
Terminal ileum	3 (6)	3	0	0	0
Total	47* (100)	19 (40)	10 (21)	16 (34)	2 (4)

Note. Distal = site of transition between rectum and splenic flexure; Proximal = site of transition proximal to the splenic flexure; TCH = total colonic Hirschsprung's disease. Numbers in parentheses are percentages. AC = ascending colon. * In 46 patients the age ranged from 1 day to 8 weeks, and 1 patient was 4 months old.

Clinical Presentation After the Neonatal Period

The low frequency with which HD is diagnosed after the neonatal period means that we have to be more demanding in our knowledge of its clinical manifestations in order for the delay in diagnosis to be as short as possible. The situation has gone from diagnosing more

HD cases in children older than 5 years than in those of less than 1 month [49-51] to one in which diagnosis of the disease after the neonatal period is now rare, close to 10%, and almost exceptional after infancy [18,52,53]. Nonetheless, these exceptions still arise in isolated cases in older children, and even in adolescents and adults [54]. Logically, the average age at diagnosis of HD has declined to about 3 months in age, with the vast majority of patients in the neonatal period or close to it [52,55,56].

The clinical presentation of most patients diagnosed with HD after the neonate period is similar to the neonate case, but always with the symptoms secondary to the difficulty in eliminating fæces. The commonest is constipation, often accompanied by abdominal distension, crises of intestinal obstruction, recurrent abdominal pain, and vomiting. Also diarrhœa from enterocolitis, as described in the newborn, may result from the fæcal retention. The possibility of chronic malnutrition in children with HD diagnosed after the neonate period is cited by virtually all publications referring to the disease's clinical manifestations [10].

The symptoms referred to may present in patients with constipation secondary to other causes [1], but HD in this age group is usually distinguishable from those other causes in the form set out in Table 5.

Table 5. Frequency of presentation of clinical peculiarities of constipation of different causes as against being secondary to Hirschsprung's disease.

Clinical peculiarities	Constipation	Hirschsprung's disease
Abdominal distension	Rare	Frequent
Intestinal obstruction crises	Rare	Occasional
Delayed growth	Rare	Occasional
Recurrent abdominal pain	Occasional	Frequent
Repeated enterocolitis	Rare	Frequent
Encopresis	Frequent	Rare
Delayed meconium passage	Rare	Frequent
Rectorrhagia	Occasional	Rare
Voluntary fæcal retention	Frequent	Rare
Fæcal volume	Large	Normal
Palpable fæcalomas	Frequent	Rare
Fæces in rectum	Frequent	Rare
Rectal ampulla configuration	Normal	Narrow
Anal fissures	Rare	Frequent

Undoubtedly, the fundamental symptom is constipation, present in the vast majority of patients diagnosed with HD after the neonatal period, and more so the older the patient [51,53,57]. HD has been diagnosed in 14% of patients undergoing rectal biopsies for constipation of unknown cause, and the authors of that study recommend considering the existence of HD in any child of any age with severe constipation, although they believe it unlikely if the onset was post-neonatal [53]. Other authors report HD in 17% of children with constipation, as detected by anorectal manometry and rectal biopsy [51]. They consider HD to be more likely if the constipation started before one year of age, and that most diagnoses correspond to ultrashort aganglionic segments. In an ample series published on ultrashort segments, it was emphasized that the typical onset of constipation was during the second semester of life, compared with an earlier onset, during the first weeks or after weaning, in patients with longer aganglionic segments [58]. In patients in whom constipation began later, that the incidence of HD is very low or null has been described as seeming to advise against resorting to manometry or rectal biopsy [59]. In our experience, however, we believe that anorectal manometry is useful in any patient with severe chronic constipation because of the safety of the test and its undoubted value if positive for HD as an indication for rectal biopsy. This is applicable at any age for children, and even for the adult patient [10,57].

The greater the association of the constipation with one or more symptoms that are also considered frequent in HD, such as chronic abdominal distension (Figure 2), vomiting, crises of intestinal obstruction, recurrent abdominal pain, enterocolitis, and a history of delayed passage of meconium, the more likely is the existence of aganglionosis [1,12,49,51,52,54].

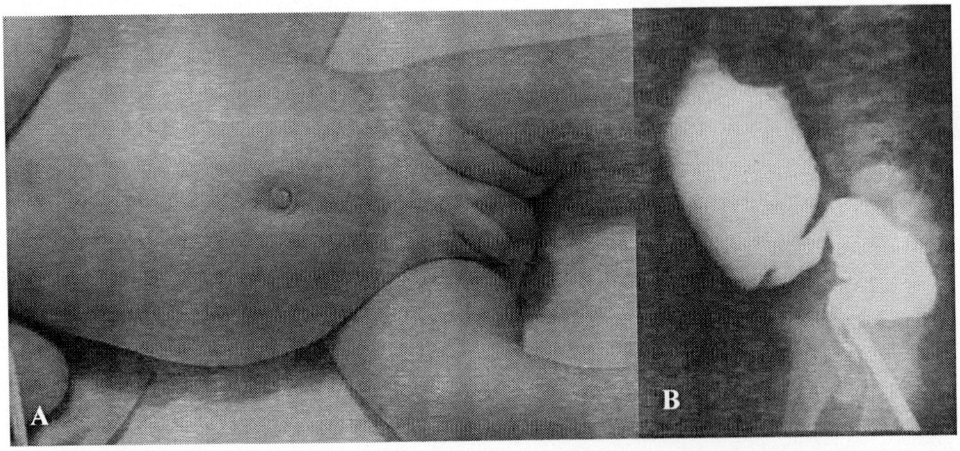

Figure 2. A. Infant of 5 months with chronic abdominal distension due to HD. B. The opaque enema of this patient shows a rectosigmoidal aganglionosis.

Even though chronic malnutrition has a higher incidence in patients with HD than in others with different causes of constipation, it is still only present in just a few patients – 5% for some authors. It is probably one of the least studied aspects of this pathology, although it has been recommended that a nutritional study be carried out prior to any surgery in these patients [60].

The incidence in the constipated patient of such symptoms as encopresis or rectorrhagia make it less likely that the ætiology is HD. This is also the case for the elimination of voluminous stools, or disorders of defæcation that condition fæcal retention [1,57].

When the physical examination detects fæcalomas in the abdomen by palpation, or in the rectum together with a large rectal ampulla by rectal digital examination, as well as anal fissures, HD is more unlikely. HD usually presents an empty rectum that fits snugly around the examining finger [1,57].

As has been shown in Chapters 5 and 6, the probability that a patient who presents the clinical manifestations referred to above has HD is greater when there is a family history of the disease, or when there exist certain chromosomal anomalies (especially trisomy 21) or neurocristopathies (particularly if they are accompanied by pigmentation defects, deafness, mental retardation, or central hypoventilation, among other defects). HD should also be suspected in patients with difficulty in defæcating who present other congenital defects or syndromes with which HD has been identified occasionally or even rarely (see Chapters 5 and 6).

References

[1] De Lorijn F, Bœckxstæns GE, Benninga MA. Symptomatology, pathophysiology, diagnostic work-up, and treatment of Hirschsprung disease in infancy and childhood. *Curr Gastrœnterol Rep* 2007;9:245-53.

[2] Puri P. Pathophysiology of Hirschsprung's disease In: Holschneider AM, Puri P (eds). *Hirchsprung's Disease and Allied Disorders*. Third Edition. Berlin, Heidelberg: Springer-Verlag; 2008. pp. 94-106.

[3] Kaiser G, Bettex M. Clnical Generalities. In: Holschneider AM, editor. *Hirschsprung's disease.* Stuttgart-New York: Hippokrates Verlag, Thieme Stratton. Inc; 1982. p. 43-54.

[4] Puri P, Lake BD, Nixon HH, Mishalany H, Clairesux AE. Neuronal colonic dysplasia: an unusual association of Hirschsprung's disease. *J Pediatr Surg* 1977;12:681-5.

[5] Schärli AF. Intestinal neuronal dysplasia. *Cir Pediatr*. 1992;5:64-5.

[6] Langer JC. Persistent obstructive symptoms after surgery for Hirschsprung's disease: development of a diagnostic and therapeutic algorithm. *J Pediatr Surg* 2004;39:1458-62.

[7] Kobayashi H, Hirakawa H, Surana R, O'Briain DS, Puri P: Intestinal neuronal dysplasia is a possible cause of persistent bowel symptoms after pull-through operation for Hirschsprung's disease. *J Pediatr Surg* 1995;30:253-7.

[8] Sandgren K, Larsson LT, Ekblad E. Widespread changes in neurotransmitter expression and number of enteric neurons and interstitial cells of Cajal in lethal spotted mice: an explanation for persisting dysmotility after operation for Hirschsprung's disease? *Dig Dis Sci* 2002;47:1049-64.

[9] Estivao-Costa J, Fragoso AC, Soares Oliveura M, Carvalho JL: An approach to minimize postoperative enterocolitis in Hirschsprung's disease. *J Pediatr Surg* 2006;41:1704-7.

[10] Puri. Montedonico S: Hirschsprung's disease: Clinical Features. In: Holschneider AM, Puri P (eds). *Hirchsprung's Disease and Allied Disorders*. Third Edition. Berlin, Heidelberg: Springer-Verlag; 2008. p. 107-13.

[11] Klein MD, Coran AG, Wesly JR, Drongowski RA: Hirschsprung's disease in the newborn. *J Pediatr Surg* 1984;19:370-4.

[12] Singh SJ, Croaker GDH, Manglick P, Wong CL, Athanasakos H, Elliott E et al. Hirschsprung's disease: the Australian Pædiatric Surveillance Unit's experience. *Pediatr Surg Int* 2003;19:247-50.

[13] Fraser GC, Berry C: Mortality in neonatal Hirschsprung's disease with particular reference to enterocolitis. *J Pediatr Surg* 1967;2:205-11.

[14] Vieten D, Spicer R: Enterocolitis complicating Hirschsprung's disease. *Semin Pediatr Surg* 2004;13:263-72.
[15] Godbole K. Many faces of Hirschsprung's disease. *Indian Pediatr* 2004;41:1115-23.
[16] Moore SW, Zaahl MG: A review of genetic mutation in familial Hirschsprung's disease in South Africa: towards genetic counseling. *J Pediatr Surg* 2008 F;43:325-9.
[17] Vermesh M, Mayden KL, Confino E, Giglia RV, Gleicher N. Prenatal sonographic diagnosis of Hirschsprung's disease. *J Ultrasound Med* 1986;5:37-9.
[18] Eliyahu S, Yanai N, Blondhein O, Reich D, Siplovich L, Shaley E. Sonographic presentation of Hirschsprung's disease. A case of an entirely aganglionic colon and ileum. *Prenat Diagn* 1994;14:1170-2.
[19] Belin B, Corteville JE, Langer JC. How accurate is prenatal sonography for the diagnosis of imperforate anus and Hirschsprung's disease? *Pediatr Surg Int* 1995;10:30-32.
[20] Núñez R, Cabrera R, Moreno C, Agulla E, Vargas I, Blesa E: Utilidad de la manometría anorrectal en el diagnóstico neonatal de la enfermedad de Hirschsprung. *Cir Pediatr* 2000;13:16-9.
[21] Guo W, Zhang O, Chen Y, Hou D: Diagnostic scoring system of Hirschsprung's disease in the neonatal period. *Asian J Surg* 2006;29:176-9.
[22] Dasgupta R, Langer JC: Hirschsprung disease. *Curr Probl Surg* 2004;41:942-88.
[23] Bekkali N, Hamers SL, Schipperus MR, Reitsma JB, Valerio PG, Van Toledo L et al. Duration of meconium passage in preterm and term infants. *Arch Dis Child Fetal Neonatal Ed* 2008;93:F376-9.
[24] 24- Lœning-Bauke V, Kimura K. Failure to pass meconium: diagnosing neonatal intestinal obstruction. *Am Fam Physician* 1999;60:2043-50.
[25] Kenny SE, Vanderwinden JM, Rintala RJ, Connell MG, Lloyd DA, Vanderhængen JJ et al. Delayed maturation of the interstitial cells of Cajal: a new diagnosis for transient neonatal pseudoobstruction. Report of two cases. *J Pediatr Surg* 1998;33:94-8.
[26] Fitzgerald JF. Constipation in children. *Pediatr Rev* 1987;8:299-302.
[27] Gryboski JD. The colon, rectum and anus. In: Gryboski JD. *Gastrointestinal problems in the infant*. Philadelphia: Saunders, 1975.p.499-564.
[28] Jenetzky E.Prevalence estimation of anorectal malformations using German diagnosis related groups system.*Pediatr Surg Int* 2007;23:1161-5.
[29] Kiely EM. Meconius ileus. In: Puri P. ed. *Newborn surgery*. Oxford: Butterworth-Heinemann, 1996.p.324-7.
[30] Lopez-Alonso M, Ribas J, Hernandez A, Anguita FA, Gomez DT, I, Martinez-Caro A. Efficiency of the anorectal manometry for the diagnosis of Hirschsprung's disease in the newborn period. *Eur J Pediatr Surg* 1995;5:160-3.
[31] Pini-Prato A, Martucciello G, Jasonni V: Rectal suction biopsy in the diagnosis of intestinal dysganglionosis: 5-year experience with solo-RBT. *J Pediatr Surg* 2006;41:1043-1048.
[32] Gil-Vernet JM, Broto J, Guillén G:Diagnóstico diferencial Hirschsprung-Neurodisplasia intestinal. Fiabilidad de las pruebas diagnósticas. *Cir Pediatr* 2006;19:91-4.

[33] Ellis D G, Clatworthy Jr. The meconium plug syndrome revisited. *J Pediatr Surg* 1966;1:54-61.

[34] van Leeuwen G, Glenn L, Woodruff C, Riley WC. Meconium plug syndrome with aganglionosis. *Pediatrics* 1967;40:665-6.

[35] Burge D, Drewett M. Meconium plug obstruction. *Pediatr Surg Int* 2004; 20:108-10.

[36] Keckler SJ, St Peter SD, Spilde TL, Tsao K, Ostlie DJ, Holcomb GW et al. Current significance of meconium plug syndrome. *J Peditr Surg* 2008;43:896-8.

[37] Teitelbaum DH, Cilley RE, Sherman NJ, Bliss D, Uitylugt ND, Ranaud EJ et al.: A decade of experience with the primary pull-through for Hirschsprung disease in the newborn period: a multicenter analysis of outcomes. *Ann Surg* 2000;232:372-80.

[38] Coran AG, Teitelbaum DH: Recent advances in the management of Hirschsprung's disease. *Am J Surg* 2000;180:382-387.

[39] Teitelbaum DH, Qualman SJ, Caniano DA:Hirschsprung's disease.Identification of risk factor for enterocolitis. *Ann Surg* 1998;207:240-4.

[40] Haricharan RN, Seo JM, Kelly DR, Mroczek-Musulman EC, Aprahamian CJ, Morgan TL et al. Older age at diagnosis of Hirschsprung disease decreases risk of postoperative enterocolitis, but resection of additional ganglionated bowel does not. *J Pediatr Surg* 2008;43:1115-23.

[41] Boley SJ, Dinari G, Cohen MI. Hirschsprung's Disease in the neonate. *Clinics in Perinatology* 1978; 5:45-60.

[42] Newman B, Nussbaum A and Kirkpatric, Jr. JA. Bowel perforation in Hirschsprung's disease. *AJR* 1987;148:1195-97.

[43] Soper RT: Hirschsprung's disease. In: Rickham PP, Soper RT and Stauffer UG: *Synopsis of Pediatric Surgery*. D-700 Stuttgart, Germany: Ed. Georg Thieme Verlag, 1975. p. 149-55.

[44] Núñez R, Cabrera R, Agulla E, Moreno C, Serrano A, Ortiz C, Blesa E: Aganglionismo cólico con afectación ileal. Plastia ileocolica. *Cir Pediatr* 2001;14:76-81.

[45] Martin LW, Perrin EV: Neonatal perforation of the appendix in association with Hirschsprung's Disease. *Ann Surg* 1967; 166:799.

[46] Soper RT, Opitz, John M: Neonatal pneumoperitoneum and Hirschsprung's Disease. *Surgery* 1963; 51:527-33.

[47] Sarioglu A, Tanyel C, Büyükpamukcu N, Hicsönmez A. Appendiceal perforation: A potentially lethal initial mode of presentation of Hirschsprung's disease. *J Pediatr Surg* 1997;32:123-4.

[48] Arliss J, Holgersen O. Neonatal appendiceal perforation and Hirschsprung's disease *Pediatr Surg* 1990;25:694-5.

[49] Swenson O, Sherman JO, Fisher JH: Diagnosis of congenital megacolon: An analysis of 501 patients. *J Pediatr Surg* 1973; 8: 587-94.

[50] Kleinhaus S, Boley SJ, Sheran M, Sieber K: Hirschsprung's disease. A survey of the members of the Surgical Section of the American Academy of Pediatrics. *J Pediatr Surg* 1979; 14: 588-97.

[51] Orr DJ, Scobie WG: Presentation and incidence of Hirschsprung's disease. *BMJ* 1983; 287:1671.

[52] Klein MD, Philippart AI: Hirschsprung's disease: Three decades' experience at a single institution. *J Pediatr Surg* 1993; 28: 1.291-94.

[53] Rajab A, Freeman NV, Patton MA: Hirschsprung's disease in Oman. *J Pediatr Surg* 1997; 32: 724-7.

[54] Wheatley MJ, Wesley JR, Coran AG, Polley TZ Jr: Hirschsprung's disease in adolescents and adults. *Dis Col Rect* 1990; 33: 622-9.

[55] Ikeda K, Goto S: Diagnosis and treatment of Hirschsprung's disease in Japan. An analysis of 1628 patients. *Ann Surg* 1984; 199: 400-5.

[56] Suita S, Taguchi T, Ieiri S, Nakatsuji T: Hirschsprung's disease in Japan: analysis of 3852 patients based on a nationwide survey in 30 years. *J Pediatr Surg* 2005; 40: 197-202.

[57] Khan AR, Vujanic GM, Huddart S: The constipated child: How likely is Hirschsprung's disease? *Pediatr Surg Int* 2003; 19: 439-42.

[58] Meier-Ruge WA, Bruder E, Holschneider AM, Piket G, Posselt HG, Tewes G: Diagnosis and therapy of ultrashort Hirschsprung's disease. *Eur J Pediatr Surg* 2004; 14: 392-7.

[59] Wales JKH: Presentation and incidence of Hirschsprung's disease. *BMJ* 1984; 288: 151.

[60] Benninga MA, Voskuijl WP,Taminiau JM: Childhood constipation: Is there new light in the tunnel? *J Pediatr Gastrœnterol Nutr* 2004;39: 448-64.

In: Hirschsprung's Disease: Diagnosis and Treatment
Ed: Ramón Núñez and Manuel López-Alonso
ISBN: 978-1-60741-349-3

Chapter IX

Manometric Diagnosis of Hirschsprung's Disease During the Neonatal Period

Manuel López-Alonso

Introduction

One of the goals of any group that treats patients with Hirschsprung's Disease (HD) is to make a diagnosis in the first few days of a baby's life, since in 80-90% of HD patients, the disease manifests itself during the neonatal period [1] and the incidence of its most serious complication, neonatal necrotising enterocolitis, increases proportionally with the delay in diagnosis after the first few days of life.

The clinical profile is varied, from a delay in the first discharge of meconium, to a greater or lesser degree of functional distal intestinal obstruction. The usefulness of anorectal manometry (ARM) as a diagnostic method for HD dates back to the 70s. However, it was not done in newborns. Current diagnostic methods continue to be the traditional ones: ARM, the conventional method of syringe suction rectal biopsy (SRB) and the contrast enema (CE). All three methods pose problems during the neonatal period, especially ARM. The first manometric results in newborns supported the existence of a delayed appearance of the anorectal reflexes due to a generalised immaturity of all the systems during this period. Therefore it was declared that ARM, although a useful diagnostic method for HD in general, was not practical during the neonatal period, when diagnostic methods should be limited to RSB and CE.

Various isolated studies attempted to disprove this statement [2-9] in the past, without managing to do so. In recent years, trends have been starting to change and ARM is gaining credibility as a diagnostic method for HD during the neonatal period [1,10-15] .

There are probably multiple reasons for the slow introduction of neonatal manometry: technical difficulties, the generalised initial criteria established is hardly reliable for diagnosis, the lack of a uniform method: with respect to the probe and perfusion pump: air-filled pressure probe system[16], micromanometric sleeve catheter[10,11,14], high-resolution manometry [13] intraluminal pressure transducer[5] or perfused side-opening catheters[6,7] . With respect to the patient's resting conditions, there are some groups in favour of carrying out the exam under sedation [6] and others in favour of carrying it out without sedation [12,14] .

Nevertheless, in our opinion, for many years this diagnostic method has been affordable, minimally invasive, and easily to be carried out. It also shows diagnostic reliability rates[2,4,5,12,15,16] which make it the diagnostic method of choice for screening HD during the neonatal period. The basic elements needed are: a pressure probe designed for a anal canal of 12-15 mm in length; a perfusion system with a steady flow of 0.05 mL/min and specialised personnel, who are specifically dedicated to this task. Obviously, there must be a sufficient guaranteed number of daily cases so that the functional digestive tests are worthwhile financially and do not become an expensive method.

The materials, methods and results obtained at the Virgen del Rocío Children's Hospital of Seville between 1984 and 2008 are as follows.

Material

Since 1984, we have used the same probe, manufactured by us [6] and the perfusion pump is basically the same with the logical updates according to how computer and electronic knowledge have been advancing.

The material used in this test is the following:

4-Chamber Probe

This probe manufactured by us is similar to that used by *Boston Scott Bowes* and *Kling* [2,3]. This probe consists of four stiffened plastic hollow catheters (Rusch Ch3 Uretric Catheters) bound to each other. The total external diameter is 2.5 mm. One of these catheters was connected to an air-inflatable small latex soft balloon (4 mm in diameter when empty) as a stimulation requirement. The balloon was obtained from a Balloon Catheter Rusch (Foley catheter) Ch/F8. The other tubes had lateral openings located 5 mm apart. The distance between the balloon and the first recording opening was 25 mm (Figure 1).

The volume of air which is blown into the balloon is not directly proportional to the diameter of inflation (Ø). With a minimum volume of 1 cc, we obtain a balloon of 12 mm in diameter, with a 2 cc volume, a 15 mm diameter balloon, with a 3 cc volume, a 17 mm diameter balloon and with a 4 cc volume, an 18 mm diameter balloon.

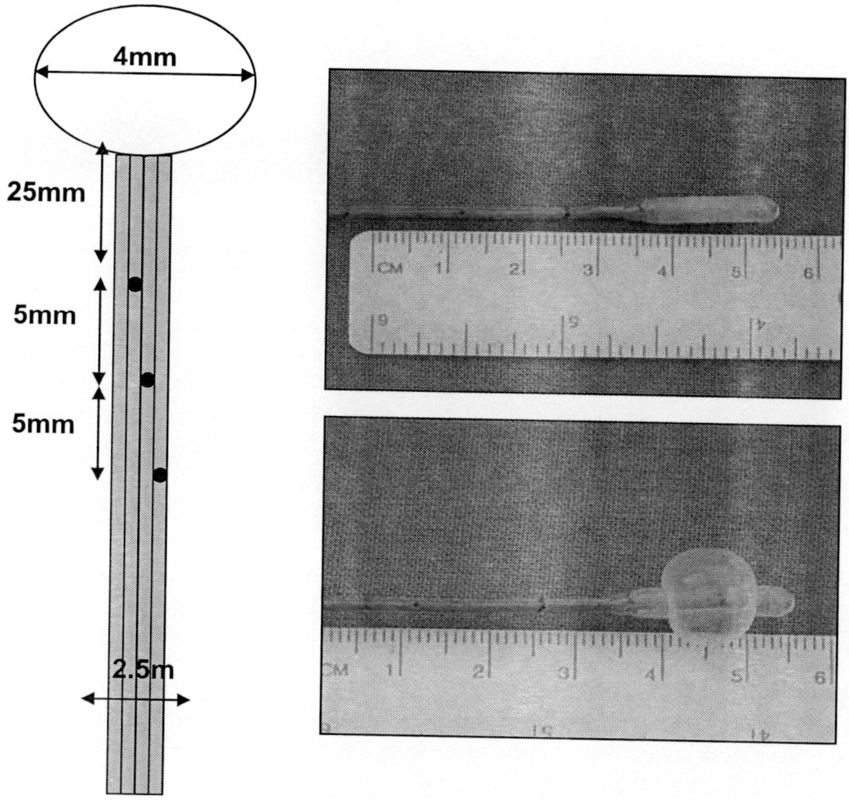

Figure 1. 4-chamber probe. Distance from balloon to proximal incision 25 mm. Distance between the incisions for taking pressure 5 mm. Exterior diameter of the probe 2.5 mm.

Perfusion

An open-distilled water perfusing system at a flow rate of 0.05 mL/min was used.

Perfusion Pump

The catheter is connected to pressure transducers and these convert pressure into an electrical signal, which is then filtered, amplified, digitalised and stored on a videotape or a CD through Siemens-Elema amplifiers, and then converted from analogue to digital in order to be stored into a videotape and an inscriptor; we also have an DAQ (Data Acquisition) Card Interface, designed by our research group which recover the data from the amplifiers and send it to a personal computer (PC) through its serial comm. In the PC there is monitoring software, also designed for us, which led us to watch the pressure measured and even calculate parameters in real time. The software is designed to make statistical analysis, once the register is ended, in order to make possible the doctor to ascertain a diagnosis for the patient (Figure 2).

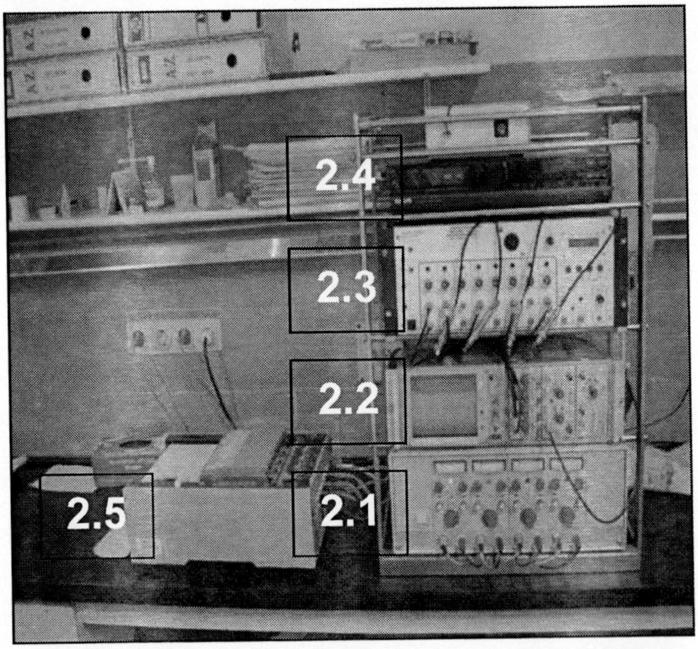

Figure 2. Perfusion pump for recording pressure. From bottom to top and right to left: amplifying and filtering stage of the signals coming from the pressure transducers (2.1); oscilloscope for the visualisation of the analogue signals coming from the transducers (2.2); 16 bit Analogue-Digital converter, converts pressure (2.3), video (2.4) and inscriber (2.5) signals to digital.

The software also acts as communication program with the Data Acquisition Card, because it led us to send commands to perform a specific task and receive digital data from the microprocessor which governs the DAQ Card in order to represent in the screen. This software is very cheap and absolutely open to our specifications because we can make several kinds of measurements, even is really suited to any requirement we ask it.

Methods

Preceding manometry exploration, the catheter and transducers are calibrated and purged. Inscription speed is one millimetre per second (1 mm/sec) so that every two consecutive and vertical lines in the inscriptor demarcate one second in the horizontal x axis; on the other hand, two consecutive and horizontal lines demarcate 2 pressure mmHg. The transducer chambers are located on the same level as the child's anal canal in order to obtain the baseline or reference line, which is given a value of zero.

In order for the exam to be illustrative, we need appropriate resting conditions and optimum manometric conditions of the anal canal. Initially we did not use sedation but we spent a long time and in some cases in spite of the great deal of time spent, we were unable to achieve good resting conditions. For this reason, we began to progressively sedate the children with midazolan and we managed to shorten the exam times and in every case achieved good resting conditions, improving results. We currently sedate all our patients of this age with intravenous or nasal midazolan [18] at a dosage of 0.1-0.3 mg/kg weight. The patient is monitored, and his heart rate and O_2 saturation recorded (pulse oximetry).

In order for the conditions of the anal canal to be optimal, we limit handling in the days prior to the exam and only in the event that they are necessary, we recommend cleaning enemas with a mild physiological serum and a number 10-12 latex urethral probe up until the day prior to the exam.

Once the child is asleep, the probe is easily inserted into the anal canal 4 or 5 cm past the last hole recording sensor for checking pressure (Figure 3). Then we carry out a gentle pull through centimetre by centimetre in order to obtain the manometric profile. Doing so we can differentiate the area of influence of the proximal internal sphincter (anorectal fluctuations) and the distal steady zone (area of influence of the external sphincter); we also measure the length, the pressure at the beginning, the maximum pressure and the pressure at the end of the anal canal. If necessary, the exam can be carried out inside an incubator (Figure 4). Next we place two hole recording sensor for measuring in the fluctuating zone and one in the steady zone (no pressure oscillations) and we begin the study of the anorectal reflexes. In order to trigger the reflex we inflate the balloon located in the rectum beginning at 1 cc. The balloon is inflated by blowing air into it with a 5 cc syringe. The minimal visible inflation of the balloon is obtained with 1 cc. The intensity of the stimulus is between 1 cc and 5 cc. The most common inflation volume is 3 ml. The duration of the stimulus varies between 5 and 30 seconds, but between 5 and 10 seconds is the most commonly used. We progressively increase the inflation until an appropriate relaxation response is obtained. During this manoeuvre we put especial care to do not reach the critical volume which causes the patient to attempt to expel the probe and could awaken him. Once settle the optimal volume of the balloon we apply a sufficient number of stimuli (20-30) in order to ensure the presence or absence of the reflex. The full exam usually takes between 60 and 90 minutes on average.

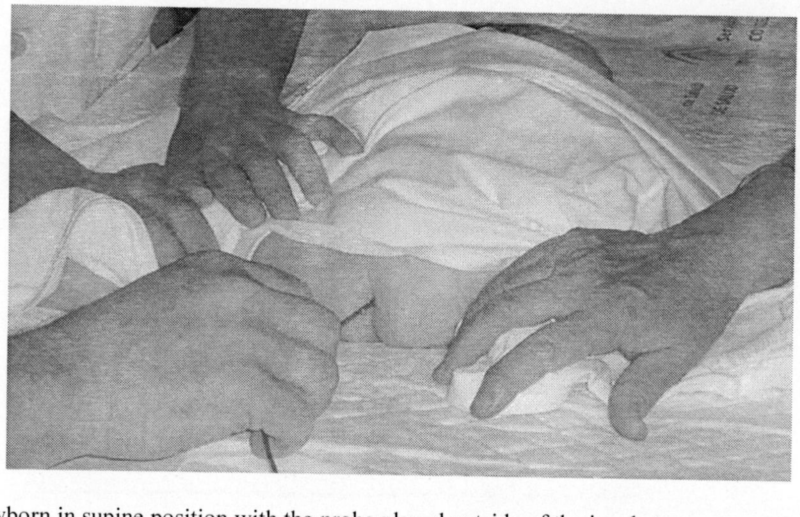

Figure 3. Newborn in supine position with the probe placed outside of the incubator.

The most laborious part of the examination is avoiding movement of the probe, which would completely change the recording. Once the appropriate recording zone is found, we pass along the fluctuating zone with enough time to carry out a series of stimuli.

In every child the number of stimuli is going to be different in both the fluctuating zone and the steady zone because of the individual behavioural characteristics of every child. That is, a set number of stimuli for every manometry cannot be established.

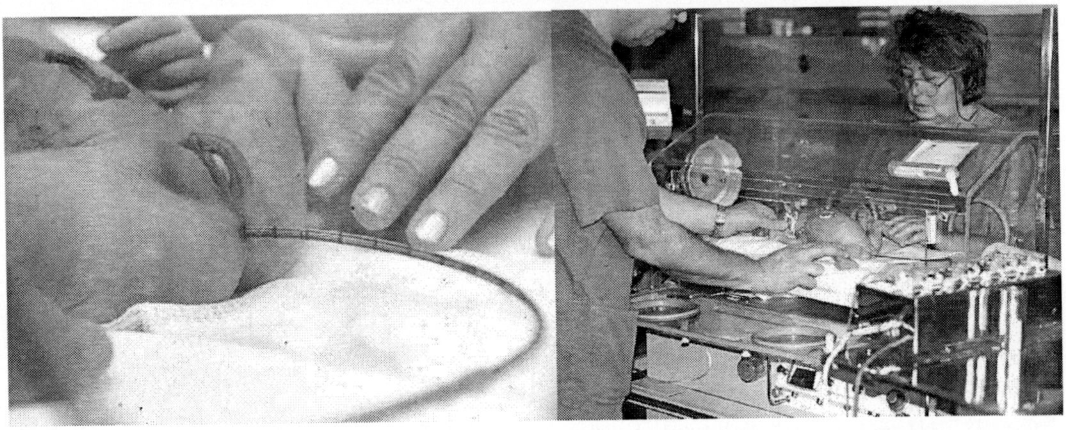

Figure 4. Exam inside the incubator.

Characteristics of the Manometric Anal Canal

If we insert a catheter to record the pressure in the rectum and we gradually remove it, we observe that at a certain point in the anal canal, a moderate rise in pressure begins, and small waves known as fluctuating waves appear at the same time. This marks the proximal (aboral) limit of the anorectal canal from the manometric point of view (Figure 5).'

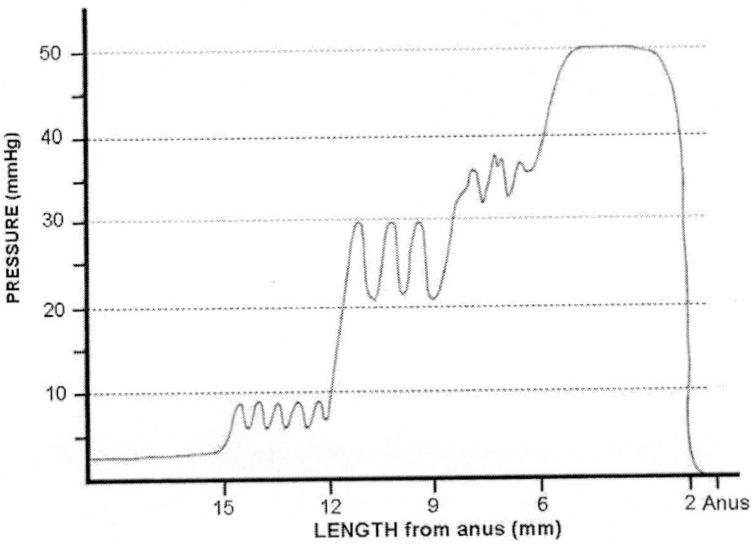

Figure 5. Graphical representation when the probe is removed using pull through cm by cm.

Reflex Zones: Fluctuating Zone and Steady Zone

Basal tone: there is an ascending pressure gradient almost until the probe pass out the anus.

Rhythmic activity: in the proximal extreme of the anorectal canal, in addition to a rise in pressure, small waves known as anorectal fluctuating waves appear. The recording scope of these waves is 11.92 (8.47 – 16.63) mmHg (median, p_{25} – p_{75}). These waves are not continuously recorded, but they appear from time to time. Their period is regular: 7.2 (6.8 – 8.0) seconds. The aboral region to the anal canal is characterised by the presence of fluctuating waves, probably the mechanical output of the pacemaker activity in the wall gut, and we named the "Fluctuating zone". In the distal direction the duration of the waves hardly varies. In contrast, the amplitude grows twofolds.

Continuing in the distal direction the fluctuations become irregular and disappear at the anus level. However, the pressure recording is a continuous line and for this reason we call it the "Steady Zone" (Figure 5).

Anorectal Reflexes

This is a relaxation wave that is recorded manometrically all along the anal canal, and is characterised by the drop in pressure which is triggered upon inflating the rectum. Preceded and followed by fluctuating waves in the fluctuating zone.

Different manometric parameters are defined and studied (Figure 6):

Stimulus

I	Intensity: (ccs of air inflated).
T	Time that balloon remains inflated.

Fluctuation Wave Preceding the Stimulus

a	Amplitude at the peak of recovery.
b	Amplitude at the peak of relaxation.
a-b	Amplitude of the fluctuating wave.
$t_{aA}=t_A-t_a$	Duration of the fluctuating wave.
100*(a-b)/a	Relaxation of the Fluctuating Wave (RFW).

Relaxation Wave Which Follows The Stimulus; Amplitudes

A	At the beginning of the wave.
B	At the lowest point.
C	At the peak of the 1st fluctuation wave following the stimulus.
100*(A-B)/A	Relaxation of the Reflex Wave (RRW).

Relaxation Wave that Follows the Stimulus for Fluctuation Zone and Steady Zone; Times

t_A-t_0	Latency.

$t_{AC}=t_C-t_A$ Duration of the relaxation wave.

Latency

Latency is the delay period between stimulation and motility responses. There are few references about this parameter in the literature. For *Bowes* [3] the latency of the rectosphincter reflex has a constant value (1.8 ± 0.15 seconds), but as Bowes states, latency is not constant throughout the anal canal.

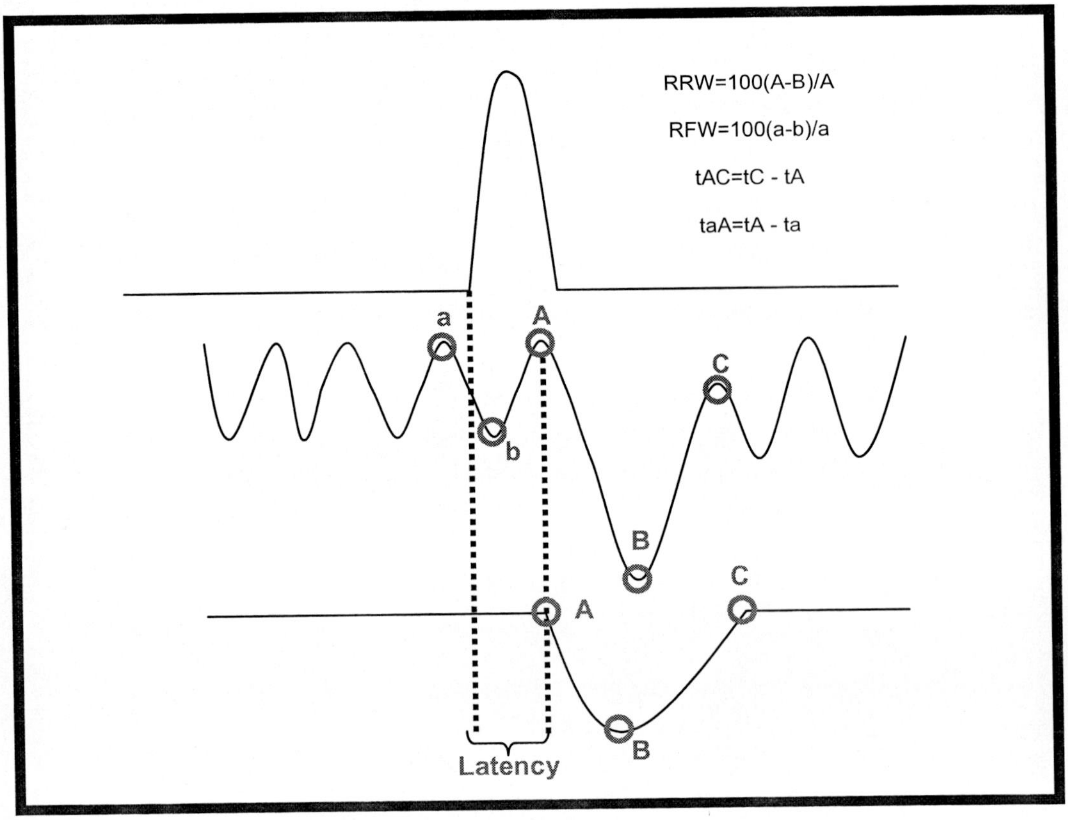

Figure 6. Diagram showing the different measurements that we take in the fluctuating zone and steady zone, both on the vertical axis (pressure) and on the horizontal (time).

Latency in the Fluctuating Zone

The fluctuating zone is characterised by rhythmic oscillations of the luminal pressure. The time course of the pressure waves increased exponentially along with the intraluminal pressure up until a peak value was reached, thereafter, an exponential decrease occurred until the resting pressure value was reached. This time period gave the fluctuating pressure recordings a wavelike appearance.

Whenever a suprathreshold stimulus was applied to the fluctuating zone of the anal canal, the anorectal wall responded with a relaxation wave. Despite the differing durations of the suprathreshold stimuli, the pressure responses were similar along the fluctuating zone.

However, the latency of the response depended on the location of the stimulus during the time course of the pressure waves.

The pressure responses showed different delays with respect to the onset of the stimulus. The shortest latencies corresponded to those stimuli delivered at the peak value of the fluctuating wave. The longest ones were seen when the stimulus was delivered just after the peak value of the fluctuating wave, during the natural rhythmic period of relaxation. Latencies with intermediate values were recorded when stimuli were applied at any time between the peak and the lowest points of the fluctuating waves. Figure 7 shows several relaxing responses with different latencies. In L_0 the relaxation is nominally instantaneous 0.23± 0.22 s; in L_1 the relaxation is 1.21 ± 0.49 s; in L_2 2. 09 ± 0.74 s. Finaly in L_3 3.16± 0.83s. Naturally, latencies varied according to the length of the interwave periods or the frequency of oscillation. The higher the frequency, the shorter the latency was.

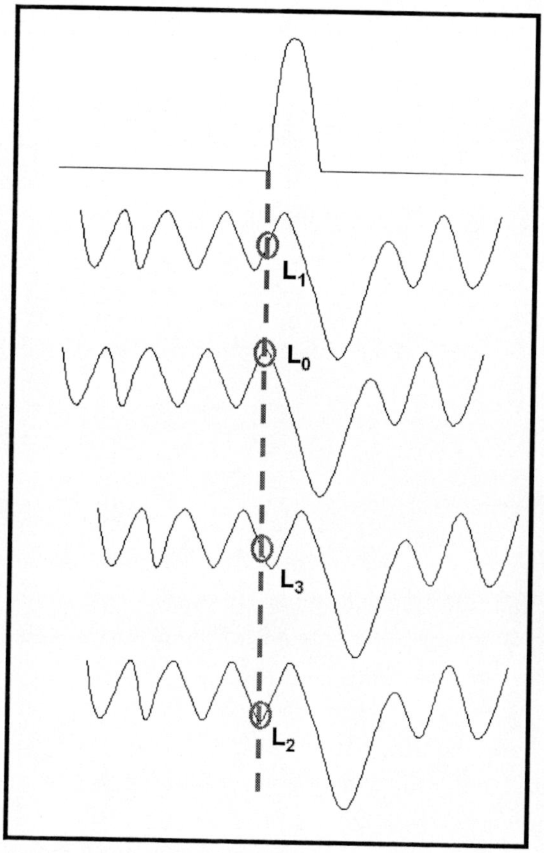

Figure 7. Diagram showing the different latencies according to the moment when the fluctuation wave coincides with the inflation of the balloon in the fluctuating zone and in the steady zone.

The most striking responses were those obtained with stimulation during the descending part of the fluctuating wave (L_3). In these cases, the fluctuating wave followed its normal course, passed by the bottom of the wave and only when pressure increased near the peak did the reflex response occur 3.16 ± 0.83 seconds later. Therefore, a great deal of time had to pass after the onset of the stimulus before the appearance of the relaxation reflex.

Latency in the Steady Zone

The main feature of this zone was the absence of pressure waves and a steady level of absolute pressure. The relaxing responses in this zone systematically appeared with a latency (L) median percentile 25, percentile 75: 0.9 (0.6, 1.2). This value was independent of those effects occurring in the fluctuating zone. Moreover, any stimulus applied during the relaxation reflex response was unable to induce a new response before complete recovery, indicating the existence of a refractory period in this zone which is absent, at least in the same manner, in the fluctuating zone (Figure 8).

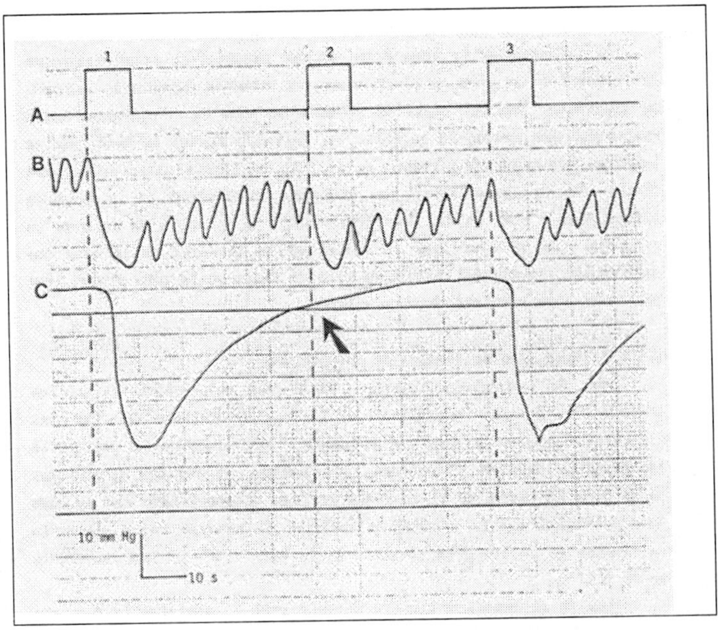

Figure 8. Refractory period in the steady zone.

Since the stimuli were delivered at a known location in the rectal ampulla and the pressure responses of both the fluctuating and/or steady zone were simultaneously recorded, it was possible to make a comparative analysis of latencies obtained in two or three different places 5 mm apart along the anal canal.

With respect to the sensitivity of the anal canal wall, normally the pressure responses were obtained from both the fluctuating zone and the steady zone with suprathreshold stimuli. However, occasionally the steady zone responses showed a lower threshold than the fluctuating zone (Figure 9).

Often two responses simultaneously recorded 5 mm apart in the fluctuating zone showed different latencies. Interestingly, the shortest latency did not always correspond to a closer location to the stimulus. In fact, the value of the latency tended to depend on the application of stimulus over the natural rhythm of fluctuation rather than on the distance to the stimulus itself.

When recordings were obtained simultaneously from two places, one in the fluctuating zone and another in the steady zone, the relationship of the latencies demonstrated interesting findings. The steady zone usually responded after a delay of 0.9 seconds. However, the response in the fluctuating zone occurred early (0.23 seconds),when the stimulus was applied during the increasing part of a pressure wave, and later than that in the steady zone when the stimulus coincided with the decreasing part of the fluctuating wave (Figure 10).

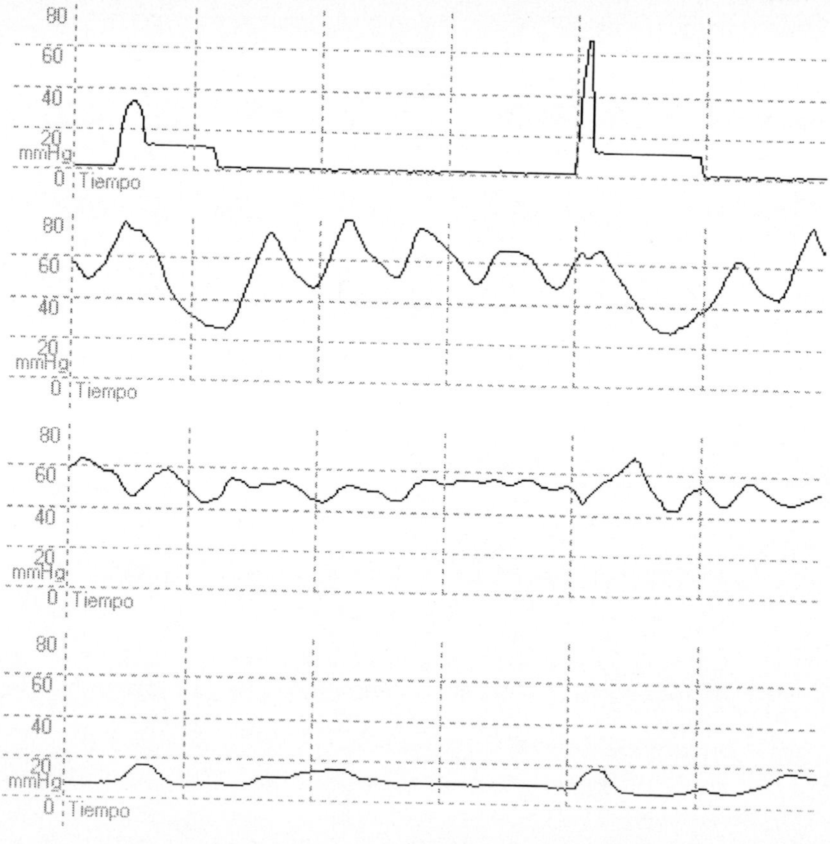

Figure 9. Relaxation wave in the fluctuating zone and absent in the steady zone.

We find references to this in other authors such as *Schuster* [19], who demonstrated by taking the pressure in the rectum and in the sphincter, that upon inflating the rectum, there was no pressure variation at the rectal level, while at the sphincter level a relaxation wave was triggered. In this way, he showed that the reflex was not a relaxation wave coming from the rectum, but rather a true intra-wall reflex with connections which run across the ganglionic cells in the myenteric plexus.

This also demonstrates that the rectosphincter reflex is not a reflex relaxation wave that begins in the proximal extreme of the anal canal and later spreads in the distal direction, taking pressure various times in the anal canal which, in accordance with the latency, the relaxation wave caused by the rectal inflation can be triggered in a distal reflex zone before in a proximal reflex zone, and in the same way it can be triggered in the distal steady zone before than in the proximal reflex zone.

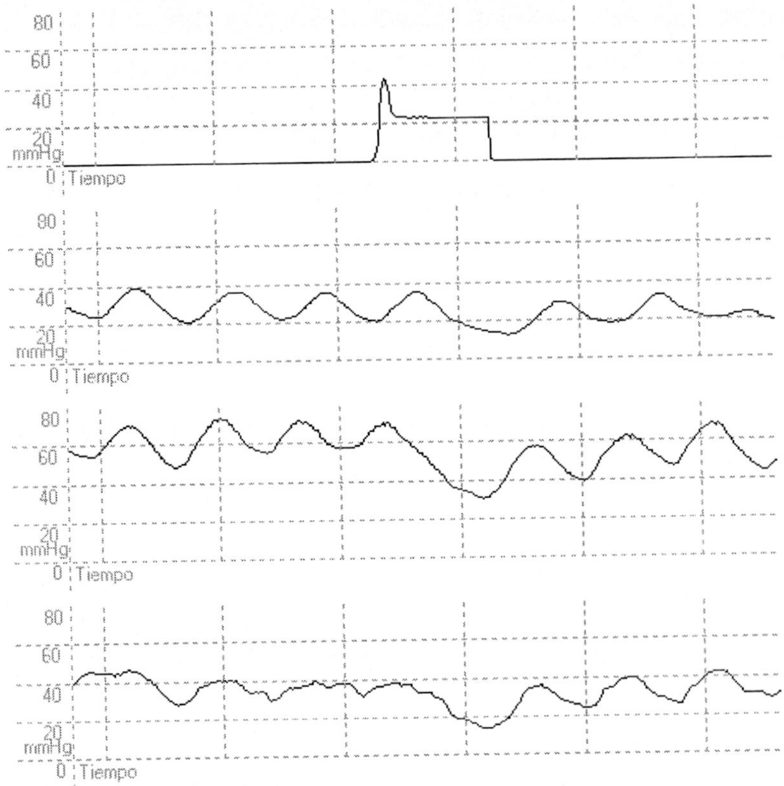

Figure 10. Example of greater latency in proximal recording zone.

Differences in the Relaxation Waves in the Reflex Zone and the Steady Zone.

Proximal Automatism Zone

This zone is characterised by a low pressure gradient, low amplitude fluctuation waves and for not having any striking differences in the graphical representation between the relaxation wave which follows rectal inflation and the fluctuation wave which precedes the reflex with regard to the % of relaxation. However, there are significant differences in the duration of the reflex wave, which is larger than the fluctuation wave (Figure 11).

Distal Automatism Zone

In this zone, the graphical representation of the reflex is clear and evident. The % of relaxation is close to 100% and the duration of the wave doubles the value of the fluctuation wave (Figure 11).

Steady Zone

In this zone, the reflex is a relaxation wave which ends when the initial amplitude is reached once more at the time the rectal balloon was inflated. In this zone there will be no supercontinence phase following the recovery curve. Duration: t_C - t_A (median percentile 25, percentile 75) is 14.6 (12.8, 16.6) seconds and the relaxation percentage: 100(A-B)/A 84.99

(69.44, 97.02). Additionally, the time that the recovery curve takes to reach the initial pressure before the reflex is longer in this zone. The recovery period in the steady zone is refractory to new stimuli, therefore, when faced with consecutive stimuli in the steady zone, a relaxation wave is not produced until total recovery is achieved (Figure 8).

Characteristics of the Reflex Relaxation Wave Depending on the Intensity and Duration of the Stimulus

The reflex is proportional to the intensity of the stimulus. There is a minimum inflation volume for the rectal balloon in order to trigger the reflex which we call the stimulus threshold, and there is a critical inflation volume. This inflation volume is uncomfortable for the child, due to the reduced size of the anal canal, causing the child to repeatedly attempt to expel the probe, which would alter the resting conditions and force the exam to come to a halt. There are no significant changes for the growing stimuli on the time axis. In contrast, the pressure drop (A-B) increases proportionally to rectal inflation. The reflex is independent of the duration of the stimulus. The relaxation waves caused by stimuli of the same intensity but with varying duration do not present significant differences.

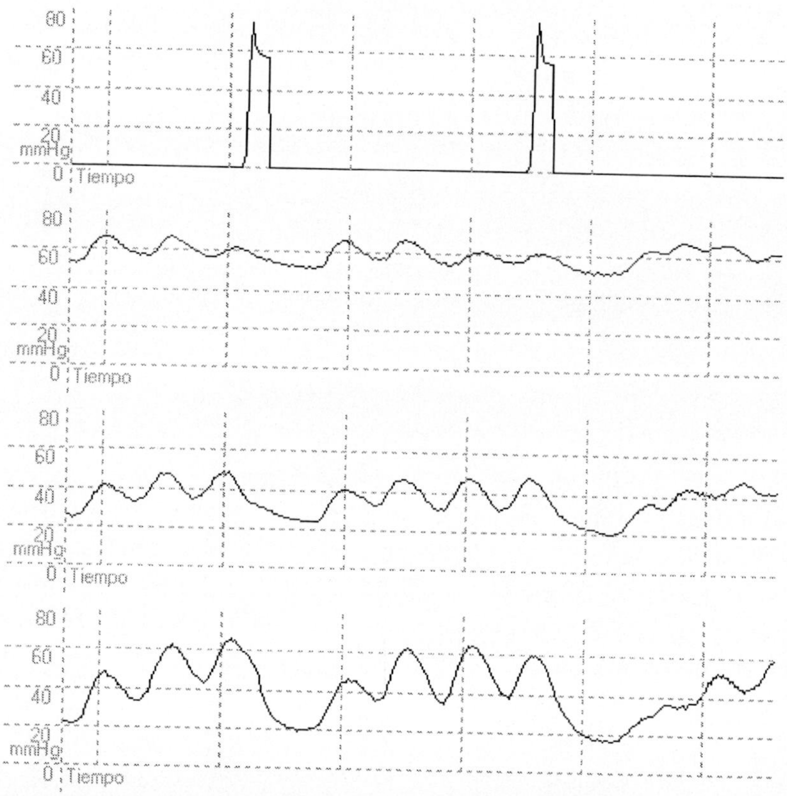

Figure 11. Difference between the relaxation wave in the proximal fluctuating zone where the most noteworthy thing is the duration of the wave, and the wave in the distal fluctuating zone in which the % relaxation is more important.

Adaptation of the Sphincter to Prolonged Stimuli

“A” shows a stimulus which is maintained for 28 secs; the sphincter recovers its tone and the fluctuation waves, in spite of the fact the rectal inflation continues (B and C) (Figure 12).

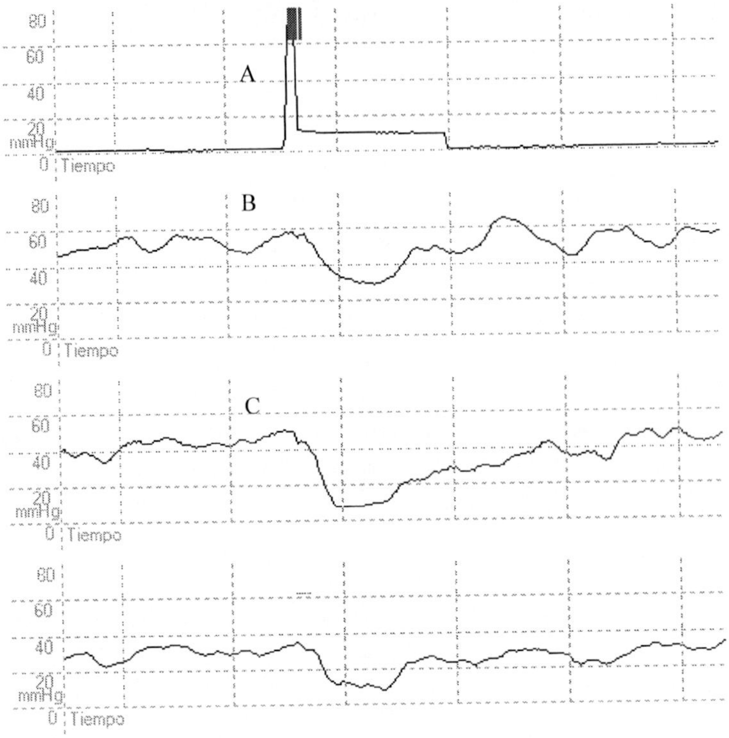

Figure 12. Adaptation of the sphincter for prolonged stimuli. Although the inflation of the balloon is maintained, pressure recovers and anorectal fluctuations appear.

False Positives

The absence of the reflex during the neonatal period is not always pathognomic of HD. We have demonstrated that the appearance of the rectosphincter reflex is independent of age, newborn weight and gestational age. On the other hand, we are not in favour of performing a rectal biopsy until the end of the neonatal period [20,21] . In our experience and that of others, there are many inappropriate diagnoses and possibilities for complications [14]. When we carry out the first exam during the child’s first week of life and there is no reflex, we usually do periodical weekly exams until the end of the neonatal period, which is when we perform the rectal biopsy. If it concurs with the manometry, we resort to surgical intervention. In some cases, for which we have not found an explanation to date, we have demonstrated the delayed appearance of the reflex and after one or more exams with the reflex absent, it appears in a subsequent exam. These cases, always during the neonatal period, are the majority of the false positives, that is, absence of the reflex which ends up not proving that the patient has HD.

Some hypotheses have been considered to explain the delay in the appearance of the reflex. The relationship of the rectoanal inhibitory reflex to the gestational age, age from birth date and newborn weight was refuted in 1992 [6]. Enterocolitis and intestinal obstruction would cause temporary achalasia which in some cases could occur at one year of age [22].

False positives do not pose any risk for the patient given that we carry out periodical weekly exams until the end of the neonatal period and we only take surgical intervention if the manometry and biopsy concur.

Non-Demonstrative Results

In newborns, whose anal canals are very affected by Digital Rectal Examinations (DREs), cleaning enemas, etc., the exam shows very low pressure in the anal canal and an absence of anorectal fluctuations; in these cases there is generally no reflex but we do not consider these as false negatives, but as non-demonstrative results due to poor conditions of the anal canal (Figure 13).

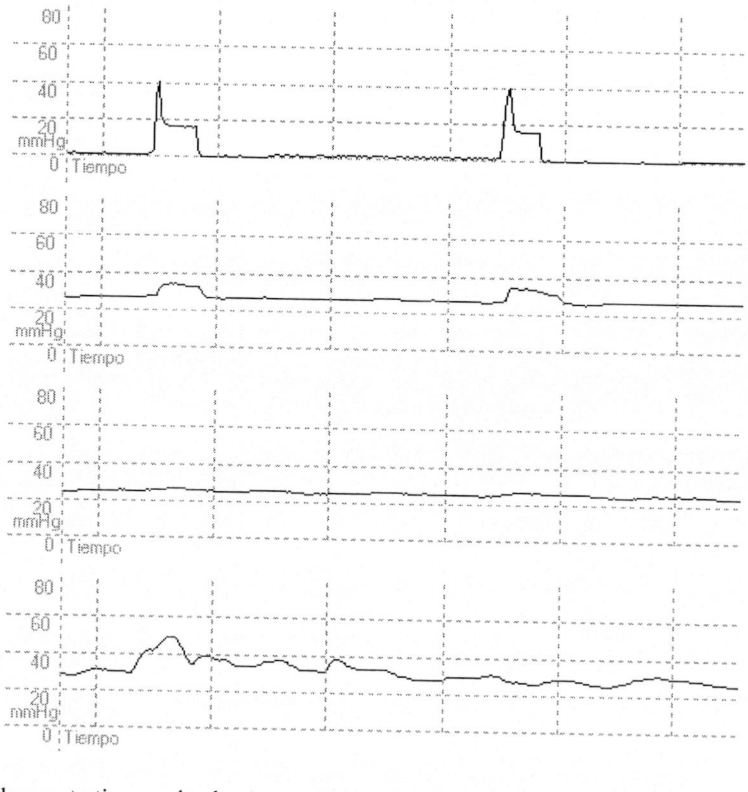

Figure 13. Non-demonstrative results, low pressure and absence of anorectal fluctuations.

Something similar occurs in newborns with sepsis (enterocolitis) and hypoxia[2,11] . In these the manometric conditions of the anal canal are similar to those of the previous group and the exam is generally non-demonstrative.

The non-functioning of the colon for a great deal of time tends to complicate both the manometric exam and the obtaining of the rectal suction biopsy. Prolonged exclusion causes an absence of anorectal fluctuations and low pressure in the anal canal. A sample containing enough submucosa is rarely obtained with forceps and suction.

False Negatives

This is when we demonstrate the presence of the reflex in patients who end up having HD. In our experience the incidence is minimal and the cause is inadvertent movements of the probe upon inflating the balloon. If we perform the exam carefully we can easily identify them. The reflex wave has two branches: one for relaxation and another for recovery. When the drop in pressure is due to movement of the probe, the latency is zero and the relaxation branch is vertical (Figure 14).

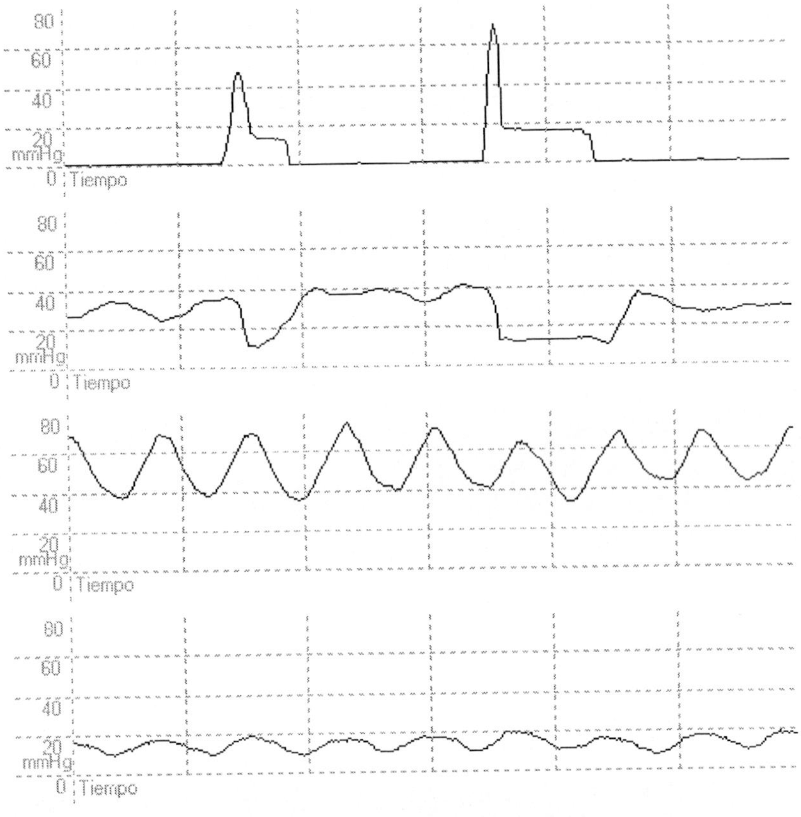

Figure 14. False negative. The drop in pressure is due to movement of the probe upon inflation of the balloon.

False negatives have serious therapeutic implications because they always delay diagnosis, increasing the incidence of enterocolitis, the most serious complication of HD [23].

Diagnostic Algorithm

In our area of influence, we perform manometry on any asymptomatic newborn with delayed meconium of more than 24 hours, and in all newborns with any symptoms of functional distal intestinal obstruction. We check those patients with an absence of the reflex (Figure 15) in the first study and we perform daily cleaning enemas with physiological serum if necessary and we repeat the study weekly until the end of the neonatal period. At this time we repeat the study and if the reflex continues to be absent (Figure 16), we perform the rectal suction biopsy and genetic study. When the biopsy report shows HD we carry out the surgical intervention, during the second month of life. This is how we have come to a correct diagnosis in all the patients we performed the surgery on. We have had no complications worth mentioning in the diagnostic method or the cleaning enemas during neonatal period, and the incidence of neonatal enterocolitis has practically disappeared.

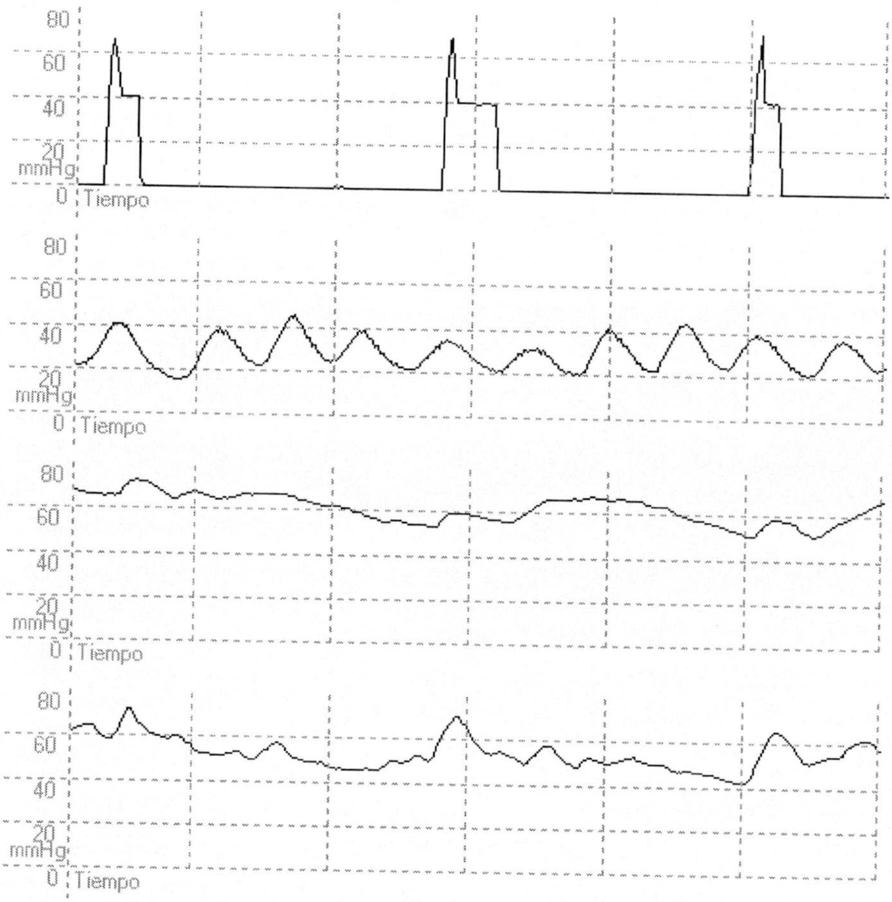

Figure 15. Anorectal reflex absent.

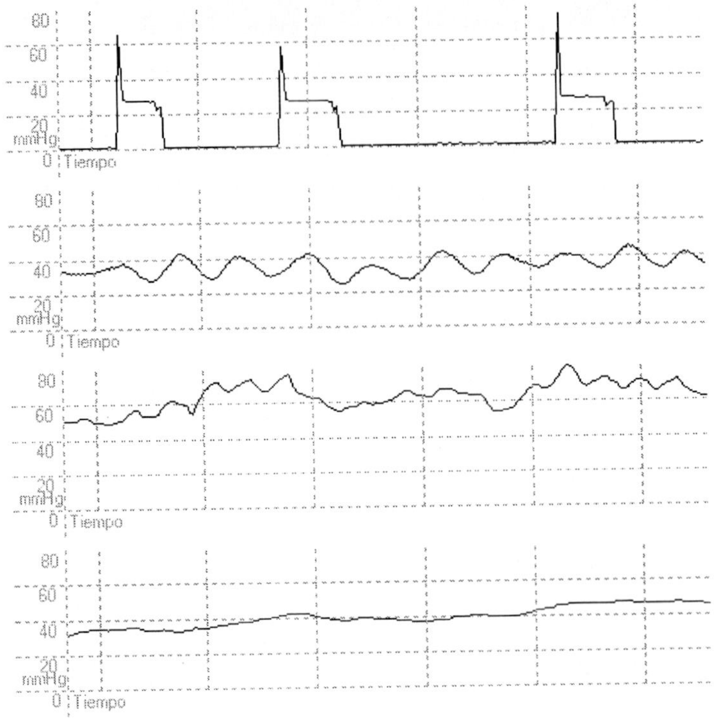

Figure 16. Anorectal reflex absent.

Results for the Period 1984-2008

During the period 10/1984 to 02/2008, we have studied 389 newborns, carrying out a total of 612 manometries, 494 of them during the first 30 days of life. 57.3% of the patients were males with an average age in the first study of 15.36 days ± 7.22 days (range: 2-29 days), a newborn weight of 3.32 ± 0.57 kg (range: 1.05-5.15 kg) and a gestational age of 39.01± 1.96 weeks (range: 29-43 weeks), with 14% of them being premature. 54.8% of them expelled meconium within the first 24 to 48 hours of life; 23.7% did so after 48 hours.

Up to 4 studies have been carried out on the same patient during the neonatal period, with results reflected in table 1, in which you can see that the percentage of children with Hirschsprung's Disease increases as we repeat the studies.

Table 1.

	Reflexes				
	Positive	Negative	Non-demonstrative	% HD	Age
Study 1	276	85	28	18 %	15.36±7.22
Study 2	36	36	3	50.7 %	19.27±7.05
Study 3	6	15	1	72.7 %	22.00±5.55
Study 4	3	5	0	62.5 %	27.75±2.43
Total	321	141	32		

The sensitivity of the manometry in our series is 99.2% with a specificity of 94.1%. The positive and negative predictive values are 85.8% and 99.7% respectively (it is easier to rule out the disease than to confirm it [16].

Therefore, only one HD patient out of every 300 manometries with the reflex being present will be erroneously recorded as not having the illness (Table 2).

Table 2.

	HD	Not HD	Total
Absent reflex	121	20	141
Present reflex	1	320	321
Total	122	340	462

Sensitivity: 121/122= 99.2 % Specificity: 320/340= 94.1 %
Positive Predictive Value: 121/141= 85.8% Negative Predictive Value: 320/321= 99.7%
Positive Likelihood Ratio: Sensitivity/1-Specificity: 16.81
Negative Likelihood Ratio: 1-Sensitivity/Specificity: 0.0085

We obtain 97.3% valid studies if we sedate the children, compared with 92.3% valid studies if the child is not sedated, with the difference being statistically significant according to the Chi-square, and there is an Odds Ratio of 2.943. Therefore, we recommend systematic use of sedation, given that the probability of obtaining a valid result is almost three times greater.

In 18 children we noted the appearance of a delayed reflex (4.63%), with the average age of the last study without a reflex being 18.06 ± 7.82 days with a range of 6-32 days. After adjusting the goodness of fit with the normality of the delayed maturation group, we did not note differences in the comparison with the Student t in weight, age, newborn weight or gestational age although greater in the delayed maturation group than in the rest of our sample. There is, however, a significant difference with respect to the corrected gestational age, which is older in these children.

We have not managed to determine any justification for this change in the clinical evolution or in the expulsion of meconium.

The existence of a delayed appearance of the reflex prevents us from making a diagnosis and pursuing definitive treatment in the first week of life. For this reason, in spite of the efficiency of neonatal manometry, we believe that the confirmation of the rectal suction biopsy is essential.

Conclusions

The usefulness of anorectal manometry in premature babies and newborns continues to be controversial. There are studies published sporadically with results that support the efficiency of manometric diagnosis during the neonatal period, but the majority doubt their efficiency during this period and the groups who carry out these exams are few and far between.

It is a diagnostic technique in which the main objective is to demonstrate the presence or absence of the relaxation reflex of the internal anal sphincter using an inflatable balloon inside the rectum. In order for the exam to be demonstrative, the reflex must be preceded and followed by anorectal fluctuations which guarantee that the pressure is being taken in the internal sphincter and that the catheter has not moved during the inflation of the balloon.

A full-time personnel is needed for these tests. This way experience, speed and safety is achieved in the exams.

Sedation shortens the time of the exam and improves the results.

We have demonstrated that neither the gestational age, nor the age from birth date or the weight of the child influence the appearance of the rectosphincter reflex. Therefore, all newborns with an absence of the reflex must be considered to have the disease.

Treatment during the neonatal period is conservative, with daily cleaning enemas and weekly manometric exams. And if the absence of the reflex persists until the end of the neonatal period, we perform the rectal suction biopsy to confirm the diagnosis. We perform definitive surgical treatment [24] during the second month of life. The incidence of enterocolitis and other complications of neonatal HD are minimal in our experience.

The absence of the reflex during the neonatal period is not pathognomic of HD. The delayed appearance of the reflex in 4.63% of our cases obliges us to repeat the exams weekly if the absence of the reflex continues, and to confirm the HD diagnosis with rectal suction biopsy at the end of the neonatal period.

False positives delay diagnosis and the cause is the inadvertent movement of the probe upon inflation of the balloon. In our experience this occurs in one out of every 300 newborn patients.

The diagnostically reliable data corresponding to our method during the period 1984-2008 are: sensitivity 99.2% (percentage of patients with HD in whom there is an absence of the reflex), specificity 94.1% (proportion of patients who do not have HD and exhibit the reflex), positive predictive value 85.8% (probability of suffering from the disease when the reflex is absent), negative predictive value 99.2% (probability of not having the disease when the reflex is present).

We confirm, that neonatal anorectal manometry with the right materials, method and specialised personnel, should always be the diagnostic method for HD and for neonatal functional distal intestinal obstruction in general in the first few days of life.

References

[1] Benninga MA, Omari TI, Haslam RR, Barnett CP, Dent J, Davidson GP. Characterization of anorectal pressure and the anorectal inhibitory reflex in healthy preterm and term infants. *J Pediatr* 2001; 139:233-7.

[2] Boston VE, Scott JE. Anorectal Manometry as a diagnostic method in the neonatal period. *J Pediatr Surg* 1976; 11:9-16.

[3] Bowes KL, Kling S. Anorectal manometry in premature infants. *J Pediatr Surg* 1979; 14:533-5.

[4] Emir H, Akman M, Sarimurat N, Kilic N, Erdogan E, Soylet Y. Anorectal manometry during the neonatal period: its specificity in the diagnosis of Hirschsprung's disease. *Eur J Pediatr Surg* 1999; 9:101-3.

[5] Loening-Baucke V, Pringle KC, Ekwo EE. Anorectal manometry for the exclusion of Hirschsprung's disease in neonates. *J Pediatr Gastroenterol Nutr* 1985;4:596-603.

[6] Lopez-Alonso M, Ribas J. Technical improvement for anorectal manometry in newborns. *J Pediatr Surg* 1991;26:1215-8.

[7] Lopez-Alonso M, Ribas J, Hernandez A, Anguita FA, Gomez dT, I, Martinez-Caro A. Efficiency of the anorectal manometry for the diagnosis of Hirschsprung's disease in the newborn period. *Eur J Pediatr Surg* 1995;5:160-3.

[8] Tamate S, Shiokawa C, Yamada C, Takeuchi S, Nakahira M, Kadowaki H. Manometric diagnosis of Hirschsprung's disease in the neonatal period. *J Pediatr Surg* 1984;19:285-8.

[9] Verder H, Krasilnikoff PA, Scheibel E. Anal tonometry in the neonatal period in mature and premature children. *Acta Paediatr Scand* 1975;64:592-6.

[10] Benninga MA, Omari TI, Haslam RR, Barnett CP, Dent J, Davidson GP. Characterization of anorectal pressure and the anorectal inhibitory reflex in healthy preterm and term infants. *J Pediatr* 2001;139:233-7.

[11] de Lorijn F, Omari TI, Kok JH, Taminiau JA, Benninga MA. Maturation of the rectoanal inhibitory reflex in very premature infants. *J Pediatr* 2003;143:630-3.

[12] de Lorijn F, Reitsma JB, Voskuijl WP, Aronson DC, Ten Kate FJ, Smets AM, et al. Diagnosis of Hirschsprung's disease: a prospective, comparative accuracy study of common tests. *J Pediatr* 2005;146:787-92.

[13] Jones MP, Post J, Crowell MD. High-resolution manometry in the evaluation of anorectal disorders: a simultaneous comparison with water-perfused manometry. *Am J Gastroenterol* 2007;102:850-5.

[14] Kawahara H, Kubota A, Hasegawa T, Okuyama H, Ueno T, Watanabe T, et al. Anorectal sleeve micromanometry for the diagnosis of Hirschsprung's disease in newborns. *J Pediatr Surg* 2007;42:2075-9.

[15] Lopez AM, Hernandez Org, Ribas SJ. Reliability index of anorectal manometry for the diagnosis of Hirschspurng disease. *Cir Pediatr* 2005;18:13-6.

[16] Aaronson I, Nixon HH. A clinical evaluation of anorectal pressure studies in the diagnosis of Hirschsprung's disease. *Gut* 1972 Feb;13:138-46.

[17] R. Núñez, I. Vargas, I. Rubio, R. Cabrera, E. Blesa: Anorectal manometry in newborn *Pediatr Surg Int* 1995; 10:105-7.

[18] Pfefferkorn MD, Croffie JM, Corkins MR, Gupta SK, Fitzgerald JF. Impact of sedation and anesthesia on the rectoanal inhibitory reflex in children. *J Pediatr Gastroenterol Nutr* 2004;38:324-7.

[19] Schuster MM, Hendrix TR, Mendeloff AI. The internal anal sphincter response: manometric studies on its normal physiology, neural pathways, and alteration in bowel disorders. *J Clin Invest* 1963;42:196-207.

[20] Cusick EL, Buick RG. Injury to the common iliac artery during suction rectal biopsy. *J Pediatr Surg* 1995;30:111-2.

[21] Rees BI, Azmy A, Nigam M, Lake BD. Complications of rectal suction biopsy. *J Pediatr Surg* 1983;18:273-5.

[22] Verder H, Krasilnikoff PA, Scheibel E. Anal tonometry in the neonatal period in mature and premature children. *Acta Paediatr Scand* 1975;64:592-6.

[23] Kleinhaus S, Boley SJ, Sheran M, Sieber WK. Hirschsprung's disease -- a survey of the members of the Surgical Section of the American Academy of Pediatrics. *J Pediatr Surg* 1979;14:588-97.

[24] De la Torre L, Ortega A. Transanal versus open endorectal pull-through for Hirschsprung's disease. *J Pediatr Surg* 2000;35:1630-2.

In: Hirschsprung's Disease: Diagnosis and Treatment
Ed: Ramón Núñez and Manuel López-Alonso

ISBN: 978-1-60741-349-3

Chapter X

Radiological Diagnosis of Hirschsprung's Disease During the Neonatal Period

Manuel López-Alonso and J.Fernando Prieto

Introduction

The barium enema was the first method for diagnosing Hirschsprung's Disease (HD) [1], and it remained the first-choice method for many years, always combined with a formal biopsy followed by a rectal suction biopsy for definite confirmation.

Over time, with the advances achieved using two other methods, rectal suction biopsy and anorectal manometry, the diagnostic reliability indices from these three methods have relegated the barium enema to third place.

Barium enema has lost favour as a diagnostic method to anorectal manometry and rectal biopsy, but has also gained favour unexpectedly due to the evolution of surgical techniques. The transrectal Soave procedure is displacing the classic Soave-Boley, Swenson, and Duhamel procedures. This procedure may be employed when the aganglionic segment is limited to the rectosigmoid area. The aid of a laparoscopy or a minilaparotomy is required when the segment reaches the descending and transverse intestine, excluding the Lester-Martin procedure, which many surgeons prefer in the case of total colonic aganglionosis.

Determining the length of the aganglionic segment before beginning the procedure is much more important now that the transrectal technique is in favour than it was when all of techniques began as laparotomies; then, the first step was to take samples from the narrow, apparently normal transition zone to determine the length of the aganglionic segment.

The relevance of the barium enema depends on what services the hospital can offer. If its capabilities include neonatal rectal manometry and rectal suction biopsy, the main use of the enema is to precisely locate the funnel-shaped transition zone (TZ) that joins the spastic segment with the narrowed distal proximal dilation [1]. If the TZ is in the rectosigmoid colon or the distal descending colon, we can choose the transrectal technique.

Unfortunately, the TZ cannot be seen in all HD patients, and secondly, when we compare the zone length indicated by the barium enema with the result of the biopsy, they do not coincide; the TZ is always longer. The results correspond more closely for short segments than for long segments, when this information is all the more crucial to the surgeon's choice of what technique to use [2].

For this reason, before choosing the surgical technique, many surgeons prefer to perform minilaparotomy or laparoscopy to do complete biopsies of the narrow segment, the transition zone and the apparently normal segment in order to know the exact length of the aganglionic segment.

Technique and Patient Preparation

The technique originated with Neuhauser, and was based on studies undertaken by Swenson [1]. During the neonatal period it is not advisable to administer cleansing enemas 24 hours previous to the barium enema, in order to avoid temporary dilation of the aganglionic segment and so as not to eliminate faeces that make the dilated area more prominent. Cleansing enemas in the newborn may make it more difficult to locate the TZ.

A *barium suspension* is used as a contrast material, which has a higher absorption coefficient than biologic tissues do. Barium, atomic number 56, atomic weight 137, is a radio-opaque heavy metal with high absorption of X-rays. The chemical used for the barium enema is *microcrystalline barium sulphate*. This salt is insoluble throughout the digestive tract, and is therefore atoxic. It is an inert substance that is not absorbed and does not alter normal physiological function.

The patient is placed in a left lateral position with the legs flexed. The suspension is introduced into the anal passage under pressure so as not to artificially distend the distal aganglionic segment, by means of a rectal probe. The probe has a stopper 1cm from its end that is connected to a *50 cc syringe* filled with warmed diluted barium.

Barium sulphate diluted in physiological saline at the approximate temperature of the anal passage (37°C) is slowly introduced until the liquid reaches the funnel-shaped transition zone. The radioscopic view at the moment when the solution enters the transition zone is more important than the static image. Once the TZ is located, solution must continue to be introduced so as to locate where the dilated part ends and the colon is normal (Figure 1 with TZ in the rectosigmoid).

Anteroposterior, oblique, and left and right lateral images are taken. The probe is removed without evacuating the contrast material and anteroposterior and lateral test radiographs are taken 24 hours later. If the barium is eliminated slowly, it is an additional sign that points to HD; also, the TZ is often seen more clearly in this radiograph than with the enema on the previous day (Figure 2, plain radiograph 24 hours later)

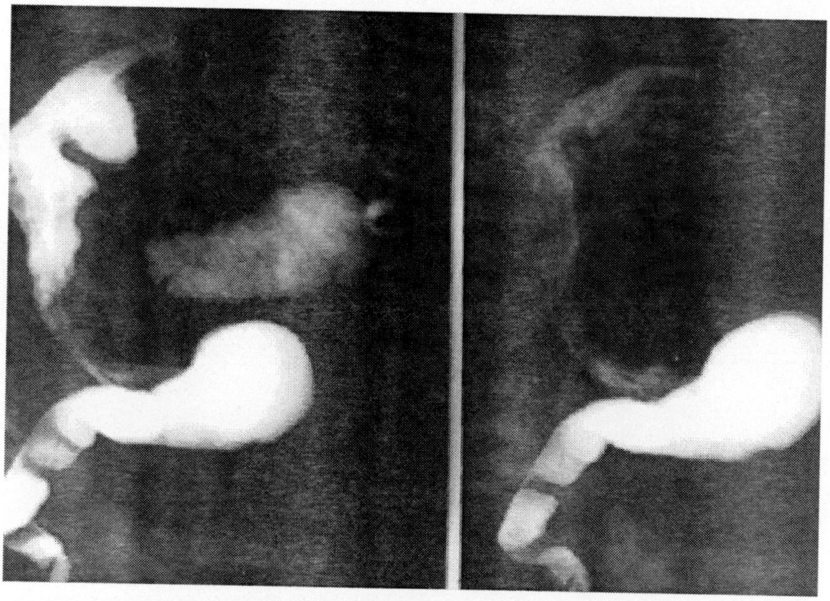

Figure 1. Barium enema: TZ located at the sigmoid level.

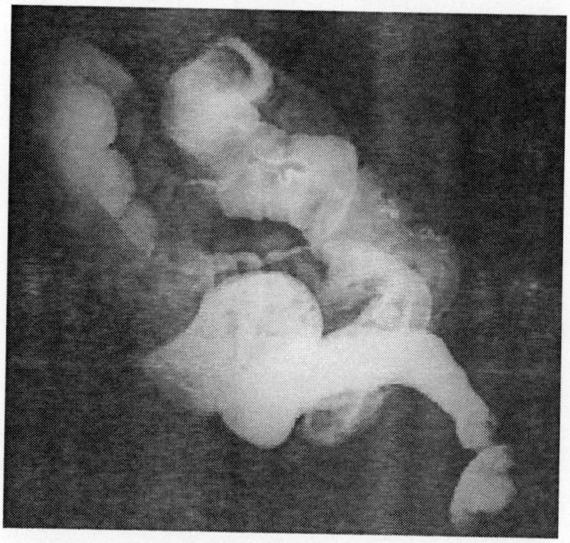

Figure 2. Plain abdominal radiograph 24 hours after administration of the barium enema.

Results Suggesting HD

Vertical, anteroposterior and lateral-view *plain abdominal radiograph*: when HD begins with a clinical profile of distal intestinal obstruction with inability to pass meconium, abdominal distention and vomiting, a plain radiograph often shows dilated loops of bowel, megacolon and absence of air distally or a narrow air-fluid image corresponding to the narrowed distal segment (Figure 3). When the clinical profile is not so apparent, we find dilated loops of bowel with absence of air distally.

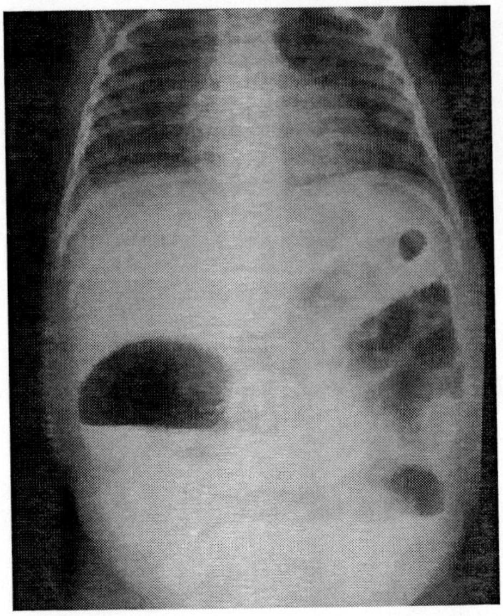

Figure 3. Vertical-beam abdominal radiograph: absence of air distally and megacolon.

Horizontal plain abdominal radiograph (PAR): In newborns, the TZ is more easily seen in horizontal radiographs than with the contrast enema. In a comparative study between the PARTZ (Plain Abdominal Radiograph Transition Zone) and the CETZ (Contrast Enema Transition Zone) in newborns, it was shown that the TZ was located by enema in 67% of the cases and using horizontal radiography in 89% of the cases, and that furthermore, the enema findings coincided with the anatomopathology in 72% of the cases, and with plain radiographs in 92% of the cases. Therefore, horizontal radiography in newborns is more precise than the enema method for locating the TZ [3] (Figure 4A and 4B).

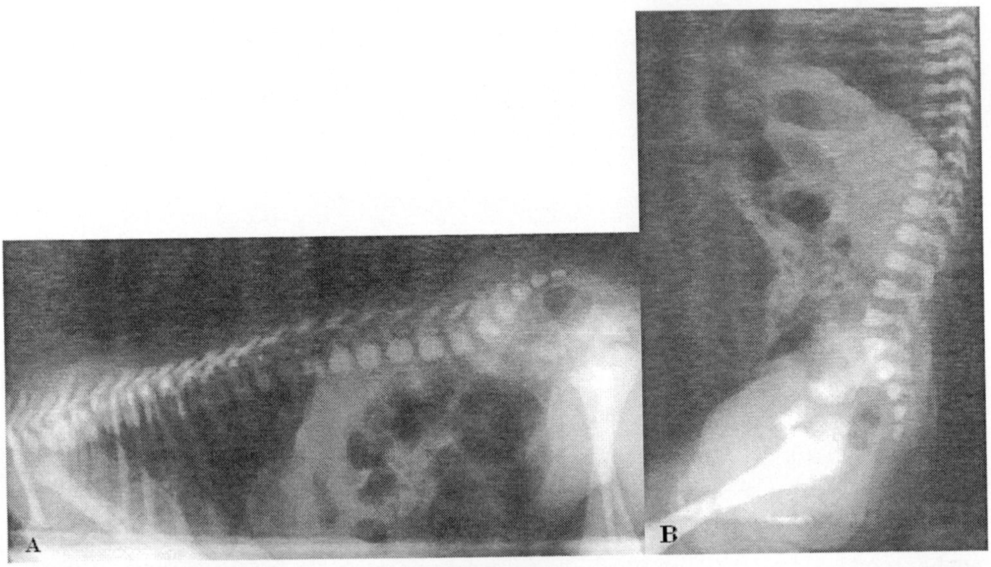

Figure 4A. Prone position. Horizontal Beam Lateral Projection. Figure 4B. Lateral vertical position.

Barium enema: Tolerance is increased upon introducing barium, which easily permits the entire colon to be filled. The barium enema procedure focuses on three highly characteristic zones: a *dilated zone*, a *transition zone* (with spiculated or serrated edges) and the *stenotic zone*, which continues to the end of the rectum. In newborns, the enema procedure tends not to be very revealing, particularly in the first two weeks of life, whereas with older children it can be used to observe these details specific to the disease.

Radiographic variables: the colon's response to the injected contrast matter is always abnormal for patients with HD, and their CE normally shows one or more of the following abnormalities: transition zone (TZ), abnormal rectosigmoid ratio, retained contrast in the postevacuation film, abnormalities of the rectal mucosal folds, and microcolon [3].

Out of the above list of radiological abnormalities, the TZ has the best diagnostic reliability index.

The TZ is a transition zone that is present between the dilated, normal proximal colon and the obstructed distal colon which is narrower because of the inability of the aganglionic intestine to relax [1]. The transition zone is not usually apparent before the first or second week of life; in the radiograph, it can be seen as an infundibular zone in the intestine, between the dilated proximal colon and the constricted distal colon.

According to the area where the TZ is located, radiology is said to show *ultrashort* segments when the TZ is present in the rectum, *typical* segments when in the sigmoidal loop, and so on, followed by the descending colon, splenic angle, transverse colon, hepatic angle, ascending colon, caecum (long-segment) and total segments when the terminal ileum is affected. The aganglionic segment may show irregular, saw-tooth borders (Figure 5).

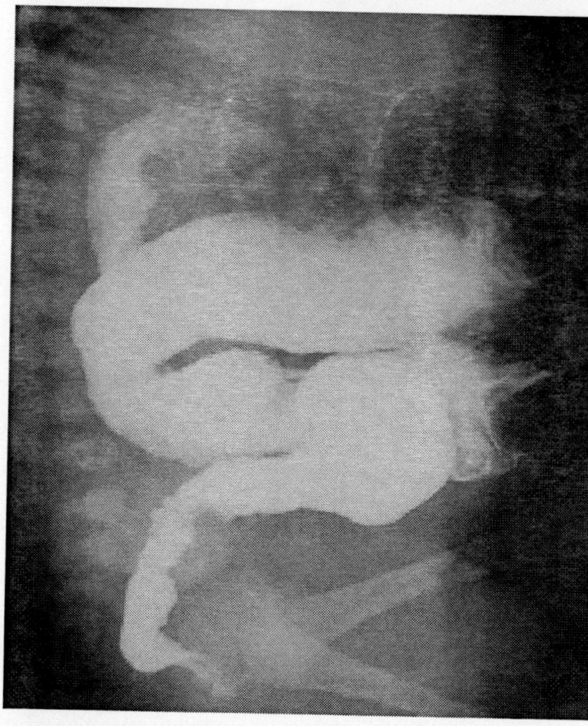

Figure 5. Saw-tooth appearance of the aganglionic segment.

Additionally, we should stress the usefulness of radiographies taken 24 hours after injecting the contrast material, as they provide a clearer image than the first one. Furthermore, if a significant quantity of barium remains in the colon after 24 hours, it may be another indication of HD, even when no transition zone was identified. Evacuation of the barium solution may take up to 14 days in children with Hirschsprung's disease.

Abnormal rectosigmoid ratio: The Pochaczeusky's index is usually employed [4]. The widest diameter of the rectum is divided by the widest diameter of the sigmoid; both measurements are taken when the colon is full of barium and without using a balloon, which would distend and obstruct the anus. The diameter of the rectum is measured at any point distal to the third sacral vertebra, and the diameter of the sigmoid, at any point along the sigmoidal loop. The projections are normally taken in anteroposterior, right and left oblique posterior and lateral positions. The highest value obtained from any projection is used. When the ratio is less than 0,8, HD is diagnosed (Figure 6).

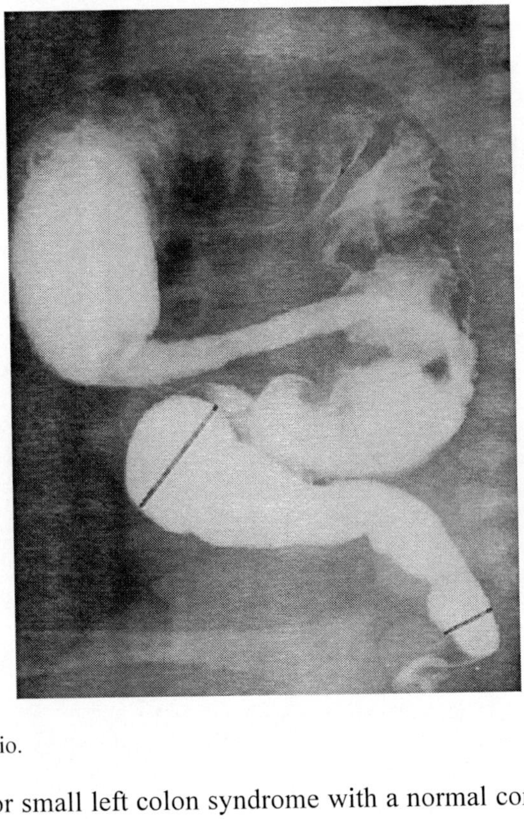

Figure 6. Rectosigmoid ratio.

In meconial plug or small left colon syndrome with a normal contrast enema, the ratio is greater than or equal to 1. It is not useful in the case of total colonic aganglionism [5].

The diagnostic reliability indices for the CE range between 50 and 80%, clearly inferior to rectal manometry (RM) and rectal suction biopsy (RSB) with indices above 90%.

The RTZ described by Swenson is a variable-length, funnel-shaped zone situated in the normally dilated, innervated area and the narrow distal aganglionic zone. It is the best radiological indicator for diagnosing HD. It is present in 50-90% of the patients. It is not identified in all HD patients and it is found in a significant number of patients with idiopathic constipation, although it is more common in HD patients (80%) than in those with idiopathic constipation (IC) [6,7] (45%).

When the RTZ is in the rectosigmoid, the sensitivity is at 62% and the specificity 100%. If we consider all points, the sensitivity increases to 70% and the specificity drops to 80%, which indicates a higher percentage of false positives when the RTZ is located outside of the rectosigmoid [7].

Currently, the TZ is not important for the diagnosis of HD, since, as we have seen, it is far less reliable than RM and RSB; rather, it is an important pre-intervention indicator of the length of the aganglionic segment. 79% of all of the RTZ correspond with the level of the aganglionic segment. When the RTZ is in the rectosigmoid, this percentage reaches 90%. This means that the error rate is at best 10% and that for long segments, it is much higher [7].

Until the last decade this was of no importance because all surgical procedures used in the definitive correction of HD, Swenson, Duhamel or Soave, the first step was to do a laparotomy and complete biopsies of the narrow, transition and dilated zones in order to locate the aganglionic segment.

In the last decade, a new transrectal technique emerged that made the laparotomy unnecessary in cases where the aganglionic segment did not reach the descending colon. This procedure clearly offered benefits to the patient, such as fewer complications, less hospital stay time, and excellent results. For these reasons it has become popular and is currently performed in most centres.

However, if this technique is initiated and it is discovered later that the aganglionic zone extends further, a laparoscopy/minilaparotomy will also be needed; in the case of total colonic aganglionism, a surgeon who prefers the Lester-Martin procedure may not carry it out.

The CE has lost favour as a method of diagnosing HD because of its low reliability indices compared with RM and RSB, but is now on the rise due to the general preference for the transrectal technique and the need to know the length of the aganglionic segment.

As we have seen, the TZ error rate is at best 11%, which is high enough for some surgeons to prefer using a biopsy to confirm the length of the aganglionic segment before beginning the transrectal intervention.

For short segments, the concordance between the aganglionic segment and the RTZ ranges between 70-90%, and for long segments, it is only 25%; it is in these cases where the transrectal technique may cause problems.

The discordance between the length indicated by the RTZ and the diseased segment is not due to the radiologist's interpretation of the RTZ, since different radiologists coincide in the reading of the same CE 90,6% of the time.

Total colonic aganglionism (TCA): The aganglionic segment may appear serrated or irregularly-shaped in local projections. This finding is particularly useful for recognising long-segment aganglionosis, because, apart from a certain shortness of the colon which causes the caecum to be displaced upward, this shape may be the only anomaly. There is no narrow segment, and the colon has a uniform width which is smaller than usual. The colonic frame is rounded, with less definition of the splenic and hepatic angles (Figure 7 A, B).

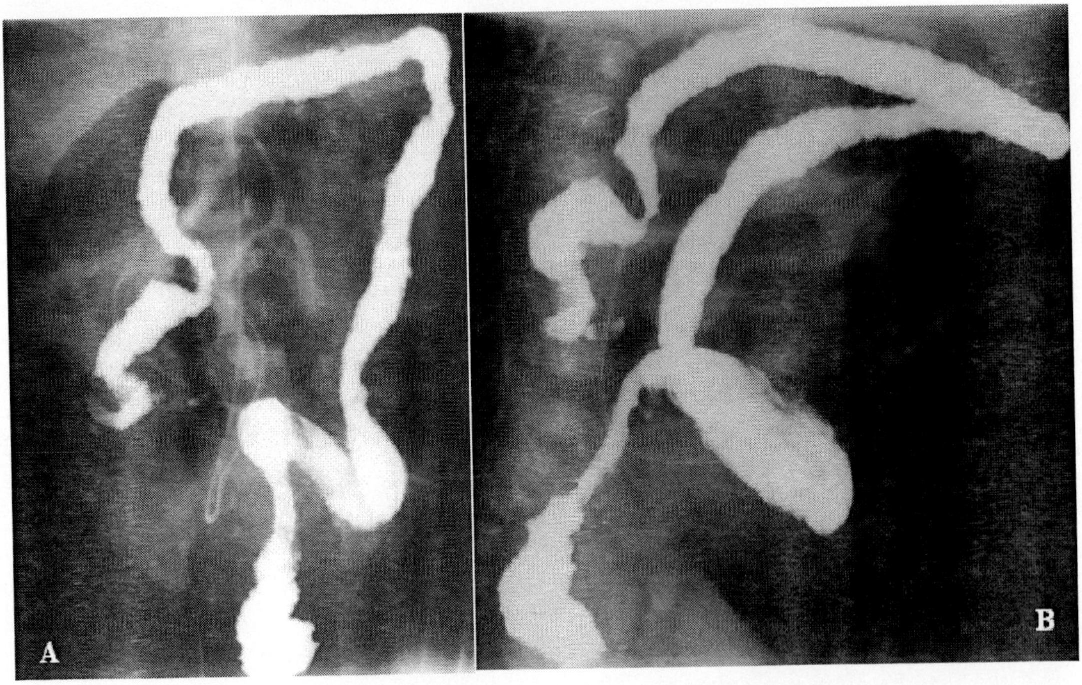

Figure 7. A, B Total colonic aganglionism. Poorly-defined hepatic and splenic angles. Smaller and no narrow segment.

In this variety, the small intestine is normally dilated and similar in appearance to one affected by meconium ileum, with meconium masses filling the loops of the terminal ileum or the caecum. The incidence of these cases ranges from 5 and 15 % of all HD patients; the length of the aganglionic segment affects the entire colon as well as 30-50 cm of the terminal ileum.

For these cases, many surgeons prefer the Lester Martin procedure. This intervention is ruled out if, given the diagnosis of HD, the transrectal intervention is initiated and the biopsy results confirm the existence of TCA. For this reason, it is especially important to know the segment length before beginning the intervention.

Unfortunately, radiological findings for TCA in the neonatal period are neither specific nor pathognomonic [8]. In most cases, the colon is of normal diameter; in 23%, it is short; in 23% it is a microcolon; in 46%, there are irregularities in the colon wall, and in 33% there is a contrast material reflux into the ileum. All of these findings are present in HD and allied disorders in neonates[9].

Basic Considerations When Interpreting the CE

The CE is more useful as an initial way of knowing the length of the aganglionic segment than for diagnosing HD [10]. The diagnosis reliability indices from anorectal manometry and rectal suction biopsy are higher than those from the CE. Inject the contrast material under low pressure using a syringe connected to a rubber probe with a small stopper at the 1cm mark.

Locate the funnel-shaped area: it is the transition point between the distal aganglionic zone and the dilated proximal zone.Note the difference in diameter between the aganglionic segment and the transition zone.

The TZ is identified in 50-90% of CE; in 80% of those patients with HD and in 45% of those with idiopathic constipation (IC). The TZ is not seen in cases of total colonic aganglionism. With respect to biopsy readings in the best possible cases (where the TZ is located in the rectosigmoid), the TZ is located with a precision of 90%. In long segments, this percentage drops to 25%.

Horizontal radiography identifies TZ in neonates more accurately than a CE. Other data observable in the CE that may increase its value as a diagnostic tool for HD, other than the TZ, are a serrated appearance and irregularities along the outline of the colon, a rectosigmoid index below 0,8, a 24-hour delay in the elimination of contrast material, shortened colon, and lastly, ileocecal valve incompetence with contrast flux to the terminal ileum. However, the best indicator is the TZ.

If the surgeon prefers the transrectal technique for surgical correction of HD and the Lester Martin procedure for TCA, he or she should perform biopsies before initiating the transrectal procedure so as to be sure of the length of the piece to be resected.

Results

We examined 137 patients whom we had diagnosed with HD and corrected surgically, excluding those with total colonic aganglionism. 123 cases, or 89%, showed a TZ.

The most common TZ location was the rectosigmoid in 61 cases, 64,7% (Table 1). We compared the length shown by radiology with the length proven by anatomical pathology and the concordance coefficient (Kappa index) is 0,1059 (95% CI: 0-0,2185), with the agreement to consider an index below 0,20 as indicating poor concordance

Table 1. Transition zone in 123 cases

		Length of segment:							
		Rectum	Rectosigmoid	Descending colon	Splenic angle	Transverse colon	Hepatic angle	Ascending colon	Total
Radiological Transition Zone	Rectum	**1**	21	6	1	0	0	0	29
	Rectosigmoid	0	**38**	17	1	3	1	1	61
	Descending colon	0	3	**4**	0	3	2	2	14
	Splenic angle	0	3	2	**2**	3	1	4	15
	Transverse colon	0	0	2	0	**1**	0	0	3
	Hepatic A.	0	0	1	0	0	**0**	0	1
	Ascending colon	0	0	0	0	0	0	**0**	0
	Total	1	65	32	4	10	4	7	123

The best relation between the TZ and the affected segment is when the TZ is located in the rectosigmoid with a coefficient of agreement of 43,18% (moderate concordance).

Concordance table for Radiology vs. Anatomical Pathology: On the diagonal and in bold: those cases in which there is concordance between both tests, which should be in the majority if there is good concordance. Note the large number of enemas with a radiological diagnosis of the rectum (29/123), which is not the case for pathology (1/123).

References

[1] Svenson O, Neuhauser EBD, Pickett LK. New concepts of the etiology, diagnosis and treatments of congenital megacolon (Hirschsprung's disease). *Pediatrics* 1948;4:201-9.

[2] Jamieson DH, Dundas SE, Belushi SA, Cooper M, Blair GK. Does the transition zone reliably delineate aganglionic bowel in Hirschsprung's disease? *Pediatr Radiol* 2004;34:811-5.

[3] Pratap A, Gupta DK, Tiwari A, Sinha AK, Bhatta N, Singh SN, et al. Application of a plain abdominal radiograph transition zone (PARTZ) in Hirschsprung's disease. *BMC Pediatr* 2007;7:5.

[4] Pochaczevsky R, Leonidas JC. The "recto-sigmoid index". A measurement for the early diagnosis of Hirschsprung's disease. *Am J Roentgenol Radium Ther Nucl Med* 1975; 123:770-7.

[5] Siegel MJ, Shackelford GD, McAlister WH. The rectosigmoid index. *Radiology* 1981; 139:497-9.

[6] O'Donovan AN, Habra G, Somers S, Malone DE, Rees A, Winthrop AL. Diagnosis of Hirschsprung's disease. *AJR Am J Roentgenol* 1996;167:517-20.

[7] Proctor ML, Traubici J, Langer JC, Gibbs DL, Ein SH, Daneman A, et al. Correlation between radiographic transition zone and level of aganglionosis in Hirschsprung's disease: Implications for surgical approach. *J Pediatr Surg* 2003;38:775-8.

[8] De Campo JF, Mayne V, Boldt DW, De Campo M. Radiological findings in total aganglionosis coli. *Pediatr Radiol* 1984;14:205-9.

[9] Hayakawa K, Hamanaka Y, Suzuki M, Nakatsu M, Nishimura K, Tanaka M, et al. Radiological findings in total colon aganglionosis and allied disorders. *Radiat Med* 2003;21:128-34.

[10] Diamond IR, Casadiego G, Traubici J, Langer JC, Wales PW. The contrast enema for Hirschsprung disease: predictors of a false-positive result. *J Pediatr Surg* 2007;42:792-5.

In: Hirschsprung's Disease: Diagnosis and Treatment
Ed: Ramón Núñez and Manuel López-Alonso
ISBN: 978-1-60741-349-3

Chapter XI

Morphological Diagnosis of Hirschsprung's Disease: Rectal Suction Biopsy

Dolores I. Segura and Manuel López-Alonso

Introduction

Intestinal aganglionosis represents a heterogeneous group of anomalies of the enteric nervous system including Hirschsprung´s disease (HD), intestinal neuronal dysplasia (IND), hypoganglionosis and sphincter neurogenic achalasia, although only HD is widely acknowledged as a clinicopathologic entity.

HD is a congenital disorder of the intrinsic innervation of the gastrointestinal tract resulting from the absence of ganglion cells in the submucosal (Meissner) and myenteric (Auerbach) plexuses. The affected segment extends from the internal anal sphincter and has a variable distance, although the rectosigmoid area is usually the most affected region (75% of cases). Aganglionosis extends to the transverse colon in 15% of patients and 10% of them show complete aganglionosis of the colon. Ultrashort segment Hirschsprung´s disease (aganglionosis limited to the area of the internal anal sphincter) affects 14 – 20% of patients with aganglionosis.

HD shows a variety of clinical manifestations being constipation and functional occlusion or subocclusion of distal intestinal segments the most common. Enterocolitis and intestinal perforation are the most serious complications in the neonatal period and occasionally at onset of the disorder, with a high mortality rate.

Clinical diagnosis of HD must be immediately suspected in neonates who fail to pass meconium in the first 24 hours of life; in the presence of functional occlusion of distal intestinal segments, enterocolitis alternating with constipation periods or in the presence of constipation which does not respond to therapy.

The diagnosis is confirmed with the help of unprepared barium enema of colon showing a transition zone (region adjacent to the contracted aganglionic portion) and manometry failing to show internal anal sphincter relaxation on air-filled balloon. At present, the final diagnosis is based upon the demonstration of absence of ganglion cells in the rectal suction biopsy and the increase of positive fibers in the histochemical demonstration of Acetilcholinesterase (AchE).

Material and Methods

Material

Suction rectal biopsy for the diagnosis of Hirschsprung´s disease (HD) and in general for the diagnosis of functional occlusion of distal intestinal segments is carried out in the Unit of digestive function tests of the Children Hospital Virgen del Rocío since 1974 using Dobbins and Bill technique modified by Noblett in 1969, which is suitable for accurately establishing the presence or absence of ganglion cells in the submucosal plexus [1].

Methods

The above mentioned unit is a tertiary-level unit where HD screening for the whole of Andalusia is performed, about 10 million inhabitants. The appointment is sent to patients by mail. Patients must perform cleansing enemas with physiological serum some days before the test, depending on the age of patients, and 2-hour fasting if they are less than 7 years old.

Once the patient is examined, we determine the necessity to sedate them. But, in general, patients < 7 are always sedated. We use oral chloral hydrate 75-100 mg/K for sedation.

First of all, we carry out the manometric registry. If we do not observe rectosphincter reflex or whenever relaxation is not complete we use the conventional method of syringe suction rectal biopsy (SRB).

In order to carry out the procedure, we take advantage of the sedation and preparation of the anal canal used for manometry. Once the manometric registry is completed, the patient is placed in the lateral decubitus position and the legs are elevated in the knee-chest position (Figure 1).

We use Noblett biopsy forceps (Figure 2): a small portion of rectal mucosa and submucosa is drawn into the side aperture of a biopsy capsule by means of suction, manometrically measured. This portion is subsequently excised by the piston-like movement of a cylindrical knife enclosed within the capsule. This instrument allows 12-15 cm of suction with respect to the anal verge and it is equipped with a suction mechanism consisting in a syringe connected to a manometer which allows to control the aspiration pressure. Once the capsule is introduced into the anal canal at the convenient point, the assistant immediately applies suction of 20 to 25 mercury inches (643-700 mmHg) for 2 to 3 seconds with the syringe while the knife is rapidly closed. This method produces a mucosal biopsy specimen of 3,5-5 mm in diameter with at least 2mm of attached mucosa causing minimal distortion [1].

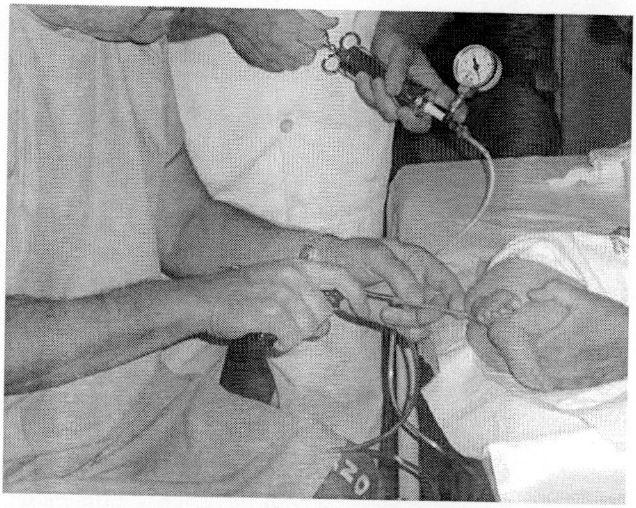

Figure 1. Patient placed in the lateral decubitus position.

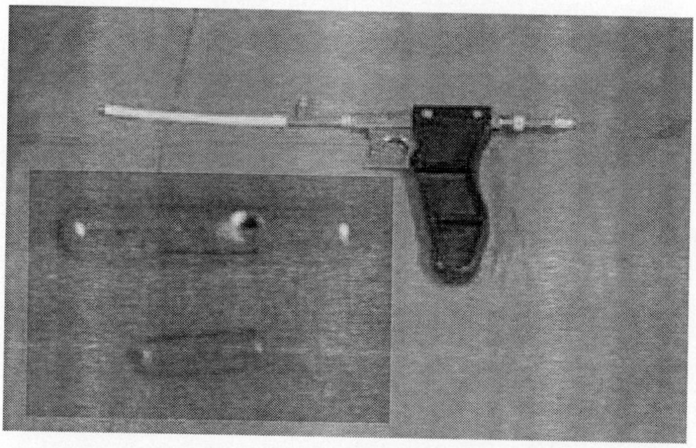

Figure 2. Noblet Biopsy forcep

We normally collect three samples at 2, 4 and 6 cms above the dentate line. Only a few complications have been described: serious bleeding, perforation, sepsis and perirectal fibrosis, always in neonates [2-4].

Biopsy is exceptionally performed in the neonatal period. Rectal suction biopsy has been widely employed by most institutions managing patients with HD for years. The review of the literature shows that few publications report complications associated with this technique. All complications occur in the neonatal period but they are serious and we even find a case of exitus. Rees et al [4] in 1983 published 5 cases of full-thickness biopsy specimens in neonates: 3 patients showed clinical signs of perforation, one of whom died of pelvic sepsis, and three suffered hemorrhage requiring transfusion. According to Rees perforation is more dangerous distal to peritoneal reflection. Cusick et al [2] report a case of a 20-day-old newborn infant who underwent biopsies at 2, 4 and 6 cm. Probably this last biopsy perforated the iliac vein provoking hypovolemic shock and putting the life of the patient at risk. It is not advisable to take biopsy specimens more than 4cm from the anal verge. A posterior approach is likely to be safer than an anterior or lateral one. Jani in 1989 [3] published a case of a 3-day-old infant with necrosis of the leg following rectal suction biopsy.

On the other hand, biopsy results in neonates reach 71% of false positives of the series according to our experience and the reports of various authors [5]. Consequently, tests must be repeated very often.

Taking into account these facts and our own experience, we do not normally carry out biopsies in the neonatal period.

In the case of preterms and neonates during their first 30 days of life, we perform anorectal manometry and opaque enema. Manometry yields a high sensitivity and specificity and allows us to choose patients and treat them until the end of the neonatal period when a suction rectal biopsy is performed in those patients who continue to show absence of rectosphincter reflex.

We recommend to continue with the cleansing enemas for 2 or 3 days after collection of biopsy sample and to wait 12-15 days to start definite treatment in case the biopsy confirms HD diagnosis. We employ Soave procedure and it is advisable to wait the period above mentioned to avoid perforation of mucosa when endorectal dissection is performed.

The following preventive measures should be taken for the adequate reception of the biopsy samples: avoid its desecation and the effect of high temperatures. The biopsy material is wrapped in sterile gauze soaked in physiologic serum stored in crushed ice and sent for examination in a wide-mouthed container. The time elapsing from the collection to the reception of the sample must not surpass 10 or 15 minutes.

Suction rectal biopsy does not require total anesthesia and if performed adequately it must yield mucosa and a superficial portion of submucosa which allows for the demonstration of presence or absence of ganglion cells in Meissner´s plexus. Samples can be collected at different levels and complications are rare. This procedure can be repeated if necessary.

The disadvantage of this type of biopsy when compared with transmural biopsy is that the sample obtained is quite small (2 – 3 mm). Sometimes the biopsy is very superficial and it does not include submucosa [6]. Submucosal plexuses are spaced out, diffuse and their study requires the collection of various samples for the demonstration of presence or absence of ganglion cells. Ganglion cells in the submucosal plexuses are more sparse, smaller and more difficult to identify. The samples must be frozen, therefore the transportation of the sample until it is frozen must be carried out carefully.

The importance of the enzymatic histochemical study for the diagnosis of HD in rectal suction biopsy is widely established. The first results of the histochemical demonstration of AchE as an adjuvant procedure in the diagnosis of HD were published by Meier-Ruge [7]. These authors highlight the value of the AChE staining method in the diagnosis of HD and this is also our opinion. In patients with HD we observe the absence of ganglion cells and an increase in AChE activity in nerve fibers of the lamina propria mucosae and submucous layers (Figure 3) whereas in normal patients AChE activity is significantly reduced in these same regions (Figure 4).

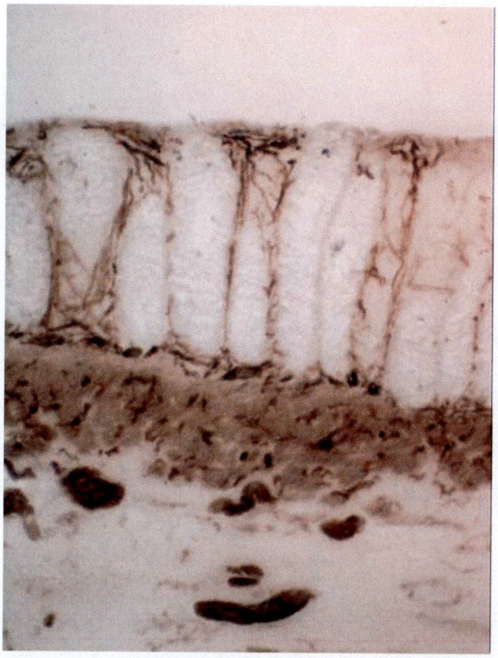

Figure 3. Rectal suction biopsy showing increase of AChE activity in parasympathetic nerve fibers of the lamina propria mucosae, muscularis mucosae and submucous layer. Aganglionosis of the rectum (HD). (AChE reaction without counterstaining; x 90).

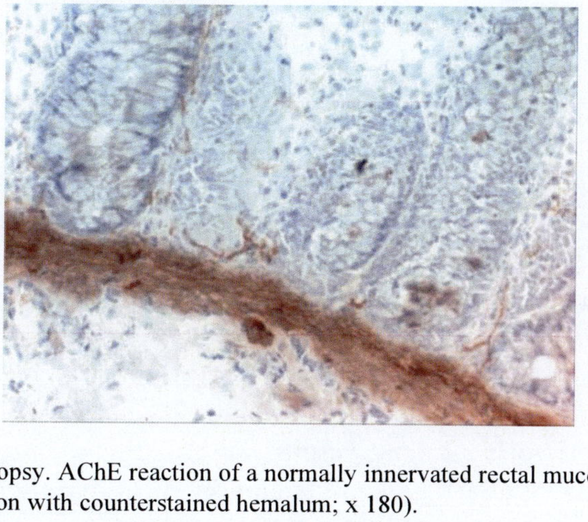

Figure 4. Rectal suction biopsy. AChE reaction of a normally innervated rectal mucosa, with slightly stained nerve fibers. (AChE reaction with counterstained hemalum; x 180).

Although AChE staining is a useful histochemical technique, it should not be used exclusively, being necessary to determine the presence of ganglion cells in seriated sections reacted for dehydrogenases. The main reason is the percentage of false negatives we obtain (at least 10%). Neonates, particularly premature infants, contribute to this percentage.

If in a biopsy sample of an adequate size which contains enough submucosa we observe a normal AChE pattern but an absence of ganglion cells in seriated sections, the diagnosis of HD cannot be discarded. Likewise, if we analyze a superficial biopsy sample without submucosa a normal AChE staining is not enough to exclude the diagnosis of HD.

Biopsy Management

Valid sample. A biopsy sample is valid for diagnosis if it contains mucosa and enough portion of superficial submucosa. Otherwise the sample will not be useful for diagnosis (Figure 5).

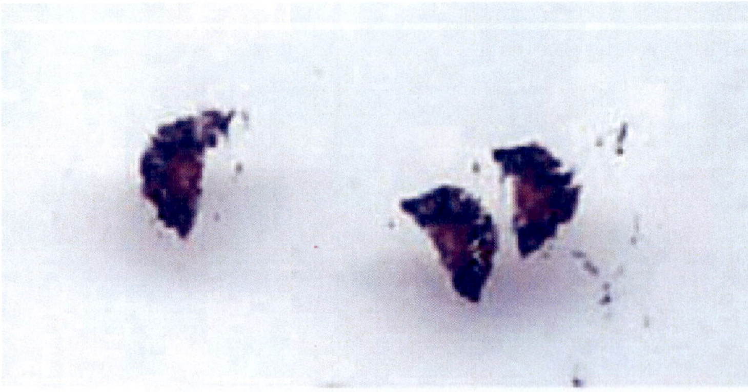

Figure 5. Rectal suction biopsy. Valid samples containing mucosa and superficial portion of submucosa. (Hematoxylin-eosine; x 40).

Lymph nodes displace the lamina propria mucosae and muscularis mucosae and may mask the characteristics of HD. Another criterion to establish the validity of a biopsy sample is to obtain it from the area above the region close to the anus, usually aganglionic.

Biopsy Transportation

The necessary preventive measures to take for the adequate reception of the biopsy sample are to avoid its desecation and the effect of high temperatures. In order to do so the sample should be wrapped in sterile gauze soaked in physiological serum and sent to Anatomopathology for examination. The time elapsing from the collection of the sample to its reception should not surpass 15 minutes. The biopsy is frozen in isopentano (methylbutano) and stored in a -80ºC refrigerator. Frozen biopsies can be stored at -25ºC.

In order to evaluate AChE staining results, we classified the degree of proliferation of AChE positive fibers as follows: (-) no proliferation of AChE positive fibers was observed in the lamina propria mucosae; (+) slight proliferation at the bottom of the lamina propria mucosae; (++) evident proliferation in the lower part of the lamina propria mucosae; (+++) significant proliferation extending to the tip of the lamina propria mucosae.

Taking into account the particular characteristics of the submucosal plexus with a low density of neural cells (about 7 neural cells per mm in colon sections) irregularly distributed, it is advisable to examine between 40 and 50 serial sections (Figure 6). The cryostat section must have a thickness of 15 μm. Neural cells are typically arranged in groups of two or three just below the muscularis mucosae and more than 7 neural cells form a giant ganglion (Figure 7).

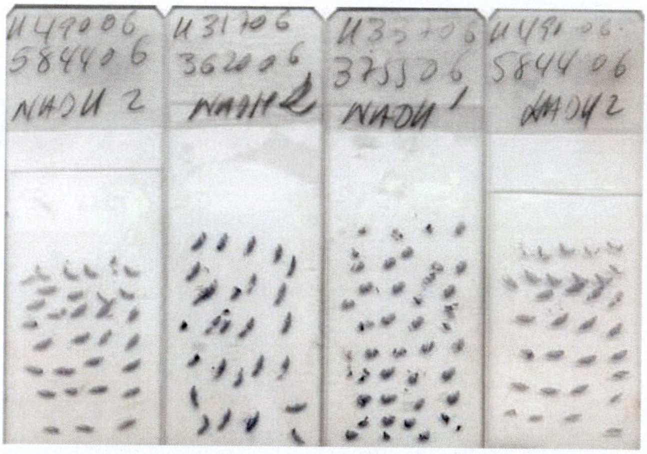

Figure 6. Microscopic slides showing 30-40 serial sections (NADH diaphorase).

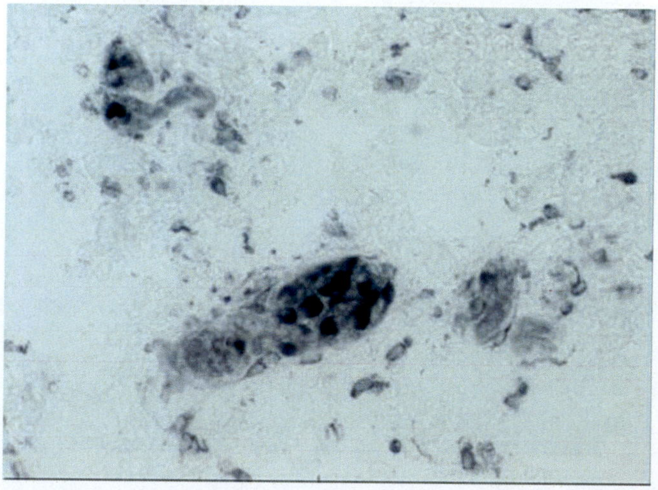

Figure 7. Rectal suction biopsy. Normal submucous ganglia in the uppermost left region. In the centre we observe a giant ganglion in a patient with IND B. (NADH diaphorase; x 480).

Diagnostic Criteria of HD in Rectal Suction Biopsy

The diagnosis of HD is based upon the presence of moderate or intense hyperplasia of AChE positive fibers in the lamina propria mucosae, muscularis mucosae and submucosa layer together with the absence of ganglion cells in the submucosa. These criteria are valid for most cases of HD. However, we can also find cases in which the hyperplasia demonstrated through AChE staining is not observed in the lamina propria mucosae but in the muscularis mucosae and submucosa (ultrashort Hirschsprung's Disease) and sometimes it is even insignificant. Then, the diagnosis is based upon the absence of ganglion cells in the submucous layer.

Results

From 1974 through 2007 we have performed a total of 1317 biopsies in 1117 patients. 173 patients underwent more than one biopsy (1,18 biopsies per patient). The age of the patients ranged from 5 days to 60 years with a mean age of 2,48 years. 372 patients were < 1 year, 241 were between 1-3 years and 474 were > 3 years (Table 1).

Table 1. Our experience 1974-2007

	Patients	Percentage
Neonates (< 30 days)	24	2,2
1-6 months	261	24
6-12 months	87	8
1-3 years	241	22,2
> 3 years	474	43,6
Total	(230 lost cases)	100

Male / female ratio: 1,87

As regards inadequate biopsies: 54 samples showed a small amount of submucosa or no submucosa. In 7 patients the first biopsy was not useful for diagnosis due to the presence of big lymphatic follicles which occupied the whole submucosa. Two samples were found to contain part of the circular muscular layer.As regards diagnosis: 342 patients showed HD (28,53%), 89 (7,42%) intestinal neuronal dysplasia type B (IND B) and 66 samples (5,50%) showed immaturity, hyperplasia of nervous trunks or hypoganglionism. In 702 cases we did not find abnormality of the enteric nervous system (Table 2).

Table 2.-Results

	Patients	Percentage
Normal	702	58,55
HD	342	28,53
IND B	89	7,42
Hyperplasia	27	2,25
Hypoganglionism	29	2,42
Immaturity	10	0,83
Total	1199	100

33 patients underwent more than one biopsy and the initial diagnosis was subsequently modified (Table 3).

During the period 1974-1984, we only employed hematoxinlin-eosin and AChE and we obtained a higher rate of errors due to the false positive results 23%. From 1984 onwards with the introduction of histochemical techniques for the demonstration of dehydrogenases this rate decreased from 23% to 1,1%. Table 4 shows reliability contingency of the whole series.

Table 3. Changes in the diagnosis of patients undergoing more than one biopsy

Initial diagnosis	Final diagnosis	Number
Normal	HD	3
	IND B	5
	Hypoganglionism	2
HD	Normal	6
	IND B	4
IND B	Normal	3
	HD	2
Hyperplasia	Normal	1
	HD	2
Hypoganglionism	Normal	4
Immaturity	Normal	1
	HD	1
Total		**33**

False negative results were observed in 28 cases (8,5%), with a mean age of 74 days (interval 23 days to 6 years). This number increased from 4,5% (3 cases) before 1984 and 7,2% (9 cases) after 2000.

Table 4.Reliability contingency of the whole series.

	Diagnosis by means of RSB		
	HD	**Not HD**	
HD	302	28	330
Not HD	40	854	894
	342	882	1224

Sensitivity value 91,5%, specificity 95,5%, positive predictive value 88,3% and negative predictive value 96,8%. From the year 2000 reliability contingency values vary as shown in Table 5.

Table 5. Reliability contingency from the year 2000

	Diagnosis by means of RSB		
	HD	**Not HD**	
HD	116	9	125
Not HD	4	313	317
	120	322	442

Sensitivity value 92,8%, specificity 98,7%, positive predictive value 96,7% and negative predictive value 97,2%.

Discussion

Enzymatic histochemical study in rectal suction biopsy is a well-established technique in the diagnosis of HD. Such diagnosis is based upon the hyperplasia of nervous trunks and the absence of ganglion cells in a valid biopsy specimen.

Inadequate samples, mainly due to the small amount or even absence of submucosa in the sample, are obtained quite often. In our experience, 4,9% of the samples were not valid. Some authors report 12% of inadequate samples when performing rectal suction biopsy and 2% using grasp technique [8,9]. In our study we have used rectal suction biopsy exclusively. Other studies on the use of rectal suction biopsy report percentages of invalid biopsy specimens ranging from 10% to more than 30% [10,11].

The absence of submucosa in the rectal suction biopsy samples is associated to age, being more frequent in patients > 3 yrs[2] [12,13].

Very few cases are explained by other reasons such as the presence of lymph nodes occupying most of the biopsy sample or hemorrhage impairing the examination and making it difficult to obtain a final diagnosis.

The incidence of intestinal disaganglionosis demonstrated by means of rectal suction biopsy has been of 41,45% in our study. A recent study carried out by other authors reports a lower percentage (31,62%). Yet, this study only considers cases of HD and IND whereas we also include patients with hypoganglionism and neuronal immaturity[14].

We have found 33 cases in which the initial diagnosis was later modified. The presence of false positives and false negatives in the diagnosis of HD after AChE staining in suction rectal biopsy is well documented in the literature [15].

In the case of 6 patients the initial diagnosis revealed HD and a second biopsy showed a normal result. Five of these cases occurred before 1984, year when we began to use dehydrogenases in the demonstration of ganglion cells. Our diagnosis was based upon AChE demonstration in hyperplasic nervous trunks. However other causes could also be responsible for this, such as IND B. A second biopsy did not reveal hyperplasic nervous trunks positive for AChE.

In two patients the initial diagnosis was normal and later on they were diagnosed of HD. The review of the literature reveals the different incidence of false positives and negatives[5,11,16-18]. False negatives are mainly reported in neonates [19,20] and it is possible to observe how AChE positive fibers increase with age [21].

Other 4 patients obtained an initial diagnosis of IND B (Figures 8, 9 and 10) and later on obtained a normal diagnosis. This supports the idea that many instances of IND B are due to the delayed maturation of the enteric nervous system. These patients were less than 1 year and at present IND B should not be diagnosed at such an early age due to the frequent presence of giant ganglia in the neonatal period [22-24] .

In another 4 patients the first examination suggested hypoganglionism which was not subsequently confirmed. The diagnosis of hypoganglionism in rectal suction biopsy is quite complicated and its confirmation requires a biopsy of the whole intestinal wall and a morphometric study [25-26].

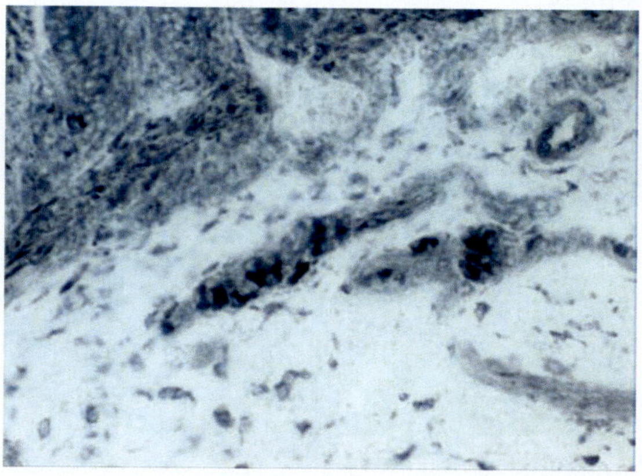

Figure 8. Rectal suction biopsy. Giant ganglia in the submucous plexus. (IND B) (NADH diaphorase; x 300).

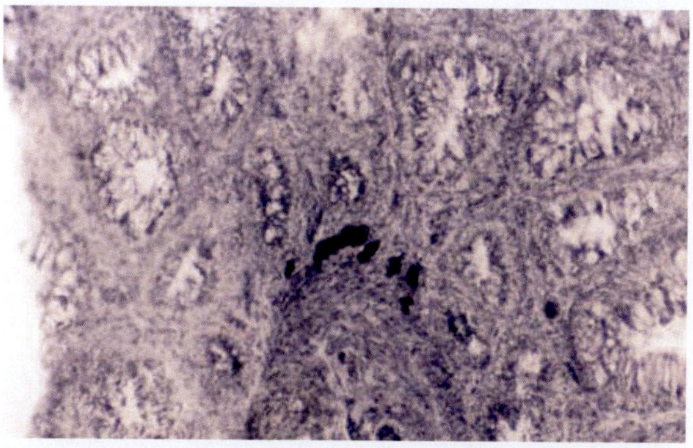

Figure 9. Nerve cells in mucosa. (IND B) (NADH diaphorase; x 480).

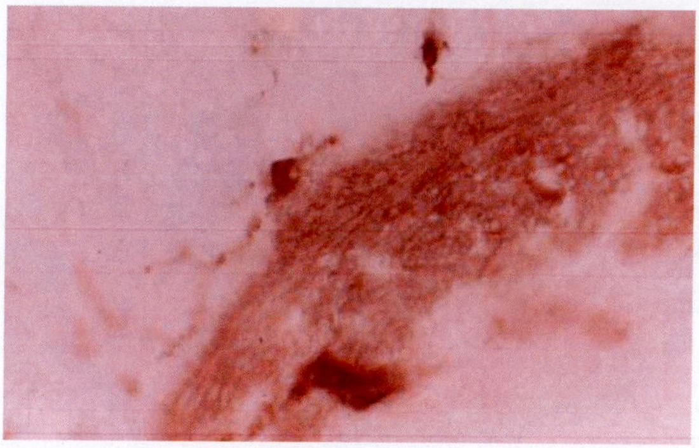

Figure 10. Nerve cells in lamina propria and muscularis mucosae. (IND B) (AChE; x 520).

In our study, the use of enzymes like AChE and dehydrogenases has been vital to obtain higher specificity and sensitivity in the diagnosis of HD, as shown by the results. Some controversy is reported in this respect in the literature. Although AChE is the technique of choice, some physicians claim that the only necessary technique is Hematoxylin –eosin staining [27-28].

In the literature we find some studies comparing the results obtained by means of different tests in the diagnosis of HD. Almost all of them agree that rectal suction biopsy is the most accurate method [29]. According to our experience, rectal suction biopsy has important advantages for patients and the use of enzymatic histochemical techniques makes an important contribution to the diagnosis.

References

[1] Noblett HR. A rectal suction biopsy tube for use in the diagnosis of Hirschsprung's disease. *J Pediatr Surg* 1969;4:406-9.

[2] Cusick EF, Buick RG. Injury to the common iliac artery during suction rectal biopsy. *J Pediatr Surg* 1995;30:111-2.

[3] Jani BR, Brereton RJ, Dillon MJ. Peripheral limb gangrene following rectal biopsy. Treatment with prostacyclin and exchange transfusion. *Clin Pediatr (Phila)* 1989;28:585-8.

[4] Rees BI, Azmy A, Nigam M, Lake BD. Complications of rectal suction biopsy. *J Pediatr Surg* 1983;18:273-5.

[5] de Mingo ML, Alvarez Bernaldo dQ, Cortes Gomez MJ, Rodriguez T, V, Garcia M, I, Colomar P, et al. [The histopathological diagnosis of Hirschsprung's disease. Our experience over 18 years]. *Cir Pediatr* 1991;4:181-4.

[6] Hirose RF, Hirata YF, Yamada TF, Kawana TF, Taguchi TF, Suita S. The simple technique of rectal mucosal biopsy for the diagnosis of Hirschsprung's disease. *J Pediatr Surg* 1993;28:942-4.

[7] Meier-Ruge W, Lutterbeck PM, Herzog B, Morger R, Moser R, Scharli A. Acetylcholinesterase activity in suction biopsies of the rectum in the diagnosis of Hirschsprung's disease. *J Pediatr Surg* 1972;7:11-7.

[8] Croffie JM, Davis MM, Faught PR, Corkins MR, Gupta SK, Pfefferkorn MD, et al. At what age is a suction rectal biopsy less likely to provide adequate tissue for identification of ganglion cells? *J Pediatr Gastroenterol Nutr* 2007;44:198-202.

[9] Ali AE, Morecroft JA, Bowen JC, Bruce J, Morabito A. Wall or machine suction rectal biopsy for Hirschsprung's disease: a simple modified technique can improve the adequacy of biopsy. *Pediatr Surg Int* 2006;22:681-2.

[10] Alizai NK, Batcup G, Dixon MF, Stringer MD. Rectal biopsy for Hirschsprung's disease: what is the optimum method? *Pediatr Surg Int* 1998;13:121-4.

[11] Athow AC, Filipe MI, Drake DP. Problems and advantages of acetylcholinesterase histochemistry of rectal suction biopsies in the diagnosis of Hirschsprung's disease. *J Pediatr Surg* 1990;25:520-6.

[12] Croffie JM, Davis MM, Faught PR, Corkins MR, Gupta SK, Pfefferkorn MD, et al. At what age is a suction rectal biopsy less likely to provide adequate tissue for identification of ganglion cells? *J Pediatr Gastroenterol Nutr* 2007;44:198-202.

[13] Ali AE, Morecroft JA, Bowen JC, Bruce J, Morabito A. Wall or machine suction rectal biopsy for Hirschsprung's disease: a simple modified technique can improve the adequacy of biopsy. *Pediatr Surg Int* 2006;22:681-2.

[14] Pini-Prato A, Martucciello G, Jasonni V. Rectal suction biopsy in the diagnosis of intestinal dysganglionoses: 5-year experience with Solo-RBT in 389 patients. *J Pediatr Surg* 2006;41:1043-8.

[15] Pacheco M, Bove K. Variability of Acetylcholinesterase Hyperinnervation Patterns in Distal Rectal Biopsy Specimens in Hirschsprung Disease. *Pediatr Dev Pathol* 2008;11:274-82.

[16] Ariel I, Vinograd I, Lernau OZ, Nissan S, Rosenmann E. Rectal mucosal biopsy in aganglionosis and allied conditions. *Hum Pathol* 1983;14:991-5.

[17] Bagdzevicius R, Vaicekauskas V, Bagdzeviciute S. Experience of acetylcholinesterase histochemistry application in the diagnosis of chronic constipation in children. *Medicina (Kaunas)* 2007;43:376-84.

[18] Bonham JR, Dale G, Scott DJ, Wagget J. A 7-year study of the diagnostic value of rectal mucosal acetylcholinesterase measurement in Hirschsprung's disease. *J Pediatr Surg* 1987;22:150-2.

[19] Moore SW, Johnson G. Acetylcholinesterase in Hirschsprung's disease. *Pediatr Surg Int* 2005;21:255-63.

[20] Nakao M, Suita S, Taguchi T, Hirose R, Shima Y. Fourteen-year experience of acetylcholinesterase staining for rectal mucosal biopsy in neonatal Hirschsprung's disease. *J Pediatr Surg* 2001;36:1357-63.

[21] Goto S, Ikeda K, Toyohara T. An improved staining technique for acetylcholinesterase activity using rubeanic acid in the diagnosis of Hirschsprung's disease. *Jpn J Surg* 1984;14:135-8.

[22] Bruder E, Meier-Ruge WA. [Intestinal neuronal dysplasia type B: how do we understand it today?]. *Pathologe* 2007;28:137-42.

[23] Meier-Ruge WA, Ammann K, Bruder E, Holschneider AM, Scharli AF, Schmittenbecher PP, et al. Updated results on intestinal neuronal dysplasia (IND B). *Eur J Pediatr Surg* 2004;14:384-91.

[24] Koletzko S, Jesch I, Faus-Kebetaler T, Briner J, Meier-Ruge W, Muntefering H, et al. Rectal biopsy for diagnosis of intestinal neuronal dysplasia in children: a prospective multicentre study on interobserver variation and clinical outcome. *Gut* 1999;44:853-61.

[25] Scharli AF, Sossai R. Hypoganglionosis. *Semin Pediatr Surg* 1998;7:187-91.

[26] Tomita R, Munakata K, Howard ER, Fujisaki S. Histological studies on Hirschsprung's disease and its allied disorders in childhood. *Hepatogastroenterology* 2004;51:1042-4.

[27] Martucciello G, Pini PA, Puri P, Holschneider AM, Meier-Ruge W, Jasonni V, et al. Controversies concerning diagnostic guidelines for anomalies of the enteric nervous system: a report from the fourth International Symposium on Hirschsprung's disease and related neurocristopathies. *J Pediatr Surg* 2005;40:1527-31.

[28] Park WH, Choi SO, Kwon KY, Chang ES. Acetylcholinesterase histochemistry of rectal suction biopsies in the diagnosis of Hirschsprung's disease. J *Korean Med Sci* 1992;7:353-9.

[29] de Lorijn F, Kremer LC, Reitsma JB, Benninga MA. Diagnostic tests in Hirschsprung disease: a systematic review. *J Pediatr Gastroenterol Nutr* 2006;42:496-505.

In: Hirschsprung's Disease: Diagnosis and Treatment
Ed: Ramón Núñez and Manuel López-Alonso
ISBN: 978-1-60741-349-3

Chapter XII

Differential Diagnosis of Hirschsprung's Disease in the Neonatal Period

José Mª Gil-Vernet, Marta De Diego and Jesús Broto

Introduction

In recent years the value of early diagnosis of Hirschsprung's Disease (HD) has gained importance as a means to initiate a fast response to intestinal management thereby favouring surgical treatment in early ages thus minimizing the risk of enterocolitis.

The 99% of healthy full-term newborns produce meconium in the first 24 hours of birth, the remaining 1% do so within 24 hours [1]. Any delay in the evacuation of meconium raises the suspicion of an intestinal obstruction or disfunction. In such cases it is imperative to conduct a thorough anamnesis and complementary studies to differentiate HD from other causes of lower intestinal obstruction – be it functional or mechanical.

Complementary studies of radiology (image), anorectal manometry (physiological study) and biopsy by suction (hystological-immunological/hystochemical) are generally used to obtain a definitive diagnosis. Radiology shows up any occlusive or subocclusive patterns on account of air-fluid levels. The contrast studies (contrast enema upon postevacuation image) confirm whether there is an area of narrow distal transition: this is vital for the radiological diagnosis of HD and also allows us to discover the length of the area affected by aganglionism [2]. Anorectal manometry allows us to detect whether or not the anal reflex is working – the absence of anal reflex is an indicator of HD [3-5], with a sensitivity factor of 98% and a specific factor of 97%. Biopsy by suction must be sufficiently deep to obtain samples of mucosa and submucosa in order to report on acetylcholinesterase activity (AChE), hyperplasia of the nerve fibers, presence or absence of ganglion cells and the quality of the same.

Differential Diagnosis

Various diseases must be considered when a neonate is being evaluated for HD. Table 1 gives a list of the more common differential diagnoses of HD in the newborn.

Table 1. Differential diagnosis of Hirschsprung's disease in in the newborn.

FUNCTIONAL OBSTRUCTIONS
Pre-term newborn
Prematurity/Immaturity
Necrotizing enterocolitis/sepsis
Fetal exposure to alcohol
Maternal drug addiction
Full-term newborn
Meconium plug syndrome
Small left neonate colon syndrome
Meconium ileus
Intestinal neuropathies and myopathies
Neuronal intestinal dysplasia and hypoganglionosis
Megacystis-microcolon-intestinal hypoperistalsis syndrome
Derived from other processes
Hydroelectrolytic alterations
Viral infections
Intra-craneal hemorrhage
Adrenal hemorrhage
Hypothyroidism
Allergy to cow's milk protein
Functional constipation
MECHANICAL OBTRUCTIONS
Distal ileal atresia or stenosis
Colonic atresia or stenosis
Low imperforate anus
Intestinal malrotation
Intestinal intussusception
Incarcerated hernia, intestinal duplication, etc.

Functional Obstructions in Preterm Newborns

Prematurity/Immaturity

In the normal premature newborn stools can be scarce or even absent for two weeks. In general, the first passage of meconium takes place between the first and the eighth day. In 1979 was published the first description ever of meconium obstruction in some extremely low-birth-weight infants [6-7]. The average weight of these patients was under <1250g and their gestation age was 27± 2 weeks. In more than 50% of the cases factors of maternal origin which affect the perfusion of the placenta were present: factors such as preeclampsia, eclampsia, chronic hypertension, diabetes mellitus with arterial involvement, oligohydramnios and chronic placenta abruption. Observations also confirm a higher incidence amongst mothers undergoing treatments involving magnesium sulphate [8-9].

Clinically speaking there is abdominal distension without peritonitis. Radiologically speaking, there is a presence of distended intestinal loops without air-fluid levels, and with little or hardly any rectal gas. Inspissated meconium is most frequently found in the distal ileum. In a contrast enema a microcolon may appear [10]; this disappears in later radiological controls as the obstruction becomes solved. At around 28-32 weeks of gestation organised motility begins and as such Rectoanal Inhibitori Response (RAIR) may already be present [11-12]. The (13C) octanoic acid breath test can also be used to measure gastric emptying in preterm patients [13-14].

In the differential diagnosis other pathologies such as meconium plug syndrome or cystic fibrosis must be discarded. In some cases radiological examination may lead to the erroneous diagnosis of necrotizing enterocolitis.

Treatment includes rectal stimulation, saline enemas, oral and rectal gastrograffin and oral N-acetylcysteine [15]. Some patients continue to have obstruction for days or show signs of perforation and peritonitis on account of a delayed diagnosis. Such patients require surgical disimpactation by means of enterotomies and intraluminal washing or even intestinal resections with or without temporary stomas. The pathological anatomy, in such cases, gives rise to the definitive diagnosis that differentiates necrotizing enterocolitis [9].

Once the process of obstruction has been solved, all patients present a high rate of normal stooling patterns.

Necrotizing Enterocolitis

This condition mainly affects premature low-birth weight infants. Only 7% of full-term newborns and 10% of newborns who are small for gestational age are affected by enterocolitis (NEC) [16]. It is a multifactorial etiology and includes a combination of prematurity, a breaching of the epithelial intestinal mucosa barrier function as a result of intestinal ischemia, pathogenic bacteria and enteral feeding all of which produce intestinal injury and set off the inflammatory cascade.

The initial clinical presentation is not specific and includes recurring apneas, bradycardia, hypoglycemia, temperature instability, lethargy and shock. The gastrointestinal presentation includes abdominal distension (up to 98%), bloody mucoid stool which can be macroscopic (up to 63%) or occult (up to 59%), an increase in postprandial gastric retention (less than 70%), vomiting (less than 70%) or diarrhea (up to 26%) [17-18].

Radiological evidence includes nonspecific bowel distention, pneumatosis intestinalis, portal vein gas, pneumoperitoneum, intraperitoneal fluid and persistently dilated, fixed loops [19].

Normally clinical presentation and radiology suggest NEC, but in some patients with presentation of obstruction and absence of intestinal pneumatosis, the differential diagnosis of HD can become difficult. The contrast enema is not recommended on account of the risk of perforation in the acute phase of NEC. It is, on the other hand, the preferred method to study stenosis that may appear in the terminal ileum or in the colon 3-6 weeks after a NEC episode. If the differential diagnosis is not clear then a manometry and a rectal suction biopsy need to be carried out.

Fetal Exposure to Alcohol

There is a pattern of anomalies occurring in children born to alcoholic women. The main features of this pattern are pre and/or postnatal growth retardation, characteristic facial abnormalities, and central nervous system dysfunction, including mental retardation [20-21]. A few children with fetal alcohol syndrome have neuropathic forms of pseudo-obstruction [22]. Long-chain fatty acid ethyl esters (FAEEs) in meconium are potential biomarkers of fetal alcohol exposure, particularly ethyl linoleate and ethyl arachidonate [23-24].

Maternal Drug Addiction

As with alcohol some children born to narcotic-abusing mothers present neuropathic forms of pseudo obstruction [22].

On the other hand, the neonatal abstinence syndrome (NAS) is a generalized disorder presenting a clinical picture of central nervous system (CNS), hyperirritability, gastrointestinal dysfunction, respiratory distress and vague autonomic symptoms. It can be due to intrauterine exposure to heroin and methadone. Other less potent opiates or non-opiate CNS depressants have also been cited as causes of NAS [25]. The onset of symptoms depends on the type of drug, the amount, frequency and duration of fetal exposure and the time elapsed between the last dosage and the birth. As a rule the clinical presentation appears between 24-48 hours after birth, although in some cases it can take as long as ten days for symptoms to appear. The gastrointestinal symptoms include excessive sucking, uncoordinated suction, regurgitation or vomiting reduced digestion time and dyspeptic stools.

Functional Obstructions in Full-Term Newborns

Meconium Plug Syndrome

This pathology is the mildest but most frequent colon obstruction in full-term neonates. Described in 1956 as intestinal obstruction due to the inability of the colon to rid itself of the meconium residue after 9 months of fetal life [26]. There is considerable clinical and radiological overlap between meconium plug obstruction and small left colon syndrome. It is a lower obstruction with the absence of passing meconium in the first 24 hours of life. It is believed to be caused by immaturity in the myenteric nervous system which causes an ineffective peristalsis; it can also be the first sign of HD [27], and for this reason a radiological study, anorectal manometry and rectal biopsy by suction are appropriate to rule out this pathology. The meconium in meconium plug syndrome is reported to have an elevated protein content with altered enzymatic activity, suggesting that the obstruction is caused by an immobile luminal obstruction rather than mural constriction and diminished peristalsis [28]. A water-soluble contrast enema is usually both diagnostic and therapeutic. The enema does not reveal a microcolon, although the colon is frequently smaller than normal. Anorectal manometry and biopsy are normally reserved for patients who remain constipated.

This may also be the first symptom of cystic fibrosis, which is why possible metabolic illnesses in the newborn infant must be discarded: a genetic study and a sweat test are used to perform this differential diagnosis.

Neonatal Small Left Colon Syndrome

In 1974 Davis defined the neonatal small left colon syndrome (NSLCS) based on a description of 20 patients [28-29]. In 40 – 50% of the cases the mother had diabetes and nearly all of them were insulin-dependent. The pathogenesis seems to be a result of the hypoglycemia-induced release of glucagon. The left colon of the newborn seems to be particularly sensitive to he smooth muscle constrictive effects of glucagon and other substances [30].

The clinical presentation includes failure to pass meconium in the first 24 hours, progressive abdominal distension and bilious vomiting. In a small number of cases of distension, this leads to early perforation, normally of the cecum. [31]. In many symptoms coincides with that of the meconium plug syndrome, but in this case there is no plug in the small distal colon, not does the meconium of the patients present alterations in terms of composition.

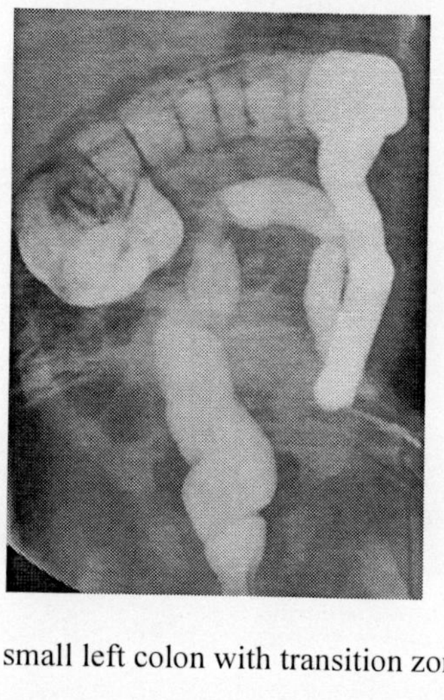

Figure 1. Gastrografin enema shows a small left colon with transition zone. The rectum is normal sized.

Simple radiology does show up signs of distal obstruction, with air-fluid levels. Very rarely there is pneumoperitoneum, a result of cecal perforation. The contrast enema (Fig. 1) shows up a small left colon with an area of transition in the splenic flexure but with no contrast in this area. The rectum is normal-sized.

Because Hirschsprung's disease with a splenic flexure transition zone is clinically and radiologically indistinguishable from NSLCS, all infants must have a suction rectal biopsy performed to exclude aganglionosis [32]. Cystic fibrosis producing a colonic variant of meconium ileus should be considered, and the appropriate DNA testing as well as a sweat chloride test should be performed, when the infant is older, if appropriate [33].

In the majority of cases the contrast enema is both diagnostic and therapeutic, although some cases may need rectal irrigation. Surgical treatment is reserved for cases with intestinal perforation or those that cannot be solved by more conservative treatments.

Meconium Ileus

Meconium ileus is often a symptom of cystic fibrosis (for 15% it is the first symptom) [34]. The clinical presentation is an obstruction of the thin distal intestine (lower small bowel), secondary to the intraluminal impact of meconium viscosity. At birth the newborn has abdominal distension which develops, as the hours pass by, until bilious vomiting occurs. Frequently, movement of the intestinal bends is observed through the abdominal wall. Normally, the intestine has no injuries, although there may be a meconial pseudocyst, meconial peritonitis with or without secondary ileal atresia. Pain and erythema in the walls are signs of complications.

Radiographs show a ground-glass appearance in the abdomen, especially in the upper right abdomen. The contrast enema demonstrates a microcolon (Fig. 2).

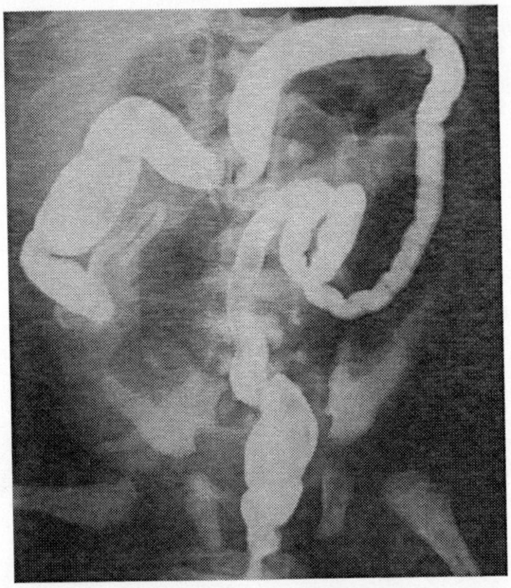

Figure 2. Gastrografin enema shows a microcolon in meconium ileus. Cystic fibrosis.

Treatment of meconial ileum consists of oral and rectal gastrograffin (diatrizoate meglumine) and oral N-acetylcysteine until the meconium has been disimpacted. If this is not effective surgery is performed and surgical cleaning is performed by way of an enterothomy. The treatment of complicated versions is always surgical and includes intestinal resections, and anastomosis or temporary stomas depending on the clinical evidence.

Intestinal Neuropathies and Myopathies

Neuronal Intestinal Dysplasia

Meier Ruge defined neuronal intestinal dysplasia (NID) in 1971 as a hyperplasia of myenteric and submucosal plexus with a resulting increase in the ganglion cells, positive AChE and malformed ganglia [35]. Later two types of NID were classified: A and B in accordance with histological and clinical criteria [36-37]. In 1999 [38] the same group of authors reached the conclusion that, provided the biopsy was performed at a sufficient depth, AChE can be useful for diagnosing HD but not NID, because the same criteria established as a diagnosis of NID can occur as a variation of normal behavior alter birth. In 2004 [39], after a study of 3984 biopsies carried out on 1328 children, the research team decided that an NID B diagnosis was controversial and a more demanding set of qualitative and quantitative diagnostic criteria was established: biopsies must be taken 8 – 10 cm above the dentate line and with sufficient submucosa and to confirm a diagnosis of NID there must be a series of 30 cuts in the submucosa (performed perpendicular to the mucosa) of 15 – 20% of the giant ganglions, with more than 8 neurons per ganglion. Last of all the increase in AChE on the slide is defined as being an age-dependant phenomenon which disappears with the increased maturity of the submucosal plexus and new criteria are established, recommending techniques such as lactic dehydrogenase, nitric oxide synthase and succinat dehydrogenase.

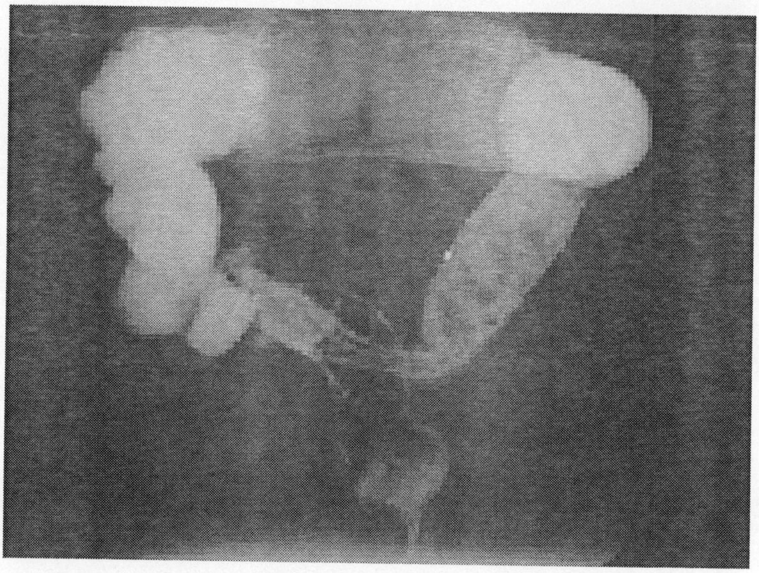

Figure 3. Neuronal Intestinal Dysplasia. Barium enema shows transitional zone.

Given the wide variety the doubt arises about whether a false diagnosis of HD can arise if radiography (Figure 3), anorectal manometry and biopsy are not performed simultaneously, resulting in radical surgery in a patient with NID, in theory an illness which is cured with maturity.

In table 2 shows an analysis of the results of studies (radiography, manometry and suction rectal biopsy) undertaken over the last five years in order to perform a differential diagnosis of the newborn suspected of having an intestinal neuropathy [40].

Table 2. Hirschsprung's disease. 26 cases diagnossed before the age of 3 months.

Clinical Features		N° of Cases
Clinical	Delayed passing/evacuation of meconium or intestinal occlusion/subocclusion	24
	Constipation	2
X-ray:	Evidence of transition zone	73%
Anorectal manometry:	Absence of RAIR	96%
Histology:	Evidence of hematoxilin-eosin and AChE	75%

RAIR: Rectoanal inhibitory reflex

Of the 26 cases, 24 started out with delayed passage of meconium and signs of occlusion/subocclusion; only two started out with constipation.

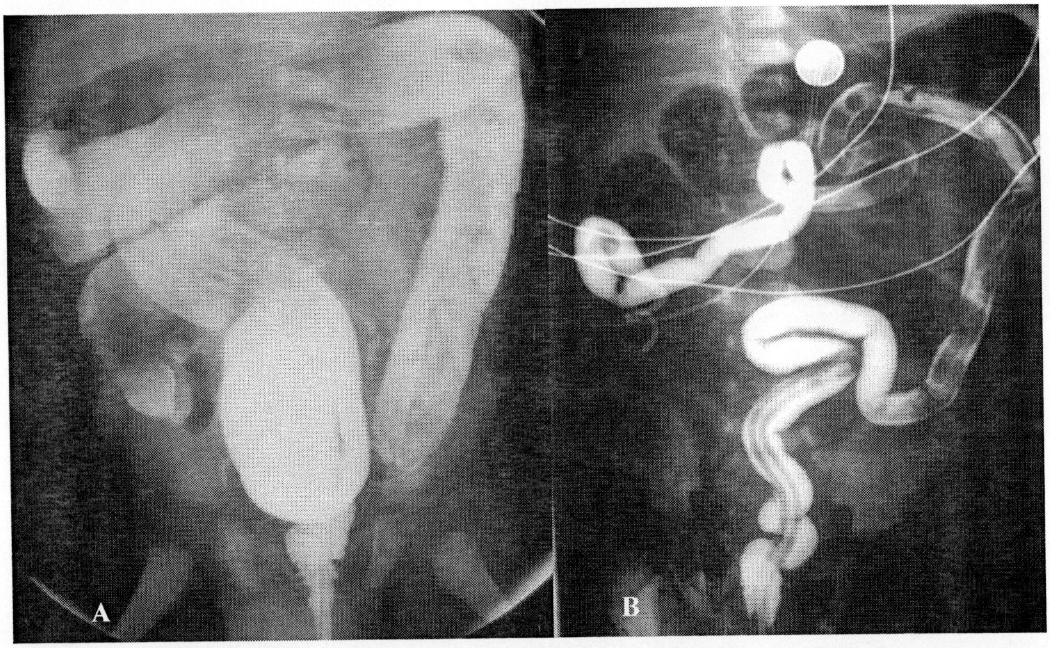

Figure 4. A. Newborn with Hirschsprung's disease. Gastrografin enema shows transitional zone at rectosigmoid. The anorectal manometry showed absence of the rectoanal inhibitory reflex and a rectal suction biopsy confirmed aganglionosis. B. Newborn with total colonic Hirschsprung`disease. Gastrografin enema shows a microcolon without transition zone. No contrast could pass through the competent ileocecal valve. The diagnosis was made at surgery.

In 73% there were clear signs (narrow distal transition zone) that indicated a diagnosis of HD (Fig. 4A). Total colonic aganglionosis cannot be confidently differentiated from ileal atresia or meconium ileus, and a definitive diagnosis may only be made histologically from frozen sections of surgical specimens (Fig 4B). The anorectal manometry indicated that there was an absence of the inhibitory anal reflex in all cases except one (96% correct HD diagnosis with manometry).

The anorectal manometry indicated that there was an absence of the inhibitory anal reflex in all cases except one which gave rise to suspect and absence of HD (96% correct HD diagnosis with manometry).

The biopsies with samples for conventional histology (hematoxilin–eosin) and hystochemical immunity (AChE) allowed the diagnosis of HD in 75% of the cases. In the remaining 25% the result was not conclusive on account of the quality of the biopsy (lack of depth and therefore insufficient biopsy).

In table 3 shows an analysis of the 9 cases of NID diagnosed before the age of 3 months. The 66% presented clinical signs of occlusion which suggested HD. In 22% of the cases there was a transition zone detected through both simple radiography and contrast studies suggesting HD.

Table 3. Neuronal intestinal dysplasia. 9 cases diagnosed before the age of 3 months.

Clinical Features		N° of Cases
Clinical	Intestinal occlusion/subocclusion	6
	Constipation	3
X-ray:	Evidence of transition zone	22%
Anorectal manometry:	Absence of RAIR	33%
Histology:	E vidence of hematoxilin-eosin and AChE	55%

RAIR: Rectoanal inhibitory reflex

Anorectal manometry demonstrated a presence of RAIR in three patients which meant discarding a diagnosis of HD, it was absent in another three and questionable in the three remaining cases. The histological and inmunohystochemical study confirmed the presence of NID in five cases; the remaining four cases did not match the required criteria, although NID was considered and for this reason there was a control of the evolution in these patients which led to discarding HD later on.

Of the 35 neonates studied in a period of 5 years, 26 had a diagnosis of HD with postoperative histological confirmation. The remaining 4 patients, who did not match all the criteria, have been considered as non HD patients and indeed their evolution confirmed this diagnosis.

There are authors who consider it sufficient to perform radiography in order to diagnose NID; our experience, however, is different and we relieve it is essential to carry out all studies described here in order to avoid erroneous diagnosis.

Hypoganglionosis

Isolated hypoganglionosis is rare, accounting for only 5% of all classified congenital innervation defects of the colon [41]. Clinically, resembles HD. The understanding of hypoganglionosis is controversial because diagnostic criteria are not strictly defined internationally [42]. Treatment of hypoganglionosis is similar to HD involving resection of the affected segment and pull-through operation.

Megacystis-Microcolon-Intestinal Hypoperistalsis Syndrome

Described by Berdon in 1976 [43], this is a visceral myopathy which mostly affects females in a 4:1 ratio. It manifests itself in the neonatal period as a severe alteration in the motility of the small intestine and the absence of stools in the colon, and microcolon. In addition, there is evidence of megacystis and hydronephrosis, laxity of the muscles in the abdominal wall and incomplete intestinal rotation. On an anatomopathological level the condition is characterized by an increase in normal intestinal ganglion cells. On an electronic microscopic level one can see a thinning of the longitudinal muscular coating with a significant quantity of connective tissue [44].

Derived from other Processes

Viral Infections

The congenital varicella syndrome can cause multiple congenital defects, i.e. neurogenic bladder and anal dysfunction [32, 45].

Hypothyroidism

The most frequent manifestations include problems with feeding, constipation, retarded growth and development, prolonged neonatal icteric and goiter. Other signs are macroglossia, puffy face, dry or mottled skin, abdominal distension, umbilical hernia and short stature [46-47].

Allergy to Cow's Milk

This affects 2-7'5% of all children. In the majority of cases the symptoms are varied and poorly-defined; they include: atopic dermatitis, infantile colic, gastro-oesophageal reflux, oesophagitis, infantile proctocolitis, food-associated enterocolitis and constipation [48]. A number of neonates present HD-like symptoms, and many are erroneously classified as benign transient non-organic ileus of neonates. The appearance of symptoms may be earlier or later as many are exclusively breast-fed and exclusively breast-fed infants seemed to have more delayed onset of symptoms than those who were not [49]. The radiological pattern of abdominal distension simulated HD and may require irrigation enemas until the patient's system becomes normalized. The diagnosis is normally a result of clinically-based suspicions and the suspension of ingestion of cow's milk and is done by way of a drug-induced lymphocyte stimulation test positive for cow's milk with a titer of more than 300%, or a positive radioallergosorbent test for cow's milk with a value higher than 0'34 U /ml [50]. In a study which followed the evolution of 86 patients on a cow milk-free diet, the percentages of tolerance of the cow's milk protein were 30%, 54.5% and 70% respectively [51].

Habit Constipation

Also know as benign transient non-organic ileus of neonates. These patients display Hirschsprung's disease-like symptoms, but respond well to conservative treatments. The symptoms occur in well-developed, well-fed infants who also have a correct pondostatural development. The stools tend to be very large and rectal touching may produce explosive defecation during examination. The radiological study will show abdominal distension with dilation of the intestinal bends and even air-fluid levels and segmentary dilations. The recto-anal inhibitory reflex is normal and the suction biopsy shows normal acetylcholinesterase activity and submucosal ganglion cells. The treatment is periodic glycerin enemas until daily spontaneous defecation; this can take between 2 and 14 months to settle [52].

Mechanical Obstructions

Neonates with complete atresia of the colon or distal small intestine will also present with a low intestinal obstruction, which may initially mimic HD. A complete obstruction, such as an atresia, will also demonstrate a microcolon on contrast enema studies. It is important to note that HD may be associated with both colonic and small intestine atresia [53, 54]. A high index of suspicion for HD should be maintained for neonates who do not seem to benefit from surgery for intestinal atresia.

There is no question that HD accompanies imperforate anus and it should always be suspected in a child with persistent constipation after definitive surgery for anorectal malformations [55, 56].

References

[1] Clark DA. Times of first void and first stool in 500 newborns. *Pediatrics* 1977;60:457-9.

[2] Jamieson DH, Dundas SE, Belushi SA, Cooper M, Blair GK. Does the transition zone reliably delineate aganglionic bowel in Hirschsprung disease?. *Pediatr Radiol* 2004;34:811-5.

[3] Gil-Vernet JM, Casasa JM, Marhuenda C, Broto J. Boix-Ochoa Manometría anorrectal en la enfermedad de Hirschsprung. *Cir Ped* 1992;5:135-40.

[4] Nuñez R, Cabrera R, Moreno C, Agulla E, Vargas I, Blesa E. Utilidad de la manometría anorrectal para el diagnóstico neonatal de la Enfermedad de Hirschsprung. *Cir Pediatr* 2000;13:16-9.

[5] López Alonso M. Hernández Orgaz A, Ribas Serna. Indices de fiabilidad de la manometría anorrectal para el diagnóstico de la enfermedad de Hirschsprung en cualquier edad. *Cir Pediatr* 2005;18:13-6.

[6] Dimmitt RA, Moss RL. Meconium diseases in infants with very low birth weight. *Semin Pediatr Surg*. 2000;9:79-83.

[7] Siegel MJ, Shackelford GD, McAlister WH. Neonatal meconium blockage in the ileum and proximal colon. *Radiology* 1979;132:79-82.

[8] Grennholz SK, Pérez C, Wesley JR, Marr CC. Meconium obstruction in markedly premature infant. *J Pediatr Surg* 1996;31:117-20.

[9] Garza-Cox S, Keeney SE, Angel CA, Thompson LL, Swischuk LE. Meconium obstruction in the very low birth weight premature infants. *Pediatrics* 2004;14:285-90.

[10] Emil S, Nguyen T, Sills J, Padilla G. Meconium obstruction in extremely low-birth-weight neonates: guidelines for diagnosis and management. *J Pediatr Surg* 2004; 39:731-7.

[11] De Lorjin F, Voskuijl WP, Omari TI, Kok JH, Taminiau JA, Benninga MA. Assessment of the rectoanal inhibitory reflex in preterm infants with delayed meconium passage. *J Pediatr Gastroenterol Nutr* 2005;40:434-7.

[12] Ito Y, Donahoe PK, Hendren WH. Maturation of the rectoanal response in premature and perinatal infants. *J Pediatr Surg* 1977;12:477-82

[13] Veereman-Wauters G, Ghoos Y, Van der Schoor S, Maes B, Hebbalkar N, Devlieger H, Eqqermont. The 13C-octanoic acid breath test: a noninvasive technique to assess gastric emptying in preterm infants. *E.J Pediatr Gastroenterol Nutr* 1996;23:111-7.

[14] Pozler O, Neumann D, Vorisek V, Bukac J, Bures J, Kokstein Z. Development of gastric emptying in premature infants. Use of the (13)C-octanoic acid breath test. *Nutrition* 2003;19:593-6.

[15] Grennholz SK, Pérez C, Wesley JR, Marr CC. Meconium obstruction in the markedly premature infant. *J Pediatr Surg* 1996;31:117-20.

[16] Kliegman RM, Fanaroff AA. Neonatal necrotizing enterocolitis: A nine-year experience. *Am J Dis Child* 1981;135:608-11.

[17] Chandler JC, Hebra A. Necrotizing enterocolitis in infants with very low birth weight. *Semin Pediatr Surg* 2000;9:63-72.

[18] Kanto WP Jr, Hunter JE, Stoll BJ. Recognition and medical management of necrotizing enterocolitis. *Clin Perinatol* 1994;21:335-46.

[19] Morrison SC, Jacobson JM. The radiology of necrotizing enterocolitis. *Clin Perinatol* 1994;21:347-63.

[20] Abel EL. Fetal alcohol syndrome: a cautionary note. *Curr Pharm Des* 2006;12:1521-9.

[21] Age-related changes in colon motility. Di Lorenzo C, Flores A, Hyman P. *J Pediatr* 1995; 127:593-6.

[22] Hyman PE, Di Lorenzo C. Chronic intestinal pseudo-obstruction. In: Wyllie R, Hyman JS eds. *Pediatric Gastrointestinal Disease*. Philadelphia, PA:WB Saunders, 1993. p. 641.

[23] Bearer CF, Lee S, Salvator AE, Minnes S, Swick A, Yamashita T, Singer LT. Ethyl linoleate in meconium: a biomarker for prenatal ethanol exposure. *Alcohol Clin Exp Res* 1999;23;487-93.

[24] Ostrea EM Jr, Hernandez JD, Bielawski DM, Kan JM, Leonardo GM, Abela MB et al:Fatty acid ethyl esters in meconium: are they biomarkers of fetal alcohol exposure and effect? *Alcohol Clin Exp Res* 2006; 30:1152-9.

[25] Finnegan L. Management of neonatal abstinence. Adapted from: *Current Therapy in Neonatal-Perinatal Medicine*, N Nelson (Ed). Ontario: B.C. Decker, Inc., Publisher; 1985.p.262-70.

[26] Clatworthy HW, Howard WH, Lloyd J. The meconium plug syndrome. *Surgery* 1956;39:131-42

[27] Burge D, Drewett M. Meconium plug obstruction. *Pediatr Surg Int* 2004;20:108-10.

[28] Davis WS, Allen RP, Favara B E, Slovis TL. Neonatal small left colon syndrome. *Am J Roentgerol. Radium Ther Nucl Med* 1974;120:322-9.

[29] David R Stewart MD, William Nixon MD, Dale G, Johnson MD, Virgil R, Condon MD. Neonatal Small Left Colon Syndrome. *Ann Surg* 1977;186:741-5.

[30] Hicks T, Turnberg LA. Influence of glucagon on the human jejunum. *Gastroenterology* 1974;67:1114-8.

[31] Philippart AI, Reed JO, Georgeson KE. Neonatal small left colon síndrome: intramural not intraluminal obstruction. *J Pediatr Surg* 1975;10:733-40.

[32] Berdon WE, Slovis TL, Campbell JB, Baker DH, Haller JO. Neonatal small left colon syndrome: its relationship to aganglionosis and meconium plug syndrome. *Radiology* 1977;125:457-62.

[33] Ellerbroek C, Smith WL. Neonatal Small Left Colon in an infant with cystic fibrosis. *Pediatr Radiol* 1986;16:162-3.

[34] Kiely EM. Meconium ileus. In: Puri P ed. *Newborn surgery*. Oxford: Butterworth-Heinemann; 1996. p. 324-7.

[35] Meier Ruge WA. Über ein erkrankungsbild des colon mit Hirschsprung-symptomatik. *Verh Dtsch Ges Pathol* 1971;55:506-7.

[36] Fadda B, Pistor G, Meier Ruge W, Hoffman-Von-Kapher S, Münterfering H, Espinoza R. Symptoms, diagnosis and therapy of neuronal intestinal dysplasia wasked by Hirschsprung'disease. Report of 24 cases. *Pediatr Surg Int* 1987;2:76-80.

[37] Fadda B, Maier WA, Meier Ruge W, Schärli A, Damm R. Neuronale intestinal dysplasie. *Z Kinderchir* 1983;38:305-11.

[38] Koletzko S, Jesch I, Faus-Kessler T, Briner J, Meier-Ruge W, Müntefering H, et al: Rectal biopsy for diagnosis of intestinal neuronal dysplasia in children: a prospective multicentre study on interobserver variation and clinical outcome. *Gut* 1999;44:853-61.

[39] Meier Ruge WA, Ammann K, Bruder E, Holschneider AM, Schärl AF, Schmittenbecher PP, Stoss F. Updated results on intestinal neuronal dysplasia. (IND B) *Eur J Pediatr Surg* 2004;14:384-9.1

[40] Gil-Vernet JM, Broto J, Guillén G. Diagnóstico diferencial Hirschsprung-Neurodisplasia intestinal. Fiabilidad de las pruebas diagnósticas. *Cir Ped* 2006;19:91-4.

[41] Meier-Ruge W: Epidemiology of congenital innervation defects of the distal colon. *Virchows Arch A Pathol Anat Histopathol*, 1992; 420:171-7.

[42] Martucciello G, Pini Prato A, Puri P, Holschneiderd A M, Meier-Ruge W, Jasonni V et al: Controversies concerning diagnostic guidelines for anomalies of the enteric nervous system: A report from the fourth International Symposium on Hirschsprung's disease and related neurocristopathies. *J Pediatr Surg* 2005;4: 1527–31.

[43] Berdon W, Baker D, Bland W. Megacystis-microcolon intestinal hypoperistalsis syndrome: a new cause of intestinal obstruction in the newborn. Report of radiologic findings in five newborns girls. *Ann Roentgenol* 1976;126:957-64.

[44] Puri P, Lake D, Gorman F, et al. Megacystis-microcolon intestinal hypoperistalsis syndrome: a visceral myopathy. *J Pediatr Surg* 1983;18:64-9.

[45] Katz G, Pfau A. Congenital varicella causing neurogenic bladder and anal dysfunction. *Urology* 1986;28:424-5.

[46] Unachak K, Dejhamron P. Primary congenital hypothyroidism: clinical characteristics and etiological study. *J Med Assoc Thai* 2004;87:612-7.

[47] Reiterer E, Borkenstein MH. Disorders of the thyroid gland in neonates and youth: latent hypothyroidism and hyperthyroidism. A*cta Med Austriaca*. 2003;30:107-9.

[48] Heine RG, Elsayed S, Hosking CS, Hill DJ. Cow's milk allergy in infancy. *Curr Opin Clin Immunol* 2002;2:217-25.

[49] Yimyaem P, Chongsrisawat V, Vivatvakin B, Wisedopas N. Gastrointestinal manifestations of cow's milk protein allergy during the first year of life. *J Med Assoc Thai* 2003;86:116-23.

[50] Kubota A, Kawahara H, Okuyama H, Shimizu Y, Nakacho M, Ida S, Nakayama M, Okada A. Cow's milk protein allergy presenting with Hirschsprung's disease-mimicking symptoms. *J Pediatr Surg* 2006;41:2056-8.

[51] Carroccio A, Montalvo G, Custro N, Notarbartolo A, Cavataio F, D'Amico D, Alabrese D, Iacono G. Evidence of very delayed clinical reactions to cow's milk in cow's milk-intolerant pacients. *Allergy* 2000;55:574-9.

[52] Stafford PW: Other disorders of the anus and rectum, anorectal function. In: O'Oneill JA, Rowe MI, Grosfeld JL, Fonkairud EW, Coran AG (eds). *Pediatry Surgery*.Fifth ed. Vol 2. St. Louis Missouri: Mosby –Year Book,Inc; 1998. p. 1449-60.

[53] Gupta M, Beeram MR, Pohl JF, Custer MD. Ileal atresia associated with Hirschsprung´s disease (total colonic aganglionosis). *J Pediatr Surg* 2005;40: E5-E7.

[54] Draus JM, Maxfield CM, Bond SJ: Hirschsprung's disease in an infant with colonic atresia and normal fixation of the distal colon.*J Pediatr Surg*. 2007;42:E5-E8.

[55] Flageole H, Fecteau A, Laberge JM, Guttman FM. Hirschsprung´s disease, imperforate anus, and Down´s syndrome: a case report. *J Pediatr Surg* 1996;31: 759-60.

[56] Oshio T: Imperforate anus, malrotation, and Hirschsprung's disease with double zonal aganglionosis: an extremely rare combination. *J Pediatr Surg*. 2008;43:222-6.

In: Hirschsprung's Disease: Diagnosis and Treatment
Ed: Ramón Núñez and Manuel López-Alonso
ISBN: 978-1-60741-349-3

Chapter XIII

Hirschsprung's Disease: Preoperative Medical Care. Enterostomies. Bowel Preparation for Pull-Through

Ramón Núñez, Isabel Vargas and Mª José Estepa

Preoperative Medical Care

The treatment of Hirschsprung's disease (HD) consists of two basic stages. The first stage is decompression of the colon by means of medical care, or with an intestinal derivation if this fails. The second stage is resection of the aganglionic segment, and the normal ganglionic intestine is brought down. In order to prevent enterocolitis, it is essential that HD is diagnosed in the first days of life, and that medical care is established for the decompression of the colon to restore the distal intestinal transit [1-3].

In the Anglo-Saxon literature, between approximately 40% and 90% of patients with HD are diagnosed in the neonatal period [4–6]. It is evident that this percentage must be improved, the aim being to diagnose almost 100% of the patients with this pathology as soon as possible after birth. What can we do to achieve this? In our experience [7] and that of other authors [8], anorectal manometry practised on all newborn in which there is a more than 24-hour delay in passing the meconium is very useful in selecting those with absence of the rectoanal inhibitory reflex (RAIR), i.e., with suspected HD. In these newborn, decompression of the colon treatment must be commenced until a rectal suction biopsy has confirmed or discarded aganglionosis [9]. The absence of RAIR in the newborn can also be due to neuronal intestinal dysplasia [9], hypoganglionosis [10], or to a transitory functional obstruction of the colon (small left colon) [7]. In the latter, enema with gastrografin is of therapeutic and diagnostic value [7, 11].

Therefore, when HD in the newborn is either suspected or definitively diagnosed, medical treatment must be commenced with saline solution rectal irrigation and daily rectal manipulation to allow evacuation of fæces.

The objectives of the preoperative medical care are:

- That the patient reaches the definitive intervention without needing a colostomy.
- To avoid the appearance of enterocolitis.
- To reduce the distension of the colon, or at least to prevent its advance.
- To ensure adequate nutrition and that the patient thrives with good height and weight development.

This treatment is especially effective in patients with rectosigmoid disease, which represents between 75% and 80% of aganglionoses [4–6], and which produces symptoms of distal functional intestinal obstruction (Fig. 1 A). In most patients, these are resolved by means of an anorectal catheter that is introduced through the anus until it surpasses the aganglionic zone and reaches the dilated segment (Fig. 1 B), which is then decompressed and cleansed, thus resolving the distal intestinal obstruction. The following paragraphs describe the medical care procedures for decompression of the distal intestine.

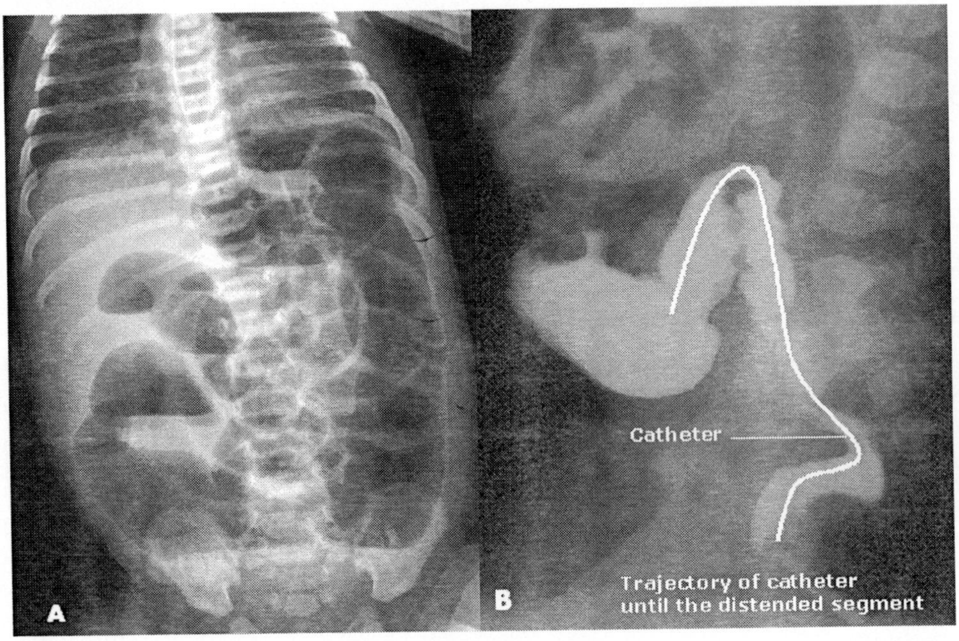

Figure 1. A Newborn of 4 days, meconial delay. Pattern of distal intestinal obstruction. B Opaque enema of the previous patient at 60 days of life: rectosigmoid aganglionosis.

Rectal Irrigation

In 1966 Shim and Swenson [12] described the effectiveness of regular rectal irrigation for the treatment of seriously ill infants with HD, since the result is to decompress the distal intestine avoiding the need for colostomy. Pellerin [13], who preferred to call the approach "nursing", described how this method allowed constipation in these children to be managed without colostomy until the time of definitive intervention. More recently, various authors [4,

5, 14–18] have referred to the effectiveness and safety of this method for controlling the neonate with HD until the time for the primary pull-through surgery.

In rectosigmoid aganglionosis, rather than rectal irrigation, the distended colon is washed out to decompress it and evacuate its entire content (fæces, liquid, and flatus). This eliminates the fæcal stasis and reduces the intraluminar pressure of the dilated intestine, avoiding the appearance of enterocolitis. These washouts (Fig.2 A) are done with lukewarm 0.9% saline solution, through a multiperforated rectal catheter (12–18 Fr) that reaches the distended colon. Table 1 lists the material used for rectal irrigation. The saline solution is injected through the catheter in the form of repeated irrigation (from 10 to 20 ml/kg), and then aspirated or left to flush out spontaneously through the catheter. Irrigation is continued until the effluent is clear. In the neonate, special care must be taken to inject only small amounts of saline each time, so as not to overcome the resistance of the ileocæcal valve and contaminate the small intestine. Also, two-or three-way Foley catheters (Rüsch 12–16 Fr) may be used. Herek [19] describes the three-way Foley catheter (16 Fr) as being very effective and safe for colon washouts of infants with HD.

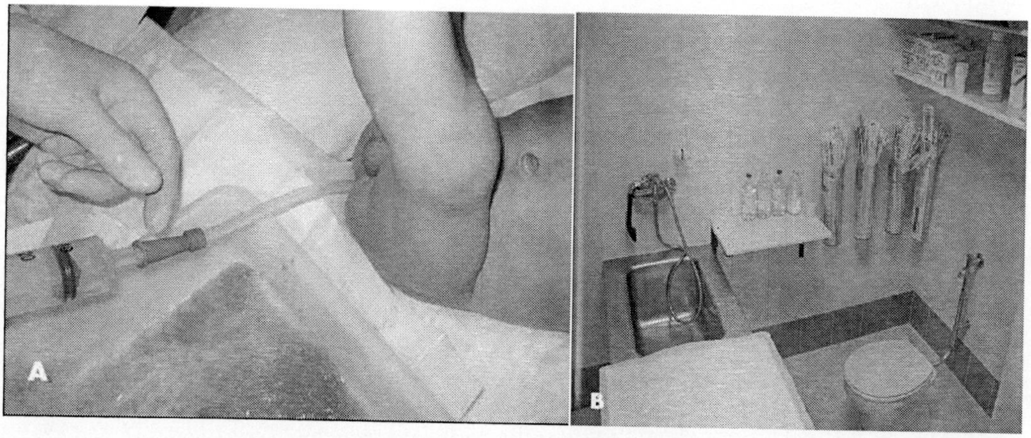

Figure 2. A. Nursing care with rectal catheter. B. Photograph of a nursing care room. (Courtesy of Dr R. Cabrera.)

Table 1. Material for rectal irrigation.

Material
• Lukewarm 0.9% saline solution
• Rectal catheter (12-18 Fr) or Foley catheter (12–16 Fr)
• 50 ml syringe
• Mineral oil
• Gloves
• Glass for mixture
• Collecting material: drainage bag or tray to receive stool

The rectal washouts must be performed once or several times a day, according to the patient's clinical evolution. The parents must learn the washout technique in the hospital, so that they can carry it out at home. Because the irrigation is with isotonic saline solution and the content is extracted immediately, there usually occur no electrolyte alterations. To this end, it is essential that all the instilled solution is evacuated. One of our infants with hypoganglionosis suffered an episode of hypertonic dehydration due to the accumulation of physiological serum within the intestine during rectal washout treatment. Steinbach [20] also reported water poisoning with circulatory overload in patients with HD, when tap-water enemas were used. Rectal perforation is another complication described [21, 22], but it is exceptional and due to the use of unsuitable catheters or their incorrect handling. In situations of gravely severe enterocolitis, especially in the neonate, rectal irrigation always requires great caution and even avoided at the beginning.

When the diagnosis of HD is made beyond the neonatal period, there usually exists fæcal retention, occasionally with large fæcalomas that require disimpaction with frequent saline enemas (10–20 ml/kg) which must be continued until the definitive intervention. We once had a patient 2 years old with Waardenburg syndrome and Hirschsprung's disease who was sent to our hospital with the erroneous diagnosis of abdominal tumour. It was an old fæcaloma of great size, that required general anæsthesia for its manual evacuation [23]. It is recommendable that hospitals should have nursing rooms such as that shown in Fig. 2 B, because the treatment more hygienic, comfortable, and effective for the patient.

For the decompression of the distal intestine, in addition to irrigation of the colon, rectal stimulation by manipulation is useful, once or several times a day, to overcome hypertonia of the rectum and the internal anal sphincter and thus facilitate fæcal evacuation.

Rectal Stimulation

This is performed by rectal manipulation, which in the newborn must always be done with the little finger so as not to cause anorectal damage [24, 25]. In the digital examination of the neonate with HD, it is possible to verify that the rectal ampulla is empty and that the rectum wall adheres to the examining finger [26, 27]. Rectal stimulation aids colon decompression because it distends the rectum and the internal anal sphincter. This reduces the anorectal hypertonia contributing to the distal intestinal obstruction [26]. In patients with short segment aganglionosis, the distended zone can be reached [25]. Occasionally, on removal of the finger there occurs a forceful discharge, typical of HD, with evacuation of flatus and fæces, and reduction or disappearance of the abdominal distension [25]. HD usually affects full-term neonates [28]. In the pre-term, rectal stimulation must be carried out using a Hegar's dilator.

For this treatment of decompression of the colon to be effective it must be performed in a correct and programmed form. The colon washouts and rectal manipulation must be done several times a day while the abdominal distension persists [15]. Once the distal obstruction has been controlled, the frequency can be reduced to once a day [15]. The patient must be evaluated in the hospital each 1–2 weeks to verify the nutritional state and that the family is managing the problem of constipation suitably [15]. The parents must be informed of possible complications that can arise during this stage of treatment. They must know how to recognize the early symptoms of enterocolitis. Thus, on the appearance of abdominal distension, rejection of food, lethargy, liquid foul-smelling fæces, vomiting, and fever, they should go to the hospital.

Although irrigation and rectal stimulation are especially indicated in rectosigmoid aganglionosis, these methods can also be used to control some neonates and infants with long segment HD or total colonic aganglionosis until the definitive intervention. It is this group of patients, however, in which stoma formation is usually necessary for intestinal decompression until the time of the pull-through surgery [29–31].

The ever earlier diagnosis of HD, together with improvements in anæsthetic techniques, and progress in neonatal care and nutrition, have contributed to one of the most important advances in the treatment of this disease – performing the definitive operation in a single stage and in the neonatal period [17, 32]. In 1980, So et al. [14] described how the diagnosis of HD in the first days of life does means that colostomy is not obligatory, and that the newborn can be managed safely with colon irrigations and rectal stimulation until the time for definitive surgery. In recent years, most patients with this disease have been operated in a single stage, in the first months of life, with techniques that are not highly invasive, at lower cost, and with shorter hospitalization times [4, 14, 16, 31–36].

There is ample evidence that the primary pull-through is effective and safe in the neonatal period, with results similar to 2-stage interventions, and with the advantage of avoiding the morbidity of the intestinal derivation [37, 38].

Table 2. The changing use of enterostomy over three decades.

Report	**Klein et al [28]**	**Sherman et al [39]**	**Suita et al [6]**	**Luis et al.[40]**	
Periods/years	1976-82	1973-85	1988-92	1992-1997	1998-2004
N° patients	26*	880 **	1121**	45 **	55**
Extensive aganglionosis	5	18	108	4	8
Enterostomy (%)	100	57,7	35.2	30	6.7

*=Newborn
**= All ages

Over the last 30 years, pre-pull-through medical care, especially irrigation and rectal stimulation, [4, 21, 30] have been replacing stoma formation which is indicated in ever fewer patients, as one observes in several series of Table 2 [6, 28, 39, 40], and as also is our experience. Thus, our last 19 neonates with rectosigmoid disease or affected up to the splenic flexure were managed with nursing care and rectal stimulation until pull-through surgery with no need for colostomy and free from episodes of enterocolitis [29]. In all newborn with total colonic aganglionosis with ileal involvement, an ileostomy was performed, although 2 patients were controlled with regular rectal irrigation and rectal stimulation for 3 and 4 months [30].

Enterostomies

In spite of the great advances in the neonatal care and surgical treatment of HD, digestive tract derivations continue to be essential for the intestinal decompression of some neonates with this pathology [21,37]. Colostomy is indicated in rectosigmoid or more proximal aganglionosis with complications that do not respond to medical treatment. Ileostomy is indicated in patients with total colonic aganglionosis with or without ileal involvement who present symptoms of intestinal obstruction [37,41–43]. An ostomy has a series of advantages, as set out in Table 3, but, being a temporary derivation, it involves one or two re-interventions and is not free of morbidity and mortality [44].

Table 3. Advantages of a decompressive stoma.

Advantages
• It resolves the intestinal obstruction
• It allows biopsies to be taken to determine the normal intestine
• It reduces the calibre of the distended intestine, and facilitates the definitive reconstruction
• Care at home is simplified and less traumatic
• Nutrition is improved, and the risk of enterocolitis is almost eliminated*

*Cases have described of enterocolitis with stoma [45]

Indications for Ostomy

The Very Sick Child with Enterocolitis

Ostomy is indicated in patients with clinical symptoms of severe enterocolitis, which can put the child's life in danger unless there is a rapid response to treatment with intravenous liquids, measures of intestinal decompression, and antibiotics [21, 37, 46].

Perforated Bowel

Perforated bowel in patients with HD is an indication for intestinal derivation [41–43]. This complication is most frequent in newborn and infants. Newman [42] describes an incidence of 4.4% of his cases (45 infants), and Surana [47] of 10.4% of 77 neonates with HD. A greater risk of this complication has been observed in the newborn with total colonic aganglionosis [48]. In most of the patients, the perforation is observed in the ganglionic intestine, but appendix perforations have also been described in the neonate [48]. The newborn with HD and perforated bowel does not usually have megacolon because the colon is decompressed through the perforation. Its diagnosis must be suspected from clinical findings and intraoperative biopsies of rectum and colon [37]. As the patient is usually very seriously ill, a simple cæcostomy or a defunctionalized ileostomy is recommended [43]. The definitive intervention must be made after the diagnostic confirmation of the aganglionosis and when the patient has recovered [37].

Perforations of the rectum needing proximal colostomy due to inadequate nursing have been described [21]. Stoma formation is indicated in patients with dehiscence of the post-pull-through coloanal anastomosis [21].

The Older Child with Massive Megacolon

Some children with a late diagnosis develop a massive distension of the proximal colon that can interfere with the pull-through procedure [37]. In some cases, the distension can be reduced with enemas and other forms of intestinal cleansing. In others, a colostomy or ileostomy must be performed to suitably decompress the distended intestine, and thus facilitate the definitive surgery [37].

Long Segment Aganglionosis

Long segment aganglionosis (ascending colon, or total colonic aganglionosis with or without ileal involvement), diagnosed by intestinal biopsies taken during a laparotomy following symptoms of intestinal obstruction, force an ileostomy prior to the definitive intervention. There are two reasons for this. On the one hand, the surgical management of these patients involves total or almost total colectomy. Any error on the part of the anatomo-pathologist in evaluating the intraoperative biopsies will complicate the patient's clinical evolution, since once the intestine has been extirpated the situation is irreversible [37]. Also, temporary ileostomy in total colonic aganglionosis allows one to see when the ileum matures and the fæces become consistent, which indicates that the definitive intervention can be performed [37].

The Child with Down Syndrome or Developmental Delay

In patients with Down syndrome and HD, there has been frequent use of colostomy prior to the definitive intervention [49]. Thus, in the series of Menezes [49] of 39 patients with Down syndrome and HD, pull-through without prior ostomy was only performed on 14. The main reason for the indication of stoma is the high risk of enterocolitis in these patients [50]. In the long term follow-up, after the pull-through procedure, the children with Down syndrome showed greater difficulty in controlling defæcation [49]. Some parents choose to return to the colostomy to improve their children's quality of life [49]. In children with mental retardation, especially in cases of total colonic aganglionosis, permanent ostomy may be a valid alternative [37].

Finally, it may be necessary to perform a colostomy in such situations as: severe under-nourishment of the patient, incorrect performance of the nursing by the parents, the hospital does not have the services of an anatomo-pathologist with experience in HD, and in difficult primary pull-through procedures in which it is desired to protect the coloanal anastomosis with stoma formation [37, 51, 52].

Placement of the Stoma

Patients in whom barium enema shows a clear transition zone in the rectosigmoid region require a limited laparotomy in the lower left quadrant, and the colostomy will be located next to the transition zone, in the dilated intestine with normal ganglionary cells [53]. The intraoperative biopsies will confirm the aganglionosis and the normal innervation of stoma that will be brought out through this wound. Colostomy next to the transition zone has several advantages: it allows the subsequent clinical confirmation of intestinal function up to the stoma, it conserves the intestinal length, and the pull-through is simplified [53].

If in the barium enema the transition zone is not clearly distinguishable, or when there are signs of intestinal obstruction, a more extensive vertical laparotomy is called for, and the intraoperative biopsies will indicate the position of the ostomy which will be brought out through a counter-incision [43]. The decompressive ileostomies are customarily located in the lower right quadrant [53]. The stomas must be placed in an anatomical position that allows the collecting bag to be put in place easily and safely.

Types of Stoma

Loop, double-barrel, and end enterostomies have been used, according to the preference and experience of the surgeon [21, 53, 54]. Some authors prefer the end ileostomy in cases of total colonic aganglionosis [21]. The present author uses loop stomas for the colostomy and ileostomy derivations in HD (Figs. 3A and 3 B) because they are performed more rapidly, are temporary, and the aganglionosis is resolved in two stages [43]

To prevent prolapse, stitches are required between the antimesenteric edges of the efferent and afferent segments of the intestinal loop within the abdomen. To avoid its retraction, the stoma must be very carefully sutured to the parietal peritoneum, muscle aponeurosis, and skin. It is important that the stoma is eased out through the wound without tension to prevent ischæmia and stenosis. With this type of stoma, there exists the risk that fæcal content can pass to the distal loop. To avoid this, the colostomy can be performed with an ample spur, using a flap of skin as a bridge between the two ends [21].

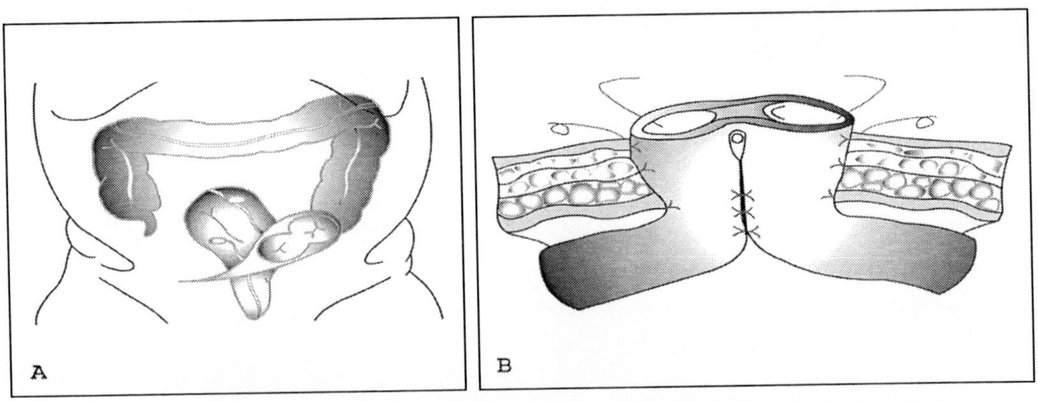

Figure 3. A. Loop Colostomy. B. Loop Ileostomy. (Modified from Gauderer [53]).

Care of the Stoma

The stoma requires special care involving the active participation of the parents, nurse, surgeon, and, if possible, a specialist in enterostomy [21, 53, 55–58]. The parents should have learnt before leaving the hospital how to handle the collecting bags to avoid the fæcal content contacting the peristomal skin [21, 53]. Ileostomies, especially the highest, usually excrete a more liquid content (which is more corrosive for the skin), so that these patients must be monitored periodically to prevent cutaneous lesions [53, 58]. Table 4 summarizes the care for ostomy.

Table 4. Care of the stoma.

- During the first 24–48 hours postoperative, the stoma is covered with vaselined gauzes.
- When the ostomy is transited, the peristomal skin is cleansed and thoroughly dried, and the bag and baseplate are put in place.
- The orifice of the baseplate through which the stoma is brought out must be the same size as the stoma so that the fæcal content does not come into contact with the skin, which is very fragile in the newborn.
- The bag will be changed as required by the rate of intestinal evacuation, and the baseplate every 4–5 days.

A great variety of collecting bags or enterostomy devices are marketed, for all ages and sizes including the small premature [53]. There are two classes of device: one-piece bags, bag and seal forming a single unit (the bags can be closed or opened at the bottom, with or without filter); and two-piece bags, formed by a plate that adheres to the skin, and a bag (opened or closed, with or without filter) that fits or sticks to the plate. This last device is more comfortable for the child. The central disc of the plate will be cut out according to the size of the stoma so that the peristomal skin does not come into contact with the fæcal content.

Among the products currently commercialized for the care of a stoma, particularly worthy of note are adhesive skin protectors, drying powders, and solutions for the control of odours [53]. The stoma will be cleansed daily with physiological serum and neutral soap, removing fæcal residue. The patient can be bathed, drying the stoma well. Occasionally, the distal end must be cleansed by irrigation with saline serum.

The parents of children with colostomy or ileostomy may find Web pages such as http://www.ostomyinternational.org/ useful. There they can obtain information about the International Ostomy Association, publications, and other resources, as well as links to commercial providers (e.g., Coloplast, Convatec, Cases, and Hollister) of stoma-related products (bags, cleansing products, etc.).

Complications of Ostomies

Colostomy and ileostomy are accompanied by high morbidity, and even mortality [53]. Table 5 summarizes the most frequent complications of colostomies performed for HD, anorectal malformations, and a group of other causes [45–48]. Transverse colon colostomies have more complications than stomas in the sigma [45, 46]. Defunctionalized colostomy is performed for anorectal malformations [39].

Table 5. Complications of colostomy.

Report Complications	Mollit et al [59] (n= 146) % HD=70	Al Salem et al [60] (n=74) % HD=34	Chandramouli et al [61] (n= 146) % HD=47	Cigdem et al [62] (n=473) % HD=117
Mortality	2.7	2.7	1.4	2.7
Morbidity	61.6	74.6	69.8	80.5
Excoriation	20	31	30.2	46.5
Prolapse	11.6	18.9	23.3	20.5
Stenosis	6.9	8.1	6.3	6.1
Bleeding	0.7	0.7	0	2.1
Revision	16.4	6.8	3.9	5

n=patients HD=Hirschsprung's disease

The morbidity of colostomy is very high and can affect up to 80% of the patients, according to a review by Cigdem [62]. Peristomal excoriation, prolapse, and obstruction/stenosis are the commonest and most important complications [59–62]. Mild prolapse is usually inconsequential, and requires no revision. Severe prolapses require rapid attention, and sometimes reconstruction of the stoma is necessary [53]. Temporizing measures for control of prolapse include a modified purse-string suture technique [63], or placement of a 'U' stitch from the lumen of the reduced intestine through the abdominal wall over an internal and external pledget [64]. This technique is based on the principle of bowel to peritoneum adhesion [64]. Stricture, if mild, may respond to dilatation [59]. However, if evacuation is decreased and the proximal intestine begins to dilate, revision is advisable [53]. Retraction of an end stoma requires revision, whereas retraction of a loop stoma interferes with proper evacuation and leads to the filling of the distal intestinal loop with fæces [53].

The morbidity of ileostomies is greater than of colostomies, because in addition to peristomal excoriation, prolapse, and obstruction/stenosis, there may occur major loss of liquids and electrolytes, and alterations in the absorption of nutrients [53, 58].

Bowel Preparation for Pull-Through

The purpose of bowel preparation for pull-through in HD must be to avoid infection of the abdominal wound, prevent dehiscence of the coloanal anastomosis, and facilitate the operation. Exclusive transanal or laparoscopic pull-through have eliminated or minimized the abdominal incision [29, 35, 65]. This technique, which can be used in the recto-sigmoid or more proximal aganglionoses, avoids infection of the wound, but the risk of dehiscence of the coloanal anastomosis persists. In a multicentre study in 2000 in the U.S., it was observed that the incidence of this complication was 2.6% in primary procedures and 9.7% in two-stage procedures [34].

In preparing the bowel for the pull-through, there are three therapeutic regimes that one can use: (1) mechanical bowel preparation with *rectal enemas* or *total irrigation of the bowel* [66–75], (2) intestinal decontamination with oral antibiotics [75–79], and (3) perioperative intravenous prophylaxis against aerobic and anaerobic germs [75, 80, 81]. The use of this therapeutic association has been reported to reduce the rates of postoperative infections in pædiatric colorectal surgery to 0–3.3% [67, 68, 70]. The current opinion is that mechanical cleansing and perioperative prophylaxis are essential in preparing the bowel for pull-through, but there is doubt about the benefits of oral antibiotics [75,82].

In the following sections, I will describe and discuss each of these therapeutic aspects of bowel preparation for pull-through.

Mechanical Bowel Preparation

The purpose here is to eliminate the fæcal content of the intestinal lumen, aid the action of oral antibiotics, and facilitate surgical manipulation of the colon and rectum [83]. Since the 1970s, this treatment has become surgical dogma for adult colorectal surgery [84–86]. Thus, in the survey by Zmora et al. [87] for the American Society of Colon and Rectal Surgeons on mechanical bowel preparation, 99% of the surgeons replied that they had used some method of intestinal cleansing before surgery. However, in recent years various randomized studies [88–92] have questioned the benefit of mechanical cleansing in reducing the postoperative morbidity of colorectal surgery. Furthermore, some recent clinical tests [93] have reported increased dehiscences of the coloanal anastomosis when practising mechanical intestinal cleansing.

In pædiatric patients, unlike in adults, there has only been one randomized study on the preparation of the bowel for elective colorectal surgery – that by Leys et al. in 2005 [94]. This pilot study included patients aged from 1 month to 20 years, and caused a certain controversy in communicating that the omission of bowel preparation in various intestinal pathologies including pull-through for HD (11 patients without preparation and 55 with preparation) does not increase the risk of infection of the wound or dehiscence of the anastomosis. Nevertheless, cleansing as preparation for pull-through in HD continues to be habitual, as is reflected in the reports of several workers [14,17,18,82, 95–99], and it is also the case for us [29]. In a survey conducted in 2007 by Breckler et al. [75] for the American Pediatric Surgical Association (136 pædiatric surgeons responded), 96% reported that they had used some method of mechanical bowel preparation for elective colorectal surgery for HD, anorectal malformations, or closure of ostomies in cases of necrotizing enterocolitis (Fig. 4). Mechanical intestinal cleansing can be carried out with rectal enemas or total irrigation of the bowel [75].

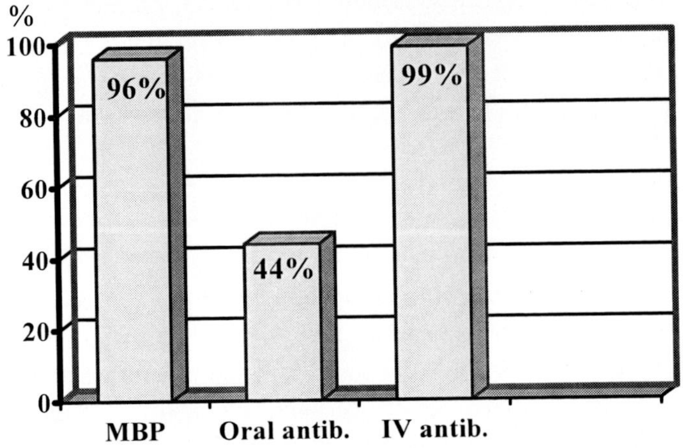

Figure 4. Survey of pædiatric surgeons on current practices of bowel preparation for elective colorectal surgery in children [75] MBP: Mechanical bowel preparation ORAL ANTIB: Oral antibiotics IV ANTIB: Intravenous antibiotics

Rectal Enemas

This is the traditional method of cleansing the colon in HD. In the survey of Breckler et al. [75], 40.7% of the surgeons responded that they had used rectal enemas to clean the colon in at least one patient. This method requires hospitalization of the child 2 days before the operation, during which time it is fed a liquid diet and given saline serum enemas through a rectal catheter (10–20 ml/kg) 2–3 times a day. Rectal enemas do not always achieve adequate cleansing of the colon [66, 82], especially in older children. Herek [19] reports, as is also our experience, that the 3-way Foley catheter is very effective and safe for preparation of the colon for pull-through in infants with HD. In neonates under a regime of daily rectal irrigation, it is in practice unnecessary to add further measures of cleansing the colon for pull-through [15].

In children with renal insufficiency or bowel dysfunction, phosphate enemas are dangerous. Even in normal children, they should not bed used under 2 years of age and with extreme caution between 2 and 5 years [100].

Total Intestinal Irrigation (TII)

This consists of total intestinal cleansing by means of the oral or nasogastric administration of an evacuant solution. It is indicated for preparation of the colon in primary pull-throughs or for pull-throughs with prior stoma [26, 75]. The latter require an additional 1 or 2 rectal enemas with saline solution.

TII as a new method of cleansing the colon was described by Hevit et al. in 1973 [101], and represented a major advance in adult colorectal surgery. Davis et al. [102] in 1980 describe the oral administration of a solution of polyethylene glycol with electrolytes and sulfate (Golytely®) to minimize the absorption of water and sodium and accelerate intestinal transit. Postuma et al. in 1982 [103] introduce TII in older children. Tuggle et al. in 1987 [66] report the safety and effectiveness of Golytely® in patients aged between 3 weeks and 14 years, and this is subsequently confirmed by other workers [70, 72–74] in neonates and infants for preoperative preparation of the colon in HD.

Electrolyte solutions (saline solution at 0.9% plus 5 mEq of KCl/l, or Hartmann's solution) have also been used with good results [68, 74]. Nevertheless the use of polyethylene glycol 3350 or 4000 (PEG-E) is recommended due to their being isotonic and iso-osmotic solutions with concentrations of Na, Cl, K, HCO3 and SO4 in amounts that do not cause their absorption or secretion when instilled through the intestine [66, 104, 105].

In the survey by Breckler et al. [75], 90.7% of the pædiatric surgeons had used PEG-E for mechanical preparation of the bowel.

Table 6 lists the trade names of some evacuant solutions with PEG-E and their composition in g/l.

Golytely® is one of the most frequently used solutions because it is well tolerated in the neonate and at other ages [26,66,68-71,73–75], although its ingestion may produce nausea, vomiting, abdominal distension, or colic abdominal pain [71, 74]. The preparation of the bowel is usually excellent in most patients [66, 68, 70, 72–75]. Engum et al. [73] administered Golytely in a regime of home-care nursing in HD patients with favourable results.

Vila et al. [71] observed, probably due to the sluicing effect of TII, a significant decline in the number of germs/ml in the colon content. This reduction was more evident in the anaerobic group ($p<0.001$) when oral neomycin and erythromycin were added.

Table 6. Evacuant solutions with polyethylene glycol for TII. Composition in g/l

	Golytely®	Lainco simple ®	Movicol Paediatric®	Bohm®
Polyethylene glycol				
type	3350	4000	3350	4000
amount	59	60.4	105	60
Sodium sulfate	5.68	5.68	-	5.6
Sodium bicarbonate	1.685	1.68	1.428	1.68
Sodium chloride	1.465	1.46	2.8	1.46
Potassium chloride	0.74	0.74	0.4	0.74
Sodium phosphate	-	-	-	0.48
Laboratory	Braintree L.	Lainco	Norgine	Bohm
Volume of water in which to dilute per sachet	4 L	1.5 L	62,5 ml	250 ml

The Method of Total Irrigation

The patient with HD about to receive bowel preparation by means of TII for pull-through is hospitalized the morning before the operation, without needing previous dietary restriction. That afternoon, fasting is commenced, and an epicutaneous catheter for fluid therapy and an 8 Fr nasogastric catheter are put in place (the gastric placement of the latter must be verified). If there is no stoma, a 12 Fr rectal catheter is well lubricated and should be passed into the transient zone, if technically possible, for distal decompression. Half an hour before beginning intestinal irrigation, metoclopramide is administered IV at 0.2 mg/kg to facilitate gastric emptying. Intestinal cleansing is begun by administering the PGE-E solution (25-30 ml/kg/h) via the nasogastric catheter until the fluid exiting the rectal catheter or the stoma is clear [26, 66, 70, 74]. The infusion rate must be adjusted to the tolerance of the patient. Between three and six hours is usually sufficient to complete intestinal cleansing.

During the procedure, arterial blood pressure, heart rate, respiratory frequency, temperature, and diuresis must be monitored with controls every half hour. If signs of discomfort such as abdominal distension, colic pain, or vomiting appear, the rate of infusion is reduced or suspended. The weight, pH, and serum electrolytes must be determined pre- and post-infusion. In bearers of an ileostomy, simultaneous IV fluid therapy must be administered because of the potential loss of electrolytes (hyponatræmia) [72]. Golytely, although well tolerated, must be used with great caution in patients with renal, cardiac, or pulmonary disease [66]. Its accidental aspiration can cause serious respiratory complications [106]. TII with PEG-E is contraindicated if there is hypersensitivity to PEG-E, risk of dehydration, or intestinal obstruction as can be the case in patients with long-segment disease who are being managed without stoma [74].

Intestinal Decontamination

This consists of the preoperative administration, orally or by nasogastric tube, of antibiotics with the purpose of reducing the number of bacteria of the normal flora of the colon. In neonates with HD, the flora that establishes itself is similar to that of healthy patients, including the formation of colonies of such anaerobes as *Clostridium difficile* [107].

The antibiotics must be fast acting, aerobic and anaerobic bactericidals, of limited absorption and with low local and systemic toxicity [83]. It has been reported that preoperative oral antibiotics reduce the infectious complications of adult colorectal surgery [79,83,108]. For that reason, although some authors have expressed doubt about its utility [109] and others [110] have observed an increase of colitis due to *C. difficile* when they have administered neomycin and erythromycin preoperatively, intestinal decontamination continues to be widely used at this age [83, 87]. Nichols et al. [86] noted that, in their survey of North American colorectal surgeons, 86.5% had used oral antibiotics for bowel preparation.

For children, different strategies have been used for oral antibiotic application in preparing the colon for pull-through: oral erythromycin and neomycin [67,72,75,97], or neomycin alone [110] and oral metronidazol [111], or neomycin at 1% added to saline serum rectal enemas [17]. There have as yet been no randomized studies that demonstrate the effectiveness of intestinal decontamination for the prevention of infections of the wound or dehiscence of the coloanal anastomosis in pull-through surgery for HD. In the survey of Breckler et al. [75] (Fig. 4), 44% of the surgeons had used oral antibiotics (33% routinely and 11% in selected cases) in preparing the bowel for surgery. Oral antibiotics reduce the microflora in the lumen and mucous of the colon before it is opened surgically but does not prevent infection, which parenteral antibiotics do [83]. For that reason, some workers [15, 26, 94, 95, 98, 112–115] do not use intestinal decontamination prior to pull-through, because they probably consider that intestinal cleansing and perioperative intravenous antibiotics constitute sufficient bowel preparation for this intervention.

Nevertheless, in spite of the lack of specific indications for its use, our practice is to perform preoperative oral decontamination in patients with risk of postoperative infections or enterocolitis, including children with Down syndrome and HD. The periods of antibiotic administration must be kept short because of the risk of bacterial resistance. Administration is started once intestinal cleansing is complete. One of the following two patterns of administration can be used: *50 mg/kg neomycin and erythromycin* orally in 3 doses of each antibiotic [72, 75, 76, 96], or the association *50mg/kg neomycin and 5mg/kg metronidazol* orally, 3 doses each drug [75, 116]. Their administration is begun at 1 p.m. and is continued at 2 p.m. and 11 p.m. of the afternoon/evening before surgery. In these cases, bowel preparation must begin at 8 a.m. of the day prior to surgery.

Antibiotic Prophylaxis

Preoperative antibiotic prophylaxis (PAP) is a therapy of proven effectiveness in preventing surgical site infections (SSI) [75,79, 80, 117]. A multicentre study found the incidence of infection of the wound in pædiatric surgery to be 4.4% [118]. Wildhaber et al. [119] report a 20% frequency of abdominal wound infection in patients with total colonic aganglionosis.

The HD pull-through is considered to be a procedure that is contaminated by Gram-negative enterobacteria and anaerobes in which PAP with broad spectrum antibiotics effective against these germs is indicated [79, 95, 96, 111]. In the survey by Breckler et al. [75] (Fig. 4), 99% of surgeons use antibiotic prophylaxis in colorectal surgery. Prophylaxis is commenced one hour before beginning surgery (at anæsthetic induction is the most advisable) so that the antibiotic has time to reach its target serum concentration and the site of potential infection [80]. Preoperative prophylaxis is begun with an initial intravenous dose of one of the following associations: *Metronidazol (7.5 mg/kg/dose), ampicillin (50-100 mg/kg/dose) and gentamicin (1.7 mg/kg/dose)* [29, 75,120,121]; *or amoxicillin–clavulanic acid (15–30 mg/kg/dose) and gentamicin (1.7 mg/kg/dose)* [79]; *or cefoxitin (80 mg/kg/dose)* [110]. During the operation, a second dose is administered if the procedure is taking longer than about 4 hours or if there is considered to be a major loss of blood. Prophylaxis is continued with 2 more doses in the first 24 hours postoperative [79]. The guidelines of the National Surgical Infection Prevention Project recommend that the prophylactic antibiotic is limited to the first 24 hours postoperative or less [122]. Nevertheless, in HD pull-throughs, most authors [26, 95, 96,114] maintain antibiotic treatment for 3-5 days postoperatively.

To summarize, colon preparation for pull-through in HD requires intestinal cleansing and perioperative prophylaxis in all patients. The possible benefits of oral antibiotics are not well known, for which reason we can not recommend their routine use. In this respect, a randomized trial would help to identify the role of oral antibiotics in colon preparation in children and to determine the optimal duration of intravenous antibiotic treatment.

References

[1] Vieten D, Spicer R: Enterocolitis complicating Hirschsprung's disease. *Semin Pediatr Surg*, 2004;13:263-72.

[2] Menezes M, Puri P: Long-term outcome of patients with enterocolitis complicating Hirschsprung's disease. *Pediatr Surg Int*, 2006;22:316-8.

[3] Teitelbaum DH, Qualman SJ, Caniano DA:Hirschsprung`disease.Identification of risk factor for enterocolitis. *Ann Surg*, 1998;207:240-4.

[4] Langer JC, Durrant AC, De LA Torre L, Teitelbaum DH, Minkes RK, Caty MG, Wildhaber BE, Ortega SJ, Hirose S, Albanese CT.One-stage transanal Soave pullthrough for Hirschsprung disease: a multicenter experience with 141 children. *Ann Surg*, 2003;238:569-83.

[5] Dasgupta R, Langer JC: Transanal pull-through for Hirschsprung disease. *Semin Pediatr Surg*, 2005;14:64-71

[6] Suita S, Taguchi T, Ieiri S, Nakatsuji T: Hirschsprung's disease in Japan: analysis of 3852 patients based on a nationwide survey in 30 years. *J Pediatr Surg*, 2005;40:197-202.

[7] Núñez R, Cabrera R, Moreno C, Agulla E, Vargas I, Blesa E:Utilidad de la manometría anorrectal en el diagnóstico neonatal de la enfermedad de Hirschsprung. *Cir Pediatr*, 2000;13:16-9.

[8] Lopez-Alonso M, Ribas J, Hernandez A, Anguita FA, Gomez de Terreros I, Martinez-Caro A: Efficiency of the anorectal manometry for the diagnosis of Hirschsprung's disease in the newborn period. *Eur J Pediatr Surg*, 1995;5:160-3.

[9] Pini-Prato A, Martucciello G, Jasonni V: Rectal suction biopsy in the diagnosis of intestinal dysganglionosis: 5-year experience with solo-RBT. *J Pediatr Surg*, 2006;41:1043-8.

[10] Zhang HY, Feng JX, Huang L, Wang G, Wei MF, Weng YZ. Diagnosis and surgical treatment of isolated hypoganglionosis. *World J Pediatr*. 2008;4:295-300.

[11] Loening-Baucke, kimura K: Failure to pass meconium: Diagnosing neonatal intestinal obstruction. *Am Fam Phsician*, 1999:60:2043-50.

[12] Shim WKT, Swenson O: Treatment of congenital megacolon in 50 infants. *Padiatrics*, 1966;38:185-93.

[13] Pellerin D: Visión sobre la enfermedad de Hirschsprung. *Cir Pediatr*, 1992;5:57-66.

[14] So HB, Schwartz DL, Berker JM, Daum F, Schneider KM: Endorectal "pull-through" without preliminary colostomy in neonates with Hirschsprung's disease. *J Pediatr Surg*. 1980;1:470-1.

[15] Ghinelli C, Del Rosi C: Treatment of Hirschsprung`disease without colostomy. *Peadtr Surg Int.* 1993;8:27-30.

[16] So HB, Becker JM, Schwartz DL, Kutin ND: Eighteen years' experience with neonatal Hirschsprung's disease treated by endorectal pull-through without colostomy. *J Pediatr Surg*. 1998;33:673-5.

[17] Coran AG, Teitelbaum DH: Recent advances in the management of Hirschsprung`disease. *Am J Surg*, 2000;180:382-7.

[18] Somme S, Langer JC: Primary versus staged pull-through for the treatment of Hirschsprung disease. *Semin Pediatr Surg*. 2004;13:249-55.

[19] Herek Ö: A new colonic lavage meted for infants with Hirschsprung' disease. *Pediatr Surg Int*, 2001;17:671.

[20] Steinbach HL, Rosenberg RH, Grossman M, Nelson TL: The potential hazard of enemas in patients with Hirschsprung's disease. *Radiology*, 1955;64:45-50.

[21] Casasa JM, Broto J, Jimenez AI, Boix-Ochoa J: Derivaciones intestinales en el tratamiento de la enfermedad de Hirschsprung. *An Esp Pediatr*, 1987;281-3.

[22] Handley DV, Rieger NA, Rodda DJ; Rectal perforation from colonic irrigation administered by alternative practitioners. *Med J Aust*. 2004;15:575-6

[23] Vázquez Rueda F, Blesa Sánchez E, Núñez Núñez R, Galán Gómez E: Síndrome de Waardenburg y enfermedad de Hirschsprung: *An Esp Pediatr*. 1998;48:306-8.

[24] El Hadad M, Corkery JJ: The anus in the newborn. *Pediatrics* 1985 Dec;76:927-8.

[25] Cabrera García R: *Estudio morfológico y funcional anorrectal en el recién nacido.* [Tesis doctoral]. Badajoz. UEx. 1998.

[26] Teitelbaum DH, Coran AG, Weitzman JJ, Ziegler MM, Kane T: Hirschsprung' disease and related neuromuscular disorders of the intestine. In O'Neill JA, Rowe MI, Grosfeld JL, Fonkairud EW, Coran AG. (Eds). *Pediatry Surgery*. Fifth Edition. St Louis: Mosby;1998. p. 1381-1424.

[27] Belkind-Gerson J, Coello-Ramirez P, Garcia-Aranda JA, Heller S,Larrosa A: Enfermedad de Hirschsprung. *Bol Med Hosp Infant Mex*, 2002:59:1665-6.

[28] Klein MD, Coran AG, Wesly JR, Drongowski RA: Hirschsprung's disease in the newborn. *J Pediatr Surg*, 1984;19:370-4

[29] Núñez R.Utilidad de la Manometría anorrectal para el diagnóstico neonatal de la Enfermedad de Hirschsprung. Comunicación Personal. *Symposium Neonatológico.* Badajoz, Spain. 2009.

[30] Núñez R, Cabrera R, Agulla E, Moreno C, Serrano A, Ortiz C, Blesa E:Aganglionismo cólico con afectación ileal. Plastia ileocolica. *Cir Pediatr*. 2001;14:76-81

[31] Anupama B, Zheng S, Xiao X: Ten-year experience in the management of total colonic aganglionosis. *J Pediatr Surg* 2007;42:1671-6.

[32] Wilcox DT, Bruce J, Bowen J, Bianchi A: One-stage neonatal pull-through to treat Hirschsprung's disease. *J Pediatr Surg*., 1997;32:243-5.

[33] Santos MC, Giacomantonio JM, Lau HY: Primary Swenson pull-through compared with multiple-stage pull-through in the neonate. J.*Pediatr Surg*. 1999;34:1079-81.

[34] Teitelbaum DH, Cilley RE, Sherman NJ, Bliss D, Uitylugt ND, Ranaud EJ et al. A decade of experience with the primary pull-through for hirschsprung disease in the newborn period: a multicenter analysis of outcomes. *Ann Surg*, 2000;232:372-80.

[35] De la Torre L, Ortega A: Transanal versus open endorectal pull-through for Hirschsprung`disease. *J Pediatr Surg*.2000;35:1630-2.

[36] Mir E, Karaca I, Gunsar C, Sencan A, Fescekoglu O: Primary Duhamel-Martin operations in neonates and infants. *Pediatr Int*. 2001;43:405-8.

[37] Somme S, Langer JC: Primary versus staged pull-through for the treatment of Hirschsprung disease. *Semin Pediatr Surg*. 2004;13:249-55.

[38] Ramesh JC, Ramanujam TM, Yik YI, Go DW: Management of Hirschsprung's disease with reference to one-stage pull-through without colostomy. *J Pediatr Surg*, 1999;34:1691-4

[39] Sherman JO, Zinder ME, Weitzman JJ, Jona JZ, Gillis DA, O`Donnell B et al.: A 40-year multinational retrospective study of 880 Swenson procedures. *J Pediatr Surg*. 1989;24:833-8.

[40] Luis LA, Encinas JL, Avila LF, Andrés AM, Burgos L, Fernández A, et al.:Enfermedad de Hirschsprung: Enseñanza de los últimos 100 casos. *Cir Pediatr*, 2006:19:167-72.

[41] Soper RT, Opitz JM: Neonatal pneumoperitoneum and Hirschsprung`disease. *Surgery* 1962:51:527-33.

[42] Newman B, Nussbaum A, Kirkpatrick JA: Bowel perforation in Hirschsprung's disease. *AJR AM J Roentgenol*. 1987;148:1195-7.

[43] Komuro H,Urita Y, Hori T, Hirai M, Kudou S, Kawamai H, Kaneko M: Perforation of the colon in neonates. *J Pediatr Surg*. 2005;40:1916-19.

[44] Nour S, Beck J, Stringer MD: Colostomy complications in infants and children. *Ann R Coll Surg Engl*. 1996;78:526-30.

[45] Surana R, Quinn FMJ, Puri P: Evaluation of risk factors in the development of enterocolitis complicating Hirschsprung`disease. *Pediatr Surg Int*, 1994; 9:23-6.

[46] Teitelbaun DH, Coran A:Enterocolitis. *Semin Pediatr Surg*.1998;7:162-9.

[47] Surana R, Quinn FMJ, Puri P: Neonatal intestinal perforation in Hirscsprung`disease. *Pediatr Surg Int*er.1994;9:501-2.

[48] Sarioglu A, Tanyel FC, Buyukpamukcu N, Hicsonmez A: Appendiceal perforation: a potentially lethal initial mode of presentation of Hirschsprung's disease. *J Pediatr Surg*. 1997;32:123-4.

[49] Menezes M, Puri P: Long-term clinical outcome in patients with Hirschsprung`disease and associated Down´s syndrome. *J Pediatr Surg*, 2005;40:810-2.

[50] Caniano DA, Teitelbaum DH, Qualman SJ: Management of Hirschsprung's disease in children with trisomy 21. *Am J Surg*. 1990;159:402-4.

[51] Shayan K, Smith C, Langer JC:Reliability of intraoperative frozen sections in the management of Hirschsprung's disease.*J Pediatr Surg*. 2004;39:1345-8.

[52] Langer JC: Repeat pull-through surgery for complicated Hirschsprung's disease: indications, techniques, and results. *J Pediatr Surg*. 1999;34:1136-41.

[53] Gauderer MWL: Stomas of the small and large intestine. In O'Oneill JA, Rowe MI, Grosfeld JL, Fonkairud EW, Coran AG. (Eds). *Pediatry Surgery*. Fifth Edition. St Louis: Mosby; 1998. p. 1345-59.

[54] Yamagiwa I, Obata K, Okuyama N, Ouchi T, Suzuki R, Shimazaki Y: An ileostomy at the aganglionic ileum for total colon aganglionosis.*Eur J Pediatr Surg*, 2000;10:62-4.

[55] Cooney DE, Grosfeld JL:Care of the child with a colostomy. *Pediatrics*. 1977;59:469-72.

[56] Davies A: Children with ostomies: parents helping parents. *J ET Nurs*. 1992;19:207-12.

[57] Turnbull RW, Turnbull GB: The history and current status of paramedical support for the ostomy patient. *J ET Nurs*. 1993;20:102-4.

[58] Bower TR, Pringle KC, Soper RT: Sodium deficit causing decreased weight gain and metabolic acidosis in infants with ileostomy. *J Peditr Surg* 1988;23:567-72.

[59] Mollit DL, Malangoni MA, Ballantine TV, Grosfeld JL: Colostomy complications in children. An analysis of 146 cases. *Arch Surg*, 1980;115:455-8.

[60] Al-Salem AH, Grant C, Khawaja S: Colostomy complications in infants and children. *Int Surg*. 1992;77:164-6.

[61] Chandramouli B,Srinivasan K, Jagdish S, Ananthakrishnan N:Morbidity and mortality of colostomy and its closure in children. *J Pediatr Surg*. 2004;39:596-9.

[62] Cigdem MK, Onen A, Duran H, Ozturk H, Otcu S: The mechanical complications of colostomy in infants and children: analysis of 473 cases of a single center.*Pediatr Surg Int*. 2006;22:671-6.

[63] Krasna IH: A simple purse string suture technique for treatment of colostomy prolapse and intussusception. *J Pediatr Surg*. 1979;14:801-2.

[64] Gauderer MWL, Izant RJ Jr: A technique for temporary control of colostomy prolapse in children. *J Pediatr Surg*. 1985;20:653-5.

[65] Georgeson KE, Robertson DJ: Laparoscopic-assisted approaches for the definitive surgery for Hirschsprung's disease. *Semin Pediatr Surg*. 2004;13:256-62.

[66] Tuggle DW, Hoelzer DJ, Tunell WP, Smith EI: The safety and cost-effectiveness of polyethylene glycol electrolyte solution bowel preparation in infants and children. *J Pediatr Surg*. 1987;22:513-5.

[67] Vila JJ, Gutierrez C, García-Sala C, Ruiz S: Whole bowel irrigation: experience in pediatric patients. *J Pediatr Surg*. 1987;22:447-50.

[68] Postuma R: Whole bowel irrigation in pediatric patients: a comparison of irrigating solutions. *J Pediatr Surg*. 1988;23:769-70.

[69] Millar AJ, Rode H, Buchler J, Cywes S: Whole-gut lavage in children using an iso-osmolar solution containing polyethelene glycol (Golytely). *J Pediatr Surg*, 1988 S;23:822-4.

[70] Wheeler RA, Davies N, Griffiths DM, Burge DM: The use of golytely for bowel cleansing in the first 3 months of life. *Pediatr Surg Int*. 1992;7:364-6.

[71] Vila Carbó JJ, García-Sala C, Gutierrez C, Ruiz Company S, Camps B: Irrigación digestiva en el paciente pediátrico: Estudio comparativo. *Cir Pediatr*, 1992:5:3-11.

[72] Donahue MC, Evangelista JK, Shamberger RC: Effect of Golytely on serum electrolytes and hydration status of infants. *J Pediatr Surg*. 1994;29:1095-6.

[73] Engum SA, Carter ME, Murphy D, Breckler FM, Schoonveld G and Grosfeld JL: Home bowel preparation for elective colonic procedures in children: Cost saving with quality assurance and improvement. *J Pediatr Surg*,2000; 35:232-4.

[74] Chattopadhyay A, Prakash B, Vepakomma D, Nagendhar Y,Vijayakumar: A prospective comparison of two regimes of bowel preparation for pediatric colorectal procedures: normal saline with added potassium vs. polyethylene glycol. *Pediatr Surg Int*. 2004;20:127-9.

[75] Breckler FD, Fuchs JR, Rescorla FJ: Survey of pediatric surgeons on current practices of bowel preparation for elective colorectal surgery in children. *Am J Surg*, 2007;193:315-8.

[76] Nichols RL, Broido P, Condon RE, Gorbach SL, Nyus LM: Efficacy of preoperative antimicrobial preparation of the bowel. *Ann Surg*; 1972;176:227-32.

[77] Nichols RL, Broido P, Condon RE, Gorbach SL, Nyus LM: Effect of preoperative neomycin-erythromycin intestinal preparation on the incidence of infectious complications following colon surgery. *Ann Surg*, 1973;178:453-62.

[78] Clarke JS, Condon RE, Bartlett JG, Gorbach SL, Nichols RL, Ochi S: Preoperative oral antibiotics reduce septic complications of colon operations: results of prospective, randomized, double-blind clinical study. *Ann Surg*, 1977;186:251-9.

[79] Lewis RT: Oral versus systemic antibiotic prophylaxis in elective colon surgery: a randomized study and meta-analysis send a message from the 1990s. *Can J Surg*. 2002; 45:173-80

[80] Cisneros JM, Rogriguez-Bano J, Mensa J, Trilla A, Cainzos M: Profilaxis con antimicrobianos en cirugía. *Enferm Infecc Microbiol Clin*. 2002;20:335-40.

[81] Kesler RW, Guhlow LJ, Saulsbury FT: Prophylactic antibiotics in pediatric surgery. *Pediatrics*. 1982;69:1-3

[82] Jasoni V, Pini Preto A, Martucciello G: Soave`s extramucosal endorectal pull-through procedure. In Holschneider AM, Puri P (Eds). *Hirschsprung's disease and Allied Disorders*. Third Edition. Berlin Heidelberg: Springer-Verlag; 2008. p. 337-88.

[83] Nichols RL, Choe EU, Weldon CB: Mechanical and Antibacterial Bowel Preparation in Colon and Rectal Surgery. *Chemotherapy*, 2005;51:115-21

[84] Beck DE, Fazio VW: Current preoperative bowel cleansing methods. Results of a survey. *Dis Colon Rectum*, 1990;33:12-5.

[85] Platell C, Hall J: What is the role of mechanical bowel preparation in patients undergoing colorectal surgery?. *Dis Colon Rectum*. 1998;41:875-82.

[86] Nichols RL, Smith JW, Garcia RY, Waterman RS, Holmes JW: Current practices of preoperative bowel preparation among North American colorectal surgeons. *Clin Infect Dis*. 1997;24:609-19.

[87] Zmora O, Mahajna A, Bar-Zakai B, Rocín D, Hershko D, Shabtai M et al.: Colon and rectal surgery without mechanical bowel preparation: a randomized prospective trial. *Ann Surg*, 2003;237:363-7.

[88] Bucher P, Mermillod B, Morel P, Soravia C: Does mechanical bowel preparation have a role in preventing postoperative complications in elective colorectal surgery?. *Swiss Med Wkly*, 2004;134:69-74.

[89] Memon MA, Devine J, Freeney J, From SG: Is mechanical bowel preparation really necessary for elective left sided colon and rectal surgery? Int J Colorectal Dis, 1997;12:298-302.

[90] Miettinen RP, Laitinen ST, Makela JT, Paakkonen ME: Bowel preparation with oral polyethylene glycol electrolyte solution vs. no preparation in elective open colorectal surgery: prospective, randomized study. *Dis Colon Rectum*, 2000;43:669-75.

[91] Fa-Si-Oen P, Roumen R, Buitenweg J, van de Velde, van Geldere D,Putter H et al: Mechanical bowel preparation or not? Outcome of a multicenter, randomized trial in elective open colon surgery. *Dis Colon Rectum*, 2005;48:1509-16.

[92] Zmora O, Mahajna A, Bar-Zakai B, Hershko D: Is mechanical bowel preparation mandatory for left-sided colonic anastomosis? Results of a prospective randomized trial. *Tech Coloproctol*, 2006;10:131-5.

[93] Bucher P, Mermillod B, Gervaz P, Morel P: Mechanical bowel preparation for elective colorectal surgery: a meta-analysis. *Arch Surg*, 2004;139:1359-64.

[94] Leys CM, Austin MT, Pietsch JB: Elective intestinal operations in infants and children without mechanical bowel preparation: a pilot study. *J Pediatr Surg*. 2005;40:978-81.

[95] De La Torre-Mondragón L, Ortega-Salgado JA: Transanal endorectal pull-through for Hirschsprung's disease. *J Pediatr Surg*, 1998;33:1283-86.

[96] Rintala R, LindhalH: Transanal endorectal coloanal anastomosis for Hirschsprung`disease. *Pediatr Surg Int*, 1993;8:128-31.

[97] Gao Y, Li G, Zhang X, Xu Q, Guo Z, Zheng B et al.: Primary transanal rectosigmoidectomy for Hirschsprung's disease: Preliminary results in the initial 33 cases. *J Pediatr Surg*,2001;36:1816-19.

[98] Teeraratkul: Transanal one-stage endorectal pull-through for Hirschsprung's disease in infants and children. *J Pediatr Surg*, 2003;38:184-7

[99] Egun Q, Celik A, Dokumucu Z, Balik E: Submucosal pressure-air insufflation facilitates endorectal mucosectomy in transanal endorectal pull-through procedure in patients with Hirschsprung's disease. *J Pediatr Surg*, 2003;38:188-90.

[100] Soumoy MP, Bachy A:Risk of phosphate enemas in the infant. *Arch Pediatr*, 1998;5:1221-23.

[101] Hewit J, Reeve J, Rigby J: Whole-gut irrigation in preparation for large-bowel surgery. *Lancet*, 1973;18:337-40.

[102] Davis GR, Santa Ana CA, Morawski SG, Fordtran JS: Development of a lavage solution associated with minimal water and electrolyte absorption or secretion. *Gastroenterology*, 1980;78:991-5.

[103] Postuma R: Whole bowel irrigation in pediatric patients. *J Pediatr Surg*. 1982;17:350-2.

[104] Swartz ML: NuLYTELY (PEG 3350, sodium chloride, sodium bicarbonate and potassium chloride for oral solution). *Gastroenterol Nurs*, 1992;14:200-3.

[105] Bichet-Sicard A, Rose E, Schmitt M, De Miscault G, Perrier JF: Biological effects of golytely in children. *Chir Pediatr*. 1988;29:181-3.

[106] Narsinghani U, Chadha M, Farrar HC, Anand KS: Life-threatening respiratory failure following accidental infusion of polyethylene glycol electrolyte solution into the lung. *J Toxicol Clin Toxicol,* 2001;39:105-7.

[107] Wilson-Storey D: Microbial studies of enterocolitis in Hirschsprung`disease. *Pediatr Sur Int*, 1994;9:248-50.

[108] Konishi T, Watanabe T, Kishimoto J, Nagawa H: Elective colon and rectal surgery differ in risk factors for wound infection: results of prospective surveillance. *Ann Surg*. 2006;244:758-63

[109] Espin-Basany E, Sánchez-García JL, Lopez-Cano M, Lozoya-Trujillo R, Medarde-Ferrer M, Armadans-Gil L et al.: Prospective, randomised study on antibiotic prophylaxis in colorectal surgery. Is it really necessary to use oral antibiotics. *Int J Colorectal Dis*, 2005;20:542-6.

[110] Wren SM, Ahmed N, Jamal A, Safadi BY: Preoperative oral antibiotics in colorectal surgery increase the rate of Clostridium difficile colitis. *Arch Surg*. 2005;140:752-6.

[111] Gaztambide Casellas J, Sánchez Diaz F, García Soldevilla N, Argos Rodríguez MD, Pérez Rodríguez J: Rectosigmoidostomía y anastomnosis término-terminal coloanal con sutura mecánica para el tratamiento de la enfermedad de Hirschsprung, *Cir Pediatr*.2004;17:61-4.

[112] Khan O, Nixon HN: Metronidazole prophylaxis elective large bowel ssurgery in children: a prospective trial. *Br J Surg*, 1978;65:804-7.

[113] Hadidi A: Transanal endorectal pull-through for Hirschsprung's disease: experience with 68 patients. *J Pediatr Surg*, 2003;38:1337-40.

[114] Kumar R, Mackay A, Borzi P: Laparoscopic Swenson procedure--an optimal approach for both primary and secondary pull-through for Hirschsprung's disease. *J Pediatr Surg*. 2003;38:1440-3.

[115] Juliá V, Castañón M, Torrado X, pinzón JC, Morales L:Descenso transanl exclusivo para el tratamiento de la enfermedad de Hirschsprung. *Cir Pediatr*, 2004;17:85-8

[116] Debo Adeyemi S, Tai da Rocha-Afodu J: Clinical studies of 4 methods of bowel preparation in colorectal surgery. *Eur Surg Res*, 1986;18:331-6.

[117] Gorecki W, Grochowska E, Krysta M: A prospective comparison of antibiotic usage in pediatric surgical patients: the safety, advantage, and effectiveness of the Surgical Infection Society guidelines versus a common practice. *J Pedatr Surg*, 2002;37:1430-4.

[118] Horwitz JR, Chwals WJ, Doski JJ, Suescun EA, Cheu HW, Lally KP: Pediatric wound infections: a prospective multicenter study. *Ann Surg*, 1998;227:553-8.

[119] Wildhaber BE, Teitelbaum DH, Coran AG: Total colonic Hirschsprung's disease: a 28-year experience. *J Pediatr Surg*, 2005;40:203-6.

[120] Giachetto G, Alvarez C, Arnaud H, Bruno P, Da Silava E, De Salterain H, Tamosiunas G et al:Uso de antibióticos en servicios de internación pediátrica. *Rev Med Uruguay*, 2001:17:55-62.

[121] Puri P: Swenson`s procedure. In Holschneider AM, Puri P (Eds). *Hirschsprung`disease and Allied Disorders*. Third Edition. Berlin Heidelberg: Springer-Verlag; 2008. p. 331-35.

[122] Bratzler DW, Houck PM: Surgical infection prevention guidelines writers workgroup. Antimicrobial prophylaxis for surgery: an advisory statement from the National Surgical Infection Prevention Project. *Clin Infect Dis*, 2004;38:1706-15.

Part III: Hirschsprung's Disease: Classical Surgical Treatment (Swenson, Duhamel, Soave, and Rehbein), Laparoscopy in Hirschsprung's Disease, Exclusive Transanal Pull-Through, Total Colonic Aganglionosis, A Critical Review of the Different Operations for Hirschsprung's Disease

In: Hirschsprung's Disease: Diagnosis and Treatment
Ed: Ramón Núñez and Manuel López-Alonso
ISBN: 978-1-60741-349-3

Chapter XIV

Swenson's Technique

Luis Lassaletta

Introduction

Orvar Swenson, one of the greatest paediatric surgeons of the XX century, reported, in 1950, a new technique for the surgical treatment of the Hirschsprung disease. Twenty years later he wrote: "On the basis of our studies of the abnormal pathophysiology in Hirschsprung disease published in 1948, we proposed removal of the aganglionic segment. This could only be accomplished by a pull-through technique since an anterior resection would leave several centimetres of aganglionic rectum in place. Consequently, the operation that we have performed now for twenty years seems best suited to accomplish a cure on the basis of the known pathophysiology of the disease. In our experience it is the most difficult operation that we encounter in paediatric surgery. It is a tedious one and consumes four to five hours." [1,2].

In these days we perform the operation in about two hours thanks to our greater knowledge of regional anatomy and the improvement of anaesthesia together with the use of better surgical instruments.

The Swenson technique is still one of the procedures chosen by many paediatric surgeons and many Paediatric Surgical Departments in the world, and a great number of surgeons defend it against other techniques such as Soave, Rehbein or Duhamel [3].

According to Swenson this procedure is the most physiological one, but as every technique may have complications, especially if it is not perfectly done. This kind of pullthrough must be done by a well trained surgeon. One mistake in the perirectal dissection can be followed by consequences related to rectal continence or genital function [4].

In 1960 Julio Monereo, a Spanish paediatric surgeon from Madrid, learned the technique from Robert Gross in Boston. In the following years he modified some steps from the original procedure. Since 1965 he was in charge of the Department of Paediatric Surgery of the Children's Hospital La Paz in Madrid. This hospital with more than 100 paediatric surgical beds was one of the most important paediatric hospitals in the country, and is still a reference for many paediatric pathologies. He developed the Swenson technique for Hirschsprung disease, and taught his team how to perform it. After his death in 1977 we called this technique as the Swenson-Monereo technique [5,6].

Age of the Operation

In his first description of the operation, Swenson considered the best time to perform the pullthrough was when the baby was one year old or weighed about ten kilogrammes, in order to find pelvic structures large enough. In those years we always performed a colostomy before the pullthrough generally on the right side or the hepatic angle of the colon, to protect the operation. For the past few years, the age of the operation has been reduced and we have performed the pullthrough without colostomy in many cases. We think that the best age for the pullthrough is around 4-6 months. Most cases wait until this time without a colostomy. The perirrectal dissection at this age, or even before, is easier and it is possible to perform the operation correctly.

In cases of intercurrent enterocolitis we are forced to make a diversion before the operation but our idea is to do it as little as possible.

Preoperative Care

If the baby has a previous colostomy, the preoperative care is very simple. The colostomy on the right side will protect the pullthrough in the postoperative period. If the colostomy is located in the distal ganglionic colon, we must prepare the bowel with evacuation solutions and enemas in order to clean the intestinal tract. The same happens if the baby has no diversion. In this case an intestinal preparation must be completed. We also add an antibiotic prophylaxis to prevent secondary contamination.

Patient Position

The patient must be in the Fowler position with the perineal area slightly elevated and with minimum Trendelemburg. Nasogastrical drainage and vesical sondage are necessary for the operation. Both remain in the postoperative period. As the bladder and the uretra in the male have close relations with the rectum, it is normal to suffer hematuria during the days following the operation.

We perform the operation in two different fields, abdominal and perineal. The abdominal field is entered by three surgeons and the perineal field is entered by two surgeons. It is necessary to prevent contamination and there must be no contact between both fields.

Most surgeons prefer to operate from the right side of the baby, but some of them prefer to operate from the other side to improve control of the rectum dissection. The second assistant is located between the legs of the patient.

Laparotomy and Biopsies

We prefer to perform a large laparotomy in the middle of the abdomen to make easier the dissection of the rectum and the liberation of the colon in case of long aganglionism. We use the Denis Bronw retractor which is an ideal instrument to dissect the pelvis.

Before the operation, all patients undergo a barium enema, a manometry and suction biopsies which are made at the time of diagnosis.

At the time of the laparotomy we repeat biopsies in at least three locations, including rectum, sigma, and left colon, in order to confirm the diagnosis and also to evaluate the size of the aganglionism. Biopsies are extramucosal and are inmediately sent to the pathologist. We usually receive the report during the rectal dissection. The location of the biopsies are sutured with long silk stitches to be recognized later at the time of the resection. It is important to delimitate the three zones: the narrow segment, the transition zone and the dilated segment, to be able to evaluate the pullthrough. We prefer to remove the transition zone, the narrow one and also a part of the dilated zone. In cases without diversion, the postoperative period is more successful if the distal portion of the normal dilated segment is removed.

Rectal Dissection

The rectal dissection starts with the ligature of the rectal superior artery, the end of the inferior mesenteric artery. Artery and vein must be divided separately, close to the rectal wall. We then move to one cm above the peritoneal reflection, where we start the rectal dissection and we advance distally, coagulating small vessels with monopolar or bipolar electrocoagulation. The dissection around the rectal wall must be performed close to this wall all the time. This is the best way to avoid injuring small branches of the perirrectal inervation.

Down to the peritoneum, rectal dissection shows the longitudinal muscle fibres of the rectal wall, which at this place has no serosa. The dissection is easier at the posterior wall because the irrigation goes through the haemorrhoidal middle artery, which is lateral in both sides. It is more difficult at the anterior wall because the urethra is very close in males. The urethral tube may be palpated in the dissection of the anterior wall. It is easier in females because the vagina wall is not so close.

All vessels must be coagulated, so the dissection is very slow. We usually put some stitches all around the peritoneum in order to have some references for the pullthrough later on. When the dissection is close to the anus, it is necessary to coagulate the middle hemorroideal artery in both sides of the rectal wall. The dissection must be finished about 2cm close to the anus. Bimanual palpation is very useful, one finger around the rectal wall and another one in the anus. We must feel the proximity of both fingers (Figure 1) [5].

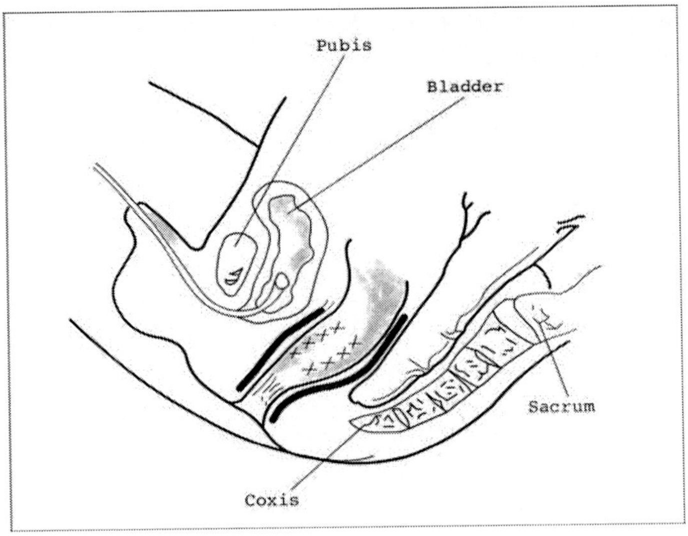

Figure 1. Dissection of the rectum

Following the rectal dissection we must perform the vascular time. At this time we will have the results of the biopsies and we must plan the extent of the resection.

Vascular Time

The pullthrough is planned according to the biopsie´s results. If the normal biopsy is located at the proximal part of the sigma, we choose the left colical artery to irrigate the colon. Then we must liberate and ligate the sigmoid arteries, leaving the peripherical arcs which are well irrigated through the left branch of the left colical artery. This artery is a very good choice, because its branches leave the irrigation of the distal colon in very good condition (Figure 2) [5].

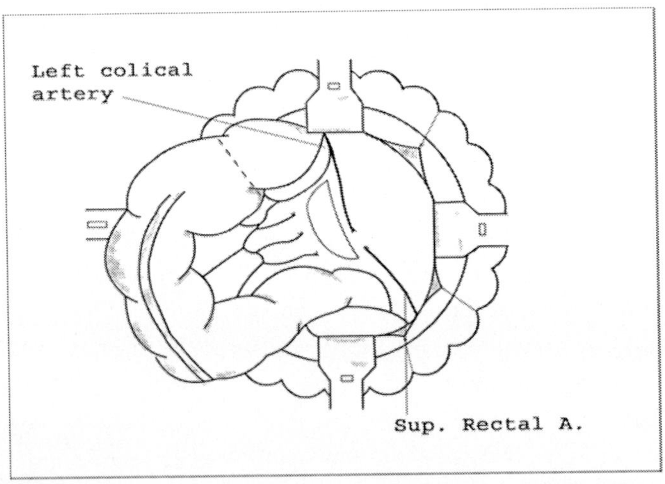

Figure 2. Vascular time. The level of transection of the colon is shown

If the left colon has no ganglionar cells, we must ligate the left colical vessels, and try to move down to the anus the splenic angle of the colon, irrigated trough the Riolano arch which is located between the middle colical artery and the left colical artery. Sometimes this procedure may be difficult. In cases of aganglionism of the tranverse colon, the only available procedure is also to ligate the middle colical artery, and perform the pullthrough with the right colon, irrigated by the ileo- ceco colic artery. In these cases the colon must rotate at the frontal plane to preserve its irrigation (Deloyer technique).

If all the colon is affected with the disease, a pullthrough must be performed with the terminal ileum irrigated by the same artery.

Abdomino Perineal Pullthrough

Two surgeons with two different sets of surgical instruments perform the perineal time, in order to avoid abdominal contamination. We start with an anal dilatation and clean the rectal cavity with serum and sponges. The pullthrough is performed with a long forceps introduced through the anus to pull and evert the colon. We prefer not to open the colon in the abdominal cavity, so we open the colon outside the abdomen, close to the anus. We open it at 2 cm. from the anus and pull the colon from inside until we can see the normal biopsy zone. Then we finish the opening of the around rectum going in to the posterior part until the anus as a sphincterotomy cutting the internal sphincter (Figure 3) [6].

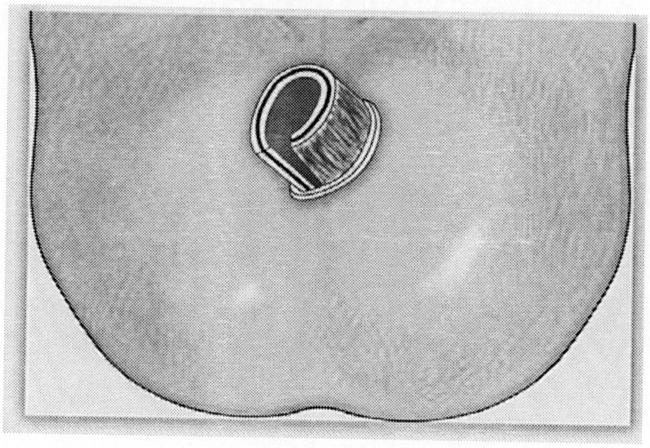

Figure 3. Posterior sphincterotomy

After that, we perform an end to end anastomosis in two layers between rectum and colon and we reintroduce the anastomosis inside the cavity.

According to the first description of Swenson, we used to perform an anterior hemianastomosis, leaving a prolapse of the descended colon to evaluate its irrigation. After ten days we performed the complete anastomosis cutting the prolapse. Nowadays we do not think it is necessary to leave a prolapse, and in most cases we perform the complete anastomosis. We leave a rectal tube for five days to allow feces and gases out.

Postoperative Care

Ten days after operation we evaluate the rectal caliber. Some patients need dilatations but they very seldom have severe stenosis. Dilatations with the finger or with other instruments usually improve the caliber of the anastomosis. We advise the child´s mother to perform rectal sondage with her finger everyday for the first six months after the operation, to facilitate the exit of air and feces, especially if the patient is very young and must adjust to a normal diet in the following months.

Histological Study

The biopsies and the resected colon are studied after the operation to find out what kind of Hirschsprung disease it is, and if the ganglionar cells are normal or displasic. We study again the suction biopsies performed at the time ot the diagnosis. It is important to have normal intestine in the proximal end of the resection and, as mentioned above, we prefer to remove the transitional segment which in the most cases has hypoganglionism. The more of the dilated segment we remove, the better the postoperative period will be, and the earlier the intestinal transit will be restored.

Postoperative Complications

Skin infections, leaks, stenosis of the anastomosis, and perineal fibrosis are the most frequent immediate complications. Skin infection may be followed by an abscess of the wall. When the infection affects the perineal anastomosis and the patient has no diversion, a colostomy must be performed as soon as possible in order to facilitate the remission of the infection. A leak in the anastomosis is usually followed by an abscess, which makes the diversion necessary. In case of severe stenosis of the anastomosis it is always better to start with dilatations ten to twelve days after the operation. In case of perineal fibrosis a new pullthrough must always be performed after a previous colostomy.

The most important long term complications of the Swenson operation are rectal incontinence, and lesion of the genital inervation in the male, this leading to impotence [10]. Fecal soiling has the greatest negative impact on the quality of life in children with Hirschsprung´s disease. Distinctions between occasional soiling and incontinence sometimes are difficult.

Constipation and evacuation fecal disorders can be seen during the first years, but most patients improve and have a normal life [7].

Methods

In our Department of Surgery the Swenson procedure was performed between 1965 – 1990 in 85% of the cases of Hirschsprung disease. Between 1990-1995 we introduced some other techniques (laparoscopy and Soave) and the Swenson was performed in 70% of the cases. Between 1995 and 2005 the Swenson technique was reduced to 60% due to the use of the transanal approach.

One hundred children who underwent consecutive pull through operations for Hirschsprung's disease between 1990 and 2005 were followed up. The average follow-up was 8 years (range 1-16 years). The location of the aganglionism was: Rectosygmoid 75 cases, Left colon 8, Transverse colon 5,Total colonic 8 and Intestinal total 4 cases.

The Swenson procedure was performed in 60 cases, another 24 cases were operated with the Soave technique, 11 cases with transanal approach and 5 with other techniques. Sixty three per cent of the patients had had a previous colostomy. In some of them the diversion had been performed before they were treated in our Department. Eighty patients had the colostomy at the hepatic angle of the colon, ten of them at the splenic angle and five of them had an ileostomy.

Sixteen per cent of the cases had associated anomalies: Down Syndrome 6 cases, Smith L. Opitz syndrome 1, Wandemburg Syndrome 1, Gastrointestinal anomalies 5,Congenital Diaphragmatic Hernia 1 and Heart anomalies 2 cases.

Postoperative Complications

We had 5 cases of intestinal obstruction secondary to adhesions that needed laparotomy. One case had evisceration, and two cases had a fistula of the anastomosis which required diversion in the postoperative period. Three patients died, one in the neonatal period because of a sepsis, one of enterocolitis, and the other one, a patient with an extensive intestinal aganglionism, died of a sepsis, after three years with parenteral nutrition. Three cases had severe stenosis secondary to isquemia, but they were cured with dilatations.

We reoperated four patients performing a new pullthrough using the Swenson technique again. All the patients are in very good condition at present. One of the patients had an insufficient pullthrough because of a pathology mistake. The other three were referred from another hospital because the operation had failed [8].

Long Term Results

According to the Holschneider scale we asked the operated patients about their rectal disorders (Tabble I). Eighty six per cent of the cases enjoy normal life and have very good continence. Eleven per cent of the cases have occasional problems and three per cent have stooling disorders. No one has genital disorders. We are aware that when we ask the patients about their functions after the pullthrough, the possibility of "social continence" is present in almost all the cases. Older patients achieve good continence, sometimes better than before [9,10,11,12].

Table I. Long term results of the Swenson's technique

Nº patients	Good results	Occasional problems	Stooling disorders	Genital disorders
60	86 %	11%	3%	0%

References

[1] Swenson. O. Early history of the therapy of Hirschsprung´s disease: facts and personal observations over 50 years. *J Pediatr Surg* 1996,31:1003-8

[2] Swenson. O. *Pediatric Surgery*.Third Edition. London: Butterworths; 1969.

[3] Swenson. O. A new surgical treatment for Hirschsprung disease. *Surgery* 1950,28: 371-83

[4] Swenson O. Hirschprung´s disease: a review. *Pediatrics* 2002;109:914-8

[5] Lassaletta L. Tratamiento quirúrgico de la Enfermedad de Hirschsprung. In *Enfermedades Anorrectales.Diagnóstico y tratamiento*. Lopez Ríos F. (ed). Harcourt Brace of Spain; 1999. p. 385-93.

[6] Monereo J.Nuevos aspectos clinico-patologicos y terapeúticos en la enfermedad de Hirschsprung. In "*Seminarios de Cirugía Pediátrica 1968-1969*". INP; Madrid 1969. p.643-61

[7] Bai Y., Chen H., Hao J., HuangY., Wang W.Long-term outcome and quality of life after the Swenson procedure for Hirschsprung's disease. *J Pediatr Surg*. 2002;37:639-42.

[8] Luis AL., Encinas JL.,Avila LF, Andres AM, Burgos L, Fernandez A, Queizán A., Olivares P., López Santamaría M., Burgos E., Hernández F., Lassaletta L., Tovar J.A. Enfermedad de Hirschsprung: lecciones aprendidas en los últimos 100 casos. *Cir Pediatr* 2006, 19:177-81

[9] Weidner BC, Waldhausen JH Swenson revisited; a one stage transanal pull-through procedure for Hirschprung disease. *J Pediatr Surg*. 2003;38:1208-11

[10] Weitzmann JJ. Swenson's procedure: In: Welch KJ, Randolph JG, Ravitch M M, O'Neill JA, Rowe MI (eds). *Pediatric Surgery*. Fourth Edition.Vol 2. Chicago: Year Book Medical Publishers INC;1986. p.1016-7.

[11] Sherman JO, Snyder ME, Fisher et al."A 40 year multinational retrospective study of 880 Swenson procedures" *J Pediatr Surg* 1989;24:833-8.

[12] Puri P: Swenson´s procedure. In Holschneider AM, Puri P (Eds). *Hirschsprung`s disease and Allied Disorders*. Third Edition. Berlin Heidelberg: Springer-Verlag; 2008. p. 229-48.

In: Hirschsprung's Disease: Diagnosis and Treatment
Ed: Ramón Núñez and Manuel López-Alonso

ISBN: 978-1-60741-349-3

Chapter XV

Duhamel's Technique

Piyawan Chiengkriwate

Introduction

The goal of surgical management for Hirschsprung's disease is to remove the aganglionic bowel and reconstruct the intestinal tract by bringing the normally innervated bowel to the anus, while preserving normal sphincter function. Surgical practice for Hirschsprung's disease has changed significantly over the past few decades, as multistaged surgical therapy has been replaced by a single-stage procedure [1-4]. With the method we now know as Duhamel's technique, Bernard Duhamel first described this technique for dealing with Hirschsprung's disease in 1956 as a modification of the Swenson procedure [5]. The procedure consisted of a retrorectal approach, whereby a significant portion of the aganglionic rectum was preserved and anastomosed to a the ganglionic proximal colon. The initial operative approach actually avoided an anastomosis, using instead a crush-clamping of ganglionated to aganglionic intestine.[6,7] The advantages of this procedure include ease of performance, reduction of anastomotic leaks and strictures, retention of anal sensory receptors, and preservation of the nervi erigentes. The Duhamel procedure is widely used around the world, and excellent long-term results have been published [8].

Over the years since it was first introduced, there have been a number of modifications of the Duhamel procedure, the most widely adopted of which has been the placement of the anastomosis above the internal sphincter to avoid incontinence.[9] An additional modification involves eliminating the proximal rectal pouch "spur" in the aganglionic rectum, which can trap large accumulations of stool, as, for instance, with Martin and Altemeier[10] and Martin and Caudill[11] who suggest careful clamp placement can entirely eliminate the rectal pouch. Another modification of Duhamel pull-through uses a gastrointestinal anastomosis (GIA) stapling technique, with the rationale that a retrorectal pull-through requires less pelvic dissection and the avoidance of anterior dissection leads to better preservation of the anal sphincter complex and reduces the possibility of injuring the genitourinary organs.[12-14] In the past, many infants with Hirschsprung's disease presented late with severe malnutrition, sepsis, and colonic distension, and in these patients a colostomy was a lifesaving procedure. A colostomy has always been an essential component of the standard treatment of Hirschsprung's disease with two main purposes: decompression of the functional obstruction and protection of the neorectum. Moreover, in some institutes where rapid pathologic diagnosis is not available, a colostomy serves to verify the functioning portion of the colon planned for pull-down. In addition, a staged surgical approach was advocated because the operation was believed to be technically easier when performed in an older child.

The primary pull-through is accepted as applicable for most colorectal anastomosies. With the possibility of early diagnosis, reliable frozen section service [15] and advancements in modern pediatric anesthetic practice, a child with Hirschsprung's disease may undergo a definitive colorectal pull-through safely in his or her first few months of life without any need of temporary stoma. It has been recently reported that the single-stage pull-through operation for Hirschsprung's disease is probably safer and may offer better functional outcomes compared with a multistage procedure [16,17]. The one-stage procedure, moreover, avoids the complications of colostomy and the costs of staged therapy [1,18]. Any previous colostomy, established at the time of diagnosis, usually during the neonatal period, is taken down at the time of the pull-through operation.

More recently, the Duhamel procedure has been performed using a laparoscopic technique, with excellent results. Because minimally invasive surgery is also playing a larger role as medical procedures advance, it seems likely that the standard Hirschsprung's procedure will ultimately end up as a one-stage transanal or laparoscopic-assisted pull-through [19-22]. However, in the developing world, the problem of late diagnosis leading to severe dilatation of the proximal colon and malnutrition still exists. For this reason, adopting the new treatment technology for this group of patients has to be carefully managed.

Operative Technique

The Duhamel operation leaves the native rectum in situ, and the normally innervate colon is moved behind the rectum to the presacral space [23]. An end-to-side anastomosis is then done, and the two lumens are joined. The procedure is conventionally used in infants between 9 and 12 months of age, although several groups have reported primary Duhamel pull-throughs in younger patients or newborns.[24-27] For these latter procedures, a smaller endo-GIA stapler is used for the anastomosis. In patients considered unsuitable for a 1-stage modified Duhamel pull-through, the initial surgical intervention consists of a laparotomy and formation of a leveling stoma in the ganglionic bowel, confirmed by histologic examination. The pull-through procedure is performed electively at a later stage, usually 4 to 6 weeks later or when the child became well nourished and/or the associated anomalies are corrected.

Bowel Preparation

Before the pull-through operation, all patients undergo mechanical bowel preparation [28]). Care must be taken to give adequate rectal and colonic washouts as stool is often inspissated in the distal rectum. Erythromycin and neomycin are used for intraluminal prophylaxis. A combination of gentamicin and metronidazole are commenced on induction of anesthesia.

Position

Excellent exposure is obtained by assistants supporting and flexing the lower extremities at the hips during the anal anastomosis. So in preparation, the patient is placed in a supine lithotomy position, with the buttocks brought to the end of the operating table and prepared for surgery from the nipples to the knees (Figure 1). The operating table is placed in a slight Trendelenburg position. Stockinets are placed around each leg to maintain warmth. Most patients receive adjunctive epidural anesthesia, and all receive an indwelling urinary bladder catheter. A nasogastric tube is placed after induction of anesthesia.

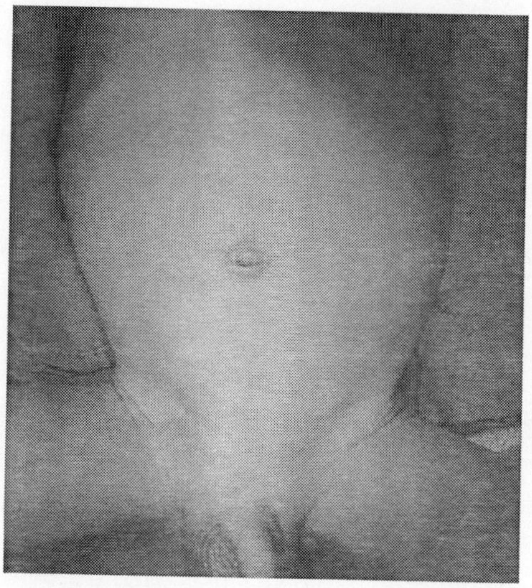

Figure 1. The patient is placed in the lithotomy position.

Incision

A low midline abdominal incision is made for excellent exposure of the rectosigmoid area. If there is an existing colostomy, a circumferential incision is made incorporating the colostomy takedown.

Procedure

After the abdomen is opened, the intestine is examined to evaluate the disease extension, and histologic confirmation of the ganglionic bowel is performed by frozen section examination. In cases with a previously established sigmoid colostomy, the stoma is usually taken down and used for the pull-through. Colon mobilization is begun in the rectosigmoid mesocolon just proximal to the rectosigmoid junction. The division of the mesocolon is accomplished using an absorbable material ligature. The aganglionic distal rectum is mobilized below the peritoneal reflection, carefully protecting the adjacent organs such as the ureters, bladder, seminal vesicle and duct. The colon is decompressed by milking the colonic content to a transition colon, where umbilical tape can be applied to ligate above the aganglionic rectum and also used for upward traction.

The aganglionic colon and ganglionic colon are divided and closed at each end with 2-0 silk. The ganglionic colon is labeled as mesenteric or antimesenteric by the use of different silk sutures, allowing the surgeon working on the pulled through segment to maintain correct orientation of the bowel as it is pulled into the anus. The pull-through ganglionic colon should look like a normal colon including having a serosal texture, a normal colonic diameter, a normal ganglionic colon and show good blood support; if these features are present, a tension-free pull-through should follow.

Anterior traction on the rectum then exposes the presacral retrorectal space. The retrorectal space is created bluntly, with dissection carried out directly in the midline. Dissection can be facilitated by using a curved Hegar dilator of appropriate size, but is also easily and safely performed with the index finger. This dissection is carried down to the pelvic floor and adequately enlarged so that another surgeon's finger can be felt when inserted 1 to 1.5 cm into the anus. At this point the surgeon's attention is directed to the perineum. For the author's practice, the operative instrument has two completely different set-ups. Also, all the instruments used in the perineal portion of the procedure are treated as dirty and exchanged for fresh instruments, and gloves are changed at the end of the anastomosis. A narrow anal retractor, or a nasal speculum is placed and held in position by the assistant still working on the abdomen. No separate field is created which allows improved communication and keeps surgeon and assistant on the same operative field.

In preparation for the second stage of the procedure, rectal cleaning is performed until the field is clear by using gauze soaked with betadine solution. Four-quadrant tacking silk sutures are placed at the dentate line from the posterior wall-six o'clock, to the right wall-nine o'clock, to the anterior wall-twelve o'clock, and turn to the left wall-three o'clock; this maneuver brings the dentate line into the operative view. After this, a curved Hegar dilator is placed in the retrorectal space to act as a cutting block. Using a scalpel, a full-thickness rectal incision is made 0.5 to 1 cm proximal to the dentate line posteriorly. Care is taken to maintain this distance by curving the incision as one moves laterally in each direction. This procedure connects the lumen of the aganglionic rectum with the retrorectal space. Full-thickness traction sutures are placed on both edges of this incision. First a lower group of three 4-0 absorbable sutures(polydioxanone) are placed on the inferior aspect of this incision, one in the midline and one each on both left and right sides, and the second group is made of three additional absorbable sutures placed on the upper portion of this incision in similar positions (Fig.2A).

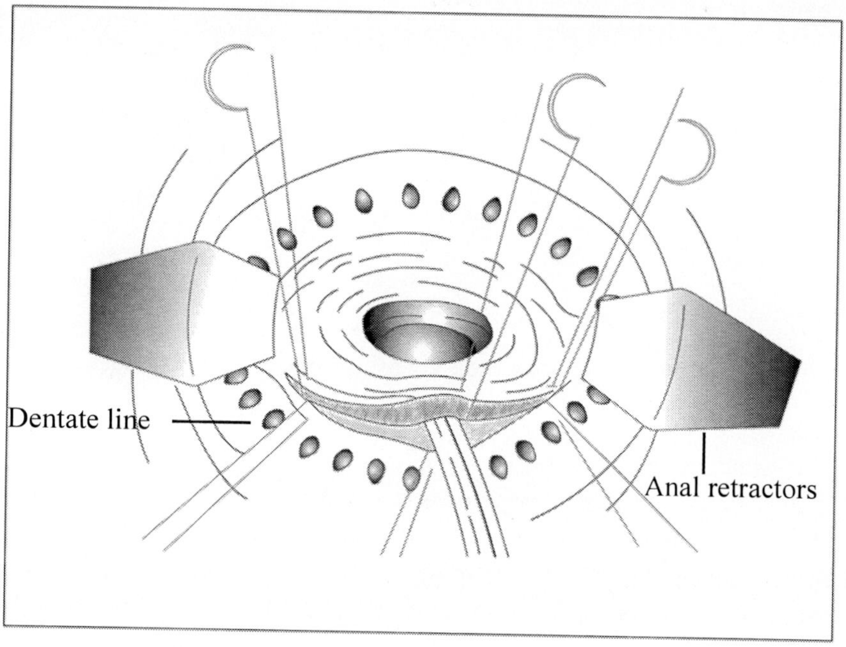

Figure 2. A. Posterior full-thickness rectal wall incision 0.5 to 1 cm proximal to the dentate line and a group of three 4-0 absorbable sutures are placed on the inferior aspect and the upper portion of this incision.

Each suture is held in place with marker hemostats. The different marker types prevent confusion of orientation once the ganglionic bowel is pulled through. The surgeon operating on the anus inserts a long clamp into the retrorectal space towards the abdominal field. The two tacking sutures on the distal ganglionic bowel are fed into this clamp and pulled down. The surgeon remaining in the abdominal field makes sure that the bowel does not rotate as it is brought down.

Once the bowel is pulled through, the suture line is excised on the anterior half of the colon and a single-layered anastomosis is created, starting with the three previously placed absorbable sutures and additional stitches (Fig.2B).

Care is taken with each stitch so that the anterior wall of the anus is not incorporated into any of the sutures. The suture tail should be kept for a tacking suture when an automatic GIA stapling device is applied. After the anterior half of the anastomosis is completed, the remainder of the suture line is excised and the anastomosis is finished with additional stitches as required (Fig.2 C).

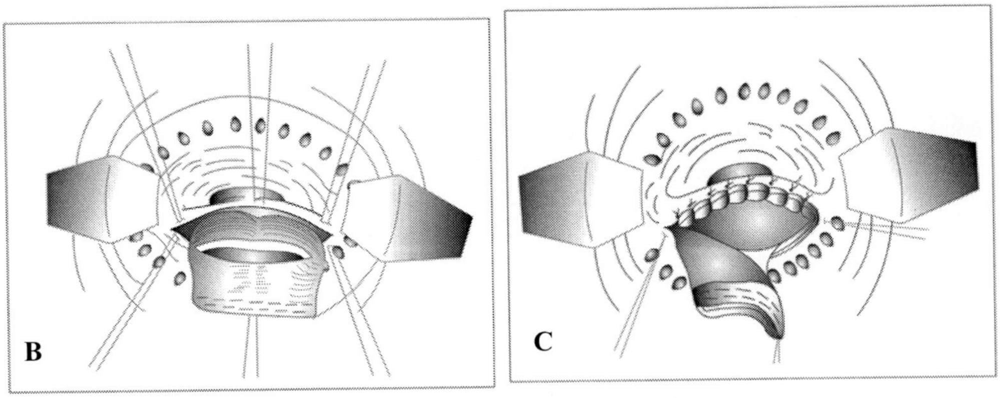

Figure 2 B. The bowel is pulled through, the suture line is excised on the anterior half of the colon and a single-layered anastomosis is created. C.The anterior half of the anastomosis is completed, the remainder of the suture line is excised and the anastomosis is finished with additional stitches as required.

An end-to-back anastomosis between the pulled-through segment and the rectum is performed by using polydioxanone. An automatic GIA stapling device, or an endo-GIA stapler in smaller infants, is placed with one arm in the native anal canal and the other in the neorectum to create a posterior-to-anterior anastomosis between the rectum and the pull-through bowel for a length of 55 to 75 mm; the proper size and length must be determined to fit the size of the infant's pelvis and to ensure that the desired length of colorectal anastomosis can be achieved (Fig.2 D).

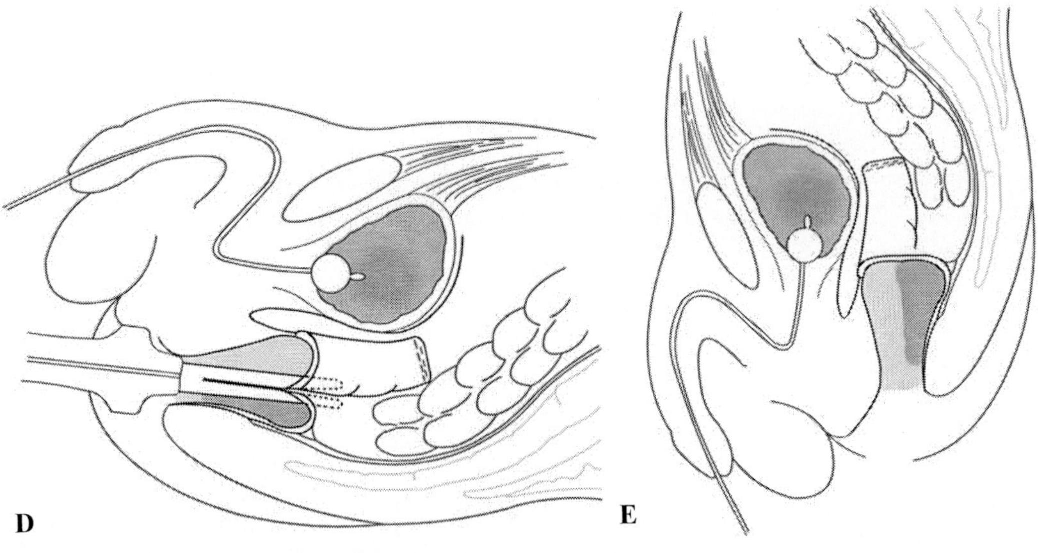

Figure 2 D. An automatic GIA stapling device is placed with one arm in the native anal canal and the other in the neorectum to create a posterior-to-anterior anastomosis. E, The two limbs of the bowel are completely anastomosed without any sign of fused septum.

Before firing the device, the surgeon ensures the orientation of both the anus and the abdomen are correct. Care must be taken to avoid interference with nearby organs such as the ureters or ovaries, bladder, or small intestine. When the desired position is safely set, the stapler is fired directly along the midline. After the stapler has been fired, complete elimination of the common rectal wall is confirmed by digital examination. It is critical for the surgeon to inspect digitally the side-to-side stapled anastomosis and make sure that the two limbs of the bowel are completely anastomosed without any sign of fused septum. Hemostasis along the suture line is checked. All retracting and holding sutures are removed. The operation from the anus is complete at this point (Fig.2 E).

The surgeon's gloves are changed. The surgeon turns to the transabdominal operation. Attention is then redirected to the pelvis. The excess remaining aganglionic rectum is finally resected.

The rectal stump is clamped and cut in the oblique line, usually 0.5 to 1 cm proximal to the GIA anastomosis. And then, the stump is closed at the level of the pelvic brim by using two layers of 3-0 absorbable running sutures. The truncated rectal spur is below the peritoneal reflection (Fig.2F). (This last step is critical. In the past, a proximal spur left between the bowel segment often resulted in the eventual formation of huge fecolomas.) At this point the anastomosis is completed. The neorectum may or may not be reperitonealized and the abdomen is closed (Fig.2 G).

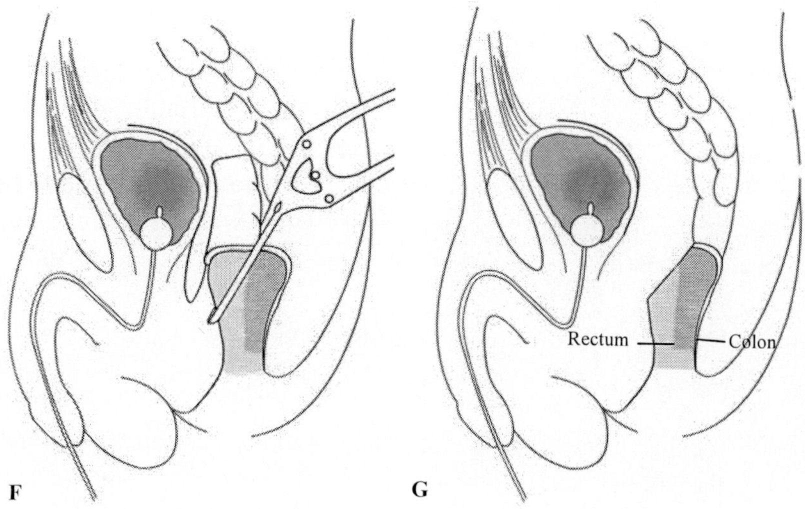

Figure 2 F: After returning to the abdominal field, the rectal stump is clamped and cut in the oblique line. G,:The stump is closed at the level of the pelvic brim by using two layers of 3-0 absorbable running sutures. The truncated rectal spur is below the peritoneal reflection. The neorectum may or may not be reperitonealized and the abdomen is closed.

Postoperative Care

Postoperatively, the urinary catheter is removed on the third postoperative day. Because bladder may be contused, a digital rectal examination or rectal irrigation should not be performed at this time. The nasogastric tube is removed once gastrointestinal activity returns.

Oral feeding is started when signs of colonic movement are observed, usually within 48 to 72 hours. Antibiotics are continued for 5-7 days after the surgery.

The potential complications of surgery for Hirschsprung's disease include the general group of complications of any abdominal surgery, including bleeding, infection, injury to adjacent organs, and the risks of anesthesia.[29]

Great attention is placed on examining the perineal region for the development of erythema or cellulites, as this is an early sign of an anastomotic leak. Investigation of a leak consists of a computed tomographic scan with contrast medium. Although fairly uncommon, should a leak be found a diverting colostomy must be performed immediately.

The patient is discharged when they have resumed full enteral feeding and need no intravenous analgesia. Parents are given thorough instructions on proper nutritional support, perineal care and the potential development of enterocolitis.

A gentle rectal examination is performed on the third week after surgery to ensure patency of the rectal anastomosis. Children should be followed up for several years for evaluation of long term outcome and growth status. The parents are regularly reminded to continue proper care.

Results

Fifty patients (80% males) underwent a modified Duhamel pull-through procedure at Prince of Songkla University Hospital over a 5-year period [27]. The patients were divided into 2 groups according to the operative approach. Group I consisted of 30 patients who underwent a 1-a stage modified Duhamel pull-through operation, whereas group II comprised 20 patients who received a definitive pull-through operation after the establishment of a colostomy (2-stage approach).

Choice of surgical management was the surgeon`s preference with agreement of the parents. However, it was generally agreed in our group that patients with 1) large dilatation of the proximal colon, 2) severe malnutrition, 3)moderate to severe enterocolitis and/or peritonitis or 4) an associated congenital anomaly necessitating correction or stabilization with a higher priority than colonic aganglionosis, were not suitable candidates for primary pull-through. Group II also included patients referred from other hospitals with an established colostomy.

Characteristics of the groups are shown in table 1. Eighteen patients presented with neonatal bowel obstruction, 22 with constipation, 9 with enterocolitis, and 1 with peritonitis. The time from diagnosis to the pull-through ranged from 2 to 435 days (median, 27 days). Operative time, including positioning, rectal irrigation, and frozen sections, ranged from 120 to 300 minutes (median, 200 minutes). Postoperative complications are summarized in table 2

Table 1. Demographic characteristics of the patients according to groups

Group	I (n = 30)	II (n = 20)
Age at pull-through (d)	72(5-10,977)	144 (64-3836)
0-12 mo	21 (70)	16 (80)
>12 mo	9 (30)	4 (20)
Weight at pull-through (kg)	5.3 (2.8-82)	5.5 (3.3-24.5)
0-5 kg	14 (47)	7 (35)
>5 Kg	16 (53)	13 (65)
Transition zone		
Rectum/Rectosigmoid	21 (70)	6 (30)
Sigmoid	7 (23.3	7 (35)
Descending colon	0	4 (20)
Splenic colon	1 (3.3)	2 (10)
Transverse colon	1 (3.3)	1 (5)

Table 2.Postoperative complications

Group	I	II	Total
Acute complications	**(n= 30) %**	**(n=20) %**	**(n=50) %**
Wound infection	2 (6.67)	3 (15)	5 (10)
Wound dehiscence	1 (3.33)	0	1 (2)
Peritonitis	1 (.33)	0	1 (2)
Hypoxic spell and death	0	1 (5)	1 (2)
Late complications	**(n= 30) %**	**(n= 17) %**	**(n= 47) %**
Partial septal fusion	1 (3.33)	0	1 (2)
Enterocolitis	11 (36.67)	7 (41.17)	18 (38.2)
Grade 1*	7 (2.1-5	5 (1.1-3)	
Grade 2	5 (2.1-2)	4 (2.1-3)	
Grade 3	1 (1)	0	
Soiling	1 (3.33)	0	1 (2)

* Presented as number of cases (median of episode per 1 case, range).

The functional results were categorized as excellent, good, fair, and poor according to published criteria with some modification [23]. The median follow-up period was 12 moths for group I and 16 moths for group II. Bowel function results are summarized en table 3.

Table 3. Functional outcomes by groups of patients

Group	I (n = 30) (%)	II (n = 17) (%)
Excellent	14 (47)	4 (23.5)
Good	13 (43	12 (70.5)
Fair	3 (10)	1 (6)

Discussion

Early postoperative Duhamel pull-through complications include wound infection, of which the incidence is similar to that in most colorectal operations, approximately 10% to 15% [27]. Reported mortality rates of 1.1% [30], 1.3% [23], 2% [27,31] have not been directly related to the operations.

Anastomotic complications, although uncommon, can be seen after any of the pull-through procedures. Anastomotic leak occurs infrequently and can be avoided by close attention to adequate blood supply of the pulled-through bowel and to minimizing tension on the anastomosis [29]. For Duhamel's technique, a long intrapelvic anastomosis between the neorectum and the native rectal stump leads to a concern that a primary pull-through with an inadequately prepared colon may result in a higher risk of anastomotic complications. Many studies have demonstrated the safety of applying the primary pull-through concept to Duhamel's technique. The crucial factors affecting this success are adequacy of mechanical colonic preparation, careful control of intraoperative contamination, and security of the anastomosis using a well-designed automatic GIA stapling device. Other studies have provided further data demonstrating the feasibility of performing primary definitive surgery in neonates and infants [1,17,27,32]. Anastomotic stricture is also generally throught to be less common with the Duhamel's procedure and in patients undergoing a one-stage reconstruction.[29]

Constipation is a frequent complaint of children after a pull-through procedure. In the literature, reported incidences of constipation after a Duhamel's procedure vary from 0% [27] to 7.7% [30] to 9% [33] to 31% [23]. Considerable soiling has also been reported, from 2% [27] to 17% [33] to 20% [23]). Lower incidences may be explained by greater care to truncating the rectal stump to a short length.

Postoperative enterocolitis has been the main problem with this procedure, with overall incidences, considering similar criteria of enterocolitis grade according to the criteria of Elhalaby and colleagues[34], ranging from 17% [31] to 21.4% [34] to 24% [33] and 38%[27]. A recent study observed that the incidence of Hirschsprung-related enterocolitis was higher in patients with trisomy-21 [35]. In addition, mental retardation may be associated with a negative impact on the functional outcomes [36].

Reoperation is often mentioned as a treatment of rectal stricture, anastomic leak, persistent rectal septum, retained aganglionic segment, and recurrent enterocolitis. In the study of Weber et al. [37], reoperation was required in 34% of the Soave pull-through cases and in 38% of Duhamel's procedure cases. In another series, the reoperation rate was 4%[27]. Stricture, megarectal pouch, fistula, and retained aganglionic bowel are preventable complications. Enterocolitis is partially preventable but can occur after a technically correct procedure. Fecal incontinence from anal canal damage is a preventable complication.[38]

Summary

The fundamental principle of the Duhamel's pull-through is to keep the dissected plane for the normally innervate neorectum within the retrorectal space, leave the native rectum in situ, make an end to side anastomosis, and joint the two lumens. The primary pull-through can be performed in patients who are younger than one year, including newborns.

The results of previous studies encourage primary definitive surgery in selected cases of Hirschsprung's disease. The modified Duhamel's procedure has the advantages of a functional outcome with no perianal excoriation, anastomotic stricture, or general tendency to reserve anal dilatation.

References

[1] Langer JC, Fitzgerald PG, Winthrop AL, Srinathan SK, Foglia RP, Skinner MA et al. One-stage versus two stage Soave pull-through for Hirschsprung's disease in the first year of life. *J Pediatr Surg* 1996;31:33 - 7.

[2] Shankar KR, Losty PD, Lamont GL, Turnock RR, Jones MO, Lloyd DA et al. Transanal endorectal coloanal surgery for Hirschsprung's disease: experience in two centers. *Pediatr Surg* 2000;35:1209- 13.

[3] De la Torre L, Ortega A. Transanal versus open endorectal pullthrough for Hirschsprung's disease. *J Pediatr Surg* 2000;35:1630-2.

[4] Minford JL, Ram A, Turnock RR, Lamont GL, Kenny SE, Rintala RJ et al. Comparison of functional outcomes of Duhamel and transanal endorectal coloanal anastomosi for Hirschsprung's disease. *J Pediatr Surg* 2004;39:161- 5.

[5] Duhamel B. New operation for congenital megacolon: retrorectal and transanal lowering of the colon, and its possible application to the treatment of various other malformation. *Press Med* 1956;64:2249-50.

[6] Duhamel B. A new operation for the treatment of Hirschsprung's disease. *Arch Dis Child* 1960;35:38-9.

[7] Duhamel B. Retrorectal and transanal pull-through procedure for the threatment of Hirschsprung's disease. *Dis Colon Rectum* 1964;7:455-8.

[8] Stockmann PT, Philippart AL. The Duhamel procedure for Hirschsprung's disease. *Semin Pediatr Surg* 1998;7:89-95.

[9] Grob M. Intestinal obstruction in the new born infant. *Arch Dis Child* 1960;35:40-50.

[10] Martin L, Altemeier W. Clinical experience with a new operation(modified Duhamel procedure) for Hirschsprung's disease. *Ann Surg* 1962;156:678-81.

[11] Martin L, Caudill D. A method for elimination of the blind rectal pouch in the Duhamel operation for Hirschsprung's disease. *Surgery* 1967;62:951-3.

[12] Hirobe S, Doody DP, Ryan DP,Kim SH, Donahoe PK. Ectopic class II major histocompatibility antigens in Hirschsprung's disease and neuronal intestinal dysplasia. *J Pediatr Surg* 1992;27:357-62.

[13] Soper G. Surgery for Hirschsprung's disease. *AORN J* 1968;8:69-81.

[14] Talbert J, Seashore J, Ravitch M. Evaluation of a modified Duhamel operation for correction of Hirschsprung's disease. *Ann Surg* 1974;179:671-5.

[15] Shayan K, Smith C, Langer JC. Reliability of intraoperative frozen sections in the management of Hirschsprung's disease. *J Pediatr Surg* 2004;39:1345- 8.

[16] Pierro A, Fasoli L, Kiely EM, Drake D, Spitz L. Staged pull-through for rectosigmoid Hirschsprung's disease is not safer than primary pullthrough. *J Pediatr Surg* 1997;32:505- 9.

[17] So HB, Becker JM, Schwartz DL, Kutin ND. Eighteen years' experience with neonatal Hirschsprung's disease treated by endorectal pullthrough without colostomy. *J Pediatr Surg* 1998;33:673- 5.

[18] Bufo AJ, Chen MK, Shah R, Gross E, Cyr N, Lobe TE. Analysis of the cost of surgery for Hirschsprung's disease: one-stage laparoscopic pull-through versus two-stage Duhamel procedure. *Clin Pediatr (Phila)* 1999;38:593- 6.

[19] De la Torre-Mondragon L, Ortega-Salgado JA. Transanal endorectal pull-through for Hirschsprung's disease. *J Pediatr Surg* 1998;33:1283- 6.

[20] Langer JC, Minkes RK, Mazziotti MV, Skinner MA, Winthrop AL.Transanal one-stage Soave procedure for infants with Hirschsprung's disease. *J Pediatr Surg* 1999;34:148 - 52.

[21] Langer JC, Seifert M, Minkes RK. One-stage Soave pull-through for Hirschsprung's disease: a comparison of the transanal and open approaches. *J Pediatr Surg* 2000;35:820- 2.

[22] Curran TJ, Raffensperger JG. Laparoscopic Swenson pull-through: a comparison with the open procedure. *J Pediatr Surg* 1996;31:1155-6.

[23] Vrsansky P, Bourdelat D, Pages R. Principal modifications of the Duhamel procedure in the treatment of Hirschsprung's disease. Analysis based on results of an international retrospective study of 2,430 patients. *Pediatr Surg Int* 1998;13:125 - 32.

[24] Liu CS, Chin TW, Wei CF. Neonatal Duhamel's pull-through for Hirschsprug's disease. *Zhonghua Yi Xue Za Zhi* 2002;65:398-402.

[25] Mir E, Karaca I, Gunsar C, Sencan A, Fesçekoglu O. Primary Duhamel-Martin operations in neonates and infants. *Pediatr Int* 2001;43:405-8.

[26] van der Zee DC, Bax KN. One-stage Duhamel-Martin procedure for Hirschsprung's disease: a 5-year follow-up study. *J Pediatr Surg* 2000;35:1434-6.

[27] Chiengkriwate P, Patrapinyokul S, Sangkhathat S,Chowchuvech V. Primary pull-through with modified Duhamel technique: 1 institution's experience. *J Pediatr Surg* 2007;42: 1075–80.

[28] Parithan P, Chiengkriwate P, Chowchuvech V, Patrapinyokul S, Sangkhathat S. Bowel preparation for pull-through operation in Hirschsprung's disease. *Songkla Med J* 2007;25:401-6.

[29] Dasgupta R, Langer JC. Evaluation and management of persistent problems after surgery for Hirschsprung disease in a child. *J Pediatr Gastroenterol Nutr* 2008; 46:13-9.

[30] Baillie CT, Kenny SE, Rintala RJ, Booth JM, Lloyd DA. Long-term outcome and colonic motility after the Duhamel procedure for Hirschsprung's disease. *J Pediatr Surg* 1999;34:325- 9.

[31] Elhalaby EA, Hashish A, Elbarbary MM, Soliman HA, Wishahy MK, Elkholy A et al. Transanal one-stage endorectal pull-through for Hirschsprung's disease: a multicenter study. *J Pediatr Surg* 2004;39:345 - 51.

[32] So HB, Schwartz DL, Becker JM, Daum Fn Schneider KM. Endorectal pull-through without preliminary colostomy in neonates with Hirschsprung's disease. *J Pediatr Surg* 1980;15:470- 1.

[33] Mattioli G, Castagnetti M, Martucciello G, Jasonni V. Results of a mechanical Duhamel pull-through for the treatment of Hirschsprung's disease and intestinal neuronal dysplasia. *J Pediatr Surg* 2004;39:1349- 55.

[34] Elhalaby EA, Coran AG, Blane CE, Hirschl RB, Teitelbaum DH. Enterocolitis associated with Hirschsprung's disease: a clinical-radiological characterization based on 168 patients. *J Pediatr Surg* 1995;30:76- 83.

[35] Morabito A, Lall A, Gull S, Mohee A, Bianchi A. The impact of Down's syndrome on the immediate and long-term outcomes of children with Hirschsprung's disease. *Pediatr Surg Int*. 2006 Feb;22:179-81

[36] Menezes M, Puri P. Long-term clinical outcome in patients with Hirschsprung's disease and associated Down's syndrome. *J Pediatr Surg* 2005;40:810- 2.

[37] Weber TR, Fortuna RS, Silen ML, Dillon PA. Reoperation for Hirschsprung's disease. *J Pediatr Surg* 1999;34:153 -7.

[38] Pena A, Elicevik M, Levitt MA. Reoperations of Hirschsprung disease. *J Pediatr Surg* 2007;42:1008-14.

In: Hirschsprung's Disease: Diagnosis and Treatment
Ed: Ramón Núñez and Manuel López-Alonso
ISBN: 978-1-60741-349-3

Chapter XVI

Original Soave Procedure

Antonio Hernández-Orgaz A and Manuel López-Alonso

Transanal Endorectal Pull-Through with Deferred Anastomosis

At first, paediatric surgery proposed extramucosal dissection of the rectosigmoid for the treatment of high anorectal anomalies [1-3] .

In later years, the technique of separating the rectosigmoid mucosa from the seromuscular layer was introduced for Hirschsprung's disease [4-7] .

Preoperative Preparation

Neomycin 2% is administered orally to patients who have undergone a previous colostomy. For those who have not, complete fasting, fluid replacement therapy and cleansing enemas for two days before the intervention are indicated. Metronidazole, gentamicine and ampicilin are administered intravenously eight hours before surgery and continue to be administered for 5-7 days [8,9] .

Patient Position

Supine position with the lumbar region elevated so as to tip the pelvis backward, facilitating access to the rectum.

Preparation

The abdomen, thighs and perineum are cleansed and disinfected. Legs are wrapped with sterile bandages, which permit the lower limbs to be moved within the surgical area. A Foley catheter is inserted in order to empty the bladder and identify the urethra.

Abdominal Surgical Process

A midline infraumbilical laparotomy is performed; the incision is extendable if the segment is long. Rectal and pyramidal muscles are split along the midline to create proper access to the pelvis. The peritoneum is incised, and the incision is extended from one side of the bladder to the other; the bladder is held with a traction suture.

A separator, preferably a rubber retractor, is set in place. A rubber retractor is recommended because it does not harm the patient during changes of position as a rigid one might.

Three or more extramucosal biopsies (Figure 1) are taken as needed. The first one is taken in the most distal spot of the narrow segment; dissection of the rectal mucosa will begin from this biopsy site.

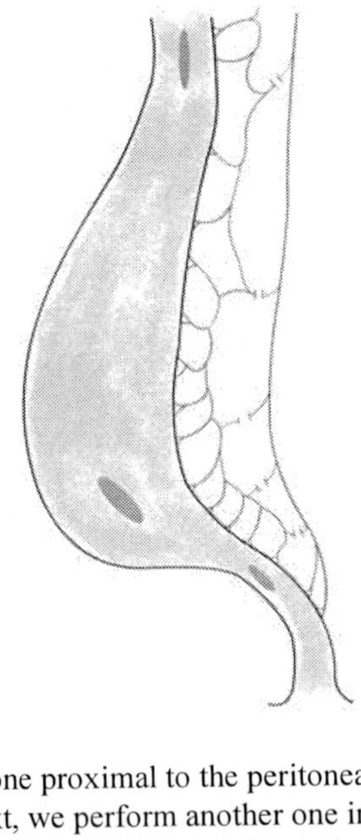

Figure 1. Distal biopsy in the narrow zone proximal to the peritoneal reflection. Extramucosa. At this level, we begin the dissection of the cuff. Next, we perform another one in the dilated zone, and lastly, the most proximal dissection in the zone that appears macroscopically normal.

The second biopsy is taken in the dilated zone, and the third one in the zone that is macroscopically normal. In all the biopsies except for the first one, the seromuscular edges are sutured shut to stop the bleeding.

Rectosigmoidal vessels are dissected, with the exception of the superior haemorrhoidal artery. This is of critical importance [5-7] .

Separating the seromuscular layer from the mucosa: this dissection is often done by infiltrating the wall with saline solution containing a vasoconstrictor[7,10,11]. We do not use the infiltration method[5,6,10,12]; rather, at the site of the first biopsy, we insert a 5-0 suture on each of the edges. We traction one of the sutures and by resting the edge on the index finger of the left hand, we begin transverse dissection with a very small swab used to separate the mucosa from the muscular layer. When one or one and a half centimetres have been dissected, we section the seromuscular layer transversely and continue dissecting and incising until the seromuscular layer is sectioned around its entire circumference. Once this step is completed, the dissection is continued distally. An easy-to-dissect cleavage plane can be recognised by the presence of straight vessels in the mucosa. Dissection is very difficult and tends to tear the mucosa when done outside of this plane, so locating it is essential.

Most of the vessels are thin and break upon contact with the swab, but if they do not, an assistant should cut them with fine, blunt-tipped scissors; forcing the vessels with the swab can cause us to leave the cleavage plane.

At the level of the internal sphincter, dissection becomes more difficult, partly because of the depth of this part of the procedure, and partly because the connections between the sphincter and the mucosa are more fibrous.

After dissecting the mucosa up to 1 cm of the cutaneomucosal line, either the mesosigma or the mesocolon is dissected, depending on the height of the segment with normal biopsy results. The dissection of the mesocolon is meticulous; the sigmoidal vessels are sectioned, but vascular continuity is maintained with superior vessels that feed the mobilized colon segment (Figure 1).

During this dissection process, care must be taken with the urethra and the vas deferens in male patients.

Perineal Procedure

Sterile bandages are wrapped around the ankles of the patient. With the help of the anaesthesiologist, the bandages are attached so that the legs are maintained in stirrup position.

An round-tipped esophageal dilator is introduced by the anus until it reaches the upper part of the dissected mucosa (Figure 2). The mucosa is attached to the dilator with a tape. Once it is attached, the dilator is drawn out, and removed through the anus (Figure 2b). We section the mucosa one centimetre from the cutaneomucous line around its entire circumference. We continue tractioning the intestine until reaching the biopsy that gave the normal reading (Figure 2c).

This manoeuvre is dangerous in that the intestine that we are drawing out can twist laterally, and if this should occur without our notice, it can lead to serious complications. To avoid this occurring, an assistant with long right-angle forceps clamps the intestine segment with the normal biopsy, and follows the intestine as it descends until it appears at the anus. Once we see the tip of the forceps, we discontinue the use of the forceps and manipulate the intestine from the perineal zone.

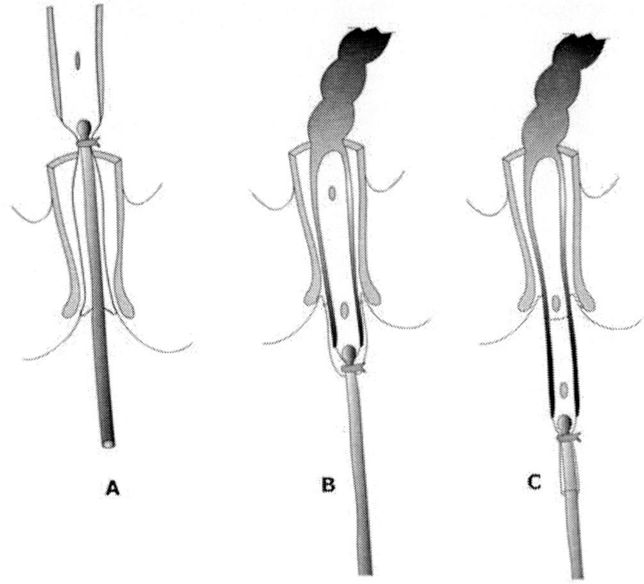

Figure 2. Anal introduction of the esophageal dilator. In (A), the mucosa is attached to the dilator with tape. In (B), it is tractioned out through the anus. In (C), the proximal segment signalled as normal in the biopsy is pulled through.

A Penrose drain is placed on the muscular cuff, leading out through a small incision below the coccyx [9-11] . It remains there for about 48 hours to drain blood.

We section the pulled-through colon 6-8 cm from the anus (Figure 3). Bleeding indicates a good vascular supply to the pulled-through colon.

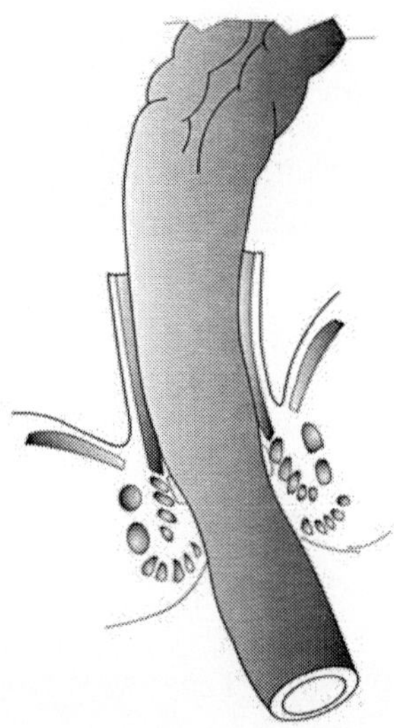

Figure 3. Sectioning the lowered colon, leaving 6-8 cm from the point of the normal biopsy.

Six to eight sutures are used between the colon and anal mucosa to close the rectal stump.

After proper hemostasis, the bandages maintaining the legs elevated are cut off, and we return to the laparotomy to attach the muscular funnel to the new rectum, close the pelvic peritoneum and close the abdominal incision.

Postoperative Care

The patient receives parenteral nutrition until peristaltism is checked, after which enteral nutrition is employed. As stated previously, the drain is moved within 24 hours and removed after 48 hours.

The rectal stump is subject to edema, which can sometimes cause obstruction at that level. This can be avoided by inserting a thick rectal tube.

Resection of the Rectal Stump

The resection of the rectal stump and the deferred coloanal anastomosis are performed 15 to 20 days later.

To avoid performing a second intervention, shortly afterwards Boley proposed primary coloanal anastomosis [10,12] .

Soave-Boley Procedure for Hirschsprung's Disease

The most important difference between the two operations is the primary coloanal anastomosis.

This presents the following advantages:

1. Decrease in infection and dehiscence of the coloanal anastomosis.
2. Coloanal anastomosis is straighter and more distal.
3. Increased patient comfort.

Soave-Boley Technique

Endorectal Pull-Through Operation with Primary Anastomosis

The technique is the same as the original Soave procedure, except that it includes a primary anastomosis.

When we started using this technique in 1982, many dehiscences were reported in medical journals. To avoid dehiscence, we did an experimental study in dogs using different types of anastomosis and we chose the procedure described below.

This anastomosis has given us excellent results with no dehiscence in any of our 110 patients.

The anastomosis is done in a single plane, with individual 4-0 vicryl sutures: the sutures are placed in the colonic seromuscular layer, internal anal sphincter and anal mucosa (Figure 4). With this last suture, the colon and the anal mucosa remain perfectly anchored to the internal anal sphincter. Sutures are placed in each of the four cardinal points and the four intercardinal points. Following this step, mucosal sutures are added between the others. Another advantage of this anastomosis is that because it is attached to the internal sphincter, there is a low incidence of stenosis.

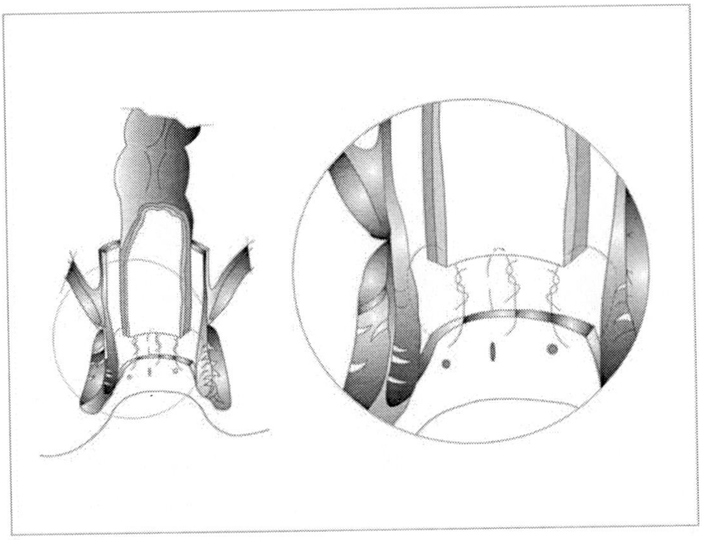

Figure 4. Coloanal anastomosis. Close-up: seromuscular layer of the lowered colon pulled through the submucosa – internal sphincter and anal mucosa.

After finishing the procedure, the height of the anastomosis is verified by rectal examination.

Eight or nine days after the surgery, the rectum is calibrated, since there may be edema in the descending colon above the anastomosis creating a stricture in the anal canal. In these cases we use dilators until the edema subsides. If this is not done, faecal stagnation may occur, which can then lead to enterocolitis.

Principal Errors In Technique

Not using prophylactic antibiotics [7,8,11] . Even under the best conditions, a pull-through procedure will always be contaminated by e-coli. Intravenous antibiotics during the intervention and during the following 48h offer maximum protection with a minimum of risk associated with prophylactic antibiotic use.

Beginning endorectal dissection proximal to the peritoneal reflection. The shorter the funnel above the pelvic floor, the better.

Perforation of the mucosa during dissection of rectal cuff increases the risk of contamination and may prolong the dissection process.

Initiating submucous transanal dissection too high in the anal canal leaves an aganglionic segment that can cause obstruction.

Incomplete mobilization of the colon causes tension on the anastomosis, leading to stenosis.

Failure to achieve hemostasis and good drainage increases the risk of infection.

Results of Surgical Intervention

Between 1974 and 1982, the authors of this chapter performed operations on 47 patients using the original Soave procedure (OS) Between 1982 and 2003, we used the Soave-Boley technique (SB) in operations performed on 110 patients.

Age of intervention: In OS patients, the mean age was 21.57 ± 27.85 P_{50} 10. In SB patients, the mean age was 16.24 ± 21.56 P_{50} 8 (Table 1). Table 2 shows that we did not operate on patients younger than 3 months using the OS technique, while 25.5% of those younger than 3 months were operated using the SB technique.

Table 1. Age at time of intervention.

	Original Soave	Soave Boley
Mean (months)	21.57 ± 27.85	16.24 ± 21.56
P_{50}	10	8
Range	6 months - 146 months	11 days - 104 months

Table 2. Population by age group.

	Soave Original		Soave Boley	
Under < 3 months	0	0 %	28	25.5 %
3 to 6 months	4	8.5%	22	20 %
6 to 12 months	24	51.1%	18	16.4 %
1 to 3 years	12	25.5%	29	26.4 %
Over 3 year old	7	14.9%	13	11.8%

Weight at the time of intervention: OS 11.51 ± 5.97 P_{50} 9.3. In SB 9.13 ± 4.78 P_{50} 8 (Table 3).

Length of Aganglionic Segment: Barium Enema

Both groups are similar as shown in Table 4, with the aganglionic segment most frequently reaching the sigmoid colon. There are no significant differences between the groups.

Table 3. Weight at time of intervention.

	Original Soave	Soave Boley
Mean (kg)	11.51 ± 5.97	9.13 ± 4.78
P_{50}	9.3	8
Range	7 kg – 36 kg	3 kg – 27.6 kg

Table 4. Localization of the narrow segment: Contrast enema

	Soave Original	Soave Boley
Rectosigmoid	30 (63.83%)	60 (54.54 %)
Colon descendens	1 (2.13%)	14 (12.72%)
Left flexure	6 (12.76%)	9 (8.19%)
Transverse colon	1 (2.13%)	3 (2.73%)
Colon ascendens	-	-
Ileum	-	-
No narrow segment	7 (14.89%)	8 (7.28%)
Uncertain Diagnosis	2 (4.26%)	16 (14.55%)

Early Complications

There are fewer early complications in the SB group than in the OS group (Table 5). There are more high-anastomosis procedures in the OS group. The difference between the two groups was statistically significant. The odds ratio is 2.90 (1.256-6.75); that is, those in the SB group are 2.90 times more likely to not present early complications than those in the SO group.

Table 5. Acute Complications.

	Soave Original	Soave Boley
ACUTE		
None	33 (70.2%)	96 (87.3%)
Ischemic Colitis	1 (2.1%)	0 (0%)
Abscess	1 (2.1%)	2 (1.8%)
High Anastomosis	5 (10.6%)	3 (2.7%)
Edema	3 (6.4%)	7 (6.4%)
Stenosis	1 (2.1%)	0 (0%)
Ileus	0 (0%)	1 (0.9%)
Sepsis	0 (0%)	1 (0.9%)
Ligate Superior Haemorrhoidal Artery	1 (2.1%)	0 (0%)
Wound Dehiscence	2 (4.3%)	0 (0%)

Later Complications (Table 6)

There were fewer total complications in the SB group. There was more occasional spotting in the SO group, and more enterocolitis in the SB group. Regarding the 17 cases of post-pullthrough enterocolitis in the SB group, in 10 cases the proximal end of the resectioned segment displayed an abnormality; in most of the cases, this was neural colonic dysplasia, and in two cases, hipoganglionism. In any case, there are no significant differences between the two groups. The odds ratio is 1.66 (0.82-3.34).

Table 6. Later Complications.

	Soave Original	Soave Boley
LATE		
None	26 (55.3%)	74 (67.3%)
Abscess	0 (0%)	1 (0.9%)
Adhesions	2 (4.3%)	2 (1.8%)
Enterocolitis	5 (10.6%)	20 (18.2%)
Stenosis	0 (0%)	1 (0.9%)
Constipation	4 (8.5%)	5 (4.5%)
Occasional Soiling	7 (14.9%)	7 (6.4%)

Discussion

The two procedures that we are comparing, SO and SB, share some identical factors, but another particular factor sets them apart The two groups underwent procedures performed in the centre by the same surgeons using the same means. The crucial difference is that the SB procedure is performed on patients younger than those operated using OS. This should be taken into account when evaluating results, including complications.

The age of intervention is lower in the SB group because, in our personal experience, the younger the patient, the easier the intervention. Since 1984 the diagnosis of HD in newborns showing symptoms was done at the end of the neonatal period. Logically, the younger age corresponds to the lower weight.

Both techniques lead to few complications and provide good results; however, they are technically difficult. The most difficult step is the dissection of the funnel-shaped rectal mucosa avoiding mucosal rupture.

High anastomoses were more frequent in the OS group. In our cases, the motive was necrosis of the distal cuff or the ascent of the cuff. With the SB procedure, this cannot occur except for a short dissection of the funnel-shaped mucosa with a high anastomosis, which has not presented itself among our cases.

Neither of the two groups presents cases of incontinence. We have had patients with occasional spotting and this is more frequent in the OS group.

We consider as enterocolitis a clinical profile that requires admission, fluid replacement therapy and antibiotic treatment, even if it had only been one episode.

Because the OS interventions were less recent, recording the episodes of enterocolitis has been more difficult and the study of the resected segment has been less precise; as a result, the number of cases of enterocolitis as well as the cases of incomplete resection have been underestimated.

The incidence of enterocolitis in our cases is linked to incomplete resection. Incomplete resection leads to disturbances of peristalsis, progressive distal retention, and episodes of enterocolitis. In our experience these symptoms are common in the first months after the pull-through and they improve over time.

Summary

We believe that both OS and SB are good techniques which provide excellent results, although they are technically difficult, requiring experienced surgeons and a significant number of cases per year. The SB technique is an improvement upon the OS technique, as it reduces the length of the hospital stay, the number of procedures, and the risk of complications.

Starting in 2003 and using our experience as a base, we began surgical treatment of HD using the Soave transanal endorectal technique [13]. It presents the same advantages as the SB technique, but leads to a much easier dissection of the endorectal mucosa. In normal cases in which the rectosigmoid is affected, laparotomy is not necessary.

When the symptoms or the enema suggest that a long segment may be affected, we recommend initiating intervention by minilaparotomic / laparoscopic biopsy to determine the length of the aganglionic segment. In the case of total colonic aganglionism we prefer an ileocolic loop attached to the abdominal wall and when formed feces are passed through the ostomy, we perform the endorectal pull-through.

If total colonic aganglionism is not suspected and we begin an endorectal transanal pull-through, the ileocolic loop and the pull-through are performed during the same surgical procedure.

References

[1] Romualdi P. *Una nuova técnica operativa per la cura di alcune malformación del retto*. Soc Romana Chir Maggio 1955.

[2] Romualdi P. [A new technic for surgical treatment of some rectal malformations.]. *Langenbecks Arch Klin Chir Ver Dtsch Z Chir*. 1960;296:371-7.

[3] Rehbein F. Operation der anal-und rectumatresie mit rectourethral fistel. *Chirurg* 1959;30:417-8

[4] Soave F. La colon-ano-stomia senza sutura dopo mobilizzazione e abbassamento extramucoso del rettosigma. Una nuova t,cnica chirurgica per la terapia della malattia di Hirschprung. *Osped Ital Chir* 1962;8:258.

[5] Soave F. Una nuovo tecnica chirurgica per la terapia della malattia di Hirschsprung. *Osped Ital Chir* 1963;8:285-91.

[6] Soave F. [A new surgical technic for the Treatment of Hirschsprung's Disease Coloanostomy without suture after mobilization and extra-mucous lowering of the recto-sigmoid.]. *J Chir (Paris)* 1963;86:451-64.

[7] Soave F. A new surgical technique for the treatment of Hirschsprung's Disease. *Surgery* 1964;56:1007-14.

[8] Soave F. Endorectal pull-through: 20 years experience. Address of the guest speaker, APSA, 1984. *J Pediatr Surg* 1985;20:568-79.

[9] Tariq GM, Brereton RJ, Wright VM. Complications of endorectal pull-through for Hirschsprung's disease. *J Pediatr Surg* 1991;26:1202-6.

[10] Boley SJ. New modifcation of the surgical treatment of Hirschsprung's Disease. *Surgery* 1964;56:1015-7.

[11] Krivchenya DY, Silchenko MI, Soroka VP, Pritula VP, Khursin VN. Endorectal pull-through for Hirschsprung's disease: 17-year review of results in Ukraine. *Pediatr Surg Int* 2002;18:718-22.

[12] Boley SJ. An endorectal pull-through operation with primary anastomosis for Hirchsprung's disease. *Surg Gynecol Obstet* 1968;127:353-7.

[13] De la Torre L, Ortega A. Transanal versus open endorectal pull-through for Hirschsprung's disease. *J Pediatr Surg* 2000;35:1630-2.

In: Hirschsprung's Disease: Diagnosis and Treatment
Ed: Ramón Núñez and Manuel López-Alonso
ISBN: 978-1-60741-349-3

Chapter XVII

Rehbein's Technique

José Mª Gil-Vernet, Jesús Broto and Marta De Diego

Introduction

Dr. Fritz Rehbein (1911- 1991) from Westuffeln, Hessen, (Germany), was a paediatric surgeon, researcher in several surgical fields, and a pioneer in the design of corrective techniques for congenital problems in children. His book on paediatric surgery interventions has been widely translated and published all over the world [1].

As Chief of the Paediatric Clinic of Bremen, one of his greatest achievements was the development of a new technique for the treatment of aganglionic megacolon of the newborn, or Hirschsprung's disease (HD).

The aim of Rehbein's technique is to try to simplify the surgical process into its most basic roots: Resection of the affected bowel and end to end anasthomosis.

Technique

Traditionally, this manually performed low anasthomosis in small children can pose serious technical problems. This circumstance led Dr. Rehbein to design a special set of instruments to facilitate the dissection and ligature of the perirectum vessels. The short configuration of the pelvic channel in children, together with the dissection under traction of the perirectum, allows the surgeon to perform a deeper release of the rectum than in adult patients.

The process begins with a rectal calibration with Hegar dilators up to 21 or 25 mm, performed in the operating room under general anesthesia in order to find the most appropriate instrument diameter for rectal stapling.

We then perform an infra umbilical laparotomy and confirm by biopsies the level of aganglionism. While awaiting the outcome of the biopsies, we proceed to prepare the bowel for resection. In this technique the preparation of the rectal sector is of great importance and we try to carry out this dissection as low as possible, coagulating accurately the small vessels of the perirectum (Figures A, B and C). The upward dissection must include the most dilated sections of the ganglionic bowel.

Given the special characteristics of the reduced depth of the pelvis of small infants, a precise dissection of the rectum under traction can be carried out, arriving until 2 cm. of the anus to perform at this site a colorectal anastomosis, respecting the final sector of the internal sphincter.

Since the advent of surgical staples, we consider that they offer more security in performing the lower colorectal anastomosis, and for this reason we employ them habitually after a careful and extensive dissection of the rectum.

When the biopsies confirm the exact level of the affectation, we perform the first stapling with a TL stapler at the lowest level possible and then cut the rectum. We perform the colon resection in the healthy and non dilated area. We then proceed to resect the aganglionic portion and introduce through the end of the healthy intestine the mobile press of the circular stapler, closing it with a tobacco pouch suture. Depending on the child's size a circular 21 or 25 mm intraluminal stapler is introduced through the anus. The end of the mobile press is connected with the pin of circular stapler and the final end to end anastomosis is then carried out, (Figure 1 D and Figure 2). The circular stapler is withdrawn through the anus and the intervention is completed [2].

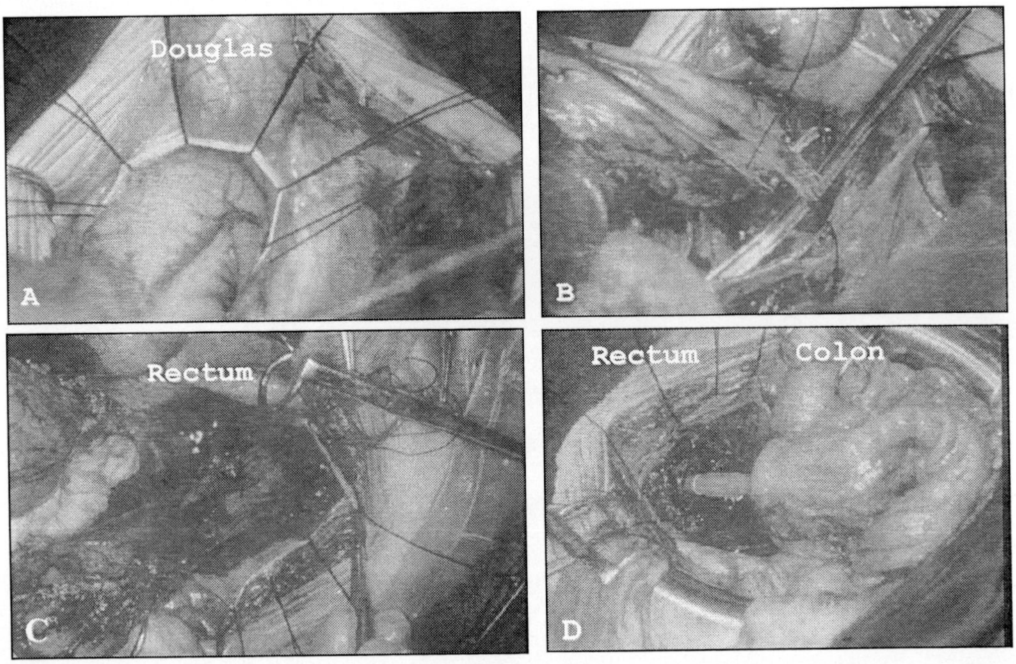

Figure 1. A: Douglas under traction. B: Perirectum dissection. C: Final dissection of the rectum. D: Stapler anastomosis.

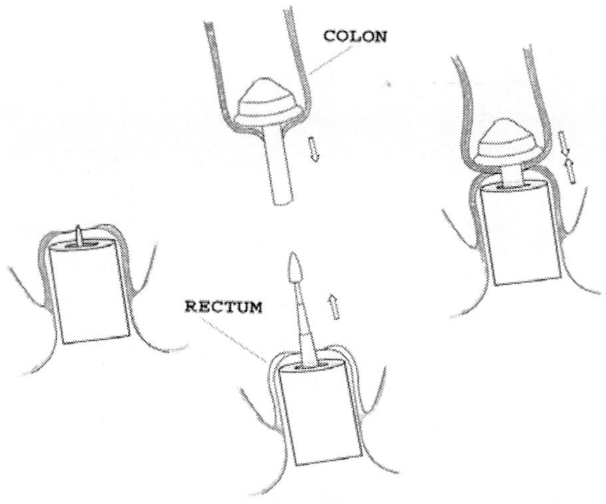

Figure 2. Adapted from Hedlund H [3]. The two parts of the device are approximated mechanically and the stapler is fired.

This procedure provides good results but requires periodic post op calibrations of the suture to prevent possible stenosis. Our experience shows that circular stapler sutures must be closely controlled, given that some cases develop a long term tendency to generate stenosis of the line of suture.

A simple rectal exploration allows us to identify this problem which can be solved by a rectal calibration with Hegar dilators.

Since the advent of laparoscopy in paediatric surgery, Rebhein's technique can also be performed using this approach.

Experience

Over the course of the years, the systematic application of early diagnosis techniques (radiology, manometry, and histochemical studies) [4-7], the intensive neonatal care units, and the standardization of nursing have allowed us to reduce the need for intestinal derivations and to perform surgery earlier.

Surgery in HD must fulfill two prerequisites: 1) To eliminate the aganglionic segment and the dilated part above it, and 2) to resolve the spasm of the internal sphincter with its incapacity of relaxation [8,9].

Rehbein's technique as employed by our group over many years correctly resolves the first objective of the treatment. However, despite technical modifications added during the course of time such as the standard use of surgical staplers, it only partially resolves the second given that an affected portion of rectum aganglionic with acalasia always remains.

The technical modifications introduced over time led us to present our experience in two time periods (see table 1).

The first from 1967-1993, published by Prof. Dr. J.Boix Ochoa, and the second until this publication in 2008.

One hundred and sixty one HD patients were diagnosed in the first period. In 105 was applied Rebhein's technique.

Of this first group of 161 patients, 61 required intestinal derivations, 42 due to intestinal occlusion, 10 for enterocolitis, 2 for rectal perforation, and 7 for intestinal caliber discordance.

In the second period, 46 patients were treated, the first 36 cases using Rebhein's technique. Twenty nine presented sigmoid affectation, 5 reached the left colon, 1 affected transversal colon, and another had total colonic affectation.

Of this group, 3 needed colostomy, two newborns by intestinal occlusion, and the other with transversal affectation due to complications that arose from the nursing period.

The remaining 10 cases were treated by endoanal pull-through.

Results

Of the 105 patients treated in the first phase using Rebhein's technique, 76 (72.4%) evolved favorably without complications.

In 29 cases (27.6%) diverse complications were found. Anal achalasia was present in 12 cases (11.4%), stenosis in 5 (4.7%), enterocolitis in 4(3.8%), suture failure in 3 (2.3%), and relaparotomies due to intestinal adhesions in 3 (2.3%).

Two patients (1.9%) died from enterocolitis and sepsis in the postoperative.

In the second study period involving 36 patients, 9 (25%) presented complications (Table 1).

These included 6 (16,6%) cases with anal achalasia, 1case of mild suture line bleeding, 1 required relaparotomy due to intestinal invagination, and 1 stapling failure that required colostomy and subsequent reparation by posterior sagital anal rectoplasty.

Upon comparing both series, the first interesting feature is that the rate of complications is very similar.The early complications like stenosis of suture line are not present in the second series due to the use of staplers of caliber 25 after six months of life.

The anal achalasia remains frequent in this type of intervention because of the remaining portion of the aganglionic internal sphincter. Among late complications, enterocolitis appeared in 5% of cases in the second series.

Table 1. Own results with Rebhein's technique

Study Period	No. of Patients	Without Complications (%)	Anal Achalasia (%)	Stenosis Anastomosis (%)	Enterocolitis (%)	Anastomotic leak (%)
1994-2008	36*	75	16,6	0	5	2,7

*Stapler anastomosis

Evolution

Rehbein's technique does not fulfill the premise of totally eliminating the spasticitiy of the internal aganglionic sphincter. Nevertheless it does achieve a adequate continence although parents must be warned of the possibility of episodes of abdominal distention and fecal retention that can be resolved by the simple introduction of a rectal catheter.

If these episodes persist, a forced anal dilatation is performed under general anesthesia which resolves the problem in the majority of cases [8-11].

Normally these episodes are not so frequents in patients of older age with sufficient self-control in which the defecation is controlled in a voluntary manner.

Complications reported by other authors such as fecal or urinary incontinence have not been present in our series [9,10,12,13].

Conclusions

In surgical treatment of Hirschsprung's disease, all techniques seek the same objective:

To suppress the aganglionic portion of the affected bowel and reestablish the intestinal continuity [8].

Rebehin's technique tries to achieve this in the most physiological manner through a resection and end to end anastomosis [9,10,13].

The ideal age for the intervention is between 6 –18 months and is preferably carried out in patients with long- length affected intestinal segments, unsuitable for the De la Torre pull-trough and without colostomy, that have been maintained under regimen of nursing with enemas [14,15].

This kind of resection in the lower rectal channel often poses technical problems which have been simplified with the advent of staplers [2].

Over the last 20 years our team has employed the "triple staple" in Rebhein's technique which has facilitated the performance of the anastomosis and dramatically reduced the complications derived from leaks in the sutures.

The appearance of constipation, most likely due to the remaining rectal aganglionic small sector, can be easily controlled by a forced anal dilatation.

Our extensive experience in this technique, comprising more than 30 years, has shown that the cases of long affectation of HD can not be adequately resolved by this technique [8-10,12].

From 1967 different techniques have been used in our center for the treatment of HD. Over time, approaches ranging from anal dilatations and sphincterectomy for short segments, to pull through Duhamel -type, Duhamel –Roviralta, and Rehbein have been employed.

In total colonic aganglionism we prefer the modified Lester Martin technique.

In the last years, the technique of endoanal pull through described by De la Torre has become the technique of choice for the sigmoid segments [14,15].

References

[1] Rehbein F. *Kinderchirurgische Operationen*. Stuttgart: Hipokrates;1976.

[2] Wester T, Hochner J, Olsen L. Rehbein's anterior resection in Hirschsprung's disease, using a circular stapler. *Eur J Pediatr Surg* 1995;5: 358-62.

[3] Hedlund H: Colorectal resection and anal anastomosis with an intraluminal stapler in Hirschsprung's disease. *Pediatr Surg Int* 1997;12:142-4

[4] Gil-Vernet JM, Casasa JM, Marhuenda C, Broto J. Boix-Ochoa Manometría anorrectal en la enfermedad de Hirschsprung. *Cir Peiatr* 1992;5:135-40.

[5] Nuñez R, Cabrera R, Moreno C, Agulla E, Vargas I, Blesa E. Utilidad de la manometría anorrectal para el diagnóstico neonatal de la Enfermedad de Hirschsprung. *Cir Pediatr* 2000;13:16-9.

[6] López Alonso M. Hernández Orgaz A, Ribas Serna. Indices de fiabilidad de la manometría anorrectal para el diagnóstico de la enfermedad de Hirschsprung en cualquier edad. *Cir Pediatr* 2005;18:13-6.

[7] Gil-Vernet H. J M, Broto J,Guillen G.Diagnóstico diferencial Hischsprung-Neurodisplasia intestinal. Fiabilidad de las pruebas diagnósticas. *Cir Pediatr*, 2006;19:91-4.

[8] Holschneider AM, Rassouli R: Rehbein's procedure (Deep Anterior Resection). In Holschneider AM, Puri P (Eds). *Hirschsprung`s disease and Allied Disorders*. Third Edition. Berlin Heidelberg: Springer-Verlag; 2008. p. 349-58.

[9] Rassouli R, Holschneider AM, Bolkenius M, Menardi G. et als. Long-term results of Rehbein's procedure: a retrospective study in German-speaking countries. *Eur J Pediatr Surg* 2003; 13: 187-94.

[10] Fuchs O, Boob D. Rehbein's Procedure for Hirschsprung´s Disease. An Appraisal of 45 years. *Eur J Pediatr Surg* 1999;.9:389-91.

[11] Wester T, Zetterlind L, Fredin K, Olsen L. Postoperative obstructive Symptoms are common after Rehbein's procedure for Hirschsprung's Disease. *Eur J Pedistr Surg.* 2006;16:100-03.

[12] Snyder CL, Ashcraft KW. Late complications of Hirschsprung's disease. In: Holschneider AM, Puri P (eds). *Hirschsprung's disease and allied disorders.* Amsterdam: Harwood Academic Publishers; 1982. p. 431-9.

[13] Dübbers M, Holscneider AM, Meier-Ruge W. Results of total and subtotal Colon Resections in Children. *Eur J Pediatr Surg*, 2003;13:195-200.

[14] De la Torre Mondragón L,Ortega-Salgado JA. Transanal endorectal Pull-Through for Hirschsprung's Disease. *J Pediatr Surg*,1998;33:1283-86.

[15] De la Torre L, Ortega A. Transanal versus open enorectal Pull-Through for Hirschsprung's Disease. *J Pediatr Surg*, 2000;35:1630-2.

In: Hirschsprung's Disease: Diagnosis and Treatment
Ed: Ramón Núñez and Manuel López-Alonso
ISBN: 978-1-60741-349-3

Chapter XVIII

Laparoscopic-Assisted Transanal Pull-Through for Hirschsprung's Disease

Atsuyuki Yamataka and Akihiro Shimotakahara

Laparoscopy Assisted Colon Suction Biopsy During Transanal Pull-Through

Laparoscopy assisted colon suction biopsy can be used in any infant or child of any size provided the caliber change is in the recto-sigmoid colon, because the sigmoid colon can be mobilized readily to allow the tip of the suction biopsy device to reach the proposed biopsy site. However, this technique cannot be applied in long segment Hirschsprung's disease, in which the caliber change is in the descending colon, splenic flexure, or more proximally, because the tip of the device cannot reach beyond the caliber change. At our center, we use conventional laparoscopic seromuscular biopsy or deliver the colon through an umbilical incision (after removing the cannula) and perform an extra-corporeal full-thickness biopsy in long segment type cases. Fortuitously, 80% of Hirschsprung's disease cases are recto-sigmoid, and laparoscopic-assisted colon suction biopsy could find wide application because it is safe, simple, and quick compared with conventional laparoscopic colon seromuscular/full-thickness biopsy.

The suction biopsy device we use is 170 - 180 mm in length with a tissue sampling mechanism located 10 - 15mm from the tip. After identification of the region of caliber change in the colon laparoscopically by a surgeon from the laparoscopy team (laparoscopic surgeon), the suction biopsy device is inserted into the anus by a surgeon from the transanal pull-through team (perineal surgeon) (Figure 1) ensuring that the tissue sampling mechanism faces anteriorly to allow the laparoscopic surgeon to check for complications at the time of biopsy, such as perforation [1]. The device is advanced until it is proximal to the region of caliber change and the perineal surgeon takes biopsies of the mucosa and submucosa under supervision of the laparoscopic surgeon. The laparoscopic surgeon places a metal laparoscopic vessel clip at the biopsy site as a marker. Biopsy specimens are sent for rapid histopathology where they are snap-frozen by a pathologist, then stained with H&E. If the result is aganglionic, the biopsy is repeated more proximally. If ganglion cells are present, the colon is pulled-through to the level of the clip transanally, and a coloanal anastomosis is performed. Before the anastomosis is performed, an open full-thickness biopsy is taken from the clipped biopsy site that is now exposed through the anus, to confirm the presence of ganglion cells in the muscle layers of the distal end of the pulled-through colon.

To date, we have had no incidence of perforation during laparoscopic-assisted suction biopsy, indicating there is minimal risk for leakage of bowel contents. On the contrary, there is a relatively high risk for perforation during conventional laparoscopic colonic seromuscular biopsy. If perforation does occur, the defect can be closed laparoscopically with several sutures, but it is time consuming and likely to cause leakage of bowel contents.

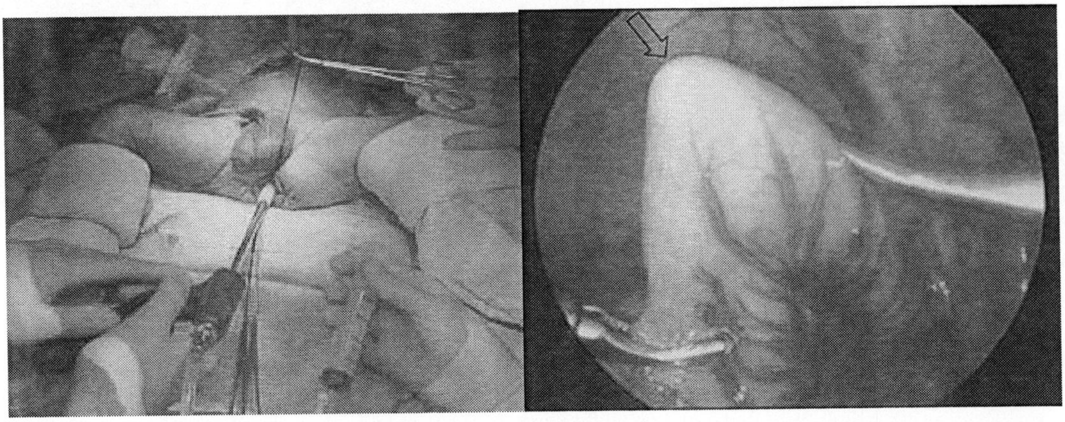

Figure 1. The suction rectal biopsy device is being advanced (left) within the colon by a surgeon from the transanal pull-through team under supervision of a laparoscopic surgeon until the tip (right: an arrow) of the device lies proximal to the caliber change.

Laparoscopy Assisted Transanal Pull-Through

Our technique similar to Georgeson's procedure and De La Torre-Mondragon's procedure, except for differences in the level at which transanal mucosal dissection is commenced and the length of the residual rectal muscle cuff.

Preoperatively, all patients are fed normally. Patients who do not require a colostomy undergo daily bowel decompression and saline bowel irrigation using a rectal tube until primary laparoscopy assisted transanal pull-through can be performed.

After induction of general endotracheal tube anesthesia, infants and small children are positioned transversely across the operating table in the supine position. The trunk and buttocks are prepared extensively, with the legs being disinfected circumferentially to the tips of the toes, and sterile stockings are placed on both legs. The laparoscopic surgeon and his/her assistant stand above the infant's head, and a monitor is positioned beyond the patient's feet. Larger children are positioned in the lithotomy position along the long axis of the table, with their legs in stirrups. The laparoscopic surgeon stands on the patient's right side. A urinary catheter is used to decompress the bladder.

A 5mm port is inserted through the umbilicus using an open technique and pneumoperitoneum is established with carbon dioxide to a pressure of 12 to 15mmHg, depending on the age and size of the child. Three additional 3.8 or 5mm ports are placed in the right upper and lower quadrants, and in the left upper quadrant. A laparoscope is placed through the 5mm port in the right upper quadrant. The surgeon's two working ports are the umbilical port for the left hand and the right lower abdominal port for the right hand. The port in the left upper abdomen can be used for either retraction of the colon, or, additionally for the surgeon's left hand.

The operation begins by identifying the level of ganglionic colon using the above-mentioned laparoscopic colon suction biopsy technique or alternative biopsy techniques. While awaiting histopathology results, the assistant from the laparoscopic team keeps the patient in the lithotomy position by flexing the legs and the perineal surgeon places circumferential 2-0 traction sutures from the anocutaneous line to the perineum 3 to 4cm outward from the anus to expose the dentate line. The crypts along the dentate line are then hooked up using a Lone Star Ring Retractor System (Lone Star Medical Products, Inc., Stafford, TX), allowing the anorectal line to be identified nicely as a ring at the top of the anal columns (Figure 2).

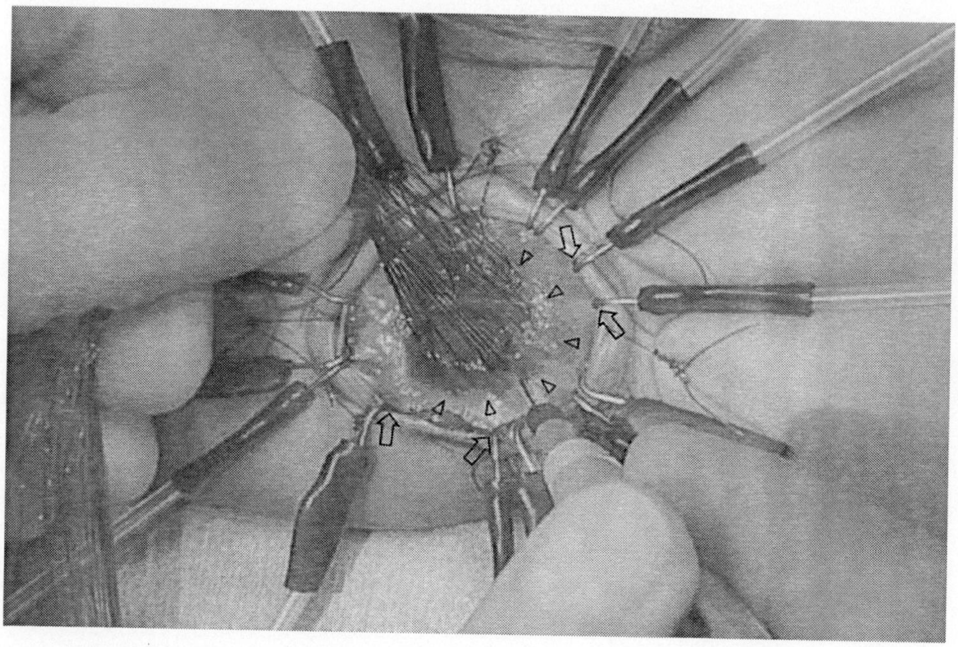

Figure 2. The anorectal line (arrowheads) can be identified by hooking the crypts (arrows) in the dentate line to expose the surgical anal canal with a ring retractor device.

By this time, histopathology results should be available. If the biopsy site is ganglionic, the perineal surgeon stops the perineal procedure and the patient is repositioned in the supine position and the laparoscopic surgeon starts dissection of the rectosigmoid colon. In most cases, the biopsy indicates the presence of ganglion cells in the distal sigmoid colon or upper rectum, that is, recto-sigmoid type Hirschsprung's disease. The laparoscopic surgeon or his/her assistant retracts the distal sigmoid colon toward the anterior abdominal wall with a grasper. Hook diathermy or a harmonic scalpel is used to open the mesocolon close to the aganglionic colon wall to mark the site from where mobilization of the colon is commenced. Mesenteric vessels are divided from the level of the caliber change proximally to the level of the peritoneal reflection distally. The surgeon should identify the location of the ureter during dissection of the mesocolon.

In cases where the ganglionic segment is proximal to the mid-sigmoid colon, it is necessary to mobilize the descending colon and splenic flexure, and the proximal inferior mesenteric artery usually needs to be ligated and divided. When dividing the arterial supply at this point, the arterial arcades (such as marginal arteries and sigmoid arteries) supplying the descending colon and splenic flexure should be left intact.

The proposed site for the coloanal anastomosis (already marked with a clip) is grasped and pushed far down into the pelvis. If there is tension on the mobilized colon at this time, especially of its vessels, further laparoscopic dissection/mobilization is required. A significant advantage of the laparoscopy assisted approach is the ability to mobilize the colon keeping marginal arteries intact to ensure a tension-free coloanal anastomosis, because with a purely transanal approach without the help of laparoscopy, the marginal arteries are likely to be damaged (Figure 3).

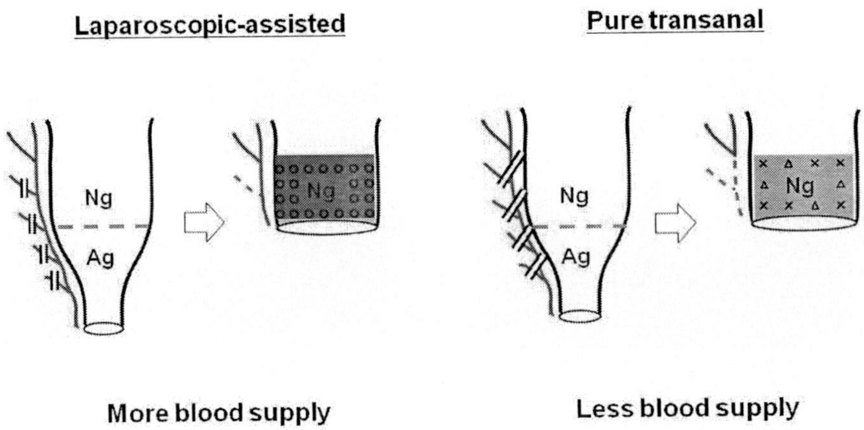

Figure 3.A significant advantage of the laparoscopy assisted approach is the ability to mobilize the colon while keeping marginal arteries intact, unlike the pure transanal approach without laparoscopy where marginal arteries in the pull-through colon are likely to be damaged. Ng: normoganglionic. Ag: aganglionic

After dissection and mobilization of the ganglionic colon, attention is turned to the perineum. The patient is again positioned in the lithotomy position by flexing the legs and securing the feet over the head to expose the anorectal line. Multiple fine traction sutures are then placed proximal to the anorectal line and the mucosa is incised just on the anorectal line circumferentially using needle-tipped electrocautery (Figure 2). The perineal surgeon commences near full-thickness rectal dissection transanally progressing cranially for 15 to 20mm in the plane of the rectal muscle layer (Figure 4), taking great care not to injure the internal anal sphincter and levator ani complex. At this stage, a large bore silicon tube is inserted into the rectal lumen (Figure 5) and the plane of dissection is changed to the submucosal plane and continued proximally between the rectal mucosa and the rectal muscle layers (Figure 4). The tube acts as a stent, greatly facilitating submucosal dissection. As mucosectomy progresses further proximally, the devascularized rectosigmoid colon begins to invaginate into the rectal muscle cuff and reaches the anus. When this happens, submucosal dissection is considered to be sufficient, the muscular wall of the rectum is divided circumferentially, and the devascularized rectosigmoid is delivered through the anus externally without tension and the proposed site for the coloanal anastomosis can be easily identified because of the metal clip.

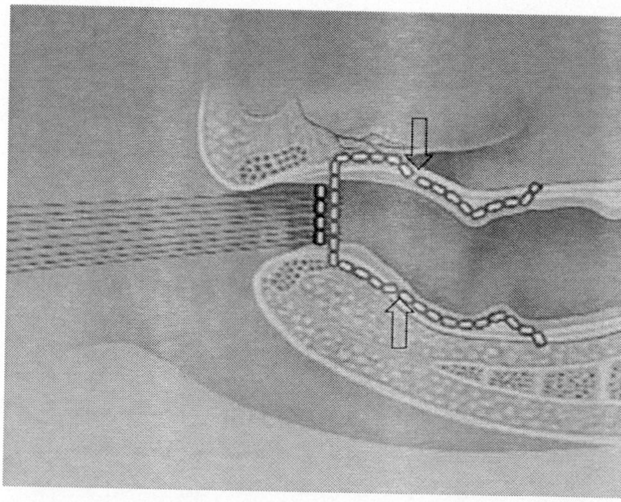

Figure 4.The perineal surgeon commences near full-thickness rectal dissection transanally progressing cranially for 15 to 20 mm in the plane of the rectal muscle layer, then the plane of dissection is changed (arrows) into the submucosa and continued proximally between the rectal mucosa and the rectal muscle layers.

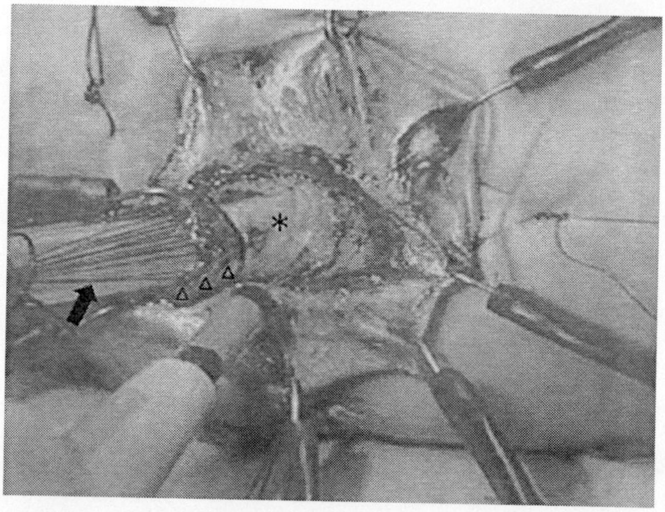

Figure 5. A photo showing a large bore silicon tube (an arrow) inserted into the rectal lumen, which greatly facilitates the transanal "submucosal" (an asterisk) dissection. Note arrowheads indicate near full-thickness rectum.

Next, the rectal cuff is excised. The posterior rectal cuff is excised distally to the level of the starting point of the rectal submucosal dissection (Figure 6 A, B and C).

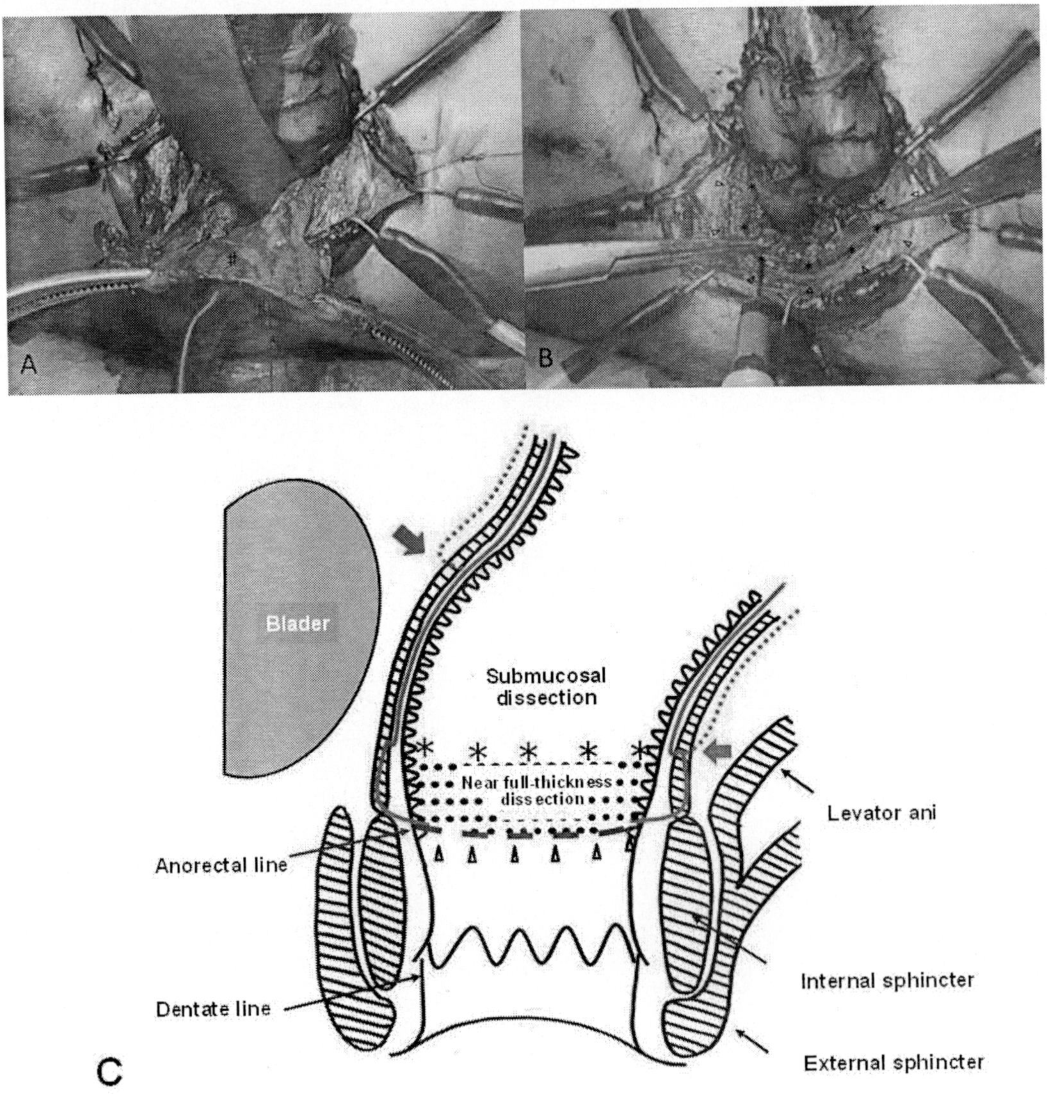

Figure 6. The posterior rectal cuff (A: #) is excised distally to the level of the starting point of the rectal submucosal dissection (asterisks). In other words, the entire posterior aganglionic rectal cuff is removed (B, compared to A), with the first 15 to 20mm (between arrowheads and asterisks) of rectal dissection from the anorectal line (arrowheads) being almost full-thickness. The anterior and posterior rectal cuffs (C: between solid and dotted lines) proximal to the arrows are removed.

In other words, the entire posterior aganglionic rectal cuff is removed, with the first 15 to 20mm of rectal dissection from the anorectal line being almost full-thickness. The anterior rectal cuff proximal to the peritoneal reflection is also excised up to and including the laparoscopically-dissected part. The pull-through colon is anastomosed to the anorectal line using interrupted sutures (Figure 7).

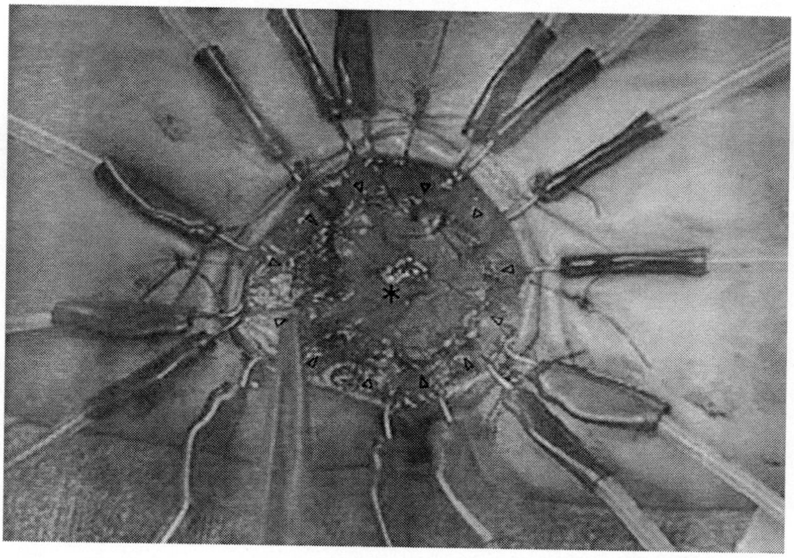

Figure 7.The pull-through colon (an asterisk) is anastomosed to the anorectal line (arrowheads) using interrupted sutures.

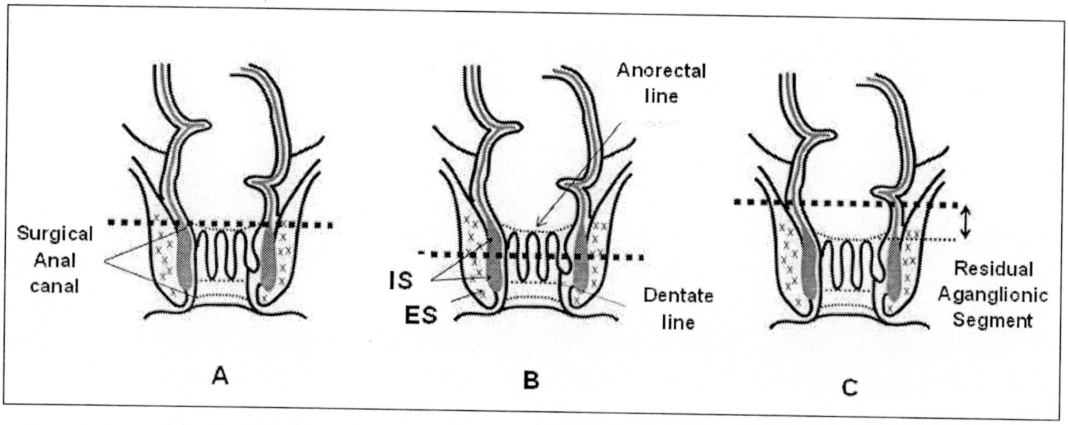

Figure 8. Bold dotted lines indicate where rectal mucosal dissection starts. When rectal mucosal dissection is commenced on the anorectal line [A], the surgical anal canal is preserved, ensuring normal sensory and motor function post-transanal pull-through, and no aganglionic segment remains to cause postoperative constipation. When the dentate line is used as a landmark, if rectal mucosal dissection is too low (i.e., below the anorectal line, [B]), there may be incontinence secondary to damage to the surgical anal canal, and if too high (i.e., above the anorectal line, [C]), there may be postoperative constipation secondary to residual aganglionic rectal segment. IS: internal sphincter, ES: external sphincter.

Traditionally, the dentate line is the landmark referred to in relation to rectal submucosal dissection. However, no surgeon can justify how far above the dentate line is appropriate (Figure 8), and distances from 5 to 20mm have been reported, although it is well known that if commenced too high, there is a tendency for constipation, and if commenced too low, there is a tendency for staining. The distance chosen above the dentate line is quite subjective, especially when the age and physique of a patient are also taken into account, with the result that postoperative outcome in patients where the dentate line is used as a landmark can be somewhat unpredictable. The anorectal line is a reproducibly recognizable landmark without any need for subjective interpretation, whereas "above" the dentate line requires subjective interpretation. With our anorectal line technique [2], the surgical anal canal between the dentate line and the anorectal line is preserved (Figure 8), ensuring that the anorectum has normal sensory and motor function, minimizing postoperative fecal staining/soiling. Furthermore, because there is no remnant of aganglionic rectum posterior to the pulled-through colon, it is unlikely that postoperative constipation and/or rectal stenosis will occur.

Comparing Laparoscopy Assisted Vs. Open Pull-Through

Laparoscopy assisted pull-through, first reported by Georgeson et al [4] in 1995, has been widely adopted as the treatment of choice for Hirschsprung's disease. However, mid- or long-term outcome following laparoscopy assisted pull-through for Hirschsprung's disease is still unclear, since there are few reports on mid-term assessment of fecal continence after laparoscopy assisted pull-through [5-9]. Functionally, laparoscopy assisted pull-through should be very similar to open pull-through, however, to the best of our knowledge, there are only two papers comparing laparoscopy assisted pull-through and open pull-through in the literature [6, 7] - which prompted us to investigate and compare postoperative outcomes after laparoscopy assisted pull-through and open pull-through.

Since 1991, we have treated 64 patients with histologically proven Hirschsprung's disease. All patients had primary endorectal pull-through without colostomy. All pull-through surgery was performed under the direct supervision of a single surgeon (the author: AY). Patients who underwent pull-through after 2003 were excluded because it was not possible to assess mid-term outcome due to the short duration of follow-up. In addition, to limit variable etiologic factors, we excluded Hirschsprung's disease patients with an aganglionic segment proximal to the descending colon, cases of re-do surgery, and patients with mental retardation or chromosomal anomalies. Furthermore, 4 open pull-through patients in whom postoperative data were incomplete were excluded, leaving 35 patients with rectal, recto-sigmoid, and sigmoid-type Hirschsprung's disease as subjects for comparison. Of the 35, 13 had open pull-through performed before 1996, and the remaining 22 had laparoscopy assisted pull-through from 1997 onwards.

The open pull-through procedure we used is a modification of endorectal pull-through involving near total excision of the posterior rectal cuff [10]. Prior to 2007 we used the dentate line as a landmark for transanal rectal dissection during laparoscopy assisted transanal pull through, but now we use the anorectal line. The steps involved in open pull-through and laparoscopy assisted pull-through, that is, ganglionic colon pull-through, and near total rectal cuff excision, are actually exactly the same because our laparoscopy assisted pull-through procedure was developed from the open pull-through procedure by the author (AY).

We used a standardized continence evaluation questionnaire (CEQ) covering 5 parameters (frequency of bowel motions, severity of staining, severity of perianal erosions, anal shape, and requirement for medications) to assess outcome [5]. Severity of staining was graded as none = 2, occasional = 1.5, often = 1, always = 0.5, and soiling = 0, with severity of staining less than or equal to 1 being defined as moderate to severe incontinence. All patients undergoing laparoscopy assisted pull-through after 1997 were evaluated prospectively by the author (AY). Patients who underwent open pull-through before 1996 were reviewed retrospectively. Annual CEQ scores were determined and used to compare the 2 groups.

To assess surgical stress, presence of fever (peak and duration), raised white blood cell count (> 10,000 /μL), and serum C-reactive protein level (> 0.3 mg/dL) were investigated, and data were compared between the 2 groups. Data were expressed as mean ± standard deviation.

Both annual CEQ scores and parameters for surgical stress were compared and analyzed using the unpaired t test and χ^2 test. A P value of less than .05 was considered to be statistically significant.

13 open pull-through patients (1991-1996) were reviewed retrospectively and 22 laparoscopy assisted pull-through (1997-2002) were reviewed prospectively. Of the 22 laparoscopy assisted pull-through subjects, 16 were boys and 6 were girls, and of the 13 open pull-through subjects, 10 were boys and 3 were girls. Types of Hirschsprung's disease were rectal in 3 (laparoscopy assisted: 2, open: 1), recto-sigmoid in 22 (laparoscopy assisted: 13, open: 9), and sigmoid in 10 (laparoscopy assisted: 7, open: 3). Mean age at pull-through was 3.81 ± 3.76 months for laparoscopy assisted pull-through and 4.18 ± 3.19 months for open pull-through. Sex ratio, type of Hirschsprung's disease and mean age at pull-through were not statistically different. Maximum duration of follow-up in the laparoscopy assisted pull-through group was 8 years, but only for 2 subjects, so direct comparison between the 2 groups was only possible for the first 7 years after pull-through. Mean annual CEQ scores for 7 years after laparoscopy assisted pull-through were 6.3, 6.9, 7.3, 7.7, 8.3, 8.9, and 9.0 and after open pull-through were 5.6, 6.4, 7.0, 7.5, 7.8, 8.3, and 8.4 (Figure 9).

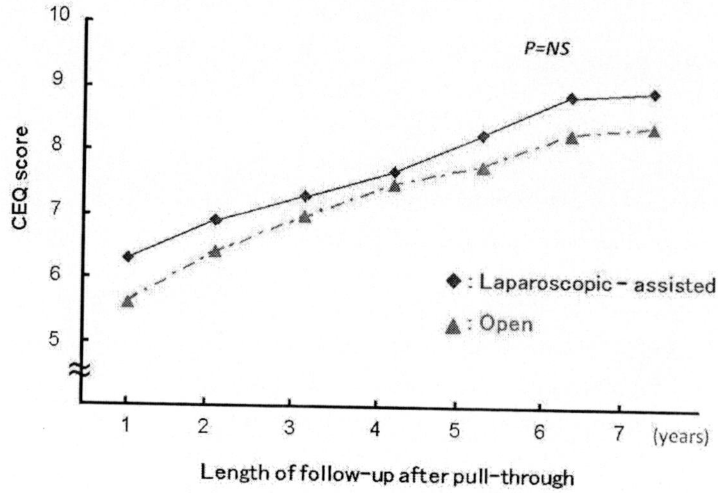

Figure 9.Continence evaluation questionnaire (CEQ) scores after laparoscopy assisted pull-through and open pull-through. Although laparoscopy assisted pull-through had higher scores, the difference was not statistically significant.

Laparoscopy assisted pull-through had higher CEQ scores throughout, but the difference was not statistically significant. The incidence of moderate to severe incontinence after 4 years was 54% (7/13) for open pull-through and 23% (5/22) for laparoscopy assisted pull-through, and after 6 years, moderate to severe incontinence was absent for laparoscopy assisted pull-through (0/10), and 23% (3/13) for open pull-through (statistically not significant in both, $P = .06$ and .10, respectively).

Mean peak white blood cell count was 13,579 ± 2,903 /μL for laparoscopy assisted pull-through and 16,264 ± 7,162 /μL for open pull-through ($P = .16$), and mean duration of raised white blood cell count was 4.2 ± 4.3 days in laparoscopy assisted pull-through and 6.9 ± 3.8 days in open pull-through ($P = .11$). Mean peak C-reactive protein for laparoscopy assisted pull-through was 3.87 ± 2.10 mg/dL and for open pull-through was 9.17 ± 4.99 mg/dL, which was statistically significant ($P < .01$). Mean duration of raised C-reactive protein for laparoscopy assisted pull-through (5.63 ± 2.1 days) was also significantly shorter than for open pull-through (10.0 ± 2.2 days, $P < .01$). Mean duration of fever was 0.9 ± 0.8 days for laparoscopy assisted pull-through and 3.9 ± 2.3 days for open pull-through and this difference was statistically significant ($P < .01$).

Postoperative complications encountered were, adhesive bowel obstruction in 2 open pull-through patients and enterocolitis in 5 open pull-through patients and 2 laparoscopy assisted pull-through patients. None of the 35 subjects we compared had enterocolitis before pull-through surgery.

Our results suggest that laparoscopy assisted pull-through is less invasive and may provide better postoperative bowel management compared with open pull-through.

Recently, we reported a prospective mid-term analysis of laparoscopy assisted pull-through for Hirschsprung's disease [5], and concluded that laparoscopy assisted pull-through was safe with acceptable outcome in the mid-term. A shortfall of past reports about fecal continence and of our own paper was that postoperative outcome was evaluated only once at the last outpatient visit [6-9]. In other words, changes in bowel habits over time were not recorded. Thus, we tried to determine what happens over time by conducting a prospective evaluation of bowel habits after laparoscopy assisted pull-through by using a CEQ with particular focus on the severity of staining/soiling, in order to more accurately assess changes in continence that might in fact provide valuable information about the effectiveness of surgical management.

There are only two reports comparing outcome of laparoscopy assisted pull-through and open pull-through in the literature [6, 7]. Kubota et al [6] reported about outcome after laparoscopy assisted pull-through by making a comparison with open pull-through, and stressed that laparoscopy assisted pull-through was less invasive and could provide a better clinical outcome compared with open pull-through in terms of postoperative staining/soiling. However, they compared voluntary defecation and staining/soiling only at 3 years after pull-through, thus we feel there could be significant shortcomings because changes in bowel habit for each subject over time were not assessed. The other report is by El-Sawaf et al [7] and is a comparative study between transanal pull-through (25% were laparoscopy-assisted transanal, 75% were pure transanal) and open pull-through. Unlike our results, their study showed significantly better continence data for open pull-through compared with transanal pull-through. The discrepancy may have arisen for the following reasons: 1) their study might have been considerably biased because patients with chromosomal anomalies, long segment Hirschsprung's disease or total colonic aganglionosis, and re-do pull-through were included;

2) 75% of patients had "pure" transanal pull-through without laparoscopic assistance where the anal sphincter must be stretched vigorously in order to select and divide the superior rectal and sigmoid vessels, especially in high recto-sigmoid type or sigmoid type Hirschsprung's disease. Overstretching of the anal sphincter could affect postoperative fecal continence. In contrast to these two reports, we aimed to keep bias to a minimum by carefully selecting patients, having all pull-through procedures supervised by the same single surgeon, and administering a CEQ to laparoscopy assisted pull-through patients prospectively. The only obvious source of bias in our study is that continence data in the open pull-through group were obtained retrospectively and in fact 4 open pull-through patients had to be excluded for insufficient information. Although we cannot say that the CEQ was administered to all subjects, our assessment of open pull-through medical records was thorough enough to provide a good picture of postoperative outcome. There were no cases of "pure" transanal pull-through in our comparison. Compared with "pure" transanal pull-through, stretching of the anal sphincter is minimal in laparoscopy assisted pull-through, since the feeding vessels to the ganglionic rectum/colon are divided laparoscopically without any need to stretch the anal canal when dividing vessels. Our findings would suggest that laparoscopy assisted pull-through appears to provide better postoperative bowel management compared with open pull-through.

Teitelbaum et al [11] investigated the early to long-term postoperative bowel habits of infants who had open pull-through for Hirschsprung's disease and found that the frequency of bowel motions went from 5-8 motions per day immediately after surgery to a mean of 3.8 ± 1.4 motions per day 6 months later. They concluded that frequency of bowel motions decreased during the first postoperative year and our experience supports this. Thus, we strongly feel that continence can in fact be evaluated nicely in patients less than 4 years of age, and invite surgeons to include our CEQ in their routine follow-up of post pull-through patients with Hirschsprung's disease because it does not include an assessment of urge to defecate, which cannot practically be assessed accurately until the ages of 3 or 4 years.

When surgical stress were compared between groups, not only were specific markers of surgical stress significantly less for laparoscopy assisted pull-through, but also laparoscopy assisted pull-through was associated with less intra-abdominal contamination because of transanal rectal dissection and less physical trauma leading to adhesion formation because of laparoscopy, although open pull-through tended to have higher risks for contamination and adhesion formation [12].

Our findings indicate that laparoscopy assisted pull-through is a less invasive procedure that results in equal or better postoperative outcome compared with open pull-through. Maximum duration of follow-up after laparoscopy assisted pull-through in our series was 8 years, which is not enough to analyze long-term outcome, but from the data we examined there is a strong indication that long-term outcome after laparoscopy assisted pull-through is most likely to be excellent, and laparoscopy assisted pull-through should be adopted as the method of choice for pull-through.

Transanal Dissection: Dentate Line Vs Anorectal Line

Rectal mucosal dissection is well known as a critical step during transanal pull-through for Hirschsprung's disease. Conventionally, the dentate line has been used as a landmark for where dissection should commence, but recently, we began to use the anorectal line instead (Figures 2 and 8) and found that patients seemed to do very well postoperatively when frequency of bowel movements, degree of staining, and anal shape were assessed using a standardized questionnaire. This prompted us to conduct a comparative study between patients who had rectal mucosal dissection commencing on the anorectal line (anorectal line group), patients who had rectal mucosal dissection commencing above the dentate line (dentate line group), and age-matched normal healthy babies without any anorectal disorders (control group).

In 2007, we began using the anorectal line as a landmark for rectal mucosal dissection during transanal pull-through and between January 2007 and April 2008 treated 11 Hirschsprung's disease patients [3]. Six of these have been followed-up for more than 6 months and were reviewed prospectively (anorectal line group). All 6 had pull-through before they were 2 months old. From 2003 to December, we treated 19 Hirschsprung's disease patients using transanal pull-through with rectal mucosal dissection commencing at various levels (0-10mm) above the dentate line. Eight of these treated before they were 2 months old formed the dentate line group. In both groups, Hirschsprung's disease patients with an aganglionic segment proximal to the descending colon and those with chromosomal abnormalities were excluded to limit variable etiologic factors. There was no aspect of the surgery performed or postoperative management that changed over time between the dentate line group and the anorectal line group except for the level of dissection. The control group consisted of 10 normal healthy babies who had their bowel habits assessed.

Details of the anorectal line technique we use can be found under laparoscopy assisted transanal pull-through earlier in this chapter. We used our CEQ [5] at each outpatient clinic visit administered by the same surgeon (the author: AY) to assess outcome. Results were collected and data were compared between the 3 groups from 2 to 6 months of age. Data were expressed as mean ± standard deviation. Mean daily frequencies of bowel movements were compared and analyzed using the unpaired Student's *t* test. A *P* value of less than .05 was considered to be statistically significant.

The anorectal line group (n=6) comprised 3 boys and 3 girls, the dentate line group (n=8) comprised 6 boys and 2 girls, and the control group (n=10) comprised 6 boys and 4 girls. Mean age at pull-through was 30.3±7.4 days for the anorectal line group and 29.5±7.1 days for the dentate line group, which was not statistically significant (*P* = NS). Mean daily frequencies of bowel movements at 2, 3, 4, 5, and 6 months of age were 9.2±2.0, 4.8±1.3, 3.7±0.8, 3.0±1.1, and 2.9±1.1 respectively in the anorectal line group; 9.1±1.8, 7.4±1.8, 6.6±1.8, 6.1±1.5, and 5.5±1.3 respectively in the dentate line group; and 5.3±2.2, 3.8±1.6, 2.9±1.2, 2.2±0.6, and 2.2±0.3 respectively in the control group, indicating that differences between the anorectal and control groups were not statistically significant after 3 months of age (*P* = NS at 3, 4, 5, and 6 months of age, respectively) (Figure 10).

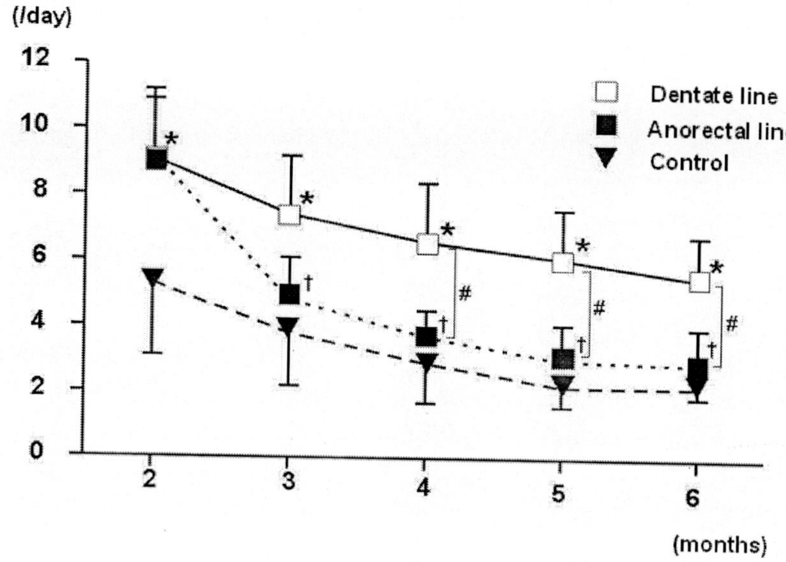

Figure 10.Daily frequency of bowel movements at 2, 3, 4, 5 and 6 months of age. Results were significantly higher in the dentate line group for every month compared to the control group (*P < .01). However, frequencies in the dentate line group were significantly higher at 4, 5, and 6 months of age when compared with anorectal line group (#P < .01). There were not significant between the anorectal and control groups after 3 months of age (†P = NS).

However, frequencies in the dentate line group were significantly higher for every month compared with the control group ($P < .01$) but only at 4, 5, and 6 months of age when compared with the anorectal line group ($P < .01$). For fecal staining, the incidence was zero by 6 months old in the control group, occasional in 1/6 (17%) of the anorectal line group, but occasional to frequent in 5/8 (63%) of the dentate line group. Anal shape at 6 months of age was basically the same without exposed anal mucosa in the anorectal line and control groups, but there was moderate exposure of the anal mucosa in 4/8 (50%) of the dentate line group. Postoperative constipation or enterocolitis did not occur in either the anorectal line group or dentate line group and there was no rectal stenosis due to a residual rectal cuff.

Our results suggest that bowel function in the anorectal line group is similar to normal and because the anorectal line is easily identifiable without the need for subjective interpretation, we recommend using the anorectal line as a landmark for rectal mucosal dissection during transanal pull-through for Hirschsprung's Disease. Further research and long-term follow-up will reveal more information about our anorectal line technique, but at this preliminary stage, it would appear to be a technique that is easy to use, predictable, with good cosmetic and functional outcome - in short a very valid alternative to conventional techniques for rectal mucosal dissection during transanal pull-through for Hirschsprung's disease.

References

[1] Yamataka A, Yoshida R, Kobayashi H, Tsukamoto K, Lane GJ, Segawa O, et al: Laparoscopy-assisted suction colonic biopsy and intraoperative rapid acetylcholinesterase staining during transanal pull-through for Hirschsprung's disease. *J Pediatr Surg*, 2002;37:1661-3.

[2] Hollwarth ME, Rivosecchi M, Schleef J, Deluggi S, Fasching G, Ceriati E, et al. The role of transanal endorectal pull-through in the treatment of Hirschsprung's disease—a multicenter experience. *Pediatr Surg Int*, 2002;18:344-8.

[3] Yamataka A, Kaneyama K, Fujiwara N, Hayashi Y, Lane GJ, Kawashima K, et al. Rectal mucosal dissection during transanal pull-through for Hirschsprung's disease: the anorectal or the dentate line ? *J Pediatr Surg*, 2009 (in press).

[4] Georgeson KE, Fuenfer MM, Hardin WD. Primary laparoscopic pull-through for Hirschsprung's disease in infants and children. *J Pediatr Surg*, 1995;30:1017-22.

[5] Ishihara M, Yamataka A, Kaneyama K, Koga H, Kobayashi H, Lane GJ, et al. Prospective analysis of primary modified Georgeson's laparoscopy-assisted endorectal pull-through for Hirschsprung's disease: short-to mid-term results. *Pediatr Surg Int* 2005; 21: 878-82.

[6] Kubota A, Kawahara H, Okuyama H. Clinical outcome of laparoscopically assisted endorectal pull-through in Hirschsprung's disease: comparison of abdominal and perineal approaches. *J Pediatr Surg*, 2004;39:1835-7.

[7] El-Sawaf MI, Drongowski RA, Chamberlain JN: Are the long-term results of the transanal pull-through equal to those of the transabdominal pull-through? A comparison of the 2 approaches for Hirschsprung's disease. *J Pediatr Surg*, 2007;42:41-7.

[8] Kumar R, Mackay A, Borzi P. Laparoscopic Swenson procedure--an optimal approach for both primary and secondary pull-through for Hirschsprung's disease. *J Pediatr Surg*, 2003;38:1440-3.

[9] Wang NL, Lee HC, Yeh ML, Chang PY, Sheu JC. Experience with primary laparoscopy-assisted endorectal pull-through for Hirschsprung's disease. *Pediatr Surg Int*, 2004; 20:118-22.

[10] Miyano T, Yamataka A, Urao M, Kobayashi H, Lane G. Modified Soave pull-through for Hirschsprung's disease: intraoperative internal sphincterotomy. *J Pediatr Surg*, 1999;34:1599-602.

[11] Teitelbaum DH, Drongowski RA, Chamberlain JN, et al: Long-term stooling patterns in infants undergoing primary endorectal pull-through for Hirschsprung's disease. *J Pediatr Surg*, 1997;32:1049-53.

[12] Georgeson KE, Cohen RD, Hebra A. Primary laparoscopic-assisted endorectal colon pull-through for Hirschsprung's disease. *Ann Surg*, 1999;229:678-83.

In: Hirschsprung's Disease: Diagnosis and Treatment
Ed: Ramón Núñez and Manuel López-Alonso
ISBN: 978-1-60741-349-3

Chapter XIX

One-Stage Transanal Endorectal Colectomy and Pull-Through for Hirschsprung Disease in Neonates and Infants

Luis De la Torre-Mondragón and J. Arturo Ortega-Salgado

Transanal endorectal approach for one-stage colectomy and pull-through (TECPT) in neonates and infants with short Hirschsprung disease (HD) has the principal benefit that it does not require an abdominal approach. Historical antecedents that have contributed to the born of this technique are the endorectal pull-through proposed by Professor Franco Soave to avoid damage to pelvic structures [1], the primary colo-anal anastomosis using this technique [2], the one stage endorectal pull-through in newborns [3], the application of endosurgery [4], and an experimental model that gave us the opportunity to observe that long segments of colon could be pulled-through by a transanal approach only [5]. After these contributions the first clinical one stage TECPT in a baby with HD was performed in October 1996 [6].

Pre-Operative Considerations

Before to perform a one-stage TECPT in a newborn with HD we strongly recommend to confirm the following determinant conditions.

Firstly, in a newborn with low intestinal obstruction syndrome (figure 1 A) and after ruled out an anorectal malformation it is important to attempt medical management to avoid a colostomy. This syndrome has different etiologies such as ileum atresia, colon atresia, intestinal malrotation, enterocolitis and other less frequent problems (figure 1 B). In this clinical condition HD should also be suspected and intestinal decompression should be try with a rectal tube and gentile warm saline rectal irrigations, if intestinal obstruction is radiologically and clinically resolved, the patient can be fed orally and it is scheduled for a rectal biopsy. However, if the rectal tube does not resolve the intestinal obstruction a colon enema can be done to demonstrate the presence of micro-colon, colon atresia, intestinal malrotation or a high transitional zone (TZ), thus abdominal exploration will be indicated when the medical management is unsuccessful or exist an evident indication.

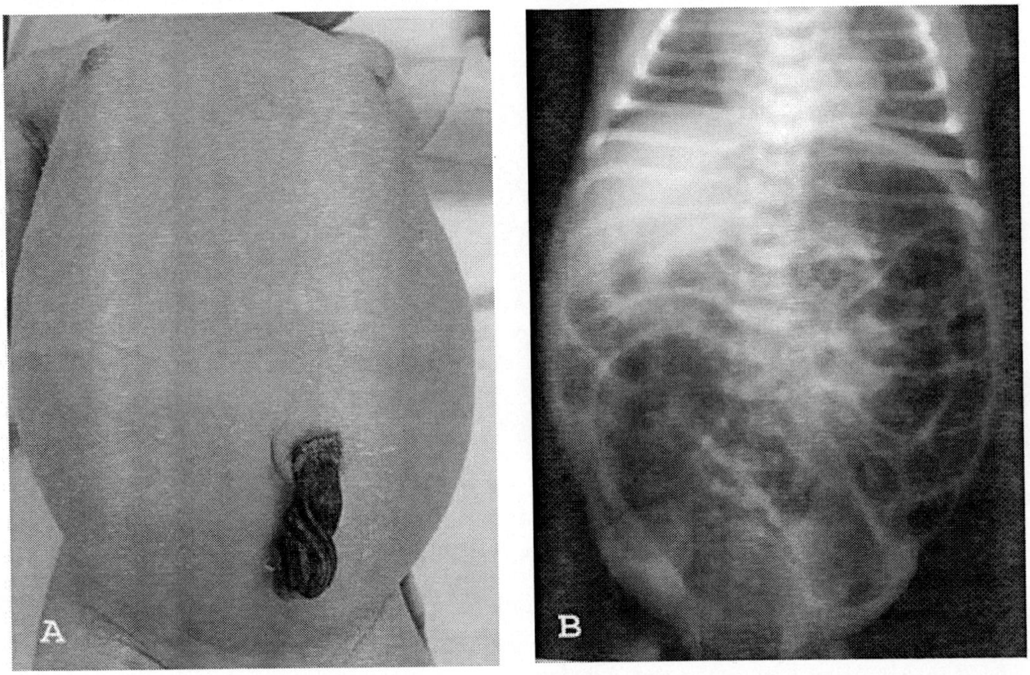

Figure 1 A. Clinical picture of a neonatal patient affected with low intestinal obstruction syndrome. Twenty days old boy who could not defecate spontaneously. He improved transitory with glycerin suppository daily. He had had occasionally gastric and bilious vomits. Three days before come to ER he could not have bowel movements. B. AP X ray film of a patient with low intestinal obstruction syndrome. Most frequent differential diagnoses in theses cases are: ileum atresia, colon atresia, intestinal malrotation, enterocolitis, and Hirschsprung disease.

The main idea of this consideration is to keep in mind that not all the newborns and infants with low intestinal obstruction will need a laparotomy as the first diagnostic or therapeutic procedure.

Secondly, we have to confirm the histological diagnosis of HD. The rectal biopsy with absence of ganglion cells in the submucosa is the gold standard study to diagnose it. However, many circumstances can provoke mistakes in this study, the most frequent misdiagnoses are biopsies informed as "aganglionic" in non-Hirschsprung babies because the obtained tissue was from a very distal place around the pectinate line where normally does not exist ganglion cells [7] (figure 2) or the sample was very superficial and did not include submucosa. Otherwise, when the tissue is appropriate in location and deepness for study, it can be inadequately processed making few disoriented sections. In this context, the lack of experience to identify immature ganglion cells in babies or either mature ganglion cells in older children is another determinant source of misdiagnosis [8,9].

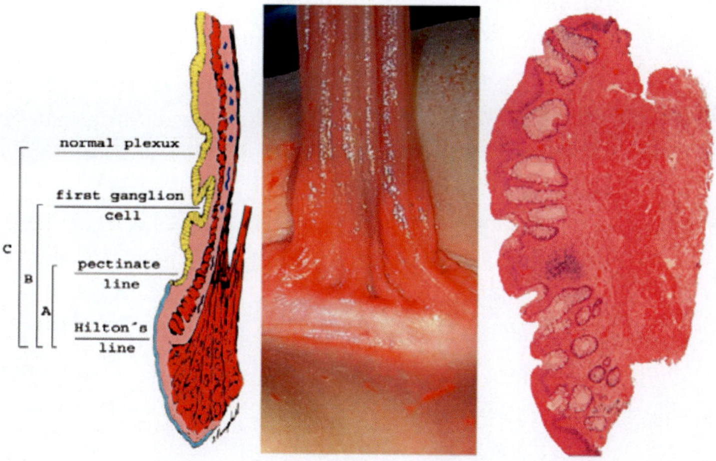

Figure 2. There are not ganglion cells in the submucosa around the pectinate line, thus a low biopsy will be normally aganglionic. The rectal biopsy should be taken 3 cm above the pectinate line. This figure shows an illustration (modified with permission from [5]), a trans-operative view and a photomicrography (courtesy from Dr. Rash Kapur) to demonstrate comparatively the location of ganglion cells and where the rectal biopsy should be taken.

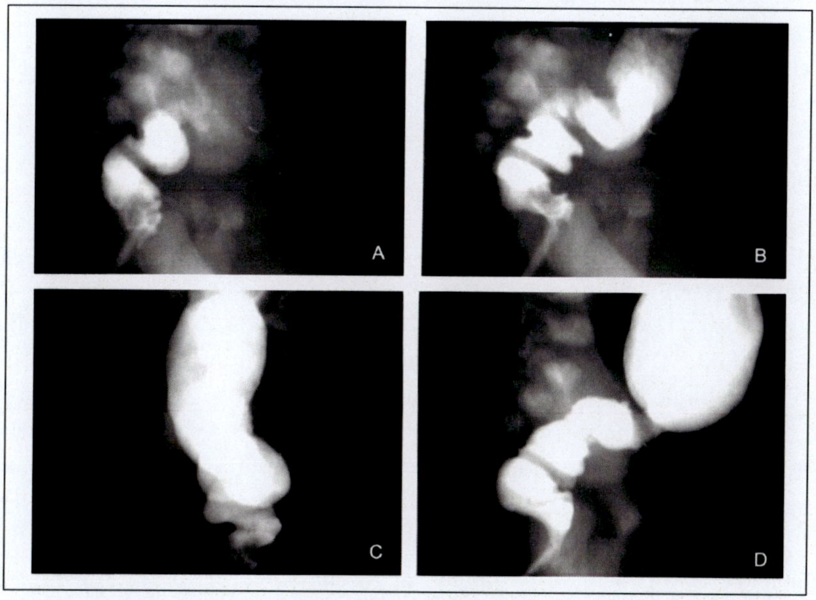

Figure 3. A. Rectogram of a histological confirmed case of Hirschsprung disease showing a fluoroscopic lateral view starting irrigation of the contrast solution (no barium), B. lateral view showing how the dilated sigmoid is being initially filled, C. frontal view shows a dilated loop, but the transitional zone can not be defined in this view, D. radiological transitional zone is clearly demonstrated in lateral view; this projection is most useful than AP views in short segment Hirschsprung.

Once we have confirmed the histological diagnosis, it is extremely important to determine the length of the affected segment before to decide a one-stage TECPT. A contrasted (none barium) rectogram is the next study that should be made. For the rectogram, it is important to wait until the patient recover the abdominal distention; this is really useful to demonstrate the radiological TZ (figure 3). This clinical condition is obtained removing the rectal tube for 48 to 72 hours, and when the baby becomes distended is scheduled for the rectogram under fluoroscopic control.

It is difficult and sometimes impossible to demonstrate the radiological TZ when the rectogram is made using a Foley (balloon) catheter or the catheter is placed above the rectum. It is also inappropriate to instill fast the contrast solution with high pressure. To observe the TZ, fluoroscopic control and lateral views are mandatory. Remember, the rectogram for HD is done after the histological confirmation, and it is for HD, not to reduce an intussusception neither to demonstrate the presence of filling defects in the entire colon [10].

The ideal candidate to perform the TECPT technique must have the following characteristics: a newborn or infant with a short aganglionic segment involving the rectum and sigmoid, and without previous abdominal surgical procedures [11,12].

Surgical Technique

The night before surgery the patient is fasted, intravenous antibiotics are given and rectal irrigation continued to maintain the colon clean and decompressed.

We prefer the prone position because the mesenteric vessels can be observed and controlled with a frontal view.

Rectal Mucosectomy

In a prone position with the pelvis elevated, the anal canal is exposed using an automatic retractor (Figure 4 A) or traction sutures fixed to the operative drapes, once the anal canal is exposed multiple 5-0 silk traction sutures are placed in the mucosa 1 cm above the pectinate line (Figure 4 B) and a (Figure 5 A). While pulling the traction sutures, a submucosal plane of dissection is developed for 1-2 cm with the electrocautery; this length of freed mucosa permitted to continue the mucosectomy using blunt dissection. A useful maneuver to separate the mucosa from the circular muscular layer is to place the tip of the index finger behind the freed mucosa, to put a dry gauze in front of it, while pulling the traction sutures, this maneuver allow the dissection with a gauze or a little ball of gauze. The inner circular layer of the muscular rectal wall should be identified to guarantee the precise plane of dissection (Figure 5 B).

During mucosectomy, firm adhesions from the mucosa to the muscular layer due to penetrating vessels are founded, these tiny vessels should be coagulated with the tip of a fine needle of electrocautery over the muscular side rather tan the mucosal side, this trick is better than a vigorous blunt dissection that sometimes cause rupture of the mucosa and intestinal spillage.

The mucosectomy continue until the peritoneal reflection to assure the entry to the peritoneal cavity. In neonates, 7-10 cm of mucosectomy is enough to get inside; in older children 15 cm may be sufficient (Figure 6 A and B). One tip-off about how to know if we are in the peritoneal reflection, it is when the muscular sleeve becomes floppy or baggy during the mucosectomy.

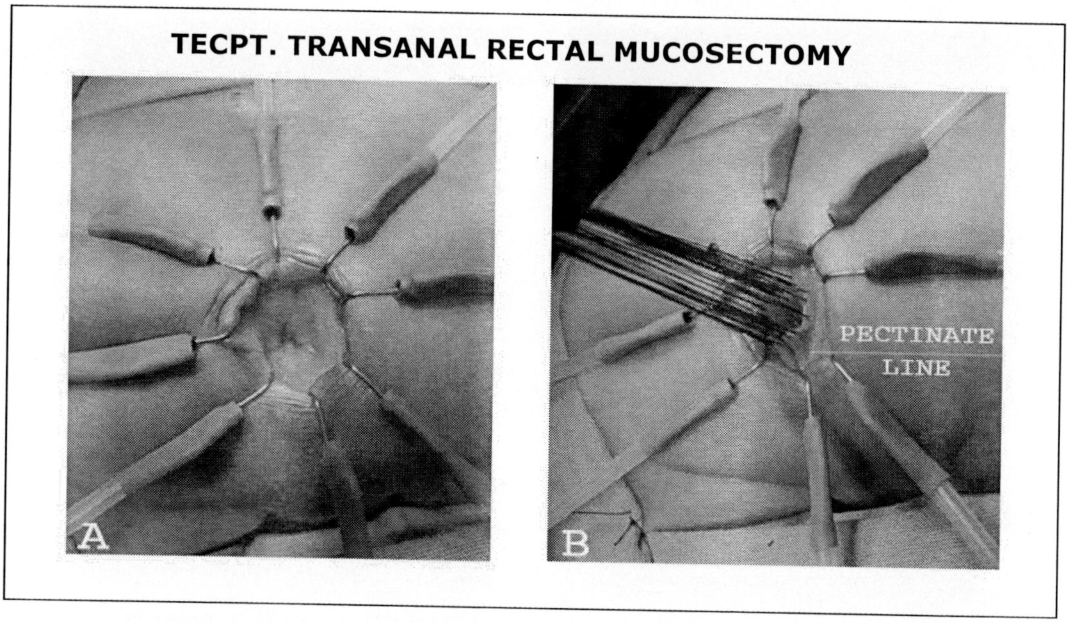

Figure 4. Prone position with the pelvis elevated offers a comfortable surgical field during a transanal approach and a good exposition of mesenteric vessels that come posterior, thus their surgical control is safer; also, other authors have used lithotomy position. A. To begin the mucosectomy an automatic retractor or fine traction sutures fixed to surgical field are placed to expose the anal canal and pectinate line. B. Trans-operative photograph shows the anal canal and pectinate line. To start mucosectomy multiple 5-0 silk traction sutures are placed in the mucosa 1 cm above from the pectinate line.

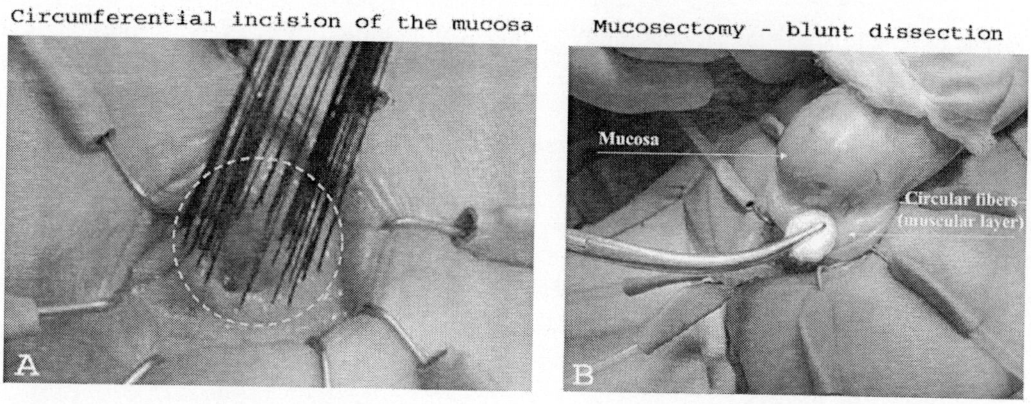

Figure 5. A. This picture shows the location where circumferential incision (yellow doted lines) is made in the rectal mucosa with electrocautery close to the traction sutures, and then pulling these sutures the submucosal plane of dissection is developed also with electrocautery B. This picture shows a useful maneuver to dissect the mucosa. The inner circular layer of the muscular rectal wall should be identified to guarantee the precise plane of blunt dissection.

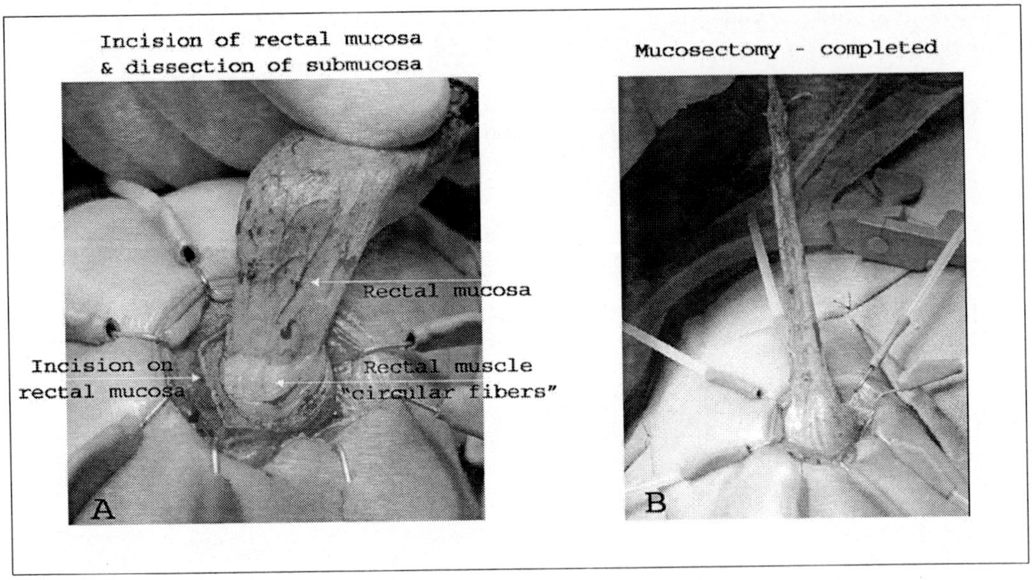

Figure 6. A. This picture shows three elements that can be identify after 6 cm of mucosectomy; the dissected rectal mucosa, the inner circular fibers of the rectum and the first incision in the mucosa proximal to the pectinate line. Also, the mucosal vessels are observed; some of them are bleeding due to the blunt dissection while others are coagulated, the last offered mayor resistance during blunt dissection and its electrocoagulation is recommended. B. The mucosectomy has finished. After 10 cm of dissection, the anatomical and vascular elements referred in figure 6 A can be recognized.

Muscular Cuff

The sleeve where the normoganglionic colon will be pulled-through is the muscular cuff, as in the classic Soave procedure; the only difference is that it is made in reverse. Surgeons that have made an endorectal pull-through are familiarized with this step.

To create the muscular cuff a circumferential incision is made with electrocautery on the denuded muscular rectal wall to separate the cuff from the whole rectal wall and entry to the peritoneal cavity. This step requires placing two stitches in four quadrants to refer the edge of the whole colon and the edge of the cuff, eight stitches in total. The first deep stitch is placed where the mucosectomy was finished; this stitch takes mucosa and denuded muscular layer. The second stitch is placed 3-5 mm from the first and it takes only denuded muscular layer. Between these traction sutures the circumferential division of the muscle fibers is done with electrocautery (figure 7A).

This circumferential section makes available the separation of two anatomical structures: the whole colon referred with the first stitches and that it will be pulled-through and, the muscular cuff referred from the second stitches. Once these structures are separated the peri-rectal tissue is reached and it is dissected all around. In this step, two peritoneal surfaces are identify, one from the muscular cuff and the other from the colon (Figure 7 B) meaning that we are into the peritoneal cavity. This verification is important to avoid dissection into pelvis and the possibility of damage to the urethra, vas deferens, vagina, or other pelvic organ [13].

The cuff is wholly split making a complete posterior myotomy (Figure 8 A), from its peritoneal end to its anal end. This posterior myotomy has the aim to relive the pressure from the aganglionic muscular cuff that is probably one of the causes of postoperative obstruction. Then, the muscular cuff is unfolded and reintroduced to the peritoneal cavity liberating the second stitches.

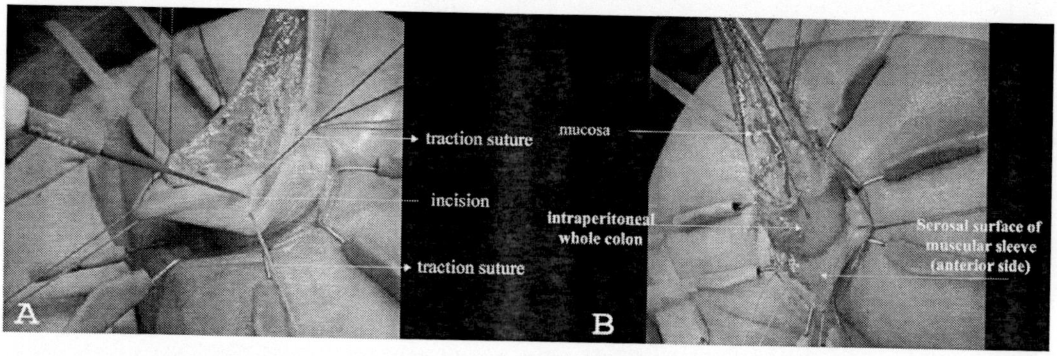

Figure 7. A. This picture shows how the muscular sleeve becomes floppy or baggy when the mucosectomy reaches the peritoneal reflection. Also, it shows the traction or reference sutures go into the peritoneal cavity and to form the rectal cuff. This illustration also shows the step (electrocautery) to go into the peritoneal cavity. B. This picture shows the peritoneal surfaces of the muscular cuff and colon after the incision on the rectal muscle has been completed.

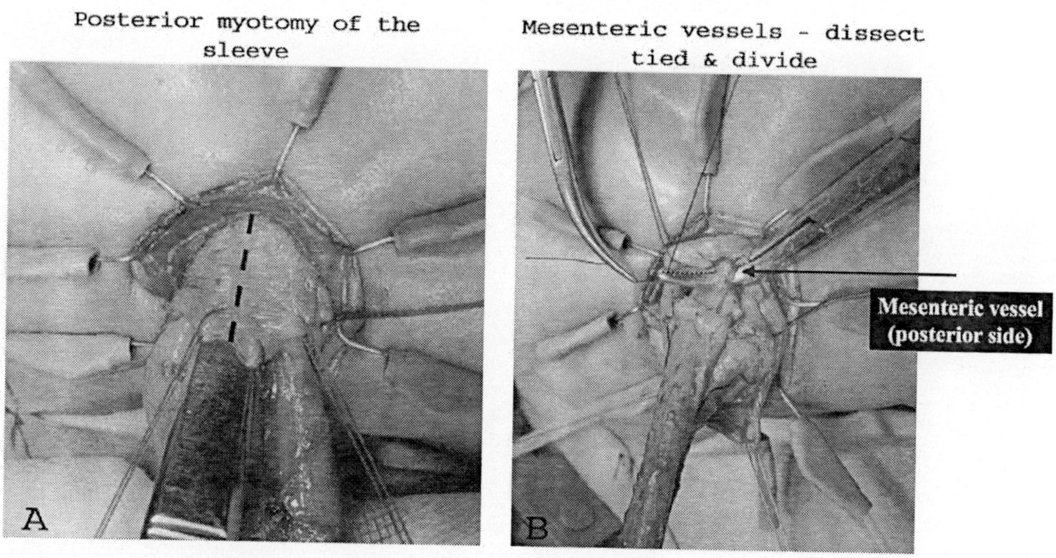

Figure 8. A. The cuff is wholly split making a complete posterior myotomy. B. To obtain colon length for pull-though, the mesenteric vessels should be clearly exposed for dissecting.

Some authors have proposed to make a shorter mucosectomy and consequently a short muscular cuff [14,15] with the same idea to relive more the postoperative obstruction. However, if the length of the muscular cuff is short (2-4 cm), extremely care should be taken to avoid going into the pelvis with the major possibility to damage pelvic structures as occur if we made a wrong Swenson procedure. The principle of the endorectal pull-through is to avoid go into the pelvic structures.

Colon Mobilization

Pulling the rectum with the initial multiple 5-0 silk traction sutures placed in the mucosa together with the four stitches placed previously to create the muscular sleeve, the peritoneal attachments of the colon are dissected; this is particularly easy in neonates and infants. At the same time, while the mesenteric vessels are exposed they are dissected, ligated and divided making available to obtain colon length for the descent (Figure 8 B). During the colon mobilization and when the macroscopic TZ is observed (Figure 9 A) a frozen section of a trans-operative full-thickness biopsy is examined it to assure normoganglionic level.

Colon Resection and Anastomosis

Until the normoganglionic colon is reached and freed without tension up to the anastomotic line, the colectomy (figure 9 B) and the anastomosis to the mucosa near to the pectinate line is performed (figure 9 C). It is advisable to include in the colectomy most of the proximal normoganglionic dilated colon; this dilated segment could be a source of postoperative motility problems. However, some authors have informed good preliminary result using this dilated segment to make the colo-anal anastomosis moreover they made urodynamic studies and did not find problems [16].

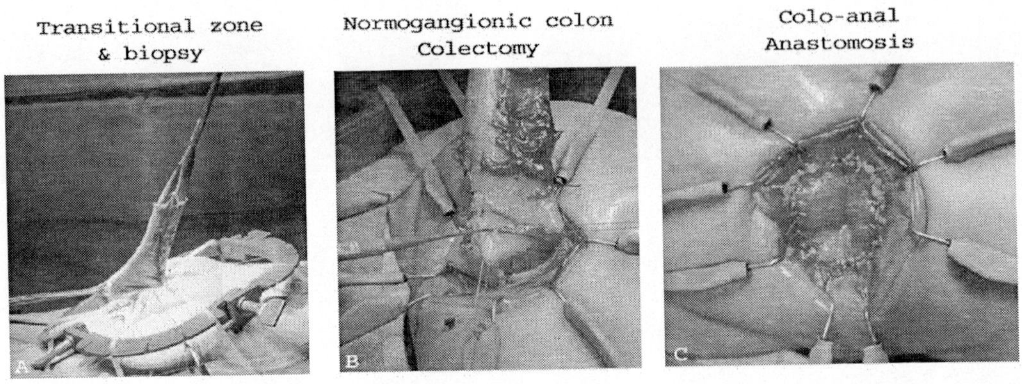

Figure 9. A. When the macroscopic TZ is observed a full-thickness biopsy is obtain for trans-operative study to assure normoganglionic level. This picture shows the macroscopic TZ exiting from the anus. B. When a normoganglionic colon is reached and freed without tension up to the anastomotic line observing an adequate irrigation the colectomy is performed with electrocautery. C. Finally, the colo-anal anastomosis to the mucosa, near to the pectinate line, is performed with absorbable suture.

Postoperative Care and Follow-up

Usually after a TECPT the intestinal activity is not affected and the patient has bowel movements during the first 24 post-operative hours and oral feed can be restarted, antibiotics are continued for a week and in all cases the mother make supervised anorectal dilatations for six months starting two weeks after the operation. We use the same dilatation program of the anorectal malformations.

During the postoperative period, many cases present perianal dermatitis due to frequent bowel movements and liquid discharges. It is important to remark the prevention and control of this clinical condition. We use skin care products such zinc oxide cream and sometimes anti-diarrhea medication for example loperamide or colestyramine. This is a transitory problem that resolved spontaneously in few weeks [13,17-19].

Most of the patients operated on TECPT have a very good postoperative outcome, however enterocolitis and residual constipation still being two unpreventable complications and we should be on alert for their opportune detection and management.

Many authors inform complications [20-22] that are common to other pull-through techniques and approaches: anastomosis dehiscence, abscesses, fecal incontinence, residual aganglionosis, fistulas and stenosis. To avoid these preventable complications we strongly recommend:

1. To avoid a pull-through in an aganglionic segment, assuring the presence of ganglion cells in the submucosal plexus and myenteric plexus in the frozen section during the operation.
2. To avoid the colo-anal anastomosis with a very dilated and hypertrophied colon.
3. To make a colo-anal anastomosis with a freed bowel, without tension and well irrigated it.
4. To make the anastomosis near the pectinate line, avoiding a very low anastomosis like a perineal colostomy or, a very high anastomosis leaving a long aganglionic segment.

Results

We have performed 58 TECPT (table 1), 80% have been males, and 48 cases were operated before the three months of age, and 10 cases were operated between 3 months and 13 years. Twelve patients suffered mild enterocolitis managed and resolved with medical treatment, 8 cases presented residual constipation medically treated. Two initial cases needed a re-operation because residual aganglionosis; in these cases a Duhamel procedure was successfully made. Also in our initial experience, seven patients with previous abdominal operations required an additional abdominal approach to free multiple intestinal adhesions that did not allow the colon mobilization through the anus. In our series we have not observed anastomosis dehiscence, abscesses, fecal incontinence, fistulas or stenosis. Thirty-nine patients have been followed for more than 8 years; the follow-up range is from 11 years to 2 months. We have lost from follow-up twelve patients.

Table 1. Our experience with TECPT.

N° patients	Age Pull-through		Mild Enterocolitis (%)	Residual Constipation (%)	Fecal Incontinence (%)
	< 3 months	3m –13 years			
58	48	10	20.6 (12)	13.7 (8)	0

Conclusions

TECPT is a safe approach to treat the most frequent form of HD mainly in neonates. TECPT allows performing the resection of the aganglionic segment, pull-through the normoganglionic colon through the pelvis downwards the pectine line to perform a comfortable anastomosis.

The fact that TECPT has been used to resect long segments and performed in older children and adolescents informing good results [23,24], we believe that an additional abdominal approach is recommended to mobilize in a safer manner the descending colon or a more proximal colonic segment. Also, we prefer to use this approach in small babies because the dissection of the mucosa and the mobilization of the colon are very easy and the operation is enjoyable. Our experience in older children as well as in adolescents were chronic colon dilatation is present this approach is really laborious being more safe and pleasured to use an abdominal approach.

Hirschsprung patients with previous abdominal surgery develop intestinal adhesions that difficult the colon dissection and mobilization during a transanal approach; in our experience, most of the patients with previous laparotomy require an additional abdominal approach.

One-stage pull-through for HD during the neonatal and infant period is an amazing procedure using Soave, Duhamel or Swenson techniques being the ideal age to perform them. However, this enthusiastic race to make one-stage operations at early ages requires experience from the surgeon and pathologist and the resources for a trans-operative frozen section study [25].

Preventable complications had their origin in a human error of judgment and we have to recognize them to take actions to prevent them. During the study, evaluation, treatment and follow of patients with HD these unintentional acts are common, in this way, when fistulas, abscess, stenosis, residual aganglionosis and fecal incontinence occur in the postoperative period may be consequence of lack of experience of the surgeon or the pathologist, but never it is consequence of an specific surgical technique.

Different modifications to Soave pull-through technique have been designed and all of them use laparotomy or laparoscopy. TECPT dose not requires an abdominal approach therefore, eliminates the risks of adhesion formation and contamination in the abdominal cavity. Also, TECPT reduces damage to pelvic structures, it is inexpensive that is an important factor in several countries [26]. Also TECPT is bloodless, expeditious and offering the best cosmetic results in the surgical correction of short segment aganglionosis. TECPT demands from the surgeon skills that can be develop using experimental models [5,27].

An uncertainty has been pointed out to the one-stage TECPT about the possible inaccurate definition of the TZ before (radiological) or during the operation (histological). Most of this misunderstanding depends on the experience to make the rectogram or colon enema as well as the experience of the pathologist to observe frozen sections, and it does not depend by the technique itself. If TZ could not be defined preoperatively, some authors before to decide for a TECPT establish the TZ using frozen sections of biopsies of the colon obtained by laparoscopy or through an umbilical incision, also preoperative endoscopic marking have been used [28,29]. When, an unexpected more proximal (higher) aganglionosis is found during a TECPT, a laparoscopy or laparotomy is used. Some authors have performed a "transanal laparoscopy" through the rectal cuff to dissect the mesenteric vessels and colon attachments as a NOTES [unpublished data and personal communication], using a vessel sealing system or other electrosurgical tool.

Since TECPT was published, it has been analyzed and compared with other techniques and approaches concluding that TECPT is a safe procedure, suitable for the most common form of HD and in some cases including long segments offering very good results or at least equal to the other previous kinds of surgical treatment for HD [30-37]. Furthermore, this approach has been applied to re-operations and other colorectal problems with favorable results [38-40].

Finally, TECPT as well as all other techniques described at the moment do not cure 100% of the Hirschsprung patients [41]; TECPT is one alternative that permits to treat successfully most neonatal and infant cases that suffer short segment HD.

References

[1] Soave, F. Hirschsprung's disease: a new surgical technique. *Arch. Dis. Child* 1964;39:116-24.

[2] Boley SJ. New modification of the surgical treatment of Hirschsprung's disease. *Surgery* 1964:54:1015-7.

[3] So HS, Schwartz DL, Becker JM, et al. Endorectal pull-through without preliminary colostomy in neonates with Hirschsprung's disease. *J Pediatr Surg* 1980;15:470-1.

[4] Georgeson KE, Fuenfer MM, Hardin WD: Primary laparosocopic pull-through for Hirschsprung´s disease in infants and children. *J Pediatr Surg* 1995;30:1017-22.

[5] De la Torre-Mondragón L, Ortega-Salgado JA, Arroyo-Fonseca A. Descenso endorrectal. Acceso anal y laparoscópico. Modelo experimental en conejos. *Cir Gen* 1997;19:151-4.

[6] De la Torre-Mondragón L, Ortega-Salgado JA. Transanal endorectal pull-through for Hirschsprung's disease. *J Pediatr Surg* 1998;33:1283-6.

[7] Winberg AG. The anorectal myenteric plexus: its relation to hypoganglionosis of the colon. *Am J Clin Pathol* 1970:54:637-42.

[8] Reyes-Múgica M. Enfermedad de Hirschsprung: neurocristopatía de la migración y la diferenciación celular. *Rev Gastroenterol Mex* 1997;62:287-92.

[9] Ridaura SC. Problemas en el diagnóstico histopatológico de la enfermedad deHirschsprung. *Acta Pediatr Méx* 2003;24:166-71.

[10] Diamond IR, Casadiego G, Traubici J, Langer JC, Wales PW. The contrast enema for Hirschsprung disease: predictors of a false-positive result. *J Pediatr Surg* 2007;42:792-5.

[11] Dasgupta R, Langer JC. Transanal pull-through for Hirschsprung disease. *Semin Pediatr Surg* 2005;14:64-71.

[12] International Pediatric Endosurgery Group. Guidelines for surgical treatment ofHirschsprung's disease. *J Laparoendosc Adv Surg Tech A*. 2005;15:89-91.

[13] Langer JC, Durrant AC, De la Torre-Mondragón L, et al. One-stage transanal Soave pullthrough for Hirschsprung disease: a multicenter experience with 141 children. *Ann Surg* 2003;238:569-76.

[14] Nasr A, Laner JC. Evolution of the technique in the transanal pull-through for Hirschsprung's disease: effect on outcome. *J Pediatr Surg* 2007;42:36-9.

[15] Rintala RJ. Transanal coloanal pull-through with a short muscular cuff for classic Hirschsprung's disease. *Eur J Pediatr Surg* 2003;13:181-6.

[16] Ateş O, Hakgüder G, Kart Y, Olguner M, Akgür F. The effect of dilated ganglionic segment on anorectal and urinary functions during 1-stage transanal endorectal pullthrough for Hirschsprung's disease. *J Pediatr Surg* 2007;42:1271–5.

[17] Van Leeuwen K, Geiger JD, Barnett JL, Coran AG, Teitelbaum DH. Stooling and manometric findings after primary pull-throughs in Hirschsprung's disease: perineal versus abdominal approaches. *J Pediatr Surg* 2002;37:1321-5.

[18] Zhang SC, Bai YZ, Wang W, Wang WL. Stooling patterns and colonic motility after transanal one-stage pull-through operation for Hirschsprung's disease in children. *J Pediatr Surg* 2005;40:1766–72.

[19] Zhang SC, Bai YZ, Wang W, Wang WL. Clinical outcome in children after transanal 1-stage endorectal pull-through operation for Hirschsprung disease. *J Pediatr Surg* 2005;40:1307-11.

[20] Pratap A, Gupta A, Shakya V, Adhikary A, Tiwari A, Shrestha P, et al. Analysis of problems, complications, avoidance and management with transanal pullthrough for Hirschsprung disease. *J Pediatr Surg* 2007;42:1869-76.

[21] Podevin G, Lardy H, Azzis O, Branchereau S, Petit T, Sfeir R, et al. Technical problems and complications of a transanal pull-through for Hirschsprung's disease. *Eur J Pediatr Surg* 2006;16:104-8.

[22] Sapin E, Centonze A, Moog R, Borgnon J, Becmeur F. Transanal coloanal anastomosis for Hirschsprung's disease: comparison between endorectal and perirectal pull-through procedures. *Eur J Pediatr Surg* 2006; 16:312-7.

[23] Hadidi A. Transanal endorectal pull-through for Hirschsprung's disease: experience with 68 patients. *J Pediatr Surg* 2003;38:1337-40.

[24] Elhalaby EA, Hashish A, Elbarbary MM, Soliman HA, Wishahy MK, Elkholy A, et al. Transanal one-stage endorectal pull-through for Hirschsprung's disease: a multicenter study. *J Pediatr Surg* 2004;39:345-51.

[25] Berrebi D, Fouquet V, de Lagausie, Carricaburu E, Ferkdadji L, Chomette P et al. Duhamel operation vs neonatal transanal endorectal pull-through procedure for Hirschsprung disease: which are the changes for pathologists? *J Pediatr Surg* 2007;42:688–91.

[26] Pratap A, Shakya VC, Biswas BK, Shina A, Tiwari A, Agrawal CS, Adhikary S. Single-stage transanal endorectal pull-through for Hirschsprung's disease: perspective from a developing country. *J Pediatr Surg* 2007;42:532-5.
[27] Takegawa B, Ortolan EP, Rodrigues AM, Chambô F, de Almeida e Paula F. Experimental model for transanal endorectal pull-through surgery. Technique of De la Torre and Ortega. *J Pediatr Surg* 2005;40:1539–41.
[28] Sauer CJ, Langer JC, Wales PW. The versatility of the umbilical incision in the management of Hirschsprung's disease. *J Pediatr Surg* 2005;40:385-9.
[29] Kohno M, Ikawa H, Fukumoto H, Okamoto S, Masuyama H, Konuma K. Usefulness of endoscopic marking for determining the location of transanal endorectal pull-through in the treatment of Hirschsprung's disease. *Pediatr Surg Int* 2005;21:873-7.
[30] De la Torre-Mondragón L, Ortega-Salgado JA. Transanal versus open endorectal pull-through for Hirschsprung's diseases. *J Pediatr Surg* 2000;35:1630-2.
[31] Hadidi A. Transanal endorectal pull-through for Hirschsprung's disease: a comparison with the open technique. *Eur J Pediatr Surg* 2003;13:176-80.
[32] Rehman Y, Emblem R, Bjørnland K. Transanal resection of colon for Hirschsprung's disease. *Tidsskr Nor Laegeforen*. 2005;125:2358-9.
[33] Till H, Heinrich M, Schuster T, V Schweinitz D. Is the anorectal sphincter damaged during a transanal endorectal pullthrough (TERPT) for Hirschsprung's disease? A 3-dimensional, vector manometric investigation. *Eur J Pediatr Surg* 2006;16:188-91.
[34] Luis LA, Encinas JL, Avila LF, Andrés AM, Burgos L, Fernández A, et al. Hirschsprung disease: lessons learned from the last 100 cases. *Cir Pediatr*. 2006;19:177-81.
[35] Aslan MK, Karam I, Karam A, Erdoğan D, Cavuşoğlu YH, Cakmak O. Our experience with transanal endorectal pull-through in Hirschsprung's disease. *Eur J Pediatr Surg* 2007;17:335-9.
[36] El-Sawaf MI, Drongowski RA, Chamberlain JN, Coran AG, Teitelbaum DH. Are the long-term results of the transanal pull-through equal to those of the transabdominal pull-through? A comparison of the 2 approaches for Hirschsprung disease. *J Pediatr Surg* 2007;42: 41–7.
[37] Tander B, Rizalar R, Cihan AO, Ayyildiz SH, Ariturk E, Bernay F. Is there a hidden mortality after one-stage transanal endorectal pull-through for patients with Hirschsprung's disease?. *Pediatr Surg Int*. 2007;23:81-6.
[38] Falcone R, Levitt MA, Peña A. Incisionless and trocarless transanal resection of the rectosigmoid for severe idiopathic constipation. *J Laparoendosc Adv Surg Tech*. 2007;17: 572-9.
[39] Hadidi A, Bartoli F, Waag KL. Role of transanal endorectal pull-through in complicated Hirschsprung's disease: experience in 18 patients. *J Pediatr Surg* 2007;42:554-8.
[40] Gobran TA, Ezzat A, Hassan ME, O'Neill J. Redo transanal endorectal pull-through: a preliminary study. *Pediatr Surg Int* 2007,23:189-93.
[41] Bax KN. Duhamel lecture: the incurability of Hirschsprung's disease. *Eur J Pediatr Surg* 2006;16:380-4.

In: Hirschsprung's Disease: Diagnosis and Treatment
Ed: Ramón Núñez and Manuel López-Alonso

ISBN: 978-1-60741-349-3

Chapter XX

Total Colonic Hirschsprung Disease

Barbara E. Wildhaber, Daniel H. Teitelbaum and Arnold G. Coran

Introduction

Total colonic Hirschsprung disease (TCH) is herein defined as aganglionosis of the entire colon with or without extension to the small intestine. Extension of aganglionosis may include the distal small bowel up to the jejunum and in rare cases, the entire small intestine is involved. In a large series reported by Escobar et al., 26/36 patients had extension of aganglionosis to the distal ileum, 8 had their level in the mid-small bowel, 1 in the mid-jejunum, and 1 included the entire bowel [1]. These reports are consistent with our own results [2].

TCH is a rare form of Hirschsprung disease, and is associated with higher morbidity and mortality rates than short segment aganglionosis [3-7]. Hirschsprung-associated enterocolitis (HAEC) represents a major problem in TCH patients, and contributes considerably to its morbidity [8]. Furthermore, TCH often requires multiple operations (9), and patients tend to have more physical, functional and emotional long-term sequelae than children with the classic form of Hirschsprung disease [9-11]. This review will summarize some of the great challenges which pediatric surgeons face in dealing with such children.

Epidemiology

TCH accounts for approximately 3% to 12% of all infants with Hirschsprung disease [12-14] with an incidence of approximately 1/50,000 live births [5]. The male to female ratio is 1.5:1, versus the 4:1 ratio in classic Hirschsprung disease [5,14].

Genetics of Total Colonic Hirschsprung Disease

Familial occurrence is much higher (15 to 20%) than is seen in the classic form of Hirschsprung disease [15] Germline mutations of the RET (REarranged during Transfection)-mediated or SOX10 (Sex determining region Y-bOX 10)-mediated signaling pathway gene [16,17], as well as accumulation of mutations in the tyrosine kinase domain [18] have been reported in TCH. The SOX10 mutations can determine a neurocristopathy (Shah-Waardenburg Syndrome) that can also be caused by EDN3 and EDNRB mutations. A large number of patients with Shah Waardenburg may have long-segment or total colonic aganglionosis. In a series of 16 patients with TCH, 11 were found to have one of the above mentioned genetic mutations, yet, this occurrence did not affect surgical results [19]

Mortality and Morbidity

The overall TCH mortality rate in the literature has been reported to be as high as 54% [20] and is closely associated with infectious complications or associated other diseases. In recent decades, however, the expected survival for TCH patients has improved dramatically due to increased awareness and knowledge of the disease and its complications, as well as an improvement in both medical and surgical care [5]. In our personal series, the pre-operative mortality rate was 13%; all of those non-surviving children being inpatients with total intestinal aganglionosis who were not surgical candidates [2]. The post-operative mortality rate currently approaches zero [2]). This may well be because of the generally increasing awareness of HAEC, with early recognition and prompt initiation of intensive medical treatment[12,21,22].

However, the morbidity associated with TCH remains high. The major morbidities of TCH are failure to thrive and fluid imbalance. These latter complications may quite often then predispose infants to catheter sepsis, further failure to thrive, stomal dysfunction, electrolyte imbalance and dehydration. The other major morbidity of TCH is enterocolitis, and this is extensively discussed in the Complication section below.

Symptoms and Diagnosis

TCH causes more diagnostic problems than classic cases of Hirschsprung disease because of a lack of specificity in not only the clinical picture but also in radiological findings. Yet, despite these challenges, TCH is most commonly recognized in the neonatal period [5]. Very few cases presenting in older childhood or adulthood have been reported [23,24].

The initial clinical presentation in a neonate is non-specific and is usually one of intestinal obstruction with bilious vomiting and abdominal distension [25]. The clinical picture and the x-ray findings of a microcolon can mimic meconium ileus. This makes the diagnosis difficult for the radiologist and surgeon. Appendiceal perforation, usually at the base of the appendix, may be a potentially lethal initial mode of presentation of TCH (26,

27). A severe form of presentation at any age is HAEC, which also may be lethal [21]. The older child usually presents with severe, intractable constipation, usually associated with failure to thrive.

Associated Syndromes and Diseases

The incidence of associated anomalies in TCH is reported as high as 15% (5). TCH may be part of the Smith-Lemli-Opitz syndrome [28] as well as Ondine's curse (central hypoventilation syndrome) [29,30]. Congenital alveolar capillary dysplasia, a rare cause of irreversible pulmonary hypertension with 100% mortality, has been associated with TCH [31]. In patients with cartilage-hair hypoplasia, a chondrodysplasia with growth failure and impaired immunity, a high incidence of Hirschsprung disease and in particular TCH has been described. In a Finish series of 147 patients with this syndrome, 13 were identified as having Hirschsprung disease, 5 of those being TCH [32].

Neuroblastoma and Hirschsprung disease are considered aberrations of neural crest cell growth, migration, or differentiation. Their coexistence, however, is rare, but cases of this association have been described [33]. TCH can be associated with the development of neuroendocrine tumors such as medullary thyroid carcinoma; the RET proto-oncogene is the major gene responsible for both Hirschsprung disease and medullary thyroid carcinoma [34].

In the literature, 19 cases of TCH have been reported to be associated with ileal atresia [35,36]. Also colonic atresia has also been reported with TCH [37,38] An early gestational colonic atresia, occurring before secondary retroperitoneal fixation of the colon at approximately 11 weeks may result in interruption of caudal migration of enteric nerves and may manifest itself as long-segment Hirschsprung disease distal to the atresia. Moreover, the aganglionosis may be predicted by a foreshortened, non-fixed colon coiled in the pelvis [37].

Imaging Studies

Even though radiological investigations are indispensable, they are often not conclusive [25,39]. A plain abdominal film, as well as a contrast enema, remain extremely helpful in making the diagnosis. Generally, in neonates a colon smaller than normal, with reflux into a distended ileum appears to be the most suggestive x-ray finding for TCH [40]. In neonates with TCH presenting with intestinal obstruction, right lower quadrant intraluminal calcifications as well as a microcolon are reported to be frequent. Thus, in a neonate with small-bowel obstruction and a microcolon, the presence of right lower quadrant intraluminal calcifications should raise the suspicion of TCH. Even if the operative findings are more typical of meconium ileus, a frozen section of the rectum above the pelvic reflection should be performed [41]. In a Japanese report a radiologist described that barium enema findings including no transition zone, a normal recto-sigmoid index, reflux of barium into a dilated ileum, and retention of barium on delayed films are frequently observed in TCH cases. In older TCH children, and sometimes in neonates a normal-sized but shortened colon with irregular contractions, and lack of redundancy may be observed [42]. Such a colon may take on a loss of well-defined hepatic and splenic flexures, and thus leave one with a classic question mark sign (Figure 1).

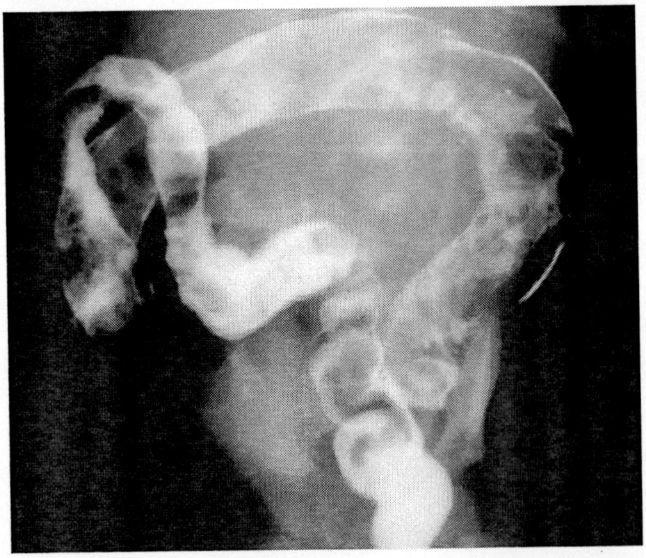

Figure 1. Typical radiograph appearance of a contrast enema in an infant with total colonic Hirschsprung disease. Note the shortened appearance, with rounded hepatic and splenic flexures. One can see that the shape almost appears to mimic a question mark sign.

The extension of TCH into the small bowel is extremely difficult to assess by radiological means. In a study performed by American pediatric radiologists, the concordance between the radiographic transition zone and pathologic extent of aganglionic bowel was 62.5% in classic colonic Hirschsprung disease; whereas, the subgroup of patients with TCH showed a concordance of only 25% [43]. In a Canadian study, a contrast-enema correctly predicted the level of aganglionosis in 89% of patients with recto-sigmoid disease, but only in 31% of those children with TCH [44]. Therefore, an accurate evaluation of the proximal extension of aganglionosis can be made only at surgery by performing leveling biopsies.

In summary, in TCH patients there are no pathognomonic contrast enema findings, and radiologic results may cover the entire spectrum of findings which can be encountered in the neonate and young infant with bowel obstruction. There may be a normal caliber colon, a micro-colon, a shortened colon, colonic wall irregularities, and significant ileal reflux [45], but the definitive diagnosis still requires surgery.

If the diagnosis is not evident before diagnostic laparotomy is performed, total colonic manometry can potentially be used as a diagnostic tool. Although performed in only a select number of centers, total colonic manometry can directly measure intraluminal pressures and contractile function along the entire length of the colon, and may help to determine suitability for primary neonatal pull-through versus a staged approach [46]. Interestingly, in a study where TCH children underwent esophageal and duodenal manometry, all children showed abnormalities on both manometries; this suggests a primary motility disorder in patients with TCH [47].

Diagnostic Laparotomy / Laparoscopy

Diagnostic surgery may be performed by laparotomy or laparoscopy. The goal of the operation is to determine 1) the diagnosis and 2) the level and extent of aganglionosis. Thus, leveling biopsies need to be performed. As alluded to above, in the majority of cases the preoperative diagnosis of TCH will be uncommon, and thus suspicion should be aroused if one does not see a gross transition zone, or once multiple biopsies of the left side of the colon fail to identify ganglion cells. In such cases, biopsies of the left and right colon as well as the appendix should be sent all at one time [39]. Additionally, biopsies of a dilated ileum should be considered. Although aganglionosis of the appendix seems to be reliable for the diagnosis of TCH, a great deal of controversy has surrounded the use of the appendix to diagnose total colonic Hirschsprung disease. The pathologist should be aware that there are significant differences in the innervation of the appendix in patients with TCH (see Histology section below). In general, however, the histologic evaluation of the appendix provides an excellent method for diagnosis of total colonic Hirschsprung disease [48,49]. There has been a case of a child with presumed total colonic aganglionosis and aganglionosis of the appendix [48,49], who subsequently was found to have normal ganglion cells in the transverse colon. This extremely rare case represents segmental Hirschsprung disease. In neonates with proximal colonic atresia, or ileal atresia, biopsies need to be performed during the neonatal operation in order to exclude TCH, since these two abnormalities are associated and well-described [38](38).

Histology

It appears that patients with TCH may have a unique pattern of innervation and histopathology compared to patients with standard length Hirschsprung disease. Puri's group has demonstrated that there are clear histopathological differences between recto-sigmoid Hirschsprung disease and TCH. In TCH there is weak or a lack of neuronal nitric oxide synthase immunoreactivity in the sparse, short nerve trunks of the myenteric and submucous plexuses and muscle layers; whereas weakly positive neuronal nitric oxide synthase nerve trunks are observed in the recto-sigmoid HD bowel [50]. Peripherin immunoreactivity is also markedly reduced in TCH specimens compared to recto-sigmoid Hirschsprung disease. In TCH specimens there is a lack of interstitial cells of Cajal in the smooth muscle layer; whereas in the recto-sigmoid aganglionic bowel interstitial cells of Cajal are only markedly reduced, but not absent. Interstitial cells of Cajal are pacemaker cells that play a key role in the motility function of the bowel [50].

Compared with both normal controls and standard length Hirschsprung disease controls, the TCH appendices show decreased numbers of nerve bundles around the muscle layers and within the submucosa. The appendix has markedly decreased numbers of smaller nerve fibers within the circular muscle, and an absence of the finer nerve fibers within the lamina propria [4]. There is no change in the overall number of epithelial neuroendocrine cells, but subepithelial neuroendocrines cells, normally found in association with mucosal nerve fibers, are totally absent [51].

Treatment

Once the diagnosis of TCH is made, several considerations need to be addressed. The first is whether a primary pull-through should be performed versus a leveling ileostomy. The second decision is whether a colectomy should be performed at the time of diagnosis of TCH. One potential difficulty with primary definitive surgical management with total colectomy is the necessity of determining the actual level of aganglionosis. As mentioned above, a frozen section of the appendix is almost always diagnostic [12]. Caution with this approach must be taken as it is possible that ganglion cells may be found in the resected colon specimen when the permanently stained histologic slides are evaluated. Thus, an experienced pediatric pathologist is absolutely indispensable during the time a patient with suspected TCH is taken to the operating room and a primary pull-through or primary colectomy is considered. To avoid too extensive or inadequate surgery, the most conservative treatment plan in children with suspected TCH is to place an initial diverting ileostomy and await histologic results. There is a risk of leaving the defunctionalized colon in place when the ileostomy is performed; the colon can become a "cesspool" from bacterial overgrowth and lead to systemic sepsis repeatedly in the baby. After ileostomy, a crucial point is the allowance of sufficient time for the small bowel to adapt its absorptive ability. Usually the majority of patients are definitely treated approximately one year after ileostomy [1,2,14].

For the definitive repair of TCH many techniques and their modifications have been suggested. Some of the techniques have been derived from operations proposed for the treatment of classic Hirschsprung disease; whereas others have been specifically designed for TCH: Soave endorectal pull-through (ERPT), Duhamel, Martin-modification of the Duhamel, Swenson, or Boley procedure, as well as J-pouch ileo-anal anastomosis may be chosen [52]. The decision to perform an open laparotomy versus a laparoscopically-assisted approach is up to the surgeon's choice, and both ways are quite acceptable [53]. Data on primary ERPT for TCH in the neonatal age period have been very uncommonly described [2]. Its clear advantage is a single operation without the potential problems of an ostomy. However, disadvantages include incorrect leveling of the aganglionic segment and an inability to adapt to the more rapid transit time. This approach can result in severe perineal excoriation. In our personal experience, 4 of 25 patients had a primary ERPT performed in the neonatal period. Of these, one patient experienced no complications, 2 developed anal strictures, 2 had severe perineal excoriation, and one child had his ERPT performed at the transition zone resulting in the need for an ileostomy [2].

The Martin procedure aimed to preserve and utilize the descending colon and used an extended ganglionic-aganglionic, left-sided channel to maximize fluid absorption [54].Figure 2 demonstrates the key technical features of the Martin modification. This modification of the Duhamel-procedure, however, has been associated with a high occurrence of complications, especially HAEC, and morbidity rate is reported to be as high as 81.8% [55]; in recent years its use has declined substantially.

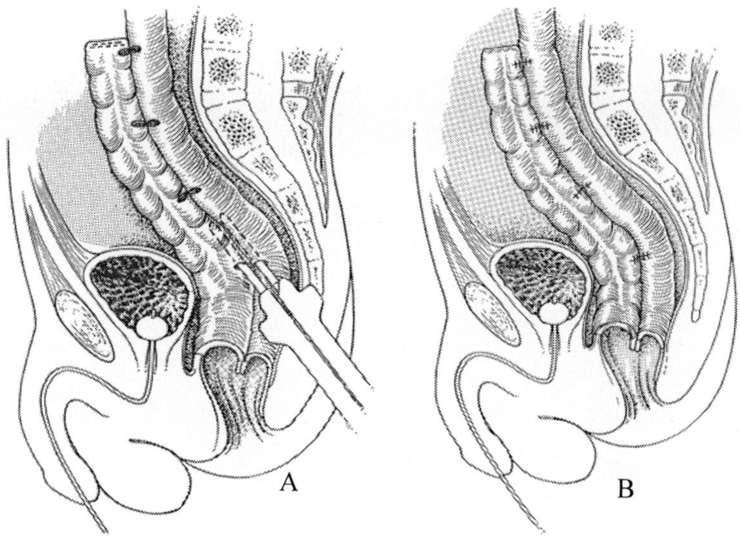

Figure 2. Martin modification of the Duhamel procedure. A. Note that using an enterotomy in both the small and large bowel, the stapler can be directed distally, and then refired proximally. The enterotomy is then closed with either a stapler or two rows of interrupted suture. B. Usually two or three additional enterotomies must be made to complete the rest of the anastomosis. Reproduced with permission by Teitelbaum, DH, Coran, AG: Hirschsprung's Disease. In: Rob & Smith's Operative Surgery, Fifth Edition, Chapman and Hall, 1995. Currently, Kluwer Academic Publishers, The Netherlands

The Kimura procedure (Figure 3) is another resourceful approach to handle TCH patients. The surgery consists of staged operations in which ganglionated small intestine is first patched onto a 10 cm segment of aganglionic terminal ileum and right colon. In the second stage, the right colon mesentery is divided and the composite intestine which has now developed a vascularization by the small intestine mesentery is prepared for pull-through [56]. An advantage of both the Martin and Kimura procedures seems to be increased water and electrolyte absorption without the risks of mechanical problems encountered with a variety of pelvic pouch creations in the young growing child [57,58]. Also an ileo-endorectal pullthrough procedure with right colon onlay patch has been described, again with the aim of facilitating the early post-operative period by increasing the surface for absorption [59].

Although these former operations may have theoretical advantages, our personal data, in concordance with those of other authors, show that the success rate with the straightforward ERPT technique [2,60] or standard length Duhamel (4) are quite favorable. Our own series, as well as other surgeon's have shown no correlation with the type of the pull-through and the eventual functional outcome [2,9,61-63]. Post-operative complications (including HAEC) were, however, more commonly observed after a Martin modification of the Duhamel procedure [1].

Thus in summary, little seems to be gained by performing a more complex procedure, such as Martin's operation [63]. It appears that any of the three standard corrective procedures for Hirschsprung disease, ERPT, Duhamel, and Swenson procedure, may be used to treat TCH with generally good results [4,12,64].

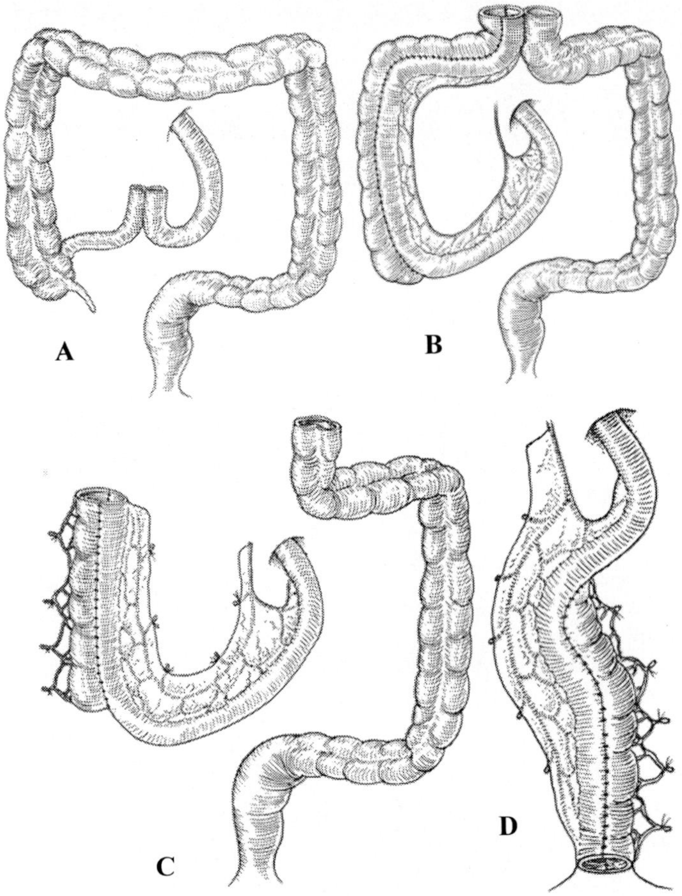

Figure 3. Kimura procedure. A. The ganglionic ileum is first decompressed with an end ileostomy. B. Several weeks later the child is returned to the operating room for an extensive longitudinal ileocolostomy, approximately 10-25 cm in length. Anastomosis is created with a two-layered suture line. Staples are avoided because they may prevent sufficient vascular growth between limbs of bowel. The end of this is used as an end stoma. C and D. The child is left alone for 6-12 months, during which time the vascular supply of the two segments joins. At the final operation the right colonic blood supply is taken down and an assessment of the blood supply to the colon is made. If the ileum has established adequate perfusion of the colon, the ileocolostomy is used for the pull-through with either a Swenson or endorectal type pull-through. If the right colonic blood supply is inadequate, the ileocolostomy may be taken down and the ileum used with a Martin modification as described above. Reproduced with permission by Teitelbaum, DH, Coran, AG: Hirschsprung's Disease. In: Rob & Smith's Operative Surgery, Fifth Edition, Chapman and Hall, 1995. Currently, Kluwer Academic Publishers, The Netherlands

In contrast, patients with extended small intestinal disease have the greatest morbidity and risk of dying from the disease process. All of these children will require long-term parenteral nutrition support, and the mortality rate is exceedingly high (some approaching 100% in those with total small bowel aganglionosis). The surgical alternatives for more extensive small intestinal Hirschsprung disease tend to be complex because the length and function of the residual ganglionated small intestine must be taken into account, and the surgeon must gauge the degree of short-bowel syndrome. For jejuno-ileal disease, a number of individuals have utilized a patch of either ileum [65] or more commonly right colon [66].

In this case, a staged approach of an initial leveling ostomy is created. The right colon is anastomosed to the functional proximal stoma. After several weeks, a pull-through of this joined side-to-side bowel is performed with preservation of the blood supply to both portions of the intestine, using either a Soave, or Swenson type pull-through.

For those infants with less than 40 cm of ganglionated small intestine, an extended myotomy or myectomy may be selected [67,68]. As described by Ziegler, the myectomy is begun at the level of transition between ganglionated and aganglionic small bowel, two antimesenteric border incisions are made parallel along the longitudinal axis of the intestine. The depth of the incision is stopped superficial to the submucosa to allow a 1-cm wide strip of seromuscular layer (with the underlying submucosal tube left intact), to be excised for an extended length. The extension onto normally ganglionated bowel should be limited, so that peristalsis in the proximal ganglionated bowel cannot push intraluminal contents distally. At the end of this segment, which is optimally estimated to be 50 to 70 cm below the ligament of Treitz, the intestine is exited as an end stoma. If any aganglionic distal intestine remains, it must be vented. Although this approach may result in some salvaging of patients, with improved techniques in transplantation, a primary intestinal or combined small intestinal, right colon and liver (in cases of liver cirrhosis due to prolonged parenteral nutrition) transplant may be the most appropriate approach (69). Recent studies suggest an excellent outcome with this latter method.

Complications

It seems that the essential issues in TCH are not only the surgical management of the disease, but also its prompt diagnosis, the management of presenting symptoms such as neonatal bowel obstruction, and the treatment of post-operative HAEC. The most frequent postoperative complication associated with TCH appears to be HAEC. It seems that the frequency of enterocolitis is significantly greater than in patients with standard length aganglionosis. In our own series [2], we noted a 55% incidence of HAEC compared to a lower incidence (approximately 15 to 35% rate) in patients with shorter lengths of aganglionosis [12,21,70,71]. In most cases HAEC is successfully treated with conservative management. However, in those children who have persistently reoccurring episodes of HAEC, it may be necessary to consider a posterior myomyectomy [2]. In cases where there is normally ganglionated bowel at the anastomotic site, a vast majority of patients will derive considerable improvement from such a procedure.

Another frequently occurring postoperative complication is anal stricture. Although in some reports, this has been treated with internal sphincterectomy [9], in our experience this may be managed quite well with repeated anal dilations. Again, no correlation between complications such as HAEC or anal strictures and type of procedure has been identified [2]. Several additional complications occur in TCH patients and are summarized in Table 1 [2]. Almost half of TCH patients require a subsequent operation, ranging in number from one to five [2].

Table 1. Complications of surgical procedures (2).

Complications	
Pre-pull-through enterocolitis	20%
Post-pull-through enterocolitis	55%
Anal strictures	25%
Wound infection	20%
Perineal excoriation	20%
Small bowel obstruction due to adhesions	10%
Rectal fistula/abscess	10%
Incorrect leveling of pull-through with subsequent ileostomy	10%

Prognosis and Long-Term Outcome

Despite the frequent occurrence of complications, follow-up of TCH patients over many years shows that TCH in the long-term has a favorable outcome. To assess functional results a standardized questionnaire may be used (Table 2). Frequency of bowel movements usually is scored within acceptable limits. Ileal adaptation shows an amazing improvement over time and stool frequency typically decreases from initially 10 to 12 liquid bowel movements per day to 1-5 daily stools. Anorectal function improves gradually over time, and the older the patients become the better they do functionally [2,13,60]. In cases where soiling is reported, it is mainly noted at nighttime. In our experience, parents and patients score the overall functional result to be good to excellent in almost 90% of all our pull-through treated patients [2]. In general, none of the patients have dietary restrictions [2,62]. If ileal involvement is distal, children follow a normal growth curve pattern in the long term [60]. However, growth retardation may appear if small bowel aganglionosis is extensive and reaches the mid- to high ileum [11]. During long-term follow-up, patients must be regularly evaluated for iron and folic acid deficiency, as well as for low levels of vitamin B12 [11,72].

Table 2. Questionnaire regarding functional outcome of TCH patients. Included in the table is the scoring system to assess objective functional outcome (2).* if > 3 years of age

Follow up Questionnaire	Score = 2	Score = 1	Score = 0
Recurrent abdominal distension	None	Mild	Severe
Frequency of defecation	1-2 / day	3-5 / day	>5 / day
Stool consistency	Normal	Loose	Liquid
Soiling	None	Occasionally	Permanently
Urgency period *	Normal	Short	Absent
Diapers required *	None	Occasionally	Permanently
Chronic use of medication *	None	Antibiotics	Anti-diarrheal
Diet	Normal	Restricted	TPN
Range of Scores **Objective functional outcome**	**11-16** **good**	**6-10** **fair**	**0-5** poor

Prognostic factors such as gestational age, sex, birth weight, ileal involvement, time to closure of the enterostomy, duration of total parenteral nutrition, and need for constant nutritional assistance may influence long-term outcome. However, the only consistent prognostic factor seems to be the length of ileal involvement. Based on a study of 26 cases treated in France, for those children with ileal involvement of more than 50 centimeters, long-term nutritional assistance was needed. In this series, the prognosis was even worse when TCH was associated with a polymalformative syndrome [73].

In our personal experience, patients typically do not feel socially impaired [2]. However, Ludman et al. [10] compared follow-up data of TCH patients with children with recto-sigmoid aganglionosis. Interestingly, in this report TCH patients rated themselves as less well adjusted to life than their matched pairs with recto-sigmoid aganglionosis. This difference in adjustment may be due to the differences between these two groups in terms of number of hospitalization days and severity of illness, especially in infancy and early childhood. In general, TCH patients develop almost normally and are socially and professionally integrated [74].

In summary, treatment of TCH is associated with a wide number of challenges and complications both after diagnosis and during the early years after their pull-through operation. The most commonly encountered being recurrent HAEC and anal stricture. Despite this difficult period during infancy and childhood, long-term functional outcome for TCH is quite favorable.

References

[1] Escobar MA, Grosfeld JL, West KW, Scherer LR, Rouse TM, Engum SA, Rescorla FJ. Long-term outcomes in total colonic aganglionosis: a 32-year experience. *J Pediatr Surg* 2005;40:955-61.

[2] Wildhaber BE, Teitelbaum DH, Coran AG. Total colonic Hirschsprung's disease: a 28-year experience. *J Pediatr Surg* 2005;40:203-6.

[3] Coran AG, Bjordal R, Eek S, Knutrud O. The surgical management of total colonic and partial small intestinal aganglionosis. *J Pediatr Surg* 1969;4:531-7.

[4] Hoehner JC, Ein SH, Shandling B, Kim PC. Long-term morbidity in total colonic aganglionosis. *J Pediatr Surg* 1998;33:961-5.

[5] Suita S, Taguchi T, Kamimura T, Yanai K. Total colonic aganglionosis with or without small bowel involvement: a changing profile. *J Pediatr Surg* 1997;32:1537-41.

[6] Rescorla FJ, Morrison AM, Engles D, West KW, Grosfeld JL. Hirschsprung's disease. Evaluation of mortality and long-term function in 260 cases. *Arch Surg* 1992;127:934-41.

[7] Levy M, Reynolds M. Morbidity associated with total colon Hirschsprung's disease. *J Pediatr Surg* 1992;27:364-6.

[8] Qualman SJ, Murray R. Aganglionosis and related disorders. *Hum Pathol* 1994;25:1141-9.

[9] Tsuji H, Spitz L, Kiely EM, Drake DP, Pierro A. Management and long-term follow-up of infants with total colonic aganglionosis. *J Pediatr Surg* 1999;34:158-61.

[10] Ludman L, Spitz L, Tsuji H, Pierro A. Hirschsprung's disease: functional and psychological follow up comparing total colonic and rectosigmoid aganglionosis. *Arch Dis Child* 2002;86:348-51.

[11] Ikawa H, Masuyama H, Hirabayashi T, Endo M, Yokoyama J. More than 10 years' follow-up to total colonic aganglionosis--severe iron deficiency anemia and growth retardation. *J Pediatr Surg* 1997;32:25-7.

[12] Coran AG, Teitelbaum DH. Recent advances in the management of Hirschsprung's disease. *Am J Surg* 2000;180:382-7.

[13] Hernandez F, Rivas S, Avila LF, Diaz M, Leal N, Martinez L, Murcia J, et al. [Extensive aganglionosis. Treatment and long term results]. *Cir Pediatr* 2003;16:54-7.

[14] Ikeda K, Goto S. Total colonic aganglionosis with or without small bowel involvement: an analysis of 137 patients. *J Pediatr Surg* 1986;21:319-22.

[15] Galifer RB, Frapier JM, Bosc O, Massip A, Rieu D, Couture A, Veyrac C, et al. [Total colonic form of Hirschsprung disease. Apropos of 6 cases]. *Chir Pediatr* 1987;28:137-44.

[16] Edery P, Lyonnet S, Mulligan LM, Pelet A, Dow E, Abel L, Holder S, et al. Mutations of the RET proto-oncogene in Hirschsprung's disease. *Nature* 1994;367:378-80.

[17] Pingault V, Bondurand N, Kuhlbrodt K, Goerich DE, Prehu MO, Puliti A, Herbarth B, et al. SOX10 mutations in patients with Waardenburg-Hirschsprung disease. *Nat Genet* 1998;18:171-3.

[18] Inoue K, Shimotake T, Iwai N. Mutational analysis of RET/GDNF/NTN genes in children with total colonic aganglionosis with small bowel involvement. *Am J Med Genet* 2000;93:278-84.

[19] Tomiyama H, Shimotake T, Ono S, Kimura O, Tokiwa K, Iwai N. Relationship between the type of RET/GDNF/NTN or SOX10 gene mutations and long-term results after surgery for total colonic aganglionosis with small bowel involvement. *J Pediatr Surg* 2001;36:1685-8.

[20] Jordan FT, Coran AG, Wesley JR. Modified endorectal procedure for management of long-segment aganglionosis. *Ann Surg* 1981;194:70-5.

[21] Teitelbaum DH, Coran AG. Enterocolitis. *Semin Pediatr Surg* 1998;7:162-9.

[22] Elhalaby EA, Coran AG, Blane CE, Hirschl RB, Teitelbaum DH. Enterocolitis associated with Hirschsprung's disease: a clinical-radiological characterization based on 168 patients. *J Pediatr Surg* 1995;30:76-83.

[23] Lall A, Agarwala S, Bhatnagar V, Gupta AK, Mitra DK. Total colonic aganglionosis: diagnosis and management in a 12-year-old boy. *J Pediatr Surg* 1999;34:1413-4.

[24] Fekete C, Ricour C, Martelli H, Jacob S, Pellerin D. Total colonic aganglionosis (with or without ileal involvement): a review of 27 cases. *J Pediatr Surg* 1986;21:251-4.

[25] Bickler SW, Harrison MW, Campbell TJ, Campbell JR. Long-segment Hirschsprung's disease. *Arch Surg* 1992;127:1047-50.

[26] Sarioglu A, Tanyel FC, Buyukpamukcu N, Hicsonmez A. Appendiceal perforation: a potentially lethal initial mode of presentation of Hirschsprung's disease. *J Pediatr Surg* 1997;32:123-4.

[27] Newman B, Nussbaum A, Kirkpatrick JA, Jr., Colodny A. Appendiceal perforation, pneumoperitoneum, and Hirschsprung's disease. *J Pediatr Surg* 1988;23:854-6.

[28] Rakheja D, Wilson GN, Rogers BB. Biochemical abnormality associated with Smith-Lemli-Opitz syndrome in an infant with features of Rutledge multiple congenital anomaly syndrome confirms that the latter is a variant of the former. *Pediatr Dev Pathol* 2003;6:270-7.

[29] Minutillo C, Pemberton PJ, Goldblatt J. Hirschsprung's disease and Ondine's curse: further evidence for a distinct syndrome. *Clin Genet* 1989;36:200-3.

[30] O'Dell K, Staren E, Bassuk A. Total colonic aganglionosis (Zuelzer-Wilson syndrome) and congenital failure of automatic control of ventilation (Ondine's curse). *J Pediatr Surg* 1987;22:1019-20.

[31] Antao B, Samuel M, Kiely E, Spitz L, Malone M. Congenital alveolar capillary dysplasia and associated gastrointestinal anomalies. *Fetal Pediatr Pathol* 2006;25:137-45.

[32] Makitie O, Heikkinen M, Kaitila I, Rintala R. Hirschsprung's disease in cartilage-hair hypoplasia has poor prognosis. *J Pediatr Surg* 2002;37:1585-8.

[33] Michna BA, McWilliams NB, Krummel TM, Hartenberg MA, Salzberg AM. Multifocal ganglioneuroblastoma coexistent with total colonic aganglionosis. *J Pediatr Surg* 1988;23:57-9.

[34] Skaba R, Dvorakova S, Vaclavikova E, Vlcek P, Frantlova M, Bendlova B. The risk of medullary thyroid carcinoma in patients with Hirschsprung's disease. *Pediatr Surg Int* 2006;22:991-5.

[35] Gupta M, Beeram MR, Pohl JF, Custer MD. Ileal atresia associated with Hirschsprung disease (total colonic aganglionosis). *J Pediatr Surg* 2005;40:e5-7.

[36] Janik JP, Wayne ER, Janik JS, Price MR. Ileal atresia with total colonic aganglionosis. *J Pediatr Surg* 1997;32:1502-3.

[37] Fishman SJ, Islam S, Buonomo C, Nurko S. Nonfixation of an atretic colon predicts Hirschsprung's disease. *J Pediatr Surg* 2001;36:202-4.

[38] Siu KL, Kwok WK, Lee WY, Lee WH. A male newborn with colonic atresia and total colonic aganglionosis. *Pediatr Surg Int* 1999;15:141-2.

[39] Jasonni V, Martucciello G. Total colonic aganglionosis. *Semin Pediatr Surg* 1998;7:174-80.

[40] Fondelli P, Martucciello G, Taccone A, Dodero P. [The radiologic picture of total colonic aganglionosis]. *Radiol Med (Torino)* 1989;77:207-10.

[41] Cowles RA, Berdon WE, Holt PD, Buonomo C, Stolar CJ. Neonatal intestinal obstruction simulating meconium ileus in infants with long-segment intestinal aganglionosis: radiographic findings that prompt the need for rectal biopsy. *Pediatr Radiol* 2006;36:133-7.

[42] Hayakawa K, Hamanaka Y, Suzuki M, Nakatsu M, Nishimura K, Tanaka M, Yamamoto E, et al. Radiological findings in total colon aganglionosis and allied disorders. *Radiat Med* 2003;21:128-34.

[43] Jamieson DH, Dundas SE, Belushi SA, Cooper M, Blair GK. Does the transition zone reliably delineate aganglionic bowel in Hirschsprung's disease? *Pediatr Radiol* 2004;34:811-5.

[44] Proctor ML, Traubici J, Langer JC, Gibbs DL, Ein SH, Daneman A, Kim PC. Correlation between radiographic transition zone and level of aganglionosis in

Hirschsprung's disease: Implications for surgical approach. *J Pediatr Surg* 2003;38:775-8.

[45] De Campo JF, Mayne V, Boldt DW, De Campo M. Radiological findings in total aganglionosis coli. *Pediatr Radiol* 1984;14:205-9.

[46] Martin MJ, Steele SR, Noel JM, Weichmann D, Azarow KS. Total colonic manometry as a guide for surgical management of functional colonic obstruction: Preliminary results. *J Pediatr Surg* 2001;36:1757-63.

[47] Faure C, Ategbo S, Ferreira GC, Cargill G, Bellaiche M, Boige N, Viarme F, et al. Duodenal and esophageal manometry in total colonic aganglionosis. *J Pediatr Gastroenterol Nutr* 1994;18:193-9.

[48] Anderson K, Chandra R. Segmental aganglionosis of the appendix. *J Pediatr Surg* 1986;21:852-4.

[49] Anderson KD, Chandra R. Segmental aganglionosis of the appendix. *J Pediatr Surg* 1986;21:852-4.

[50] Solari V, Piotrowska AP, Puri P. Histopathological differences between recto-sigmoid Hirschsprung's disease and total colonic aganglionosis. *Pediatr Surg Int* 2003;19:349-54.

[51] Shaw PA. The innervation and neuroendocrine cell population of the appendix in total colonic aganglionosis. *Histopathology* 1990;17:117-21.

[52] Rintala RJ, Lindahl HG. Proctocolectomy and J-pouch ileo-anal anastomosis in children. *J Pediatr Surg* 2002;37:66-70.

[53] Bonnard A, de Lagausie P, Leclair MD, Marwan K, Languepin J, Bruneau B, Berribi D, et al. Definitive treatment of extended Hirschsprung's disease or total colonic form. *Surg Endosc* 2001;15:1301-4.

[54] Martin LW. Total colonic aganglionosis preservation and utilization of entire colon. *J Pediatr Surg* 1982;17:635-7.

[55] Ross MN, Chang JH, Burrington JD, Janik JS, Wayne ER, Clevenger P. Complications of the Martin procedure for total colonic aganglionosis. *J Pediatr Surg* 1988;23:725-7.

[56] Kimura K, Nishijima E, Muraji T, Tsugawa C, Matsutmo Y. Extensive aganglionosis: further experience with the colonic patch graft procedure and long-term results. *J Pediatr Surg* 1988;23:52-6.

[57] Boley SJ. A new operative approach to total aganglionosis of the colon. *Surg Gynecol Obstet* 1984;159:481-4.

[58] Shermeta DW, Meller JL. Ideal treatment for total colonic Hirschsprung's disease. *J Pediatr Surg* 1989;24:88-91.

[59] Emslie J, Krishnamoorthy M, Applebaum H. Long-term follow-up of patients treated with ileoendorectal pull-through and right colon onlay patch for total colonic aganglionosis. *J Pediatr Surg* 1997;32:1542-4.

[60] Dodero P, Magillo P, Scarsi PL. Total colectomy and straight ileo-anal soave endorectal pull-through: personal experience with 42 cases. *Eur J Pediatr Surg* 2001;11:319-23.

[61] Azzis O, Fremond B, Dabadie A, Jouan J, Bracq H, Babut JM. [Total colonic form of Hirschsprung disease. Treatment and long-term follow-up in 16 cases]. *Chirurgie* 1996;121:225-9.

[62] Endo M, Watanabe K, Fuchimoto Y, Ikawa H, Yokoyama J. Long-term results of surgical treatment in infants with total colonic aganglionosis. *J Pediatr Surg* 1994;29:1310-14.

[63] Festen C, Severijnen R, v d Staak F, Rieu P. Total colonic aganglionosis: treatment and follow-up. *Z Kinderchir* 1989;44:153-5.

[64] Markham LA. Total colonic aganglionosis: a case study. *Neonatal Netw* 2001;20:23-9.

[65] Kottmeier PK, Jongco B, Velcek FT, Friedman A, Klotz DH. Absorptive function of the aganglionic ileum. *J Pediatr Surg* 1981;16:275-8.

[66] Kimura K, Nishijima E, Muraji T, Tsugawa C, Matsumoto Y. A new surgical approach to extensive aganglionosis. *J Pediatr Surg* 1981;16:840-3.

[67] Ziegler HW, Heitz PU, Kasper M, Spichtin HP, Ulrich J. Aganglionosis of the colon. Morphologic investigations in 524 patients. *Pathol Res Pract* 1984;178:543-7.

[68] Ziegler MM, Ross AJ, 3rd, Bishop HC. Total intestinal aganglionosis: a new technique for prolonged survival. *J Pediatr Surg* 1987;22:82-3.

[69] Yann R, Yves A, Dominique J, Thierry Y, Olivier G, Florence L. Improved quality of life by combined transplantation in Hirschsprung's disease with a very long aganglionic segment. *J Pediatr Surg* 2003;38:422-4.

[70] 70.Sarioglu A, Tanyel FC, Buyukpamukcu N, Hicsonmez A. Clinical risk factors of hirschsprung-associated enterocolitis. II: Postoperative enterocolitis. *Turk J Pediatr* 1997;39:91-8.

[71] 71.Hackam DJ, Filler RM, Pearl RH. Enterocolitis after the surgical treatment of Hirschsprung's disease: risk factors and financial impact. *J Pediatr Surg* 1998;33:830-3.

[72] 72.Núñez R, Cabrera R, Agulla E, Moreno C, Serrano A, Ortiz C, Blesa E. [Colonic aganglionosis with ileal involvement. Ileocolic plasty]. *Cir Pediatr* 2001;14:76-81.

[73] 73.Fouquet V, De Lagausie P, Faure C, Bloch J, Malbezin S, Ferkhadji L, Bauman C, et al. Do prognostic factors exist for total colonic aganglionosis with ileal involvement? *J Pediatr Surg* 2002;37:71-5.

[74] 74.Hengster P, Pernthaler H, Gassner I, Menardi G. Twenty-three years of follow-up in patients with total colonic aganglionosis. *Klin Padiatr* 1996;208:3-7.

In: Hirschsprung's Disease: Diagnosis and Treatment
Ed: Ramón Núñez and Manuel López-Alonso
ISBN: 978-1-60741-349-3

Chapter XXI

A Critical Review of the Different Operations for Hirschsprung's Disease

Juan A. Tovar

Introduction

Cure of Hirschsprung's Disease (HD) can be successfully achieved with several surgical techniques. All of them aim at resecting partially or totally the aganglionic segment and as much transitional and dilated colon as possible, reestablishing the continuity by a variety of colo-rectal or colo-anal anastomoses. In this way, they address the obstruction caused by the immobile bowel but they leave intact the internal sphincter which remains unable to relax. Weakening this structure by myotomy or myectomy is often used as an adjunct, although taking into account that the internal sphincter is necessary for involuntary, baseline continence. Therefore, a compromise between preservation of continence and weakening of the permanently contracted sphincter is sought and even mild insufficiencies in either direction explain why the outcome is not perfect in a proportion of cases.

The results obtained with all techniques are in general considered more satisfactory by surgeons than by patients [1]. A large comparative study of the 4 major operations in several centres around the world was carried out by Holschneider in 1982 [2] and, leaving aside the immediate postoperative complications in 426 patients, constipation persisted in 32% of them immediately after operation and in close to 10% several years later. As regards soiling, it was suffered by 30% of cases during early follow up and only in part improved with time because it persisted in more than 20% years later. Although the proportions for the 4 different procedures were not identical in his series, it is fair to say that this is what can be grossly expected from any of them and our own impressions after analyzing our recent series is not very different [3].

We will address critically the results with the different techniques by surveying the literature of the long-term results with them. However, the reader should be aware of the pitfalls of the objectivity of these reports since most of them, if not all, are retrospective, they are devoted to assess the locally preferred procedure and, when they compare different techniques, they do so with understandably uneven criteria.

Swenson Operation

This was the first procedure based on understanding of the physiopathology of HD and it attempeted at resecting radically the aganglionic, transitional and dilated bowel [4,5]. The original approach involved more often a previous colostomy followed by the pullthrough itself and completed by the closure of the diversion [6]. These three steps could be reduced to 2 by performing the colostomy just above the transitional zone and pulling down the ganglionic stoma during the rectosigmoidectomy. More recently, Swenson operation tended to be performed earlier and in one single step without diversion [7-9], except in cases with long aganglionosis or with enterocolitis. Exteriorized anastomosis was advocated for reducing the risks of pelvic leaks [10,11] and various forms of partial or total internal sphincterotomy were proposed. None of these variations changed substantially the long-term results of this operation that remains the gold standard. This procedure was early adapted to the laparoscopic approach [12,13].

However, surgeons' preferences evolved not only as a function of the results, but also of the difficulties of the operative challenge. Apparently, Swenson's procedure is considered as a demanding one because, despite its undisputable benefits, it is being progressively abandoned by recent generations of pediatric surgeons. A survey among the members of the Surgical Section of the AAP involving 5093 definitive operations for Hirschsprung showed that, although the more frequently performed was Swenson's, this was because it was the oldest one. In fact, only 23% of the 181 surgeons surveyed declared it as their favorite [14]. An equally surprising 8% of the members of the BAPS signaled Swenson pullthrough as their favorite for Hirschsprung in 1998 [15]. It is true that deep pelvic dissection may be risky for the genitourinary structures and their innervation, but many years of experience with this form of pullthrough showed that maintaining the dissection flush to the longitudinal layer of the rectal muscle, a radical resection whith preservation of these structures is possible.

One of the largest surveys of the results of this operation [16] (880 cases followed-up for an average of more than 10 years) showed outstanding results with an overall mortality of 2.4% that improved in recent years and excellent fecal emptying and continence after the first 5 years after the operation. No erection or voiding disturbances were found. It should be pointed out, however, that this survey was performed by several of the original proposers of the operation, including Swenson himself.

Another report from South Africa rated Swenson procedure behind Soave and Duhamel ones because, although 75% of the patients overall had satisfactory results, those having Swensons had more micturition disturbances, abdominal distension and strictures [17]. Results reported from China in 45 patients and from Belgium in another 45 followed up for long periods of time showed that, although in general these results are considered good by the surgeons, the proportions of patients with soiling was disturbingly high [18,19] with a tendency to improve with time.

Rehbein Operation

Rehbein proposed a new procedure in 1953 [20]. It was a radical variation of the anterior rectosigmoid resection proposed by State for adults with tumors but it was not an entirely physiological approach since it removed the intrapelvic rectum only down to (or slighly below) the peritoneal reflection [21,22]. The transitional segment and the dilated colon are resected as well and anastomosed to the aganglionic rectum (or part of it) which was therefore left in place together with the internal sphincter that cannot relax. Vigorous postoperative dilatations of the anus and rectum are a part of this treatment in an attempt to weakening the contractured smooth muscle that will otherwise remain obstructive [23].

This operation had a widespread success, particularly among Rehbein students who became leaders on this side of the Atlantic and it was progressively refined by increasing the extent of the aganglionic rectum resected and by operating earlier. Mechanical sutures contributed to this increased radicality [24,25] and those surgeons favoring this technique claim that presently the colo-rectal anastomosis is not very different from those of other apparently more radical operations.

The long term results reflect apparently the limitations of this approach. A large collective series of 200 patients from German-speaking countries followed for 5 to 10 years showed anastomotic leak in 6.6 %, rectal stricture requiring dilatation in 9.9 %, residual constipation in 22.8 %, encopresis in 4.3 % and enterocolitis in 10.6 % [26]. A recent account from Sweden showed that after a mean of 82 months of follow-up, only 29% had adequate defecatory function whereas 46% had episodes of obstruction and 27% had soiling [27].

Duhamel Operation

This procedure is apparently only in part "physiologic" but it has become very popular mainly because it works well and is technically easier than either Swenson's or Rehbein's ones. It consists of the division of the aganglionic rectum above the peritoneal reflection, the resection of the remaining aganglionic segment together with the transitional and part of the dilated colon and in the retrorectal pullthrough of healthy colon to the posterior anal margin to which it is anastomosed. The original operation included the closure of the rectal stump and the sutureless side-to-side colo-rectal anastomosis with two Kocher clamps that fell apart spontaneously several days after the procedure [28-30].

Problems with the progressively dilated rectal pouch when part of the recto-colonic septum was not taken down in its entirety prompted the introduction of several types of crush clamps to improve the anastomosis [31]. The development of stapling instruments greatly facilitated this procedure [32] which became more and more popular to the point of being one of the more widespread techniques. Its simplicity makes it applicable to young infants without previous diversion [33] and this as been the trend, like for other procedures, in the last couple of decades [34-36]. The use of staplers was a useful adjunt as well for performing Duhamel operation by laparoscopic approach [37-39].

The normally-innervated posterior half of the recto-colonic end of the bowel suffices for providing propulsion in spite of the still aganglionic anterior half. The point of emergence (below, in the middle or above the internal sphincter) of the pulled-through colon certainly influences the quality of continence.

Early results were considered superior to those of other techniques [40], provided that the operation involved elimination of the remaining rectal septum and pouch [41] that caused constipation and soiling [41].

The long term results are, like for other techniques, better when 5 or more years after the operation had elapsed. They were considered excellent in a large collective French series of 2430 cases [42]. However, it should be pointed out again that the authors were all related to Duhamel who signed himself the article. Another series of 131 patients operated upon by a single surgeon showed that the procedure could be performed early and without colostomy. The results were good although there was postoperative enterocolitis in 10%. Bowel function was normal within 3 months in 77.3% and 1 year after operation in 91.6% [43]. Equally good results were reported from Genoa [44] and from London where the technique involved leaving a very short rectal pouch [45]. Other reports are less optimistic: In a series of 103 patients treated in the USA with this operation, only 65% had normal bowel function whereas 27% required enemas and 8% had severe constipation or soiling [46]. In another series from Norway, out of 48 patients followed up for a median of 18 years, only 60% had perfect fecal control whereas 31% had occasional staining and 8% constant soiling. In addition, 10% complained of constipation [47]. Another report from Liverpool showed that only 42% of patients had fully satisfactory results and that this proportion significantly increased to 79% after the age of 14 [48]. Other results did not show significant improvement over time [49]. In a series of 75 patients from Amsterdam, only 10 out of the 49 over 4 were continent whreas 22 had soiling and/or constipation, and 17 were incontinent [50]. Soiling in proportions of up to 30% (32) and occasional micturition disturbances were reported also from the Netherlands [38].

My personal experience with Duhamel operation is very limited, certainly because I was trained by my mentors in France and Spain in the Swenson procedure, but my impression is that, with comparable results, it is technically easier and therefore suitable for more pediatric surgeons and applicable as a primary early operation without colostomy in most cases. Stapling devices and laparoscopic approach add appeal to this ingenious operation that is, as previously stated, that with a largest acceptance worldwide [24].

Soave Operation

Soave described his own technique, based on submucosal dissection of the rectum and subsequent pullthrough of ganglionic colon to the anus in 1963 [51]. This operation involved exteriorized mucocolonic anastomosis which required a secondary minor procedure [52,53]. The concept of endorectal pullthrough had immediate acceptance [54] because it avoided any pelvic hazardous dissection. Several improvements were soon introduced and particularly primary anastomosis, performance during early infancy [55,56] and ultimately transanal, laparoscopically-assisted approach. Other variations reported are the posterior sagittal approach [57] and the oblique anastomosis with minimal myectomy [58].

When I started to operate my own Hirschsprung patients in the first months of life, I found that this approach was particularly attractive: Starting the development of the rectal muscular cuff below the peritoneal reflection and pushing the cuff downwards to separate it from the mucosa (instead of pulling the cuff upwards to work inside it) makes the dissection down to the anus quite straightforward, decreases the risk for pelvic organs and their innervation and allows for a cuff-covered anastomosis. On the other hand, the short cuff obtained by this modality of the operation reduces the risk of stenosis at this level. I never performed sphincterotomy or sphincterectomy as an adjunct to this operation [59,60] and I did not observe obstructive sphincter achalasia described in other series [61,62].

Soave operation was the most popular for the treatment of Hirschsprung's disease [14,15] even before laparoscopically-assisted, transanal modification was introduced. We will discuss these modifications later.

The results were reported as good in most series. Once again, the account by the original describers was the most optimistic [63,64]. A manometric study from Japan showed that close to 90% of patients had good function and clinical results 10 years after the operation [65]. No major unfavourable results were accounted for in a large series from Ucraine [66]. As regards continence, Soave procedure fared better than Duhamel in a series of 135 children from the USA (7% vs 12% soling) [67]. In other series, the results of Soave (and of other procedures) were less encouraging with continence problems in up to 50% of patients in the short term although with almost constant improvement in the long term [68]. The results perceived by the patient were worse than those reported by their surgeons [1] and it seems that preoperative Hirschsprung enterocolitis is an unfavourable predictor for postoperative troubles of continence [69].

Transanal Approach

This was originally developed by Georgeson to allow a colo-anal anastromosis after laparoscopic biopsy and mobilization of the colon [70] but a similar concept had been previously proposed by Telander using an open approach [71]. The pure transanal operation was later proposed by De la Torre for rectosigmoid forms of aganglionism not requiring extensive colonic mobilization [72,73]. A rapidly growing number of pediatric surgeons (including ourselves) adhered later to the principles of this ingenious procedure, consisting of the submucous dissection of the rectum from below [74-83]. Dissection is pursued up to the peritoneal reflection where the abdominal cavity is entered and the sigmoid dissection with division of the vessels is carried out close to the wall until ganglionic, non-dilated bowel suitable for anastomosis is found. This operation is particularly straightforward in newborns and can be complemented with posterior myotomy of the cuff extended or not into the internal sphincter, an adjunct that largely facilitates the intrapelvic part of the procedure. A variation of the purely transanal approach include full thickness dissection of the rectum 1 to 2 cm above the dentate line (like in a Swenson operation) [84].

The temptation to apply the purely transanal procedure to more extensive aganglionosis (that extended above the mid-sigmoid) should be resisted since it is hardly possible to bring down healthy sigmoid to the anus unless the length of this part of the colon and its vessels are increased as it happens in recto-low sigmoid forms that constitute 80 to 85% of cases overall. Additional laparoscopic or open management of the longer forms of the disease is strongly advisable in order to avoid hazardous and demanding operations.

The results are expected to be similar to those of the regular Soave operations since the principles and the dissection are identical although performed from below. However, some doubts have been cast about the possible effects of forced anal dilatation caused by the per-operative retraction of the anal margins. Early results have been good in terms of continence and also of manometric assessment [85], but a recent study comparing 2 successive series of open and transanal Soaves show less good results with the latter [86] although the follow-up for these cases was shorter.

In my opinion, and I am a firm believer in the benefits of this operation when it is well indicated, the results will not be worse than those of old-fashioned Soave. The magnitude of anal dilatation is by no means more potentially destructive than that caused by anal dilatations that are routinely indicated after Rehbein operation.

The purely transanal approach has, in my opinion, three minor setbacks: First, it requires a more or less long waiting time until the frozen sections are examined by the pathologist precisely when the dissection is already finished. Second, the resection specimens sent to the pathologist are incomplete (the muscular rectum remains on site) and may be source of confusion particularly in purely rectal forms [87] and, finally, the absence of scar and the rapid recovery transmit to parents and attending pediatricians a wrong idea about the extent and the complexity of the procedure that is certainly wellcome... except when complications arise.

Commentary

It is impossible for a critical review not to be tainted by personal judgement by the reviewer. This is why I added some comments of my own to several of the techniques analyzed and used the first person. I acknowledge that some of them might be based on incomplete experience on some of the techniques.

My review will end with some personal observations on the surgical treatment of Hirschsprung disease.

Surgeons have to struggle between conservatism and innovation. They have to maintain alive what has been demonstrated to be good while, at the same time, keeping an eye on the new possibilities offered by new concepts, approaches or techniques. A reasonably eclectic attitude would be neither being the last to abandon a good, old operation nor being the first to embrace an attractive new one of yet not proven benefits.

The surgical treatment of Hirschsprung disease illustrates well this dilemma: Swenson pullthrough in two or three steps could have remained the gold-standard because it was physiologically sound and demonstrably good. But the trends towards simplifyng pediatric operations by limiting the surgical steps and by completing the treatment at an age as young as possible prompted innovation. In addition, Swenson's is a difficult operation to be performed by everybody and alternatives that were simpler in themselves, like the Duhamel, or that went around the more difficult part of the Swenson, pelvic dissection, like the Soave, found rapidly their place. On top of that, we surgeons, like everybody else in other fields of life, are influenced by fashion. If laparoscopic approach is possible, why not trying this less invasive route for our operation and, by the same token, why not modifying the operation itself to fit it to the approach?. And once that we have proved that the operation is feasible without opening the belly, why not trying to perform it purely through the anus?.

This attitude has brought enormous progress to the treatment of Hirschsprung disease but also some new risks that should be pointed out:

1. Multiple learning curves forced by this rapid progress are superimposed in most centers (with their inherent risks) because Hirschsprung's disease is not a common condition. Most western countries do not have enough patients for adequate training of all pediatric surgeons and it is not a surprise for China, India, Mexico, Egypt or Brazil to be collecting in short time the largest experience on the new techniques.
2. Personal expertise, divided among various procedures, is decreasing for all of us.
3. Long-term evaluation, the only way of granting on solid grounds the category of gold-standard to any treatment, is being progressively delayed by the perpetual introduction of innovative procedures that are still to young for definitive assessment.
4. If the approach predominates over the rationale for any operation, gross mistakes may be made: transanal operation for a long aganglionism may generate serious complications or minimally invasive operation at any price into unexperienced hands may be more damaging than old-fashioned but safe open procedures.

Therefore, pediatric surgeons should be able to balance tradition and innovation also in this particular field and this is only possible if they remain permanently open to high quality information, if they perform often assessment of their own results and, over all, if they keep their maind open and critical.

References

[1] Yanchar NL, Soucy P. Long-term outcome after Hirschsprung's disease: patients' perspectives. *J Pediatr Surg* 1999;34:1152-60.

[2] Holschneider AM. Clinical and electromanometric studies of postoperative continence in Hirschsprung's disease: Relationship to the surgical procedures. In: Holschneider AM, editor. *Hirschsprung's disease.* Stuttgart-New York: Hippokrates Verlag, Thieme Stratton. Inc; 1982. p. 221-42.

[3] Luis LA, Encinas JL, Avila LF, Andres AM, Burgos L, Fernandez A, et al. Enfermedad de Hirschsprung: lecciones aprendidas en los últimos 100 casos. *Cir Pediatr* 2006;19:177-81.

[4] Swenson O. A new surgical treatment for Hirschsprung's disease. *Surgery* 1950;28:371-83.
[5] Swenson O. Hirschsprung's disease (aganglionic megacolon). *N Engl J Med* 1959;260:972-6.
[6] Swenson O. Early history of the therapy of Hirschsprung's disease: facts and personal observations over 50 years. *J Pediatr Surg* 1996;31:1003-8.
[7] Carcassonne M. Maladie de Hirschsprung: un commentaire. *Ann Pediatr (Paris)* 1991;38:133-6.
[8] Wilcox DT, Bruce J, Bowen J, Bianchi A. One-stage neonatal pull-through to treat Hirschsprung's disease. *J Pediatr Surg* 1997;32:243-5.
[9] Carcassonne M, Delarue A. Management of Hirschsprung's disease. The definitive operation: which, when, why and how. *Aust N Z J Surg* 1984;54:435-8.
[10] Pellerin PD. Maladie de Hirschsprung chez l'enfant. *Ann Gastroenterol Hepatol (Paris)* 1984;20:129-31.
[11] Pellerin D. Maladie de Hirschsprung. *Ann Gastroenterol Hepatol (Paris)* 1992;28:99-103.
[12] Hoffmann K, Schier F, Waldschmidt J. Laparoscopic Swenson's procedure in children. *Eur J Pediatr Surg* 1996;6:15-7.
[13] Georgeson KE, Robertson DJ. Laparoscopic-assisted approaches for the definitive surgery for Hirschsprung's disease. *Semin Pediatr Surg* 2004;13:256-62.
[14] Kleinhaus S, Boley SJ, Sheran M, Sieber WK. Hirschsprung's disease -- a survey of the members of the Surgical Section of the American Academy of Pediatrics. *J Pediatr Surg* 1979;14:588-97.
[15] Huddart SN. Hirschsprung's disease: present UK practice. *Ann R Coll Surg Engl* 1998;80:46-8.
[16] Sherman JO, Snyder ME, Weitzman JJ, Jona JZ, Gillis DA, O'Donnell B, et al. A 40-year multinational retrospective study of 880 Swenson procedures. *J Pediatr Surg* 1989;24:833-8.
[17] Moore SW, Albertyn R, Cywes S. Clinical outcome and long-term quality of life after surgical correction of Hirschsprung's disease. *J Pediatr Surg* 1996;31:1496-502.
[18] Bai Y, Chen H, Hao J, Huang Y, Wang W. Long-term outcome and quality of life after the Swenson procedure for Hirschsprung's disease. *J Pediatr Surg* 2002;37:639-42.
[19] Reding R, de Ville de Goyet J, Gosseye S, Clapuyt P, Sokal E, Buts JP, et al. Hirschsprung's disease: a 20-year experience. *J Pediatr Surg* 1997;32:1221-5.
[20] Rehbein F. Intraabdominelle Resektion oder Rectosigmoidektomie bei der Hirschsprung'schen Krankheit. *Chirurg* 1958;29:366-9.
[21] Rehbein F, Nicolai I. Operation der Hirschsprung'schen Krankheit. *Dtsch Med Wochenschr* 1963;88:1595-7.
[22] Rehbein F, Halsband H. Maladie de Hirschsprung: Technique de résection intra-abdominale de Rehbein. *Ann Chir Infant* 1970;11:92-3.
[23] Rehbein F. Megacolon congenitum Hirschsprung. In: Rehbein F, editor. *Kinderchirurgische Operationen.* Stuttgart: Hippokrates Verlag; 1976. p. 309-49.

[24] Meier H, Willital GH. [Modified Rehbein surgical procedure using a surgical staple--progress in the treatment of Hirschsprung disease in children]. *Langenbecks Arch Chir* 1987;372:751-3.

[25] Holschneider AM. Experience with Rehbein's Technique. In: Holschneider AMaP, P, editor. *Hirschsprung's disease and allied disorders.* 2nd ed. London-New York: Taylor & Francis; 2000. p. 366-74.

[26] Rassouli R, Holschneider AM, Bolkenius M, Menardi G, Becker MR, Schaarschmidt K, et al. Long-term results of Rehbein's procedure: a retrospective study in German-speaking countries. *Eur J Pediatr Surg* 2003;13:187-94.

[27] Wester T, Zetterlind L, Fredin K, Olsen L. Postoperative obstructive symptoms are common after Rehbein's procedure for Hirschsprung's disease. *Eur J Pediatr Surg* 2006;16:100-3.

[28] Duhamel B. Une nouvelle opération pour le Mégacolon Congénital: abaissement retrorectal and transanal et son application posible au traitement de quelques autres malformations. *Presse Med* 1956;64:2249-50.

[29] Duhamel B. A new operation for the treatment of Hirschsprung's disease. *Arch Dis Child* 1960;35:38-9.

[30] Duhamel B. Retrorectal and Transanal Pull-through Procedure for the Treatment of Hirschsprung's Disease. *Dis Colon Rectum* 1964;7:455-8.

[31] Louhimo I, Rintala R. Duhamel-Sulamaa operation for Hirschsprung's disease--early and late results in forty-eight patients. *Z Kinderchir* 1985;40:97-100.

[32] van der Zee DC, Bax KN. One-stage Duhamel-Martin procedure for Hirschsprung's disease: a 5-year follow-up study. *J Pediatr Surg* 2000;35:1434-6.

[33] Chiengkriwate P, Patrapinyokul S, Sangkhathat S, Chowchuvech V. Primary pull-through with modified Duhamel technique: 1 institution's experience. *J Pediatr Surg* 2007;42:1075-80.

[34] Yanagihara J, Iwai N, Tokiwa K, Deguchi E, Shimotake T. Results of a modified Duhamel Operation for Hirschsprung's disease using the GIA stapler. *Eur J Pediatr Surg* 1997;7:77-9.

[35] Mattioli G, Buffa P, Martinelli M, Ivani G, Jasonni V. All mechanical low rectal anastomosis in children. *J Pediatr Surg* 1998;33:503-6.

[36] Vrsansky P, Bourdelat D, Pages R. Principal modifications of the Duhamel procedure in the treatment of Hirschsprung's disease. Analysis based on results of an international retrospective study of 2,430 patients. *Pediatr Surg Int* 1998;13:125-32.

[37] de Lagausie P, Berrebi D, Geib G, Sebag G, Aigrain Y. Laparoscopic Duhamel procedure. Management of 30 cases. *Surg Endosc* 1999;13:972-4.

[38] Boemers TM, Bax NM, van Gool JD. The effect of rectosigmoidectomy and Duhamel-type pull-through procedure on lower urinary tract function in children with Hirschsprung's disease. *J Pediatr Surg* 2001;36:453-6.

[39] Travassos DV, Bax NM, Van der Zee DC. Duhamel procedure: a comparative retrospective study between an open and a laparoscopic technique. *Surg Endosc* 2007;21:2163-5.

[40] Khan O, Nixon HH. Results following surgery for Hirschsprung's disease: a review of three operations with a reference to neorectal capacity. *Br J Surg* 1980;67:436-8.

[41] Livaditis A. Hirschsprung's disease: long-term results of the original Duhamel operation. *J Pediatr Surg* 1981;16:484-6.

[42] Bourdelat D, Vrsansky P, Pages R, Duhamel B. Duhamel operation 40 years after: a multicentric study. *Eur J Pediatr Surg* 1997;7:70-6.

[43] Jung PM. Hirschsprung's disease: one surgeon's experience in one institution. *J Pediatr Surg* 1995;30:646-51.

[44] Mattioli G, Castagnetti M, Martucciello G, Jasonni V. Results of a mechanical Duhamel pull-through for the treatment of Hirschsprung's disease and intestinal neuronal dysplasia. *J Pediatr Surg* 2004;39:1349-55.

[45] Antao B, Radhwan T, Samuel M, Kiely E. Short-pouch and low-anastomosis Duhamel procedure results in better fecal control and normal defecation pattern. *Dis Colon Rectum* 2005;48:1791-6.

[46] Rescorla FJ, Morrison AM, Engles D, West KW, Grosfeld JL. Hirschsprung's disease. Evaluation of mortality and long-term function in 260 cases. *Arch Surg* 1992;127:934-41.

[47] Bjornland K, Diseth TH, Emblem R. Long-term functional, manometric, and endosonographic evaluation of patients operated upon with the Duhamel technique. *Pediatr Surg Int* 1998;13:24-8.

[48] Baillie CT, Kenny SE, Rintala RJ, Booth JM, Lloyd DA. Long-term outcome and colonic motility after the Duhamel procedure for Hirschsprung's disease. *J Pediatr Surg* 1999;34:325-9.

[49] Conway SJ, Craigie RJ, Cooper LH, Turner K, Turnock RR, Lamont GL, et al. Early adult outcome of the Duhamel procedure for left-sided Hirschsprung disease--a prospective serial assessment study. *J Pediatr Surg* 2007;42:1429-32.

[50] Heij HA, de Vries X, Bremer I, Ekkelkamp S, Vos A. Long-term anorectal function after Duhamel operation for Hirschsprung's disease. *J Pediatr Surg* 1995;30:430-2.

[51] Soave F. Une nouvelle technique pour le traitement de la Maladie de Hirschsprung. Coloanstomie sans suture après mobilisation et abaissement extra-muqueux du recto.sigmoïde. *J Chir (Paris)* 1963;86:451-64.

[52] Soave F. A New Surgical Technique for Treatment of Hirschsprung's Disease. *Surgery* 1964;56:1007-14.

[53] Soave F. Hirschsprung's Disease: A New Surgical Technique. *Arch Dis Child* 1964;39:116-24.

[54] Singh SJ, Croaker GD, Manglick P, Wong CL, Athanasakos H, Elliott E, et al. Hirschsprung's disease: the Australian Paediatric Surveillance Unit's experience. *Pediatr Surg Int* 2003;19:247-50.

[55] Langer JC, Fitzgerald PG, Winthrop AL, Srinathan SK, Foglia RP, Skinner MA, et al. One-stage versus two-stage Soave pull-through for Hirschsprung's disease in the first year of life. *J Pediatr Surg* 1996;31:33-6.

[56] Sidler D, Millar AJ, Rode H, Brown RA, Franck M, Cywes S. Neonatal Soave endorectal pull-through for Hirschsprung's disease. *S Afr J Surg* 1999;37:47-9.

[57] Liem NT, Hau BD, Son HT. Modified Soave procedure through the posterior sagittal approach for Hirschsprung's disease. *J Pediatr Surg* 2005;40:547-50.

[58] Li AW, Zhang WT, Li FH, Cui XH, Duan XS. A new modification of transanal Soave pull-through procedure for Hirschsprung's disease. *Chin Med J (Engl)* 2006;119:37-42.
[59] Kimura K, Inomata Y, Soper RT. Posterior sagittal rectal myectomy for persistent rectal achalasia after the Soave procedure for Hirschsprung's disease. *J Pediatr Surg* 1993;28:1200-1.
[60] Miyano T, Yamataka A, Urao M, Kobayashi H, Lane GJ. Modified soave pull-through for Hirschsprung's disease: intraoperative internal sphincterotomy. *J Pediatr Surg* 1999;34:1599-602.
[61] Millar AJ, Steinberg RM, Raad J, Rode H. Anal achalasia after pull-through operations for Hirschsprung's disease -- preliminary experience with topical nitric oxide. *Eur J Pediatr Surg* 2002;12:207-11.
[62] Wildhaber BE, Pakarinen M, Rintala RJ, Coran AG, Teitelbaum DH. Posterior myotomy/myectomy for persistent stooling problems in Hirschsprung's disease. *J Pediatr Surg* 2004;39:920-6.
[63] Dodero P, Magillo P, Moran Penco JM, Borella F, Giorgini F, Martinelli M, et al. Tratamiento con la técnica de Soave y resultados a largo plazo en 270 casos de Enfermedad de Hirschsprung. *An Esp Pediatr* 1984;20:571-8.
[64] Soave F. Endorectal pull-through: 20 years experience. Address of the guest speaker, APSA, 1984. *J Pediatr Surg* 1985;20:568-79.
[65] Morikawa Y, Matsufugi H, Hirobe S, Yokoyama J, Katsumata K. Motility of the anorectum after the Soave-Denda operation. *Prog Pediatr Surg* 1989;24:67-76.
[66] Krivchenya DY, Silchenko MI, Soroka VP, Pritula VP, Khursin VN. Endorectal pull-through for Hirschsprung's disease: 17-year review of results in Ukraine. *Pediatr Surg Int* 2002;18:718-22.
[67] Marty TL, Seo T, Matlak ME, Sullivan JJ, Black RE, Johnson DG. Gastrointestinal function after surgical correction of Hirschsprung's disease: long-term follow-up in 135 patients. *J Pediatr Surg* 1995;30:655-8.
[68] Fortuna RS, Weber TR, Tracy TF, Jr., Silen ML, Cradock TV. Critical analysis of the operative treatment of Hirschsprung's disease. *Arch Surg* 1996;131:520-4.
[69] Murthi GV, Raine PA. Preoperative enterocolitis is associated with poorer long-term bowel function after Soave-Boley endorectal pull-through for Hirschsprung's disease. *J Pediatr Surg* 2003;38:69-72.
[70] Georgeson KE, Fuenfer MM, Hardin WD. Primary laparoscopic pull-through for Hirschsprung's disease in infants and children. *J Pediatr Surg* 1995;30:1017-21.
[71] Saltzman DA, Telander MJ, Brennom WS, Telander RL. Transanal mucosectomy: a modification of the Soave procedure for Hirschsprung's disease. *J Pediatr Surg* 1996;31:1272-5.
[72] De la Torre-Mondragon L, Ortega-Salgado JA. Transanal endorectal pull-through for Hirschsprung's disease. *J Pediatr Surg* 1998;33:1283-6.
[73] De la Torre L, Ortega A. Transanal versus open endorectal pull-through for Hirschsprung's disease. *J Pediatr Surg* 2000;35:1630-2.
[74] .Morikawa Y, Hoshino K, Matsumura K, Yoshioka S, Yokoyama J, Kitajima M. Extra-anal mucosectomy: laparascopic-assisted endorectal pull-through using a prolapsing technique. *J Pediatr Surg* 1998;33:1679-81.

[75] Albanese CT, Jennings RW, Smith B, Bratton B, Harrison MR. Perineal one-stage pull-through for Hirschsprung's disease. *J Pediatr Surg* 1999;34:377-80.

[76] Langer JC, Minkes RK, Mazziotti MV, Skinner MA, Winthrop AL. Transanal one-stage Soave procedure for infants with Hirschsprung's disease. *J Pediatr Surg* 1999;34:148-51.

[77] Langer JC, Seifert M, Minkes RK. One-stage Soave pull-through for Hirschsprung's disease: a comparison of the transanal and open approaches. *J Pediatr Surg* 2000;35:820-2.

[78] Shankar KR, Losty PD, Lamont GL, Turnock RR, Jones MO, Lloyd DA, et al. Transanal endorectal coloanal surgery for Hirschsprung's disease: experience in two centers. *J Pediatr Surg* 2000;35:1209-13.

[79] Gao Y, Li G, Zhang X, Xu Q, Guo Z, Zheng B, et al. Primary transanal rectosigmoidectomy for Hirschsprung's disease: Preliminary results in the initial 33 cases. *J Pediatr Surg* 2001;36:1816-9.

[80] Hollwarth ME, Rivosecchi M, Schleef J, Deluggi S, Fasching G, Ceriati E, et al. The role of transanal endorectal pull-through in the treatment of Hirschsprung's disease - a multicenter experience. *Pediatr Surg Int* 2002;18:344-8.

[81] Ekema G, Falchetti D, Torri F, Merulla VE, Manciana A, Caccia G. Further evidence on totally transanal one-stage pull-through procedure for Hirschsprung's disease. *J Pediatr Surg* 2003;38:1434-9.

[82] Hadidi A. Transanal endorectal pull-through for Hirschsprung's disease: experience with 68 patients. *J Pediatr Surg* 2003;38:1337-40.

[83] Langer JC, Durrant AC, de la Torre L, Teitelbaum DH, Minkes RK, Caty MG, et al. One-stage transanal Soave pullthrough for Hirschsprung disease: a multicenter experience with 141 children. *Ann Surg* 2003;238:569-83.

[84] Rintala RJ. Transanal coloanal pull-through with a short muscular cuff for classic Hirschsprung's disease. *Eur J Pediatr Surg* 2003;13:181-6.

[85] Till H, Heinrich M, Schuster T, D VS. Is the anorectal sphincter damaged during a transanal endorectal pull-through (TERPT) for Hirschsprung's disease? A 3-dimensional, vector manometric investigation. *Eur J Pediatr Surg* 2006;16:188-91.

[86] El-Sawaf MI, Drongowski RA, Chamberlain JN, Coran AG, Teitelbaum DH. Are the long-term results of the transanal pull-through equal to those of the transabdominal pull-through? A comparison of the 2 approaches for Hirschsprung disease. *J Pediatr Surg* 2007;42:41-7.

[87] Berrebi D, Fouquet V, de Lagausie P, Carricaburu E, Ferkdadji L, Chomette P, et al. Duhamel operation vs neonatal transanal endorectal pull-through procedure for Hirschsprung disease: which are the changes for pathologists? *J Pediatr Surg* 2007;42:688-91.

Part IV: Enterocolitis in Hirschsprung's Disease, Long-Term Results, Variant Hirschsprung's Disease, Intestinal Transplant, and Nutrition in Hirschsprung's Disease

In: Hirschsprung's Disease: Diagnosis and Treatment
Ed: Ramón Núñez and Manuel López-Alonso
ISBN: 978-1-60741-349-3

Chapter XXII

Enterocolitis in Hirschsprung's Disease

Ramón Núñez, Ana Torres and J.Ignacio Santamaría

Hirschsprung's-associated enterocolitis (HAEC) remains the most frequent cause of this disease's morbidity and mortality [1–4]. It is characterized by explosive diarrhœa, abdominal distension, pyrexia, colicky abdominal pain, lethargy and the passage of blood-stained stools [3]. It may be the first clinical manifestation of Hirschsprung's disease (HD) in the newborn, or it can present at any time during the course of the disease, i.e., before or after surgery [5]. Despite great advances in understanding the disease's pathophysiology and genetics, and in its surgical treatment, little is known about the ætiopathogenesis of its greatest complication – enterocolitis – or how it can be prevented [6, 7].

Antecedents

In 1886, Harald Hirschsprung described two infants with the disease which subsequently carried his name. One patient died of HAEC. In this early work, Harald Hirschsprung referred to various histopathological aspects related to HAEC: "There is full-thickness ulceration penetrating to the serosa, abscess formation in the submucosa, and mottled submucosal spaces containing pus" [8]. Nonetheless, despite the long-standing knowledge of this complication, over the following 70 years HAEC did not receive the attention it deserved [6, 7, 9–11].

The concept of HAEC was alluded to in the literature in 1950 by Burnad [12], Fisher and Swenson [13] in 1956 and Dorman [14] in 1957. The same year, Swenson [15] reported a follow-up of 200 patients operated due to HD over a period of 10 years. Some patients presented recurring diarrhœa. Swenson et al. in 1960 [16] referred to the "diarrhœa following rectosigmoidectomy for Hirschsprung's disease". Nonetheless, it was not until 1962 that Bill and Chapman [17] presented the first definitive description of the condition. They considered that the cause was partial mechanical obstruction of the aganglionic segment. To prevent

HAEC, colostomy was performed on all patients after the diagnosis of aganglionosis. In 1964, Swenson [18] suggested that HAEC should be treated by decompression of the colon with a rectal catheter and partial sphincteromyotomy of the internal sphincter. That author and co-workers reported in 1975 [19] their experience with this disease over a period of 25 years. They referred to the incidence of neonatal enterocolitis (24%) and postoperative enterocolitis (16%). Kleinhaus et al. [20] in 1979, in a survey of members of the Surgical Section of the American Academy of Pediatrics, noted that HAEC was present in 15% of patients at the time of diagnosis of HD, and the greatest increase in frequency of this complication was observed in the first 3 months of life.

In the 1980s and 1990s, different hypotheses were put forward on the pathogenesis HAEC, since the mechanical obstruction mentioned above [16,17] did not explain the presentation of this complication in patients with a digestive tract derivation, or after the definitive operation. The origin of HAEC was considered multifactorial [21-26]. Teitelbaum et al. [6] in 1988, Carneiro et al. [27] in 1992, Hackman et al. [2] in 1998, and Murphy et al. [5] in 2005 analyzed the risk factors of HAEC.

At present there is no specific treatment for the prevention of this complication of HD [28,29]. In our experience [28] and that of other authors [30–33], postoperative rectal irrigation decreases the incidence and severity of episodes of post-pull-through enterocolitis.

The aim of this chapter is to describes the epidemiology, pathology, theories of pathogenesis, clinical manifestations, diagnosis, current best practice in management and prevention of HAEC.

Epidemiology

Incidence

The incidence of HAEC ranges from 5.7% to 44.6% in the preoperative period, from 0% to 9% in the post-stoma period, and from 4.6% to 41.8% in the post-pull-through period, depending on the series analyzed [6,11,17,19,20,34–44] (see Table 1). The primary reason for the variable results of HAEC in the literature is attributed to different criteria to diagnose HAEC in different centres.

The period prior to the diagnosis of HD is considered to be that of greatest risk for HAEC [3]. The observation of this complication at the time of diagnosis of HD ranges from 5.7 to 24% of patients (mean 12.9%), according to various series [6,11,19,20,27,34,36,37,39]. The HAEC tends to be more severe in this group of patients [6]. In the study of Carneiro et al. [27], 10 patients (13%) had enterocolitis at the time of diagnosis of HD. Of these 5 neonates, 4 of whom were premature, suffered necrotizing enterocolitis with radiological evidence of intestinal pneumatosis. Bill and Chapman [17] observed that the presentation of 87.5% of HAEC cases was pre-enterostomy, and that this complication was the most frequent cause of death. In our experience [28] and that of other authors [45, 46], early diagnosis of HD in the first week of life, and the commencement at that time of daily rectal irrigation and rectal manipulation until the final intervention, virtually eliminates the risk of preoperative HAEC.

Table 1. Incidence of enterocolitis in reported series of HD.

Report	Pre-pullthrough %	Post-stoma %	Post-pullthrough %
Bill 1962 [17]	44.6	0	6.3
Swenson 1975 [19]	24	0	34.2
Kleinhaus 1979 [20]	15	0	9.8
Teitelbaum 1988 [6	16.3	2.6	5.3
Carneiro 1992 [27]	13	9	9
Rescorla 1992 [34]	5.7	0	12.3
Blane 1994 [35]	NS	NS	33
Surana 1994 [36	18.5	2.5	18.3
Elhalaby 1995 [11]	12.5	NS	26
Moore 1996 [37]	16.6	0	11
Sarioglu 1997 [38]	26	0	14
Murthi 2003 [39]	11	0	22
Elhalaby 2004 [40]	NS	NS	17.8
Suita 2005 [41]	25.2	NS	15.1
Menezes 2006 [42]	24.3	NS	41.8
Pratap 2007 [43]	30.7	NS	4.6
Haricharan 2008 [44]	6	NS	37

NS: Not stated

Despite the advances in surgical treatment of HD, enterocolitis is still its principal postoperative complication [3,29]. It can occur immediately postoperative or later, even several years after the definitive intervention [17]. But most of the episodes of HAEC occur during the two years following surgery [3]. In the series of Blane et al. [35], the HAEC attacks occurred from 1 month to 176 months following endorectal pull-through, with a mean of 29 months and a median of 18 months. According to Swenson et al. [19], the greatest risk of HAEC is in the first year after the definitive intervention, and in our series [28] the highest incidence was observed during the first month postoperative.

Recurrent HAEC has an incidence of 5 to 41% [17,27,36]. In the series of Menezes [42] of 259 patients with HD, 74 presented HAEC and 27% suffered more than 2 episodes of enterocolitis. In our experience of 37 patients with HD [28], 11 presented HAEC and 9 of them suffered more than 2 episodes of this complication. The frequency of HAEC episodes tends to decrease with age, and its observation is rare from five years postoperative onwards [28, 47]. Chronic HAEC is very common in patients with Down syndrome [3].

Morbidity and Mortality

HAEC remains the major cause of morbidity and mortality in patients with this disease [3, 48]. Periods of hospitalization can be lengthy, and in some cases HAEC may present serious complications [48]. One of our patients with Waardenburg syndrome and HD presented a severe HAEC on the 5th day postoperative. He required parenteral nutrition and digestive tract rest for 2 weeks [28]. Carneiro et al. [27] report hospitalization for patients with HAEC of between 6 and 29 days (mean, 13 days). The cost of care of an infant with HAEC is 2.5 times more than the patient with HD and without HAEC [6].

The mortality of HD in the absence of enterocolitis is very low [3]. Swenson and Davidson [49] reported a 4% mortality in patients with HD without enterocolitis compared with 33% in patients with this disease and enterocolitis. Frank and Nixon [50] analyzed the causes of death in HD and found that 56% could be attributed to HAEC. This complication was the commonest cause of preoperative, post-colostomy, and post-pull-through deaths [50]. Patients with Down syndrome have an increased risk of mortality from HAEC [6]. The mortality of HAEC ranges from 0% to 33.3% in both, in the preoperative period and in the post-pull-through period, and from 0% to 100% in the post-stoma period, depending on the series analysed [17, 43] (see Table 2).

Table 2. Mortality related to HAEC.

Report	Preoperative mortality HAEC %	Postperative mortality HAEC %	
		Post-Stoma	Post-pullthrough
Bill 1962 [17]	33.3	0	0
Swenson 1975 [19]	NS	0	9.7
Kleinhaus 1979 [20]	30	0	9.2
Teitelbaum 1988 [6]	5	0	0
Rescorla 1992 [34]	27	0	0
Carneriro 1992 [27]	0	14.2	0
Surana 1994 [36]	0	100	5
Elhalaby 1995 [11]	0	0	0
Sarioglu 1997 [38]	7.6	0	0
Murthi 2003 [39]	0	0	0
Langer 2003 [51]	0	0	0
Suita 2005 [41]	4.3	NS	5.2
Menezes 2006 [42]	0	0	3.4
Pratap 2007 [43]	0	0	33.3
Haricharan 2008 [44]	0	NS (Not stated)	0

The enterocolitis present at the time of diagnosis of HD and postoperative enterocolitis have been associated with a higher risk of mortality in some studies [20, 52,53].

The mortality of pre- and post-operative HAEC has undergone a sharp decline in the past 30 years as reflected by Suita et al. [41] in their review of 3852 cases of HD in Japan. Thus, in the period 1978–1982 preoperative mortality from this complication was 6.5% and postoperative mortality was 7.1%, and in the period 1998–2002 it was 0.7% and 3%. respectively (Fig. 1) [41].

To this declining mortality due to enterocolitis have contributed the early diagnosis of HD. and advances in its surgical treatment and in intensive neonatal care [3].

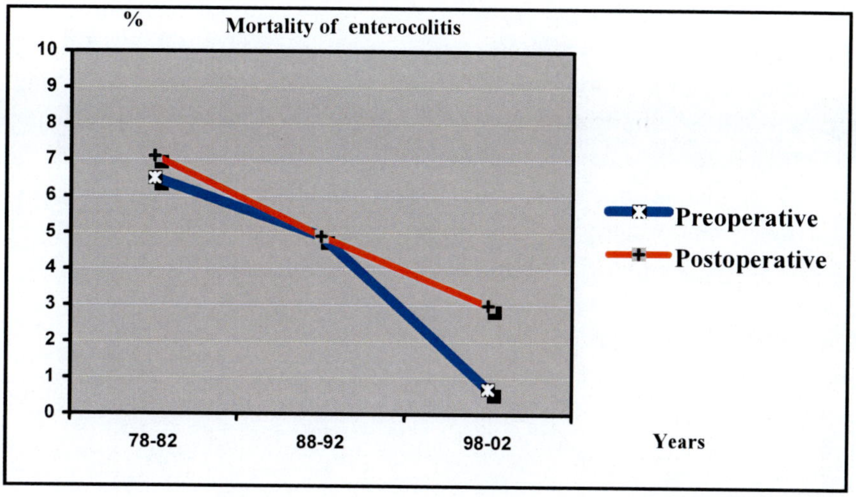

Figure 1. Mortality from preoperative and postoperative HAEC (Suita et al. [41]).

Risk Factors for Enterocolitis

Several workers [2,3,6,27,32,42,48] have analyzed the pre- and post-operative risk factors for HAEC. It is believed that delay in diagnosis, the association with Down syndrome, and mechanical obstruction are specific risk factors for HAEC.

Preoperative Risk Factors

Delay in Diagnosis

Diagnosis of HD delayed until after the first week of life is considered by many authors to be a risk factor for preoperative HAEC [3, 6, 19]. Thus, Teitelbaum et al. [6] noted that the average age of the infants with a diagnosis of HAEC was 16.6 ± 11.3 days, significantly greater ($p<0.01$) than the 4.6 ± 6.5 days average age at diagnosis of neonates with HD without enterocolitis.

Klein et al. [52] reported no enterocolitis in neonates with HD on whom an ostomy had been performed in the first two weeks of life. Surana et al. [36] found 11% of neonates with enterocolitis when the diagnosis of HD was in the first week of life compared with 24% with enterocolitis when the diagnosis was made after the first week of life. Kleinhaus et al. [20] concluded on the basis of their series that, when the diagnosis of HD was in the first month of life. the incidence of enterocolitis was minimal.

Down Syndrome

Trisomy 21 associated with HD is well known to be a risk factor for enterocolitis [3]. Carneiro et al. [27] reported an HAEC incidence of 50% in patients with Down syndrome and HD compared with 29% in patients with that disease but without trisomy 21. Vela Desojo et al. [53] also report an HAEC incidence of 50% in children suffering from Down syndrome and HD as against 8.5% in patients with that disease but without the Down syndrome. This high incidence of HAEC has been confirmed by several workers [6, 32, 54], and is due to Down syndrome children having a marked deficiency of cytotoxic T-cells and interferon production. as well as a diminished non-specific immune response which predisposes them to such infectious processes as enterocolitis [55]. To this should be added the delay in diagnosing HD in these children because of, among other things, preoccupation with the treatment of other malformations such as cardiopathies, and the constipation that these patients usually suffer due to their hypotonia or hypothyroidism [55].

Long Segment Aganglionosis

In some series, there was a higher incidence of HAEC in patients with long segment HD [30,33,45,56]. Surana et al. [36] found a 28% incidence of HAEC in patients with rectosigmoid involvement compared to 38% with long segment aganglionosis or total colonic aganglionosis. These findings are consistent with our experience [28, 57]. But other workers [6,17,20,27,38] have not confirmed these results.

Family History

A family history of HD is known to predispose to HAEC [3,58]. In the series of Carneiro et al. [27], 57% of the patients (4 out of 7) with a family history of this disease presented enterocolitis compared to 29% (20 out of 69) with no such family history. This may be because long segment aganglionosis predominates in familiar HD [3].

Associated Congenital Anomalies

Increased incidence of enterocolitis has been observed in patients with HD and associated congenital anomalies (cardiac, gastrointestinal, genitourinary, or central nervous system) [3]. In the series of Carneiro et al. [27], of 76 patients with HD, 15 had associated abnormalities (cardiopathy being the most common), and 53% of those presented HAEC compared with 26% of the patients without associated anomalies. These findings have been confirmed by Elhalaby et al. [11] who observed an HAEC incidence of 47% in patients with associated congenital anomalies compared with 29% of those without abnormalities. This increased incidence of HAEC may be because both works included many patients with Down syndrome who were not studied as a separate group. One of our patients with Waardenburg syndrome and HD, with a history of preoperative enterocolitis, presented a severe episode of HAEC immediately postoperative [59].

Previous Episodes of Enterocolitis

Previous episodes of HAEC have been regarded as a risk factor for the recurrence of this complication [17, 19, 20, 60]. It was speculated that the early appearance of enterocolitis in HD could permanently alter the bowel's defence mechanisms. and thus predispose the patient to recurrent episodes [3]. Nonetheless, other studies [6, 27, 61] have not confirmed this relationship.

Postoperative Risk Factors

Ten risk factors were evaluated by Hackman et al. [2] in patients with HAEC (n=33) and a control group without HAEC (n=56 patients). Risk factors were examined in three areas. Patient factors (gender, age at diagnosis, age and weight at pull-through), technical factors (type of repair, number of stages, location of transition zone, previous HAEC), and mechanical factors (stricture or leakage at the coloanal anastomosis, bowel obstruction requiring lysis of adhesion). Factors related to the patient (diagnosis of HD after the first week of life) and the type of surgical technique have no influence on the occurrence of postoperative HAEC [2]. But it has been shown that mechanical factors (intestinal obstruction due to adherences, neuronal intestinal dysplasia, anastomotic stenosis, or incomplete resection of the aganglionosis) are specific risk factors for the development of postoperative HAEC [2].

Menezes et al. [42], in reviewing their cases of HD (259 patients), only describe the association with Down syndrome as being a risk factor for postoperative HAEC, and noted that the greater frequency of this complication that they found in total colonic aganglionoses was not significantly different from that of other types of aganglionosis. Neither did the type of surgical technique influence the incidence of postoperative HAEC [42].

Table 3. Type of pull-through and HAEC.

Type of pull-through	% HAEC
Swenson (n=82)	21 (25.6)
Soave (n=88)	24 (27.3)
Duhamel (n=61)	19 (31.2)
Transanal (n=10)	4 (40)
	M Mnezes [42]

Table 4. Transanal pull-through and HAEC.

Author	N° patients (HD)	N° patients (EC)*	% HAEC
De la Torre [64]	10	0	0
Langer [51]	141	9	6.3
Elhalaby [40]	149	26	17.4
Zhang [65]	3	3	5.1
Antao [66]	2	2	33.3

* EC=Enterocolitis

Type of Pull-Through and Enterocolitis

Carneiro et al. [27] report a low incidence of postoperative HAEC with the Duhamel procedure. Kleinhaus et al. [20]. Ikeda et al. [45], and Bai et al. [62] describe a higher frequency of this complication with the Swenson technique. But since this technique has been modified to use a more distal colonic anastomosis, in most recent series the incidence of post-pull-through HAEC is found to have no relationship with the type of surgical technique or the timing of the definitive intervention [2, 27, 36, 61, 63]. Tables 3 and 4 present the data for the incidence of enterocolitis in HD and the type of pull-through in different studies [40, 42,51, 64, 65, 66].

Pathology

The gross pathology of HAEC was described initially by Harald Hirschsprung as follows: "There is full-thickness ulceration penetrating to the serosa, abscess formation in the submucosa, and mottled submucosal spaces containing pus" [8].

Microscopically, the HAEC is characterized by infiltration of the intestinal crypts by neutrophils (cryptitis) and abscess formation in the intestinal crypts. Retention of mucus with dilation of the crypt is often observed [67]. In the evolution of this complication there is an increase in abscesses in the crypts, ulceration of the mucosa, and eventually transmural necrosis and perforated bowel [67]. Late stages are indistinguishable from ulcerative colitis [3]. The abscesses in the crypts are observed both in the aganglionic and the ganglionic segments [67].

Teitelbaum et al. [67] proposed in 1989 a histopathological classification of HAEC, with varying degrees of evolution (Table 5) from Grade 0 = no pathological alterations observed, to Grade V = necrosis or perforated bowel. Of their patients, 88% (16 out of 18) presented grade III enterocolitis (multiple crypt abscesses) or higher. Their control group consisted of 18 patients without clinical evidence of HAEC, and 86% were classified as Grade II or lower by histological study of a rectal biopsy.

Table 5. Pathological grading of HAEC [67].

Grade	Pathological Findings
0	No abnormalities
I	Crypt dilatation and mucin retention
II	Cryptitis or < 2 crypt abscesses per high-power field
III	Multiple crypt abscesses per high-power field
IV	Fibrinopurulent debris and mucosal ulceration
V	Transluminal necrosis or perforation

Ischæmic enterocolitis is an infrequent finding in association with HD, and the reported cases concern term infants with septic shock [68]. It is possible that inadequate infusion and intestinal distension led to the ischæmic changes observed in the intestine of these patients [3]. Carneiro et al. [27] observed in 5 infants that the colitis associated with Hirschsprung's disease evolved to necrotizing enterocolitis with radiological evidence of intestinal pneumatosis.

The association of pseudomembranous colitis (PMC) and HD was originally described by Thomas et al. [69], who referred to the role of *Clostridium difficile* in the ætiology of HAEC. Brearly et al. [70] also observed this complication of HD. In their series of 72 patients with this disease, 26 presented HAEC and in 7 of them there were histological alterations consistent with PMC. The alterations were in both the aganglionic and ganglionic segments. The clinical picture of PMC is indistinguishable from that of inflammatory colitis which are more typically associated with HD, but the mortality of PMC in this series was greater (43%) than the mortality of HAEC (23%) [70]. Since the PMC of these HD patients was not related to previous administration of antibiotics, those authors considered that the disease itself predisposed to this type of colitis [70].

Theories of Pathogenesis

The possible causes of HAEC have been extensively investigated, but little progress has been made in understanding the pathogenesis of this complication [3, 5–7, 21–26]. Its origin is thought to be multifactorial [5]. Various theories have been proposed to explain its genesis – partial mechanical obstruction of the aganglionic intestine, infectious causes (*Rotavirus*, *C. difficile*), defects in the intestinal mucosal barrier, enterocyte adherence, bacterial translocation, immunological defects of the intestinal wall, alterations in intestinal motility, increased prostaglandin-E1 activity, Schwartzman-type reaction, and intestinal ischæmia [3. 5,48]. Local antigens appear to be the main stimulants of the histopathological changes [5].

Mechanical Obstruction

In 1962, Bill and Chapman [17] related HAEC with partial mechanical obstruction of the aganglionic segment causing chronic distension of the colon, fæcal stasis, and intestinal ischæmia. They based their opinion on the experience of colitis with other forms of intestinal obstruction [17]. According to this hypothesis, the HAEC would only affect the dilated proximal ganglionic segment. However this theory explains neither HAEC of the distal colon in patients with colostomy nor postoperative episodes of HAEC [5,41].

Furthermore, when Glotzer et al. [71] tried to reproduce enterocolitis experimentally in dogs by creating an artificial obstruction in the colon, they observed only two of the anatomo-pathological characteristics of enterocolitis – the local inflammation and the multiple ulceration of the mucosa. They did not find the large amount of mucosity, or the numerous abscesses in the intestinal crypts which are the typical lesions of HAEC.

Harrison et al. [72] reported that post-pull-through HAEC might be attributable in part to spasm of the internal anal sphincter, and Swenson [18] noted that partial sphinceromyotomy resolved the enteritis. In a recent study however, Rintala et al. [73] noted that none of their patients with chronic or recurrent post-pull-through HAEC presented intestinal stenosis, and the anal sphincter pressures were similar in all the children with HD, whether or not they had HAEC.

The above discussion notwithstanding, partial mechanical obstruction caused by the aganglionic segment in the period prior to surgery, and postoperative obstruction due to anastomotic stenosis, incomplete resection of the aganglionosis, intestinal adherences, or associated neuronal intestinal dysplasia, are seen as specific risk factors for HAEC. Hackman et al [2] studied the risk factors for postoperative enterocolitis and found that both the presence of anastomotic leak or stricture and the development of postoperative intestinal obstruction secondary to adhesions increased the relative risk and subsequent enterocolitis by approximately 3-fold. These risk factors increase intestinal stasis and create the cycle (stasis–bacterial overgrowth–mucosal invasion) leading to the subsequent local and systemic inflammatory response [2]. Nonetheless, other factors participate in the ætiopathogenesis of HAEC, some of them still not well known [2, 3, 5].

Infection

The ætiology of infection (bacterial and viral) has been proposed by various authors as a cause of HAEC. Thomas et al. [69] reported that the cytopathic toxin of *C. difficile* (CD) was present with higher incidence and concentrations in the fæces of children with HAEC than in healthy patients. Also, all patients with severe HAEC had positive toxin in the stool. In another study [27], all the patients with CD toxin in the stool (63% of patients with HAEC) responded to the oral or stoma administration of vancomycin.

Hardy et al. [74] found that children with HD had CD positive stool for a longer period (>12 months of age) compared to the absence of this germ in healthy patients of this age. This suggests that patients with HD have more difficulty in eliminating this germ and may be more susceptible to infections caused by it [6]. Other studies [36, 67, 73] have found, however, that few patients with HD had CD in the fæces, suggesting that these patients' susceptibility to infection was more important than the mere presence of the pathogens themselves. Furthermore, it has been found that more than 90% of healthy infants have CD in fæces, and many secrete the toxin, suggesting that the pathogen alone does not cause HAEC [75]. When intestinal motility is altered, there is an overgrowth of bacteria which could cause excessive growth of these pathogens. The entero-invasive property of an organism, which allows it to penetrate the epithelial barrier of the intestinal mucosa, may be more important than the type of germ.

Thomas et al. [76] reported that healthy infants are colonized by CD from their own intestinal flora, which changes with age. Patients with HD have greater difficulty in eliminating this germ. Those authors find that the role of CD in the ætiology of HAEC seems to be clear, especially in children under 3 years of age. It has been suggested that a secretional and motor abnormality may cause overgrowth of CD. While the colonization of the gastrointestinal tract by CD is well tolerated by healthy infants, it may pose a threat to patients with HD [70, 76].

Wilson-Story et al. [22] reported rotaviruses in the fæces of 77% of patients with HAEC. The immunological defence against rotaviruses depends on the IgA in the intestinal wall. Rotaviruses are thought to play a role in the pathogenesis of HAEC that may be related to deficiencies in the host defence mechanisms [22].

Golderman et al. [78] found that enterocyte adherence allows microorganisms to invade the epithelial barrier. In a study of patients with HAEC, histology showed enterocyte adherence in 39%, with the most frequent organisms being *Escherichia coli*, *C. difficile*, and *Cryptosporidium* [67]. Suita et al. [41], in a review of HD in Japan (3852 cases), observed a broad spectrum of germs in the fæces cultures of 69 patients with preoperative HAEC (Table 6)

Table 6. Pathogenic organisms of preoperative enterocolitis in 69 patients with HD [37].

Organism	Nº Patients	%
Escherichia Coli	21	30.4
Staphylococcus Aureus	14	20.3
Klesiella Pneumoniae	7	10.1
Enterococcus fecalis	6	8.7
Clostridium difficile	5	7.2
Pseudomonas aeruginosa	5	7.2
Klesiella oxytoca	4	5.8
Enterobacter cloacae	3	4.3
Enterophatogenic E Coli	2	2.9
Staphylococcus epidermidis	2	2.9

A wide variety of immune system abnormalities have been suggested in children with HD which can make them prone to pathogen and commensal infection [78]. These alterations include impaired white blood cell [79] and immunoglobulin S-IgA [80] function, and decreased acidic sulfomucin secretion in the intestine [81, 82]. These immune system abnormalities in children with HD could make them more susceptible to developing severe enterocolitis with more serious sequelae.

Imamura et al. [83] argue that the diversity of local alterations in response to enterocolitis reflects a multifactorial microbiological ætiology. They recommend studies of the fæcal microorganisms. including bacteria (*C. difficile*) and viruses (*Rotavirus*), in all patients with HAEC.

Defective Mucosal Barrier

The luminal surface of the intestinal tract is covered by a layer of mucous gel that acts as a lubricant, protects against mechanical trauma, and is the first line of defence against potential pathogens, toxins, and foreign bodies [84]. The mucus, which in the colon is water insoluble, is composed of many glycoproteins, 80% consisting of carbohydrates and the rest of peptides. These are responsible for the viscoelastic properties of the mucus. It also contains secretory immunoglobulin A (S-IgA) which protects the intestine against bacteria and viruses by binding and inactivating them, thus preventing their entry into the epithelial cells [48,84, 85, 86].

In patients with HD, mucus retention is observed in the glands of the aganglionic segment and in the ganglionic intestine [48]. In the initial stages of HAEC there is dilation of the mucous glands with accumulation of mucus [48]. Clearly, an abnormal barrier of mucus can contribute to enterocolitis in patients with HD [48]. Akkary et al. [81], and subsequently Teitelbaum et al. [48], observed a loss of acidic sulfomucins and an increase in neutral mucus in sections of the colon mucosa in patients with HAEC. The association of sulfate loss and inflammatory bowel processes is well known [3]. Alterations in the concentrations of sulfate and sialic acid contained in the glycoproteins of the mucus leave the mucosal barrier more susceptible to degradation by the normal intestinal flora and pathogenic bacteria [87]. Likewise, the deficient secretion of acidic sulfomucins allows increased adhesion of such enteropathic organisms as *C. difficile* or *E. coli*, causing increased susceptibility to bacterial invasion of the intestinal wall when bacterial toxins can then begin the process of HAEC [67,84,81].

Abnormalities have been observed in the protective barrier of mucus in the proximal ganglionic intestine after the definitive operation [67]. This may explain the presentation of enterocolitis after pull-through and recurrent episodes of HAEC [67]. Aslan [85], in an extensive study of the mucus barrier in patients with HAEC, noted that there were changes in the secretion of mucus in both the ganglionic and aganglionic segments of the intestine. He noted a reduction in the production of mucin (detected by metabolic markers with [35S]-sulfate and [3H]-glucosamine) in cells in the aganglionic and ganglionic intestine as compared with a control group of the same age [85, 86]. Since the production of mucin is reduced. the quality and quantity of the mucus of the intestinal barrier is compromised [87, 88]. The physical protection and immune function – the organism's first line of defence – are damaged, leaving the patient susceptible to bacterial invasion and colonization [89]. In a prospective study of patients with HD, it was observed that there persisted after the definitive intervention a decreased production of mucus in the ganglionic intestine, and that it was this that principally predisposed the patient to suffer post-pull-through enterocolitis [87].

The MUC-2 gene is located on chromosome 11p15.5 [90] and is the most important with respect to the production of mucin in the human colon [91]. Mattar et al. [92] found MUC-2 protein expression in stool samples to be significantly lowered in patients with HD compared with controls. They reported that there were no levels of it in patients with enterocolitis and HD. The deficit in MUC-2 production of may lead to pathogenic bacteria invading the intestinal mucosa [86].

As they age, the patients lose their susceptibility to recurrent HAEC. This can be explained by the fact that the defensive mucus barrier in healthy children is lower at 3 months of age than at 3 years, and that with the increase in age this barrier becomes stronger and has an increased production of mucin [89]. The older child is better prepared to resist bacterial invasion of the mucosa, and the barrier provides greater protection against toxins and foreign bodies.

The secretion of mucus is partially under the control of the autonomic nervous system [93]. Soeda et al. [94] showed a reduction of neuroendocrine cells in patients with HAEC compared with controls. The weak defensive barrier of mucus in HD may be due to abnormalities in the autonomic nervous system and a reduction of neuroendocrine cells in the ganglionic intestine. This would explain the low secretion of mucus and disturbances in motility frequently observed after surgery in patients with HD.

In a recent study, Lui et al. [95] suggested that a defect in the mucus layer may cause a loss of integrity of the mucosa due to proliferation and defective differentiation of epithelial cells. The CDX genes (CDX-1 and CDX-2) control the proliferation and differentiation of cells in the intestinal mucosa. That study found that the expression of both genes in the epithelial cells of the colon mucosa was reduced in patients with HAEC. This suggests that this reduced expression of these genes in the mucosa may be associated with the development of HAEC.

Enterocyte Adherence

The adherence of the bacteria to the intestine is the first stage in the initiation of many intestinal infections, and seems to be the main way in which microorganisms can access the epithelial barrier [96]. Teitelbaum & Coran [67] found that 39% of patients in their study (38 patients with HD) with clinical HAEC showed enterocyte adherence in the histological study of the tissues involved in the procedure. All these patients had Grade III or higher HAEC. Specific immunological and histo-chemical methods showed entero-adherent microorganisms in the dilated crypts and pseudomembrane areas. Enterocyte adherence was observed in none of the control group patients (18 patients with HD without enterocolitis). The entero-adherent organisms observed included *E. coli* (5), *C. difficile* (1), and *Cryptosporidium* (1). Serum titres of toxins were positive in two patients: *E. coli* verotoxin (1:16) and *C. difficile* cytotoxin. Five of these seven infants (71%) with enterocyte adherence died of sepsis and coagulopathy [67]. It seems that the adherent nature of the microorganism is more important than the microorganism itself [48].

Intestinal Immune Defences

Once the pathogen has adhered to the intestinal epithelium, it still has to overcome the immune defence mechanism of the mucosa to penetrate the intestinal wall [48]. This mechanism consists of humoural immunity, i.e., secretory IgA (S-IgA), and cellular immunity, i.e., the T-lymphocytes located in the epithelium, lamina propria, lymphoid follicles (Peyer's patches), and mesenteric lymph nodes [48]. In HD, alterations in both cellular and humoural immunity have been described which could be a cause of HAEC [79]. That study found decreased white blood cell counts and function in patients with HAEC compared to other patients. as well as decreased serum complement and IgA.

Wilson-Storey & Scobie [80] observed that patients with HD had apparently normal S-IgA levels in the lamina propria, but those with HAEC presented a deficient release of IgA into the intestinal lumen. Imamura et al. [83] studied the IgA, IgM, and J-chains in plasma cells of patients with HAEC, and noted increased amounts of these immunoglobulins. Nonetheless, they observed low levels of the secretory components in the lumen of the aganglionic colon in patients with HAEC, suggesting that it could be due to a defect in the release of these immunoglobulins. Another study [97] showed low levels of IgA in the lamina propria of patients with HD, and even lower in the patients with HAEC.

In an experimental model of HD in mice (the piebald lethal strain) it was observed that the animals with enterocolitis had low serum levels of S-IgA [98, 99]. This suggests that the decline in levels of S-IgA may be the result of enterocolitis and not its cause [48].

In two studies of the T-lymphocyte and natural killer cell immune system [83, 98], high intestinal levels of T-lymphocytes were found in patients with HAEC compared to other HD patients without this complication. There was a significant increase of natural killer cells in the lamina propria of the ganglionic intestine of patients with HAEC compared with HD patients without enterocolitis and control patients [83].

Nitric oxide, which has several non-specific defence actions against bacteria. Mycobacteria, and viral agents, has a reduced production in the aganglionic segment [100]. This could contribute to the development of enterocolitis. It is well known that patients with trisomy 21 and HD have a high risk of enterocolitis. An intrinsic immune deficiency has been observed, with diminished function of the cytotoxic T-lymphocytes and impaired humoural immunity [101.102].

Abnormal Bowel Motility

Intestinal peristalsis protects against bacterial translocation (bacterial invasion of the intestinal wall) because it prevents stasis and the consequent prolonged presence of bacteria in the intestinal lumen and mucus. In the absence of intestinal motility, there is an increase in the number of bacteria that adhere directly to the enterocytes.

Neuronal intestinal dysplasia (NID) has been observed in the proximal ganglionic colon in 20% to 75% of patients [29,103]. For other workers [48] and in our experience, however, this association is less frequent. There is evidence that if at the time of the pull-through the aganglionic segment and the NID segment are not completely extirpated, the patient may suffer alterations of intestinal motility and postoperative HAEC [29,48].

Suzuki et al. [104] used endothelin receptor null rats as a model for long-segment HD in which they produced a mega-ileum proximal to the aganglionic segment. They noted that the number of macrophages increased in the tunica muscularis, suggesting that they may play an important role in the inflammation of this tissue in rats. They postulated that the increased number and activation of the macrophages could injure the interstitial cells of Cajal, and cause intestinal motility disorders in the region of the intestine where the myenteric ganglia are normal. These alterations in motility may cause fæcal stasis, bacterial overgrowth, and mucus abnormalities with increased bacterial translocation.

Porras et al. [105], in a model of enteritis in rats, observed that when there occurs a bacterial invasion of the intestinal wall (bacterial translocation), intestinal motility is diminished, and there is an increase in the indicators (leukocytes) in the blood of the inflammatory process.

Schwartzman Reaction

In 1968, Berry & Fraser [106] suggested that the enterocolitis might be initiated by a Schwartzman-type reaction caused by intraluminal organisms invading the submucosa. In a rabbit experimental model of HD, they noted that injecting endotoxin directly into the bowel proximal to the obstruction led to enterocolitis in most of the animals (6 out of 9). According to this theory, patients with HD would be hypersensitive to bacterial antigens.

Figure 2 shows an algorithm representing the possible pathogenesis of HAEC.

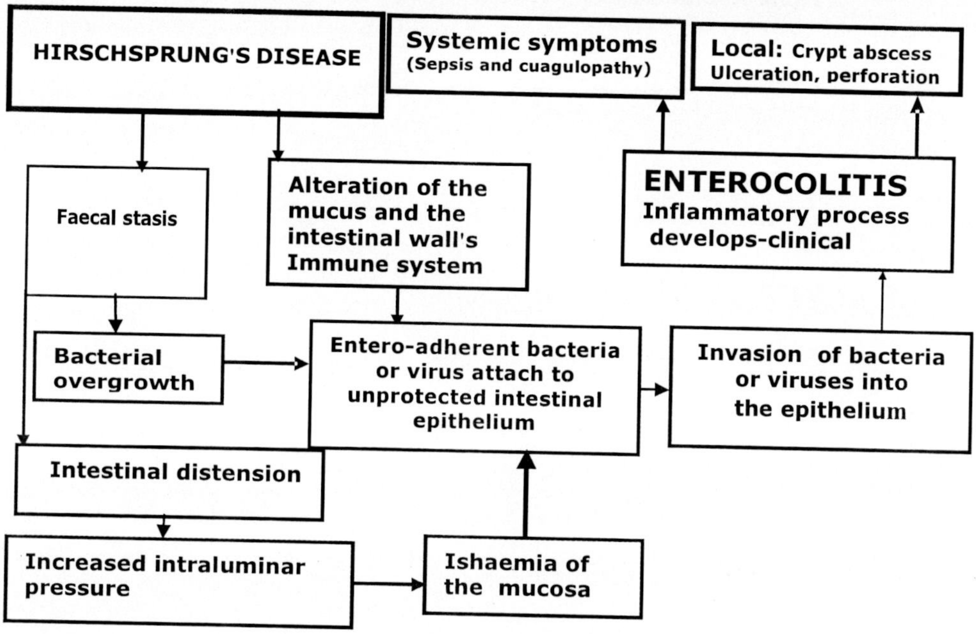

Figure 2. Possible pathophysiologic for development of HAEC.

Clinical Manifestations

The clinical manifestations of Hirschsprung-associated enterocolitis cover a spectrum of presentation that runs from mild episodes of abdominal distension to explosive diarrhœa with perforated bowel, sepsis, fulminant shock, and exitus [44]. Thus, the clinical presentation can be mild, moderate, or fulminant. Its natural, untreated, evolution is towards perforated bowel and septic and/or hypovolæmic shock.

Bill & Chapman [17] were the first to describe the clinical features of HAEC. The manifestations they described included abdominal distension, fever, and foul-smelling stool. Preoperative enterocolitis and post-pull-through enterocolitis have a similar clinical picture. In the neonate. enterocolitis may be the first clinical manifestation of HD, and is usually characterized by a more than 48-hour delay in passing the meconium, vomiting, and abdominal distension. Table 7 lists the clinical aspects of HAEC that have been reported by various workers and Table 8 gives the early and late symptoms of this complication.

Many cases of diarrhœa or abdominal distension may be misdiagnosed as gastroenteritis or the obstructing sphincter syndrome; however, most of these are cases of mild enterocolitis. Elhalaby et al. [107] proposed a grading system based on clinical criteria (Table 9) to facilitate the diagnosis of enterocolitis. Examination will show a markedly distended abdomen that is hyperresonant to percussion. Rectal examination often results in an explosive discharge of flatus and stool.

Table 7. Clinical manifestations of HAEC [27,36,38]

Clinical features	% patients
Diarrhoea (foul smelling, explosive, and watery)	80-100
Abdominal distension	30-83
Vomiting	10-77
Explosive expulsion of flatus and liquid on rectal examination	30-69
Abdominal pain	20-30
Pyrexia	11-50
Lethargy	30
Blood in stools	2.5-10
Bowel perforation	2-5

Table 8. Symptoms of HAEC [7].

Early	**Late**
Abdominal distension	Emesis
Foul-smelling, watery stool	Fever
Lethargy	Haematochezia
Poor feeding	Shock or death

Table 9. Clinical grading system for HAEC.

Grade	*Clinical symptoms*
I	Mild explosive diarrhoea; mild or moderate abdominal distension; no systemic manifestations
II	Moderate explosive diarrhoea; moderate to severe abdominal distension; mild systemic symptoms
III	Severe explosive diarrhoea; marked abdominal distension; shock or impending shock

Diagnosis

It is very important to recognize HAEC early to reduce morbidity and mortality. HAEC must be suspected in a term newborn with delayed (>48 hours) meconium passage, whose symptoms commence with abdominal distension, vomiting, and watery stools [108]. Digital rectal manipulation, at least in rectosigmoid disease, causes the forceful discharge of flatus and liquid fæces.

Although in the majority of patients the diagnosis can be made easily on clinical evaluation, plain abdominal radiographs are the most useful investigation. Simple anterior-posterior and lateral decubitus abdominal radiographs can show thickening of the bowel wall, mucosal edema, abnormal air-fluid levels, dilated bowel loops, pneumatosis intestinalis or sings of perforation (Fig.4A and 4 B) [3]. Elhalaby et al. [11] assessed 150 plain radiographs acquired during and between episodes of HAEC. Colon dilatation was the most radiologically sensitive sign (90%), but it had a specificity of only 24%. "Intestinal cut-off" sign which appears when the gaseous intestinal dilatation is abruptly cut off at the pelvic brim was both sensitive (74%) and specific (86%) for HAEC. Because of risk of perforation, a contrast enema should not be used in the presence of clinical enterocolitis. Nonetheless, it is not unusual to see findings of subclinical enterocolitis during such radiological studies.

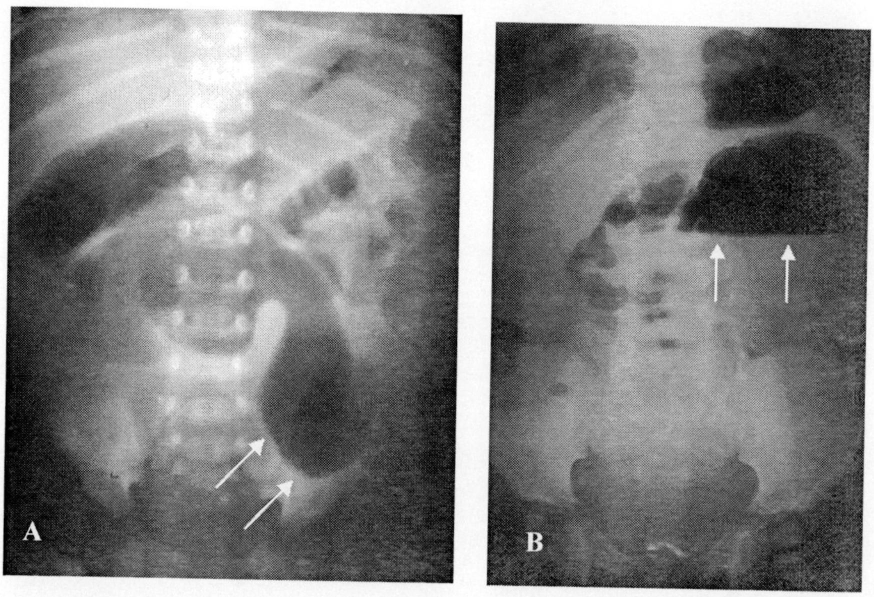

Figure 4. A. This plain abdominal x-ray film from infant with preoperative Hirschsprung's-associated enterocolitis, shows a typical intestinal "cut-off" sign (arrows) with no gas seen in the pelvis. B. Plain abdominal x-ray film. HAEC episode in a patient with Down syndrome and total colonic aganglionosis treated by the Kimura technique. One observes an air-fluid level *(arrows)* as well as the mechanical suture.

A barium enema in a patient with HAEC can demonstrate mucosal nodularity, ulceration and edema, speculation, narrowing of the anorectal junction and colonic dilatation. Typically, an irregular mucosal lining, with a resultant 'sawtooth' appearance, is seen (Fig. 5).

Rectal biopsy may be performed as part of the investigation for HAEC, but is not recommended during the fulminant phase as there is high risk of perforation [3]. The biopsy may show the classical pattern of enterocolitis, but also serves to confirm that ganglion cells are present after the pull-through procedure, and some workers have reported NID in association with HD, which may contribute to the development of enterocolitis [29,103]. Necrotizing enterocolitis (NEC) in term infants should raise suspicion, and a rectal suction biopsy should be performed. HD should also be considered in some premature infants with NEC, as this may be a presenting feature [3].

Chronic enterocolitis is characterized by persistent diarrhœa or loose stools, soiling, intermittent abdominal distension, nausea, vomiting, and poor feeding leading to failure to thrive [3]. Recurrent bouts of enterocolitis after pull-through surgery should be investigated by contrast enema, endoscopy, and rectal biopsy to exclude a mechanical cause such as obstruction in the neo-rectum or residual segment of aganglionic bowel [3].

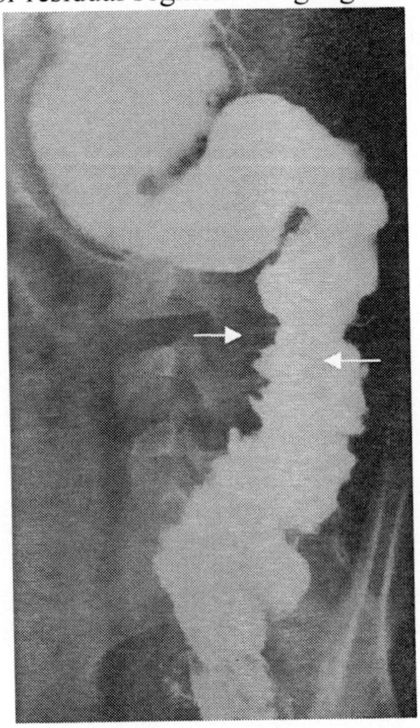

Figure 5. Contrast enema after the acute phase of HAEC. Two-year-old patient with rectosigmoid aganglionosis treated by the Rehbein technique. Sawtooth edges on the colon wall *(arrows)*. There is no evidence of anastomotic stenosis.

In patients with enterocolitis, studies should be carried out for bacteria (*C. difficile*) and viruses (*Rotavirus*) in the fæces. Wang et al. [4] recommend determining the presence of T-antigen (marker for anaerobic bacterial infection) in patients with recurrent HAEC.

The differential diagnosis of HAEC should be against acute gastroenteritis, postoperative complications such as intestinal adherences, and intra-abdominal abscesses [3].

Treatment

The treatment of HAEC must be adapted to its degree of evolution. In the initial management, decompression of the bowel by rectal washouts or a stoma are imperative. Also, in acute fulminant enterocolitis, a priority is hydrotherapy to correct electrolyte imbalance, and the administration of intravenous antibiotics against anaerobes and Gram-negative aerobes (metronidazol or vancomycin, and an aminoglucoside) [3, 5, 48,109].

In patients with HAEC, especially newborn, whose intestine can not be adequately decompressed with colon washouts, or if there is clinical worsening, immediate laparotomy is called for and the formation of a stoma (colostomy or ileostomy) proximal to the transition zone. Biopsies should be taken to ascertain whether the stoma has been situated in the ganglionic intestine [3]. In cases of very severe enterocolitis in which the colon has a gangrenous appearance. total colectomy may be necessary [3].

Orvar Swenson [12, 18, 19] was the first to suggest that the initial approach to HAEC. regardless of the patient's age, should be the placement of a rectal catheter to decompress the colon. The catheter must be soft and multiperforated to facilitate drainage, and of a large bore (12–18 Fr) according to the age of the patient. In preoperative enterocolitis, the catheter is inserted through the anus and advanced gently, simultaneously injecting a small quantity of serum, until the tip surpasses the aganglionic segment and is situated in the dilated colon. In postoperative patients, the catheter is advanced until it begins to drain flatus and liquid fæces.

The decompression of the colon is done by irrigation, using the same lukewarm saline serum with bolus of 20 to 50 ml depending on the size of the infant. to total volumes of 100 to 150 ml for this age. The serum is suctioned out or left to emerge spontaneously through the rectal catheter, the aim being for it to clean and empty the entire contents of the colon. In older children, volumes of between 500 to 1000 ml of normal saline are usually necessary for irrigation of the colon to be effective. The rectal irrigation procedure is repeated 3 or 4 times a day until complete decompression of the colon has been achieved and the patient shows clear clinical improvement.

Rectal washouts should be avoided in fulminant enterocolitis due to the risk of perforation of the colon. One should not use either phosphate enemas due to the risk of toxicity [3], or saline enemas without a rectal catheter because they may worsen the enterocolitis [3].

To reduce the morbidity and mortality of enterocolitis, it needs to be diagnosed early. The family need to know the early symptoms of enterocolitis so that. if they arise, the child is taken to their doctor or the hospital. Before the child's discharge, the parents should be instructed in the technique of rectal irrigation. so that they can do it at home. In mild and even moderate enterocolitis (Grades I-II). rectal washouts alone may be sufficient to resolve this complication.

Patients with severe acute HAEC need to be hospitalized. In addition to the bowel decompression (with nasogastric tube and colon washouts), intravenous fluids need to be administered to prevent dehydration and hypovolæmic shock. In patients with slow evolution, digestive repose and parenteral feeding may be indicated. One should administer intravenous antibiotics which cover *C. difficile* [69, 70], such as metronidazol or vancomycin. These can also be administered orally, in a rectal enema, or through the stoma if the patient has one [3].

The administration of cholestyramine resin may be useful to bind *C. difficile*, and neutralize the effect of prostaglandin E which causes water and electrolytes to be lost into the intestinal lumen [110].

There is no experience with probiotics for the treatment of HAEC. Herek [111] suggests that the association of *Saccharomyces boulardii* (S.b.) – a probiotic widely used in cases of antibiotic-associated diarrhœa [112, 113] – with the routine treatment of enterocolitis may be useful in cases of *C. difficile* toxin positive stools. This probiotic stimulates the production of S-IgA, and increases the resistance of the mucosa to enteropathogenic bacterial infections, as well as inhibiting the effects of toxins A and B of *C. difficile* in the human colon mucosa [[112–115]. Recent studies [115, 116] have shown that treatment of *C. difficile* enteritis with the combination of metronidazol or vancomycin plus S.b. eliminates the chance of recurrence. which is not the case if only the standard therapy (intravenous metronidazol or vancomycin) is used.

Mattar et al. [92] observed that *Lactobacillus casei* GG increases the epithelial expression of MUC-2, and hence mucin secretion, thereby reducing the risk of bacterial translocation and enterocolitis. Recently, Tatekawa et al. [117] reported a patient with near total intestinal aganglionosis treated by Ziegler myectomy who had recurring enteritis. They were able to control the bacterial enteritis and translocation in this patient with the symbiotic use of three agents – *Bifidobacterium breve* Yakult (BBG-1), *L. casei* Shirota (Biolactis Powder), and galactooligosaccharides (Oligomate HP).

Most patients with chronic or recurrent enterocolitis can be managed with conservative measures such as rectal washouts, oral metronidazol, and a residue- and lactose-free diet to reduce bacterial overgrowth [3, 56, 73]. Post-pull-through sugar intolerance has been observed in HD patients. due to disaccharidase deficiencies [118].

Rintala & Lindahl [73] treated 8 patients with chronic or recurrent post-pull-through enterocolitis by administering sodium cromoglycate (SCG). Four patients had Down syndrome, and two others bore chromosomal abnormalities. The doses of SCG used were: 100 mg four times a day in 6 patients. and 200 mg four times a day in the other two of 10 and 22 years in age. The duration of the treatment was 6 weeks. Five (60%) of the patients responded positively to the treatment with a decrease in the frequency of bowel motions and more solid consistency of stool leading to diminished soiling. Exacerbations of enterocolitis requiring hospital admission and antibiotics were abolished in the median follow-up period of 14 months. The 3 patients with recurrent enterocolitis responded favourably.

Nonetheless, some cases of chronic enterocolitis may be caused by stenosis of the anastomosis, the persistence of a residual aganglionic segment, or the presence of neuronal intestinal dysplasia (NID) associated with the HD [48, 119]. Investigation of these possible causes begins with an opaque enema, and if this is normal it is followed by a rectal biopsy. If the biopsy rules out the residual aganglionosis and NID. Wildhaber et al. [119] propose a posterior anal myotomy or myectomy. They also believe that non-invasive options should be tried such as the topical administration of nitric oxide or the injection of botulinum toxin into the internal sphincter [119]. With this technique (myotomy or myectomy), favourable results were obtained in 75% of patients, leaving them free of the symptoms of chronic enterocolitis. These findings are consistent with the experience of Polley et al. [120] and of Marty et al. [121] who describe favourable results from performing sphincteromyotomies in children with chronic enterocolitis. Nonetheless. these last authors recommend waiting for a significant period of time using just conservative measures, since, in most children with postoperative enterocolitis, the episodes decrease as the child gets older.

Swenson et al. [18] initially showed enthusiasm for partial anal sphincterotomy to treat enterocolitis, since it resolved the sphincter hypertonia that they observed in some of these patients. Subsequently, however, they appreciated that the results were not so favourable [19]. In one of our patients with chronic post-pull-through enterocolitis, anal sphincterotomy was not effective [28]. In others, we observed clinical improvement in enterocolitis after forced anal dilatation.

A redo-pull-through may be indicated in patients with chronic enterocolitis due to residual aganglionosis, stenosis of the anastomosis, twisted pull-through of the colon, or the presence of NID, and is as effective as the primary pull-through in terms of frequency and continence of defæcation. resolving the episodes of HAEC [5, 119]

Prevention

Despite the great advances in the treatment of HD, little is known about the ætiology of enterocolitis associated with this condition and how it can be prevented [3, 28]. Early diagnosis of HD in the first days of life, immediate and effective intestinal decompression by means of nursing care or through a stoma, and the definitive surgery in the first few months of life, have all contributed to the near eradication of preoperative enterocolitis [6, 7,28,41, 122–126]. In our experience [127] and that of other workers [128], anorectal manometry is very useful for the early suspicion of HD, which makes it possible to initiate decompression of the colon sooner. Suspicion of HD must always be confirmed by rectal suction biopsy [129].

Post-pull-through HAEC remains the greatest postoperative complication of HD, and no surgical technique can prevent it [2,27,28,42,61,66,130,131]. It has been suggested that exclusive transanal endorectal pull-through or laparoscopic pull-through to minimize the intestinal trauma decreases the risk of postoperative adherences and HAEC [2, 51,64,132-134]. Georgeson et al. [135] give an incidence of postoperative HAEC of 7.5% when they use laparoscopy for the definitive surgery in HD. Hakam et al. [2] noted that anastomotic stenosis is a specific risk factor for postoperative HAEC. They therefore consider that it is essential to routinely dilate the anal anastomosis with a Hegar's dilator to prevent its stenosis [2]. These dilations are begun at two weeks postoperative, and maintained for three to six months [2,28,44].

According to Estivao-Costa et al. [29], to minimize postoperative HAEC the aganglionic and the neuronal intestinal dysplasia (NID) segments should be resected at the time of pull-through when this anomaly is associated with HD They diagnose the NID before the definitive operation by full-thickness biopsies for histochemical colonic mapping taken by laparoscopy, or during the laparotomy if it was necessary to form a stoma [29]. They limit resection of the colon to its hepatic flexure [29].

Postoperative rectal irrigation, according to Marty et al. [30], Honchar [31], Danylov et al. [32], Teitelbaum et al. [33], and also in our experience [28], decreases the incidence and severity of episodes of HAEC. It eliminates fæcal stasis and prevents bacterial overgrowth. Marty et al. [30] begin the washouts between week 1 and week 2 postoperative, applying them twice daily for three months and once daily for a further 3 months. The volume of rectal irrigation is 10 ml/kg, although some children require more for effective evacuation. Table 10 presents the incidence and mortality of postoperative enterocolitis in 135 patients with HD, with or without rectal irrigation, according to the experience of Marty et al. [30].

Table 10: Incidence and mortality of postoperative enterocolitis in HD.

	N.° of patients in HD cohort	N° with postoperative enterocolitis	N° of deaths from postoperative enterocolitis
No irrigations	95	34	5
Postoperative irrigations	40	3*	0

P<0.001 *In these children. enterocolitis developed during the rectal irrigations.

Our method of post-pull-through rectal irrigation [28] is very similar to that of Marty et al. [30], but in patients with total colonic aganglionosis treated by ileocoloplasty we continue the treatment for 12 months or more because of the risk of enterocolitis in the first postoperative months.

Teitelbaum et al. [67] suggest that it may be useful to begin with antibiotic prophylaxis in those patients in whom the rectal biopsy showed Grade III or higher enterocolitis.

There is no experience with probiotics, prebiotics, or symbiotics for the prevention of HAEC. It is known that the bacteria that colonize the gut act as a control mechanism to prevent overgrowth of pathogenic organisms, forming a natural barrier that protects against infection [136]. Certain circumstances, such as alterations of intestinal peristalsis (aganglionosis) or intestinal stenosis, affect this balance, and there is increased susceptibility to intestinal infection. Probiotics contribute to restoring the intestinal microflora, enhance the immune response, and compete with pathogenic bacteria and sequester their toxins [137]. It would thus seem clear that they could potentially collaborate in preventing enterocolitis in HD. Herek [111] suggests that the probiotic *Saccharomyces boulardii* (a non-pathogenic yeast) might be useful for the prophylaxis of HAEC. According to Murphy & Puri [5] and Mattar et al. [92], the prophylactic use of the probiotic *Lactobacillus* GG can increase the epithelial expression of MUC-2, and reduce the risk of bacterial translocation. Nonetheless, before their use can be recommended, there need to be controlled and double-blind randomized studies.

We do not know what the future holds in terms of preventing enterocolitis in HD, but it is likely that correcting the abnormalities of the mucous barrier will play an important role. It may be that defective mucus could be replaced by a synthetic mucus, or its secretion improved by administering substances that stimulate production [3]. Also, it is to be hoped that in the future it will be possible to define the extent of the abnormal mucosa barrier of the ganglionic colon, and thus to resect during the pull-through procedure not only the aganglionic segment, but also the segment of ganglionic colon with a damaged mucus barrier. This would eliminate a probable cause of post-pull-through enterocolitis.

References

[1] Fraser GC, Berry C: Mortality in neonatal Hirschsprung's disease with particular reference to enterocolitis. *J Pediatr Surg*. 1967;2:205-11.

[2] Hackam DJ, Filler RM, Pear RH: Enterocolitis after the surgical treatment of Hirschsprung's disease: risk factors and financial impact. *J Pediatr Surg*.1998;33:830-3

[3] Vieten D, Spicer R: Enterocolitis complicating Hirschsprung's disease. *Semin Pediatr Surg*. 2004;13:263-72.
[4] Wang JS, Lee HC, Huang FY, Chang PY, Sheu JC: Unexpected mortality in pediatric patients with postoperative Hirschsprung's disease. *Pediatr Surg Int*.2004;20:525-8.
[5] Murphy F, Puri P: New insghts into the pathogenesis of Hirschsprung`s associated enterocolitis. *Pediatr Surg Int*. 2005;21:773-9.
[6] Teitelbaum DH, Qualman SJ, Caniano DA: Hirschsprung's disease. Identification of risk factors for enterocolitis. *Ann Surg*. 1988;207:240-4.
[7] Coran AG, Teitelbaum DH: Recent advances in the management of Hirschsprung's disease. *Am J Surg*.2000;180:382-7.
[8] Hirschsprung H: Stuhltragheit neugeborener infolge Dilatationen und hypertrophie des colons. *Tarbush Kinderheilkunde*. 1888;27:1-7
[9] Hiatt BR: The surgical treatment of congenital megacolon. *Ann Surg* 1951;133:321-9.
[10] Leon EE, Karshner RG: Hirschsprung's disease and congenital megacolon. *Calif Med* 1952; 76:276-80.
[11] Elhalaby EA, Coran AG, Blane CE, Hirschl RB, Teitelbaum DH: Enterocolitis associated with Hirschsprung's disease: a clinical-radiological characterization based on 168 patients. *J Pediatr Surg*. 1995; 30:76-83.
[12] Swenson O, Fisher JH: Hirschsprung's disease during infancy. *Surg Clin North Am*. 1956.36:115-22.
[13] Swenson O: Follow up on 200 patients treated for Hirschsprung's disease during a ten-year period. *Ann Surg*. 1957; 146:706-14.
[14] Wyllie GG: Treatment of Hirschsprung`disease by Swenson operation. *Lancet*. 1957; 1:850-5.
[15] Hiatt RB: A further description of pathologic physiology of congenital megacolon and results of surgical treatment. *Pediatrics*. 1958; 21:825-31.
[16] Swenson O, Fisher JH, Scott JE: Diarrhea following rectosigmoidectomy for Hirschsprung's disease. *Surgery*. 1960; 48:419-21.
[17] Bill AH, Chapman ND: The enterocolitis of Hirschsprung`disease. Its natural history and treatment. *Am J Surg*. 1962; 103:70-4.
[18] Swenson O: Partial internal Sphincterotomy in the treatment of Hirschsprung`disease. *Ann Surg*. 1964; 160:540-50.
[19] Swenson O. Sherman JO. Fisher JH. Cohen E: The treatment and postoperative complications of congenital megacolon: A 25 year followup. *Ann Surg*. 1975; 182:266-73.
[20] Kleinhaus S, Boley SJ, Sheran M, Sieber WK: Hirschsprung's disease -- a survey of the members of the Surgical Section of the American Academy of Pediatrics. *J Pediatr Surg*. 1979:14:588-97.
[21] Thomas DF, Fernie DS, Bayston R. Spitz L. Nixon HH: Enterocolitis in Hirschsprung's disease: a controlled study of the etiologic role of Clostridium difficile. *J Pediatr Surg*. 1986; 21:22-5.
[22] Wilson-Story D, Scobie WG, McGenity KG: Microbiological studies of the enterocolitis of Hirschsprung's disease. *Arch Dis Child*. 1990; 65:1338-9.

[23] Akkary S, Sahwy E, Kandil W, Hamdy MH: A histochemical study of the mucosubstances of the colon in cases of Hirschsprung's disease with and without enterocolitis. *J Pediatr Surg*. 1981; 16:664-8.

[24] Aslam A, Spicer RD, Corfield AP: Biochemical analysis of colonic mucin glycoproteins in children with Hirschsprung disease show disease specific alterations. *Biochem Soc Trans*. 1997;25:8S.

[25] Armstrong GR, Raafat F: Humoral reaction in the inflamed colon in Hirschsprung's disease and ulcerative colitis. *J Clin Pathol* 1988; 41:975-7.

[26] Moore SW, Jhnson G, Schneider JW: Elevated tissue immunoglobulins in Hirschsprung's disease--indication of early immunologic response. *Eur J Pediatr Surg*. 2000; 10:106-10.

[27] Carneiro PMR, Bereton RJ, Drake DP, Kiely EM, Spitz L, Turnock R: Enterocolitis in Hirschsprung's disease. *Pediatr Surg Int*. 1992;7:356-60.

[28] Núñez R, Torres A, Agulla E, Moreno C, Marín D, Santamaría I: La irrigación rectal y descontaminación digestiva para la profilaxis de la enterocolitis postoperatoria en la enfermedad de hirschsprung. *Cir Pediatr*. 2007; 18:96-100.

[29] Estivao-Costa J, Fragoso AC, Soares Oliveura M, Carvalho JL: An approach to minimize postoperative enterocolitis in Hirschsprung's disease. *J Pediatr Surg*. 2006; 41:1704-7.

[30] Marty TL, Seo T, Sullivan JJ, Matlak ME, Black RE, Johnson DG: Rectal irrigations for the prevention of postoperative enterocolitis in Hirschsprung's disease. *J Pediatr Surg*. 1995; 30: 652-4.

[31] Honchar VV: The prevention and treatment of enterocolitis in children with Hirschsprung's disease *Lik Sprava*. 2000; 2:69-72.

[32] Danylov OA, Iurchenko MI, Honchar VV, Rybal'chenko VF: The prolonged intestinal irrigation in a child with Hirschsprung disease complicated by enterocolitis *Klin Khir*. 2000; 5:59-60.

[33] Teitelbaum DH, Cilley RE, Sherman NJ, Bliss D, Uitylugt ND, Ranaud EJ. Kirstioglu I. Bengston T. Coran AG:A decade of experience with the primary pull-through for hirschsprung disease in the newborn period: a multicenter analysis of outcomes. *Ann Surg*. 2000; 232:372-80.

[34] Rescorla FJ, Morrison AM, Engles D, West KW, Grosfeld JL: Hirschsprung's disease. Evaluation of mortality and long-term function in 260 cases. *Arch Surg*. 1992; 127:934-41.

[35] Blane CE, Elhalaby E, Coran AG: Enterocolitis following endorectal pull-through procedure in children with Hirschsprung's disease.*Pediatr Radiol*. 1994; 24:164-6.

[36] Surana R, Quinn FM, Puri P.: Evaluation of risk factors in the development of enterocolitis complicating Hirschsprung`s disease. *Peditr Surg Int*. 1994; 9:234-6.

[37] Moore SW, Albertyn R, Cywes S: Clinical outcome and long-term quality of life after surgical correction of Hirschsprung's disease. *J Pediatr Surg*. 1996; 31:1496-502.

[38] Sarioglu A. Tanyel FC. Buyukpamukcu N. Hicsonmez A: Clinical risk factors of Hirschsprung-associated enterocolitis. I: Preoperative enterocolitis. *Turk JPediatr*. 1997; 39:81-9.

[39] Murthi GV, Raine PA: Preoperative enterocolitis is associated with poorer long-term bowel function after Soave-Boley endorectal pull-through for Hirschsprung's disease. *J Pediatr Surg*. 2003; 38:69-72.

[40] Elhalaby EA, Hashish A, Elbarbary MM, Soliman HA, Wishahy MK, Elkholy A et al.: Transanal one-stage endorectal pull-through for Hirschsprung's disease: a multicenter study. *J Pediatr Surg*. 2004; 39:345-51.

[41] Suita S, Taguchi T, Ieiri S, Nakatsuji T: Hirschsprung's disease in Japan: analysis of 3852 patients based on a nationwide survey in 30 years. *J Pediatr Surg* 2005;40:197-202.

[42] Menezes M, Puri P: Long-term outcome of patients with enterocolitis complicating Hirschsprung's disease. *Pediatr Surg Int*. 2006; 22:316-8.

[43] Pratap A, Gupta DK, Shakya VC, Adhikary S, Tiwari A, Sherestha P et al: Analysis of problems, complications, avoidance and management with transanal pull-through for Hirschsprung disease. *J Pediatr Surg*. 2007; 42:1869-76.

[44] Haricharan RN, Seo JM, Kelly DR, Mroczek-Musulman EC, Aprahamian CJ, Morgan TL et al. Older age at diagnosis of Hirschsprung disease decreases risk of postoperative enterocolitis. but resection of additional ganglionated bowel does not. *J Pediatr Surg*. 2008; 43:1115-23.

[45] Ikeda K, Goto S: Diagnosis and treatment of Hirschsprung's disease in Japan. An analysis of 1628 patients. *Ann Surg*. 1984; 199:400-5.

[46] Lopez-Alonso M, Hernández Orgaz A, Ribas Serna J: Índices de fiabilidad de la manometría anorrectal para el diagnóstioc de la enfermedad de Hirschsprung a cualquier edad. *Cir Pediatr* 2005; 18:13-6

[47] Fortuna RS, Weber TR, Tracy TF Jr, Silen ML, Cradock TV: Critical analysis of the operative treatment of Hirschsprung's disease. *Arch Surg*. 1996; 131:520-4.

[48] Teitelbaum DH. Coran AG: Enterocolitis. *Semin Pediatr Surg*. 1998; 7:162-9.

[49] Swenson O, Davidson FZ: Similarities of mechanical intestinal obstruction and aganglionic megacolon in the newborn infant: a review of 64 cases. *N Engl J Med*. 1960 14; 262:64-7.

[50] Frank JD, Nixon HH: auses of death in Hirschsprung's disease: analysis and conclusions for therapy. *Prog Pediatr Surg*. 1979; 13:199-205.

[51] Langer JC, Durrant AC, De La Torre L, Teitelbaum DH, Minkes RK, Caty MG et al: One-stage transanal Soave pullthrough for Hirschsprung disease: a multicenter experience with 141 children. *Ann Surg*. 2003; 238:569-83.

[52] Klein MD, Coran AG, Wesly JR, Drongowski RA: Hirschsprung's disease in the newborn. *J Pediatr Surg*. 1984; 19:370-4

[53] Vela Desejo E, Gonzalo Alonso E, López Álvarez.Buhillo P, Bobo Gumpert C, Cotero Lavín A, Centeno Monterrubio C: Enfermedad de Hirschsprung y malformaciones asociaadas: Revisión casuística. *Rev Esp pediatr*. 1998; 54:229-33.

[54] Quinn FM, Surana R, Puri P: The influence of trisomy 21 on outcome in children with Hirschsprung's disease. *J Pediatr Surg*. 1994; 29:781-3.

[55] Wilson-Storey D, Scobie WG: Impaired gastrointestinal mucosal defense in Hirschsprung's disease: a clue to the pathogenesis of enterocolitis? *J Pediatr Surg*. 1989; 24:462-4.

[56] Wildhaber BE, Teitelbaum DH, Coran AG: Total colonic Hirschsprung's disease: a 28-year experience. *J Pediatr Surg*. 2005; 40:203-7.

[57] Núñez R, Cabrera R, Agulla E, Moreno C, Serrano A, Ortiz C, Blesa E:Aganglionismo cólico con afectación ileal. Plastia ileocolica. *Cir Pediatr*. 2001;14:76-81

[58] Passarge E: The genetics of Hirschsprung's disease. Evidence for heterogeneous etiology and a study of sixty-three families. *N Engl J Med*. 1967;276:138-43

[59] Vázquez Rueda F, Blesa Sánchez E, Núñez Núñez R, Galán Gómez E: Síndrome de Waardenburg y enfermedad de Hirschsprung: *An Esp Pediatr*. 1998;48:306-8.

[60] Lifschitz CH, Bloss R: Persistence of colitis in Hirschsprung's disease. *J Pediatr Gastroenterol Nutr*. 1985; 4:291-3.

[61] Sarioglu A, Tanyel FC. Buyukpamukcu N. Hicsonmez A: Clinical risk factors of hirschsprung-associated enterocolitis. II: Postoperative enterocolitis. *Turk J Pediatr* 1997; 39:91-8.

[62] Bai Y, Chen H, Hao J, Huang Y, Wang W: Long-term outcome and quality of life after the Swenson procedure for Hirschsprung's disease. *J Pediatr Surg*. 2002;37:639-42.

[63] Rintala RJ: Transanal coloanal pull-through with a short muscular cuff for classic Hirschsprung's disease. *Eur J Pediatr Surg*. 2003; 13:181-6.

[64] De La Torre L, Ortega A: Transanal versus open endorectal pull-through for Hirschsprung`disease. *J Pediatr Surg*.2000; 35:1630-2.

[65] Zhang SC, Bai YZ, Wang W, Wang WL: Clinical outcome in children after transanal 1-stage endorectal pull-through operation for Hirschsprung disease. *J Pediatr Surg*. 2005; 40:1307-11.

[66] Antao B, Roberts J: Laparoscopic-assisted transanal endorectal coloanal anastomosis for Hirschsprung's disease. *J Laparoendosc Adv Surg Tech A*. 2005; 15:75-9.

[67] Teitelbaum DH, Caniano DA, Qualman SJ: The pathophysiology of Hirschsprung's-associated enterocolitis: importance of histologic correlates. *J Pediatr Surg*. 1989; 24:1271-7.

[68] Teich S, Schisgall RM, Anderson KD: Ischemic enterocolitis as a complication of Hirschsprung's disease. *J Pediatr Surg*. 1986; 21:143-5.

[69] Thomas DF, Fernie DS, Malone M, Bayston R, Spitz L: Association between Clostridium difficile and enterocolitis in Hirschsprung's disease. *Lancet*. 1982; 1:78-9.

[70] Brearly S, Armstrong GR, Nairn R, Gornall P, Currie AB, Buick RG et al: Pseudomembranous colitis: a lethal complication of Hirschsprung's disease unrelated to antibiotic usage. *J Pediatr Surg*. 1987; 22:257-9.

[71] Glotzer DJ, Gpihl BG: Experimental obstructive colitis. *Arch Surg*. 1966; 92:1-8.

[72] Harrison MW, Deitz DM, Campbell JT. Campbell DT: Diagnosis and management of Hirschsprung's disease. A 25 year perspective. *Am J Surg*. 1986; 152:49-56.

[73] Rintala RJ, Lindahl H: Sodium cromoglycate in the management of chronic or recurrent enterocolitis in patients with Hirschsprung's disease. *J Pediatr Surg*. 2001; 36:1032-5.

[74] Hardy SP, Bayston R, Spitz L: Prolonged carriage of Clostridium difficile in Hirschsprung's disease. *Arch Dis Child*. 1993;69:221-4.

[75] Rietra PJ, Slaterus KW, Zanen HC. Meuwissen SG: Clostridial toxin in faeces of healthy infants. *Lancet*. 1978; 2:319.

[76] Thomas DF, Fernie DS, Bayston R, Spitz L, Nixon HH: Enterocolitis in Hirschsprung's disease: a controlled study of the etiologic role of Clostridium difficile. *J Pediatr Surg.* 1986; 21:22-5.

[77] Golderman L, Kaplan B, Rubinstein E: Escherichia coli adherence to the intestine of mice. *Isr J Med Sci.* 1985; 21:410-4.

[78] Wilson-Storey D: Microbial studies of enterocolitis in Hirschsprung`disease. *Pediatr Sur Int.* 1994;9:248-50.

[79] Wilson-Storey D, Scobie WG, Raeburn JA: Defective white blood cell function in Hirschsprung's disease: a possible predisposing factor to enterocolitis. *J R Coll Surg Edinb* 1988; 33:185-8.

[80] Wilson-Storey D, Scobie WG: Impaired gastrointestinal mucosal defense in Hirschsprung's disease: a clue to the pathogenesis of enterocolitis? *J Pediatr Surg.* 1989; 24:462-4.

[81] Akkary S, Sahwy E, Kandil W, Hamdy MH: A histochemical study of the mucosubstances of the colon in cases of Hirschsprung's disease with and without enterocolitis. *J Pediatr Surg.* 1981;16:664-8.

[82] Fujimoto T, Puri P: Persistence of enterocolitis following diversion of faecal stream in Hirschsprung`disease. A study of mucosal defence mechanisms. *Pediatr Surg Int.* 1988:3:141-6.

[83] Imamura A, Puri P, O'Brillan DS, Reen DJ: Mucosal immune defence mechanisms in enterocolitis complicating Hirschsprung's disease. *Gut.* 1992; 33:801-6.

[84] Smith AC, Podolsky DK: Colonic mucin glycoproteins in health and disease. *Clin Gastroenterol.* 1986; 15:815-37.

[85] Aslam M: Hirschsprung's disease: Complications including enterocolitis. In: *The formation and development of the colonic mucus defensive barrier in normal children and those with Hirschspring's disease.* MD thesis. University of Bristol; 1998. p. 55-85. 148-154.

[86] Aslam A, Spicer RD, Corfield AP: Children with Hirschsprung's disease have an abnormal colonic mucus defensive barrier independent of the bowel innervation status. *J Pediatr Surg.* 1997; 32:1206-10

[87] Aslam A, Spicer RD, Corfield AP: Turnover of radioactive mucin precursors in the colon of patients with Hirschsprung's disease correlates with the development of enterocolitis. *J Pediatr Surg* 1998; 33:103-5.

[88] Aslam A, Spicer RD, Corfield AP: Histochemical and genetic analysis of colonic mucin glycoproteins in Hirschsprung's disease. *J Pediatr Surg.* 1999; 34:330-3.

[89] Corfield AP, Wagner SA, O´Donnell LJ, Durdey P, Mountford RA, Clamp JR: The roles of enteric bacterial sialidase. sialate O-acetyl esterase and glycosulfatase in the degradation of human colonic mucin. *Glycoconj J.* 1993; 10:72-81.

[90] Gum JR, Hicks JW, Kim YS: Identification and characterization of the MUC2 (human intestinal mucin) gene 5'-flanking region: promoter activity in cultured cells. *Biochem J.* 1997; 325:259-67.

[91] Buisine MP, Devisme L, Saavidge TC, Gespach C, Gosselin B, Porchet N et al: Mucin gene expression in human embryonic and fetal intestine. *Gut.* 1998; 43:519-24.

[92] Mattar AF, Coran AG, Teitelbaum DH: MUC-2 mucin production in Hirschsprung's disease: possible association with enterocolitis development. *J Pediatr Surg*.2003;38:417-21.

[93] Forstner G: Signal transduction. packaging and secretion of mucins. *Annu Rev Physiol.* 1995;57:585-605.

[94] Soeda J, O'Briain DS, Puri P: Regional reduction in intestinal neuroendocrine cell populations in enterocolitis complicating Hirschsprung's disease. *J Pediatr Surg*. 1993; 28:1063-8.

[95] Lui VC, Li L, Sham MH, Tam PK: CDX-1 and CDX-2 are expressed in human colonic mucosa and are down-regulated in patients with Hirschsprung's disease associated enterocolitis. *Biochim Biophys Acta*. 2001;1537:89-100

[96] Golderman L, Kaplan B, Rubinstein E: Escherichia coli adherence to the intestine of mice. *Isr J Med Sci*. 1985; 21:410-4.

[97] Turnock RR. Spitz L. Strobel S: A study of mucosal gut immunity in infants who develop Hirschsprung's-associated enterocolitis. *J Pediatr Surg*. 1992; 27:828-9

[98] Caniano DA, Teitelbaum DH, Qualman SJ, Shannon BT: The piebald-lethal murine strain: investigation of the cause of early death. *J Pediatr Surg*. 1989; 24:906-10.

[99] Fujimoto T: Natural history and pathophysiology of enterocolitis in the piebald lethal mouse model of Hirschsprung's disease. *J Pediatr Surg*. 1988; 23:237-42.

[100] MacMicking J, Xie QW, Nathan C: Nitric oxide and macrophage function. *Annu Rev Immunol.* 1997;15:323-50

[101] Nair MP, Schwartz SA: Association of decreased T-cell-mediated natural cytotoxicity and interferon production in Down's syndrome. *Clin Immunol Immunopathol*. 1984; 33:412-24.

[102] Schärli AF: Neuronal intestinal dysplasia. *Pediatr Surg Int*. 1992; 7:2-7.

[103] Kobayashi H, Hirakawa H, Surana R, O'Briain DS, Puri P: Intestinal neuronal dysplasia is a possible cause of persistent bowel symptoms after pull-through operation for Hirschsprung's disease. *J Pediatr Surg*. 1995;30:253-7;

[104] Suzuki T, Won KJ, Horiguchi K, Kinoshita K, Hori M, Torihashi S et al.: Muscularis inflammation and the loss of interstitial cells of Cajal in the endothelin ETB receptor null rat. *Am J Physiol Gastrointest Liver Physiol*. 2004;287:638-46

[105] Porras M, Martín MT, Soler M, Vergara P: Intestinal motor disorders associated with cyclical bacterial overgrowth in a rat model of enteritis. *Am J Physiol Gastrointest Liver Physiol*. 2004 287:G58-64.

[106] Berry CL, Fraser G: The experimental production of colitis in the rabbit with particular reference to the Hirschsprung`disease. *J Pediatr Surg*. 1968;3:36-42.

[107] Elhalaby EA, Teitelbaum DH, Coran AG, Heidelberger KP: Enterocolitis associated with Hirschsprung's disease: a clinical histopathological correlative study. *J Pediatr Surg*. 1995;30:1023-6;

[108] Parsons J, Fenton E, Dargaville P: Clostridium difficile associated severe enterocolitis: a feature of Hirschsprung's disease in a neonate presenting late. *J Paediatr Child Health*. 2005;41:689-90.

[109] Chiengkriwate P, Patrapinyokul S, Sangkhathat S, Chowchuvech V: Primary pull-through with modified Duhamel technique: 1 institution's experience. *J Pediatr Surg*. 2007;42:1075-80.

[110] Lloyd-Still JD, Demers LM: Hirschsprung's enterocolitis, prostaglandins and response to cholestyramine. *J Pediatr Surg*. 1978;13:417-8.

[111] Herek O: accharomyces boulardii: a possible addition to the standard treatment and prophylaxis of enterocolitis in Hirschsprung's disease? *Pediatr Surg Int*. 2002;18:567.

[112] Buts JP, Bernasconi P, Vaerman JP, Dive C: Stimulation of secretory IgA and secretory component of immunoglobulins in small intestine of rats treated with Saccharomyces boulardii. *Dig Dis Sci*. 1990;35:251-6.

[113] Rodrigues AC, Cara DC, Fretez SH, Cunha FO, Vieira EC, Nicoli JR et al: Saccharomyces boulardii stimulates sIgA production and the phagocytic system of gnotobiotic mice. *J Appl Microbiol*. 2000;89:404-14.

[114] Castagliuolo I, Riegler MF, Valenick L, LaMont JT, Pothoulakis C: Saccharomyces boulardii protease inhibits the effects of Clostridium difficile toxins A and B in human colonic mucosa. *Infect Immun*. 1999;67:302-7.

[115] McFarland LV, Surawicz CM, Greenberg RN. Fekety R, Elmer GW, Mover KA et al: A randomized placebo-controlled trial of Saccharomyces boulardii in combination with standard antibiotics for Clostridium difficile disease. *JAMA* 1994.;271:1913-8.

[116] Surawicz CM, McFarland KV, Greenberg RN, Rubin M, Fekety R, Mulligan ME et al: The search for a better treatment for recurrent Clostridium difficile disease: use of high-dose vancomycin combined with Saccharomyces boulardii. *Clin Infect Dis*. 2000;31:1012-7.

[117] Tatekawa Y, Muraji T, Takamizawa S: A case report of a patient with near total intestinal aganglionosis followed by the role of extended myectomy and synbiotics therapy. *J Pediatr Surg*. 2007;42:E9-12.

[118] Branski D, Lebenthal E: Small intestinal changes in enterocolitis complicating Hirschsprung's disease. *J Clin Gastroenterol*. 1979;1:237-40.

[119] Wildhaber BE, Pakarinen M, Rintala RJ, Coran AG. Teitelbaum DH: Posterior myotomy/myectomy for persistent stooling problems in Hirschsprung's disease. *J Pediatr Surg*. 2004;39:920-6.

[120] Polley TZ, Coran AG, Wesley JR: A ten-year experience with ninety-two cases of Hirschsprung's disease. Including sixty-seven consecutive endorectal pull-through procedures. *Ann Surg*. 1985;202:359-55.

[121] Marty TL, Seo T, Matlak ME, Sullivan JJ, Black RE, Johnson DG: Gastrointestinal function after surgical correction of Hirschsprung's disease: long-term follow-up in 135 patients. *J Pediatr Surg*. 1995;30:655-8

[122] Somme S, Langer JC: Primary versus staged pull-through for the treatment of Hirschsprung disease. *Semin Pediatr Surg*. 2004;13:249-55.

[123] Dasgupta R, Langer JC: Transanal pull-through for Hirschsprung disease. *Semin Pediatr Surg*. 2005;14:64-71

[124] So HB, Schwartz DL, Berker JM, Daum F, Schneider KM: Endorectal "pull-through" without preliminary colostomy in neonates with Hirschsprung's disease. *J Pediatr Surg*. 1980;1:470-1.

[125] So HB, Becker JM, Schwartz DL, Kutin ND: Eighteen years' experience with neonatal Hirschsprung's disease treated by endorectal pull-through without colostomy. *J Pediatr Surg*. 1998;33:673-5.

[126] Ghinelli C, Del Rosi C: Treatment of Hirschsprung`disease without colostomy. *Peadtr Surg Int.* 1993;8:27-30.

[127] Núñez R, Cabrera R, Moreno C, Agulla E, Vargas I, Blesa E:Utilidad de la manometría anorrectal en el diagnóstico neonatal de la enfermedad de Hirschsprung *Cir Pediatr*. 2000;13:16-9.

[128] Lopez-Alonso M, Ribas J, Hernandez A, Anguita FA, Gomez de Terreros I, Martinez-Caro A: Efficiency of the anorectal manometry for the diagnosis of Hirschsprung's disease in the newborn period. *Eur J Pediatr Surg*. 1995;5:160-3.

[129] Pini-Prato A, Martucciello G, Jasonni V: Rectal suction biopsy in the diagnosis of intestinal dysganglionosis: 5-year experience with solo-RBT. *J Pediatr Surg*.2006;41:1043-8.

[130] Nasr A, Langer JC: Evolution of the technique in the transanal pull-through for Hirschsprung's disease: effect on outcome. *J Pediatr Surg*. 2007;42:36-9.

[131] Van Leeuwen K, Teitelbaum DH, Elhalaby EA, Coran AG: Long-term follow-up of redo pull-through procedures for Hirschsprung's disease: efficacy of the endorectal pull-through. *J Pediatr Surg*. 2000;35:829-33.

[132] Hadidi A: Transanal endorectal pull-through for Hirschsprung's disease: experience with 68 patients. *J Pediatr Surg*. 2003;38:1337-40.

[133] El-Sawarf MI, Drongowski RA, Chamberlain JN, Coran AG, Teitelbaum DH: Are the long-term results of the transanal pull-through equal to those of the transabdominal pull-through? A comparison of the 2 approaches for Hirschsprung disease. *J Pediatr Surg*. 2007;42:41-7;

[134] Tander B, Rizalar R, Cihan AO, Ayyildiz S, Ariturk E, Bernay F: Is there a hidden mortality after one-stage transanal endorectal pull-through for patients with Hirschsprung's disease? *Pediatr Surg Int*. 2007;23:81-6.

[135] Georgeson KE, Robertson DJ: Laparoscopic-assisted approaches for the definitive surgery for Hirschsprung's disease. *Semin Pediatr Surg*. 2004;13:256-62.

[136] Oliveira Fuster G, Gonzalez-Molero I: Probióticos y prebióticos en la práctica clínica. *Nutr Hosp*. 2007;22:26-34

[137] Ewaschuk JB, Dieleman LA: Probiotics and prebiotics in chronic inflammatory bowel diseases. *World J Gastroenterol*. 2006;12:5941-50

In: Hirschsprung's Disease: Diagnosis and Treatment
Ed: Ramón Núñez and Manuel López-Alonso
ISBN: 978-1-60741-349-3

Chapter XXIII

Long-Term Results After Treatment of Hirschsprung's Disease

Scott A. Engum. and Jay L. Grosfeld

Introduction

There have been many advances in the surgical management of Hirschsprung's disease with several operative procedures proven effective with minimal mortality and satisfactory results [1-5]. Surgical practice has transitioned from multi-staged surgical therapy (classic Duhamel [6], Soave [7], Swenson and Bill [8], and Rehbein [9], to single-staged procedures [10-14]. More recently, the totally transanal endorectal pull-through (TEPT) has gained wide popularity over the open and laparoscopic assisted one-stage procedures [15].

The pace of technical innovation has left many advances poorly understood in terms of long-term outcomes and the ultimate success of any operation can only be appreciated at adult follow-up. Analysis of long-term function after surgical management is hampered because of the inability to define normal bowel function; lack of precise definitions and objective measurements; use of different scoring and grading systems by different investigators; different study methods to assess bowel function; grouping together patients with different surgical procedures; and the influence of varying social, cultural, dietary, environmental and economic conditions on bowel function [16].

As systems study their patient cohorts more closely, it is becoming evident that many patients may have persistent bowel dysfunction. The most commonly encountered problems include constipation, incontinence, enterocolitis and the overall impact of the disease on lifestyle (quality of life).

Definitive Procedures

The classic Swenson, Duhamel, and Soave pull-through procedures are now accomplished by one-stage laparotomy [17-19] or with laparoscopic assistance [20-24] and the early results are as good or better than those procedures classically completed in two- or three-stages. In some centers, the Duhamel operation is now carried out shortly after birth to eliminate the need for bowel washouts.

Vieira Travassos [25] compared the open and the laparoscopic Duhamel pull-through procedure noting that the laparoscopic group was fed earlier (3.4 days versus 5.1 days) and had a shorter hospitalization (6 versus 7.8 days). However, the study occurred from 1987-1994 and 1994-2003 and this raised the concern for practice variations contributing to their data. Others [26] have shown that 54% of young adults still have an unsatisfactory outcome after the Duhamel procedure. The patient assessment utilized the primary outcome measure of the functional outcome score (FOS), which was first described by Rintala and Lindahl [27]. This is a multivariate scoring system based on responses to questions concerning stooling frequency, rectal sensation, fecal incontinence, and social impact of bowel function (maximum score is 20). All patients (n=78) had a Duhamel pull-through procedure at approximately 9 months of age with 81% having recto-sigmoid disease. Enterocolitis was seen in 10% of patients and they noted an operation failure rate of 11.5%. Their survey response rate was 63% and analyzing their individual paired FOS showed there was a significant improvement over time (1997 = 14.1 +/-5.1; 2005 = 16.4 +/-2.8). Satisfactory outcome (defined by FOS of >= 17, bowel continuity, and lack of requirement for an ACE procedure or major revision pull-through operation) was obtained in only 23 patients (47%) [26]. In contrast, in 1997, Bourdelat [2] described a series of 2,430 patients undergoing a Duhamel operation, and at 15 to 30 years' follow up, the majority of patients achieved good or excellent anal function.

Sherman's report [1] concerning 880 Swenson procedures demonstrated that at 5 years' or more follow-up, 89.9% of patients had normal bowel habits; and this improved to 93.7% at more than 20 years' follow-up. However, others [28] have studied 45 patients with a mean follow-up time of 9.1 years (range, 4 to 15.5) following Swenson's procedure, and noted that 51.5% of patients had long-term bowel dysfunction, with 37.8% having fecal soiling (especially at night), 6.7% had fecal incontinence, and 6.7% had evidence of constipation. The majority of patients had 1 or 2 bowel movements per day (55.6%) and a fair number had 3 to 5 bowel movements per day (24.4%). Postoperative enterocolitis occurred in 37.8% of patients with only 2 of 17 having an anastomotic stricture.

In 1995, Georgeson [20] described a minimal-access one-stage pull-through operation that involved laparoscopic mobilization of the rectum in combination with a transanal submucosal dissection (Soave), however, long-term outcome results are a continuing concern in regards to fecal continence [29,30]. Fujiwara [31] presented 35 patients (3-4 months of age) that underwent an open transanal pull-through technique (n=13) employing a modified primary Soave procedure (near total excision of the posterior rectal cuff) with an internal sphincterotomy and a laparoscopic (n=22) modification where the rectum is dissected laterally and posteriorly, but not anteriorly below the peritoneal reflection. Continence evaluation was performed using a standardized continence evaluation questionnaire (CEQ) covering 5 parameters (stool frequency, severity of staining, severity of perianal erosions, anal shape, and medication requirements). This study was limited by lack of long-term follow-up for some patients, but the cohort was compared annually for 7 years post pull-through procedure. The laparoscopic assisted PT patients had a higher CEQ, however this was not statistically significant. The incidence of moderate to severe incontinence after 4 years was 54% for the open group and 23% for the laparoscopic group, and after 6 years, these numbers improved with no laparoscopic patients experiencing any evidence of moderate to severe incontinence, and this occurrence dropped in the open group to 23%, however, this was not statistically significant. This data is helpful however; some patients early in their study had CEQ data determined from outpatient records rather than at the time of the follow -up visit.

De la Torre-Mondragon [15] and Langer [32] subsequently described a complete transanal pull-through approach that negated the need for any laparoscopic intervention (TAEPT). This transition has the benefit of a shorter hospital stay, less pain, earlier initiation of feedings, lower cost, and improved cosmesis[12,24,33,34]. As with many new procedures, the transanal pull-through has evolved as individuals address problems they have encountered. Nasr [35] has adjusted two specific areas and this includes the length of the remaining rectal cuff (shortening it from 10-15 cm to 1-2 cm) and performing routine biopsies of the intra-abdominal colon to determine the level of aganglionosis prior to beginning the transanal dissection. In their evaluation of 45 patients they showed that shortening the cuff decreased the number of patients requiring daily anal dilations as well as the number of patients with postoperative enterocolitis, however, this did not reach statistical significance. Many surgeons perform routine rectal dilations after this procedure until formed stool is present, thus, gauging the impact of cuff length may be difficult to determine. Further, their study did not document any frequency change in the location of the transition zone with the transition to intra-abdominal colon biopsies.

Some investigations have evaluated the clinical outcomes and lower colon manometry during defecation after TAEPT for short segment aganglionosis [36]. Clinical outcome was based on the requirement of enemas/suppositories, number of stools per day, severity of perianal erosions, and the incidence of enterocolitis requiring hospitalization. Manometry was evaluated at 3 locations (anal canal, 5 and 10 cm proximal to the anal canal) during defecation and without sedation or defecation stimulation. Median age at pull-through was 2 months and the follow-up median time was 58 months. Clinical data showed 19% required enemas/suppositories, the defecation rate dropped from 4-5 per day to 2-3 per day at 1 year and leveled off at this number with more follow-up. Perianal erosions were noted in 3/21 patients but disappeared within 3 years postoperatively. Enterocolitis was evident in 2/21 cases with one being secondary to a rotavirus infection. Manometry was performed in only 8 patients at a median interval from operation to 31 months. Median anal resting pressure was 29 $cmH2O$ and high amplitude contractions during defecation occurred in 83% of patients. None of the patients exhibited a normal anorectal reflex. There has been concern regarding the primary transanal pull-through and potential damage to the defecation function, however, reports have indicated that the resting anal sphincter pressure 1-2 years following surgery does not differ from that of the laparotomy group.[34] In addition, there does not appear to be any physiologic damage [37].

Risk analysis has shown that there is an increased incidence of complications based on age and the type of pull-through. Three independent predictors of complications were identified [38] and multivariate analysis of risk factors contributing to complications showed a higher enterocolitis rate in patients less than 1 month of age at surgery, undergoing a staged transanal pull-through and an increased risk of anal stenosis if the patient was less than 1 month of age at operation. Pratap noted that delayed passage of stools beyond 24 hours after pull-through and abdominal distention are signs of sphincter spasm and to overcome the spasm, gentle dilation of the anus starting on the second day and daily thereafter with the smallest, well-lubricated Hegar dilator can be beneficial[38].

Constipation

Constipation is one of the most common complaints after a pull-through procedure with the incidence noted in 6% to 60% of patients [1,39-48].These complaints may not develop for weeks or months postoperatively [49]. Rescorla [5] noted that 88% of patients that were followed for less than 5 years had difficulty stooling, however, symptoms improved with time and there was 100% patient satisfaction noted at 15 years or more. It is known that stooling patterns in patients change in the first few years after a pull-through procedure and the frequency may decrease from more than 6 bowel movements per day immediately after operation to 2 or 3 per day within the first year of follow-up [48,50]. Investigation of patients with an open procedure found that the frequency of bowel motions went from 5 to 8 motions per day immediately after surgery to a mean of 3.8 motions per day at 6 months post procedure[51].

In most cases constipation can be managed medically with laxatives and do not necessitate further workup, however, a dilated neorectum and distal colon with persistent constipation may necessitate repeat neorectum biopsy, as recurrent obstipation unresponsive to diet and laxatives can be associated with recurrent bouts of enterocolitis.

Common treatment options for unresponsive constipation include anal myectomy, use of botulinum toxin and a redo pull-through procedure. In cases where chronic and progressive distention of the pull-through segment is the etiology, Shorter has presented another option; a simple antimesenteric plication (38 cm long) of the dilated colon (8 cm dilated segment) with gratifying results at 29 months follow-up [52].

Others have evaluated a multidisciplinary treatment plan for chronic defecation problems based on a biopsychosocial approach which utilized patient self control (maximum voluntary evacuation on a regular basis results in less medication use and a more independent patient) and suggest that this can reduce the incidence and severity of postoperative chronic bowel problems and possibly the necessity for redo procedures. This method has been utilized in toddlers and preschool children [53].

Continence

Many surgeons thought that constipation was the major problem noted after a pull-through procedure; however, fecal soiling appears to be the central issue. Fecal soiling is a common and bothersome complication and may occur in as many as 32 – 80% of patients [42,54] and some [54] have shown that may be severe in as many as 12.6% of patients. Fecal soiling is a physical, emotional, and psychological problem that can disable the patient and cause social and developmental concerns and is likely underreported [42]. Fortunately, most series have shown improvement in fecal continence with age. Mills [55] noted the overall mean continence score as fair, but there was a statistically significant improvement in fecal continence scores with age. Although a poor fecal continence score was reported in 37.5% of toddlers, this dropped to only 7% in teenagers. A good fecal continence score increased from 12.5% in the toddler group to almost 80% in the teenage years. While this is somewhat reassuring, a significant number of patients still have incontinence in their teenage years (20%) [55,56].

An accurate assessment of continence has been difficult to determine and many studies either do not include this data or fail to make a distinction between occasional soiling and significant incontinence. The availability of manometric pressure profile measurements now permits a comparison of pressures between the neorectum and anus.

Unfortunately, anorectal manometric findings in patients with Hirschsprung's disease continue to be inconsistent. Holschneider [57] presented a multinational series and noted resting pressures were either increased or reduced depending on the operative method. Others [58] have reported an increased resting pressure in most of their patients. Sillen [59] and Moore [60] both noted no significant differences in resting pressures between healthy controls and patients with Hirschsprung's disease. Historical data show that in normal children the average resting rectal and anal pressures were 7.1 +/- 3.7 cm H_20 and 13.7 +/- 5.6 cm H_20, respectively. However, an earlier study showed the pressures in a patient with HD were higher at 1 month post pull-through and then similar to normal children at 3 years follow-up [61].

Current surgical procedures resect the proximal part of the internal sphincter (Swenson) or bypass it with an endorectal or retrorectal pull-through to overcome the functional obstruction caused by the disease process. A low postoperative resting pressure reflects mainly internal sphincter dysfunction. Investigators believe [62] the dysfunction of the internal sphincter caused by the surgical procedures is permanent and is a major cause of continence problems. In the adult there is a statistically significant positive correlation between the resting pressure and continence outcome and the performance of the voluntary anal sphincter remained less disturbed [62]. Some studies have suggested that the rectoanal reflex is restored postoperatively in 39-91% of patients [57,61]. It is difficult to understand how a completely aganglionic internal sphincter in Hirschsprung's disease would regain normal function after an anastomosis with proximal ganglionic colon. Functional reinnervation of the internal sphincter seems unlikely especially after operations without a full-thickness end to end anastomosis as noted in the Duhamel or Soave techniques. Overall continence is most likely salvaged by the normal function of the voluntary sphincters, which can compensate for a low resting pressure caused by surgical procedures for HD which causes a dysfunctional internal sphincter. Keshtgar [63] demonstrated an intact internal and external anal sphincter below the pull-through on endoanal sonography and noted that patients with incontinence had significantly lower resting anal pressures.

Heikkinen [62] described 54 adults that underwent pull-through procedures in childhood, (Swenson=7, State-Rehbein=4, Soave=4, Duhamel=39). The mean follow-up time was 26.5 years and the mean age at manometry was 29 +/- 7.2 years. Fourteen patients had a normal bowel function score, while 34 rated their fecal continence score as good and 6 patients were fair. Within the fair group, these patients had significant problems in bowel function including severe constipation or limitations in social life caused by fecal soiling. None of the six patients were totally incontinent. The median basal resting pressure (BRP) in patients who had normal continence was 25 cm H_20. In those with good continence, the median BRP was 20 cm H_2O and in the fair continence group 15 cm H_2O. A statistically significant difference was obtained between the normal and good groups, but not the good and fair groups. They also noted statistically significant correlations between the anal resting pressure and quantitative continence scores. All patients had a negative recto-anal relaxation reflex. The initial method of pull-through procedure had no effect on the manometric findings.

Concerns have been raised regarding the transanal pull-through procedure and the greater amount of retraction of the anorectal tissues necessary to perform the operation and its potential effects on continence. An adult manometric evaluation after rectocele repair and hemorrhoidectomy showed lower resting anal and squeeze pressures postoperatively compared to controls [64]. In the pediatric patient, the perineal and transabdominal techniques were found to be similar when comparing postoperative anal resting pressure, stool frequency, and loss or absence of the anorectal inhibitory reflex [65]. On conventional 4 channel and computerized 8 channel manometry, Till [37] has shown that the TERPT preserves the functional integrity of the anorectal sphincter complex and has a favorable clinical manometric outcome. Anal endosonography after a Duhamel procedure showed that most patients had a partial interruption in the hyperechoic band, which corresponds to the external anal sphincter in the 6th direction. This interruption was also identified with the scar tissue in the external anal sphincter [66,67] and indicates retrorectal dissection may cause partial injury to the external anal sphincter muscle. Bjornland [66] has also shown that the presence of abundant scar tissue in the internal anal sphincter had the lowest resting pressures. It is postulated that anal retraction and myotomy are likely reasons for these observations.

Because of the complexity of these postoperative concerns, some authors have proposed a more systematic method of following these patients. This involves acquiring a standardized detailed history and physical examination, anorectal manometry, profilometry, endosonography, and measuring colonic transit time [68] in an effort to demonstrate anorectal functional impairment at an early stage. However, with aging, there is no data present regarding continence and if the integrity of the voluntary sphincters maintains its integrity or decreases as it is noted that up to 46% of institutionalized elderly individuals have fecal incontinence without the diagnosis of Hirschsprung's disease.

Enterocolitis

Enterocolitis (EC) remains the most serious complication of Hirschsprung's disease and can occur both before and after operative interventions. Incidence rates can be as high as 48% [69,70] with an associated mortality rate of 3% to 30% [5,71,72]. This wide variation in occurrence rates is likely the result of various authors' definition of the condition. There has been a decline in the incidence of EC and this is likely due to improved recognition, prompt diagnosis and therapy. A 1979 survey of the members of the Surgical Section of the American Academy of Pediatrics [73] showed the incidence of pre diagnosis HD enterocolitis was 15% with a 30% mortality rate. In contrast, a follow-up report in 1997 [74] documented a 26% incidence of preoperative enterocolitis and a 7.6% mortality rate.

The proposed causes of EC include obstruction, infection, alterations in intestinal mucous, diminished immunocytes, and intestinal neuronal dysplasia[75]. Investigators have also noted certain risk factors which include age, sex, family history, presence of long segment aganglionosis, delayed diagnosis, and the association of trisomy 21 [69,70,76]. In the postoperative patient, Hackam [77] identified anastomotic leak or stricture as significant risk factors; and the development of postoperative intestinal obstruction due to adhesions increased the relative risk of subsequent enterocolitis by three-fold. In a multicenter review of primary endorectal pull-through procedures, logistic regression analysis of risk factors for the development of enterocolitis showed that stricture was a significant risk factor.[78] This suggests that partial obstruction may result in stasis, bacterial overgrowth and mucosal invasion that ultimately leads to subsequent local and systemic inflammatory response[77,79-82]. Although others [69] have shown a greater risk for EC in girls, Menezes [83] failed to demonstrate this finding. This was also true of long segment disease where they noted a 36% incidence compared to 27% and this was not significant. A 48% EC rate was noted in patients with trisomy 21 patient compared to 25% non-Down syndrome patients and this was significant and consistent with other studies [70,78]. Their evaluation in 259 patients[83] failed to show any significance in regards to the type of pull-through procedure utilized and the incidence of enterocolitis (Swenson = 25.6%, Soave = 27.3%, Duhamel = 31.2%, Transanal = 40%). Of the seventy-four of 259 patients that had enterocolitis, 24.3% of patients presented preoperatively, 41.8% presented postoperatively, and 33.7% had enterocolitis both pre and postoperatively. Most authors have noted that post-pull-through enterocolitis is primarily seen in the first two years after the definitive procedure[49,83]. Some have noted that infants that experience enterocolitis prior to operative repair have an increased risk of this post pull-through [79].

Because anastomotic stricture is an important covariate risk factor that contributes to the incidence of enterocolitis,[78] many pediatric surgeons have adopted a dilation program that provides for close surveillance and follow-up to minimize the risk. Others believe that excision of a portion of the internal sphincter to within 1 cm of the dentate line posteriorly, recognized by Swenson [84] is an important factor to prevent subsequent enterocolitis, and this is an advantage of the Soave endorectal technique[85].

Therapy for enterocolitis involves rectal tube decompression and washouts, intravenous hydration and antibiotics. If the infant fails to improve, the performance of a leveling colostomy at a site of confirmed ganglion cells will likely be necessary. Recurrent bouts of enterocolitis after a pull-through procedure will require investigation to rule out a mechanical cause of obstruction. This will likely involve a contrast enema and if normal, a rectal biopsy should be performed to rule out a residual segment of aganglionosis or the presence of intestinal neuronal dysplasia (IND) [60,86]. A normal biopsy may indicate the need to consider a posterior anal myotomy, myectomy, or internal sphincterotomy.

Anastomotic Leak / Stricture Formation

The incidence of anastomotic leak varies from 1.5% to 8% [16,46,54,87]. Most, but not all strictures are associated with an early leak[88]. Patient's treated with a Soave operation can develop a cuff abscess in as many as 5.3% of cases[89]. This occurs when there is damage to the mucosal tube, retraction of the anastomosis, or poor blood supply to the pull-through segment resulting in leakage of intestinal contents causing an inflammatory process and abscess.

Anastomotic stricture rates vary from 3% to 35% and can typically be managed by simple repeated dilations[43,46,54,87,89,90]. The etiology of most strictures is likely anastomotic ischemia or dehiscence, a circular rather than oblique anastomosis, and failure to adhere to a dilation program. Strictures can be classified into two basic types (simple and persistent). Simple strictures result in moderate narrowing at the anastomotic site and are seen within the first few weeks following a pull-through procedure and are addressed with serial dilations. Persistent strictures as seen with anastomotic leak or an ischemic segment have a higher likelihood of not responding to dilations. It is not uncommon for an advanced stricture to require surgical correction (stricturoplasty or redo pull-through). In the worst case scenario a diverting colostomy may be necessary.

Urinary Function and Impotence

Pelvic and perineal surgery may cause damage to the pelvic splanchnic nerves, the hypogastric nerves, or the pelvic nerve plexus, resulting in autonomic denervation of the lower urinary tract[91-95]. In HD, postoperative bed wetting has been documented and concern was raised for iatrogenic nerve damage [57,96]. The incidence for postoperative "enuresis" is estimated at 9.5%[57]. The observed incidence following the various pull-through procedures is Rehbein, 5.4%; Swenson, 10.4%; Soave, 15.3%; and Duhamel, 14.3% [57]. One would expect the Soave (endorectal) and Duhamel (retrorectal) procedures to have a lower incidence of this postoperative complication. In addition, because the data regarding detrusor denervation is inconsistent, some conclude that children should be screened clinically and ultrsonographically for preexisting urologic signs and symptoms related to outflow obstruction. If children present with urinary problems after their pull-through procedure, urodynamic assessment should be performed.

With the transition to a completely transanal approach for newborn pull-through procedures, one would anticipate a decreased postoperative complication rate in regards to urinary dysfunction. Ates [97] recently evaluated 7 patients that had a one-stage transanal endorectal pull-through procedure with standard urodynamic studies after at least 6 months. Patients had a post void residual of less than 20 ml, the detrusor activities of all patients were found to be normal. None of the patients developed urinary tract problems during the follow-up period.

Down Syndrome

Approximately 5 -15% of Hirschsprung's patients also have Down syndrome (DS) [70,76,98]. It has been suggested that the co-existence of DS and HD result in a poorer outcome in regards to postoperative complications, continence, and mortality and at times has favored more conservative treatment plans [99]. Some studies have shown that despite the increased risk of enterocolitis and the fact that many patients have associated complex cardiac disease, these patients can develop satisfactory continence[100] and that Down syndrome should have little influence on the outcome following a pull-through [101].

Morabito [102] studied continence outcomes using the modified Wingspread scoring system [103] in Down syndrome patients (15 patients) compared to a control group (140 patients) and noted children with DS in terms of continence did worse; (53% of DS group compared to 85% of the control group was continent). Catto-Smith [104] showed in 10 patients surveyed with HD and DS that fecal soiling is a significant long-term problem, however, their sample size was small and their patients did show significant improvement in many aspects of bowel control with increasing age. In addition, they found that food had a significant impact on bowel function. Celiac disease is more common in children with Down syndrome [105], and they noted that the patient's surveyed (vast majority of non-celiac patients) also had problems with either grains or other food groups

A national study of toilet training in children with DS conducted in the United Kingdom found that 94% of individuals had achieved full bowel control by the age of 6 years [106]. Difficulty in achieving good bowel control becomes evident in children with trisomy 21 due to their low motivation and limited abilities, and some may cope better with a permanent stoma [83]. This data is far better than what is reported in current Hirschsprung's disease patients. Despite a worse continence outcome, the mere co-existence of HD and DS should not influence the operative management for HD.

Total Colonic Aganglionosis

Total colonic aganglionosis (TCA), with our without involvement of the small intestine, is a more severe form of Hirschsprung's disease. The incidence of TCA in patients with HD is between 2% and 14% [107]. The incidence of disease extending into the small intestine is 1 case in 50,000 live births.[108] It is typically associated with a more complicated diagnosis as well as higher morbidity and mortality [109-112] Anupama [113] evaluated 25 cases of TCA with ileal involvement among 831 cases of HD from 1996-2005. There were 32% female and 68% male with none of the patients having any prior family history for TCA. Eighteen patients underwent definitive treatment (16 staged procedures) and (2 primary pull-through procedures). The procedures performed were 12 Martin procedures (10-15 cm stapled application), 4 Ikeda-Soper procedures, 1 Rehbein procedure, and 1 Soave procedure. Preoperative enterocolitis was noted in 44.4%, postoperative enterocolitis noted in 61.1%, wound infection in 22.2%, perianal excoriation 77.7%, anastomotic leak in 16.6%. In our own series [114], 81% (n=29) of patients underwent a definitive pull-through procedure (20 modified Duhamel, 4 Martin long Duhamel, and 5 Soave). Perianal excoriation was seen universally in all patients. Other complications included enterocolitis in 11 patients most frequently in the Martin long Duhamel procedure (75%), Soave (40%), and Duhamel (30%). Long-term follow-up show that 83% of our patient population exhibited growth by weight at the 25th percentile. Ninety-one percent of children older than toddler age wer potty-trained and had 4 to 6 bowel movements per day with 81% continent.

Survival for TCA has improved significantly since the condition has been recognized. An AAP survey in 1979 reported a 53% survival rate[73]. Later reports by Ikeda and Goto [111] in 1986 and by by Hoehner [115] in 1998 reported a 70% and 97% survival rate, respectively. Interestingly, Hoehner noted that neither age nor weight at presentation, diagnosis, diversion, definitive procedure or ostomy closure were determinants of long-term functional outcome. In addition, the specific length of involved ileum was not predictive. Satisfactory outcome was noted in patients whose definitive repair did not incorporate an extended ganglionic-aganglionic common channel. (Martin procedure – abandoned by most) [115]. There appears to be an advantage to leaving some of the aganglionic rectum in place to serve as a reservoir to improve water and electrolyte absorption. Some [116] believe that the standard Duhamel procedure best accomplishes these goals and does so without the need for a colon patch as described by Kimura [117], while others have described the use of an S-shaped ileal pouch to create a reservoir for the patient[118].

In instances where the aganglionic process extends to the proximal small intestine and the length of normal innervated intestine is quite short, these infants are managed similar to the short bowel syndrome patient and an intestinal lengthening procedure such as the Bianchi procedure or the STEP [119] procedure may be useful. Unfortunately, intravenous hyperalimentation carries the risk of associated intrahepatic cholestasis and intraluminal bacterial overgrowth and it is not uncommon to have repeated episodes of catheter sepsis. In rare cases, combined liver, intestine and right colon transplantation has been utilized in near total aganglionosis with associated liver failure[108]. Intestinal length less than 60 cm warrants an early family discussion about transplantation evaluation.

Intestinal Neuronal Dysplasia

Intestinal neuronal dysplasia type B (IND B) is a disease of the submucosal plexus of the intestine often associated with Hirschsprung's disease and was first described in 1971 by Meier-Ruge [120] and then described in association with Hirschsprung's disease by Lassman and Wurnig in 1973 [121]. It has been documented in the proximal ganglionic colon of 20% to 75% of patients with HD [86,122-123] and may be associated with a higher incidence of postoperative complications or stooling abnormalities[86,123-125].

In the involved intestinal segment there is an increase of ganglionic (nerve) cells in the ganglion with more than eight nerve cells per ganglion. Nerve cells are smaller than in the normoganglionic intestinal segment and are grouped into spherical giant ganglia in contrast to normal disciform ganglia. To make the diagnosis of IND B, a minimum 25 submucosal ganglia must be analyzed, more than 20% of submucosal ganglia must be giant ganglia, a giant ganglion contains more than 8 nerve cell cross sections, and the patient must be older than 1 year [126]. Unfortunately, routine hematoxylin-eosin (HE) staining of frozen section specimens does not permit a precise intra-operative evaluation of IND and it has been recommended that rapid acetylcholinesterase (AChE) staining of intraoperative frozen sections may offer more precise assessment[127,128].Others have used the application of nicotinamide adenine dinucleotide, reduced form tetrazolium reductase reaction. The advantages of this method are the quick preparation of an incubation medium, a short incubation time, and the good demonstration of ganglion cells [129].

A search for dysganglionosis seems to be indispensable in minimizing postoperative dysfunction, however, extensive resection of bowel with IND with limited understanding of the etiology, clinical consequences, and evolution of this entity is not recommended [128]. The final goal of any procedure with HD and IND is to resect the aganglionic segment and deal with the dysganglionic segment according to its function. In the combination of HD with IND B, the systematic screening for the RET proto-oncogene mutation should be a standard part of the diagnostic and treatment protocol in order to identify the risk of medullary thyroid carcinoma in the preclinical stage of the disease in patients with HD and their relatives [129]. Similarly, HD may co-exist with other neural crest related conditions including neuroblastoma, and Ondine's curse [130,131].

Transition Zone Pull-Through

Accurate historical interpretation of intraoperative seromuscular biopsies is an important factor impacting the success of a pull-through procedure. The outcome of a transitional zone pull-through is not well documented and some estimate the incidence to be approximately 14.8% [132]. Errors in sampling or interpretation may result in a transition zone pull-through. This is typically characterized by diminished numbers of ganglion cells in the myenteric and submucosal plexuses. There can also be increased irregularity and wider spacing of the polygonal network of ganglia and nerve fibers of the myenteric plexus [133,134].

The circumferential distribution of the transition zone is uneven with the maximum length of the leading edge 2.4 cm (myenteric plexus) and 2.1 cm (submucosal plexus), respectively [135]. Ganglion cells are noted at the tip of the leading edge (most often observed along the antimesenteric border) and present in clusters in contrast to an absence of cells in most of the remaining areas of the circumference [135]. This distribution peculiarity can lead to misleading results when sampling at the time of the pull through procedure [136].

Various options exist for revisional surgery for a transition zone pull-through and include rectal myectomy[137,138], but is limited by the proximal extent of residual aganglionosis [132]. A redo pull-through shows promising results [138,139], however, surgical options for children with incontinence following revision procedures are limited and typically center on the benefits of a Malone antegrade continence enema procedure or permanent stoma.

Redo Procedures

Despite numerous reports detailing excellent results following surgical correction of HD, there is a small subset of patients where their complications are insurmountable and necessitate a redo pull-through procedure. Indications for a second procedure include: retained or acquired aganglionosis, severe stricture, dysfunctional bowel segment, marked dilation of the bowel likely secondary to constipation, anocutaneous fistula, and intestinal neuronal dysplasia [139-142]. Four diagnostic procedures are beneficial prior to reoperation and include: an anorectal palpation by an experienced surgeon; biopsies and histochemical examinations by an experienced pathologist; endosonography to exhibit formation of scars surrounding the pelvic floor; and radiologic studies to show the megacolon and possibly the length of the transition zone [143]. The question one needs to ask is whether this is a primary disorder that resulted from an incomplete resection or an acquired condition.

Procedures typically fall into two categories, myomectomy or a redo pull-through procedure [49]. Most surgeons prefer to perform a Duhamel or Swenson type of procedure with a success rate varying between 33% and 94% [66,139-142]. These procedures can be associated with complications such as difficult pelvic dissection in the Swenson procedure and kinking of the pull-through bowel with the Duhamel procedure[88]. Gobran [144] recently studied the use of TEPT for redo procedures. These patients had developed persistent obstructive symptoms of Hirschsprung's disease; tight anastomotic strictures associated with enterocolitis or repeated soiling. They [144] utilized an incision 0.5 to 1.0 cm above the anastomotic line of the previous operation. After a 2 cm submucosal dissection was done, the seromuscular cuff was opened and incised circumferentially to expose the external wall of the colon. The colon was mobilized as much as possible and the colon was removed until normal innervation was noted. Of the 7 patients (age 2.5 – 6 years old) treated, in follow-up, (8-16 months), one patient developed an anastomotic stenosis relieved by twice weekly dilations for 3 weeks and obstructive symptoms were relieved in all patients with no soiling noted. Enterocolitis was noted in 2 patients and responded to conservative treatment. Gobran[144] determined that redo TEPT is a simple and feasible procedure with good functional results when compared with standard pull-through procedures [12,54].

It is important for the family and child to have realistic expectations before any reoperative procedure is performed. Continence data is not always included in studies; however, Teitelbaum [49] described an experience with 26 redo procedures and a mean follow-up of 14 years. In patients that were not neurologically impaired and older than 3 years, 92% were continent. The number of stools per day ranged from 1 to 10 with a mean of 3.2.

Quality of Life

Quality of life remains a difficulty multidimensional concept that takes into account the physical, psychological, spiritual, functional, and social well being of the individual. Possible reasons for discrepancies in the quality of life reporting following the surgical correction of HD may lie in study design, the depth of the investigation undertaken, or the lack of an objective independent observer.[46] The literature has primarily concentrated on the functional outcomes for children with HD with little focus on the psychosocial impact HD has on both the child and family. Fecal soiling has the greatest impact on the overall psychosocial functioning of children with HD [39,40,46]. Unfortunately, many patients underrate problems resulting in a false impression either because they wish to please the surgeon or because they deny the problem exists.

Emotional and psychosocial development appeared to be within normal limits in the absence of severe symptoms. With good family support, the outcome for patients with minor problems was no less favorable than for those with and excellent outcome. In the absence of a stable emotional basis, problems were magnified, and a correlation between incontinence and doing poorly in school was noted[46]. Moore has shown that physically, patients treated for HD develop within the population norms [145]. The average for those in the well-nourished group (ie, > 50th percentile weight for age) was 13 years. Those in the 10th and 50th percentile had an average age of 10 years, and patients between the 3rd and 10th percentiles had an average age of 7 years. Those patients below the 3rd percentile had an average age of 5 years.

Athanasakos[41] evaluated 72 of 131 children and of the 53% that were toilet trained, 75% were experiencing long-term fecal soiling. The majority stated that it was mild or minimal with 30% of events occurring during the day, and 55% in both the day and night. Unfortunately, 3% reported it to be severe. Seventy-five percent of the young adults with HD were satisfied with their bowel function; however, 17% still remained unsatisfied. They noted no statistical differences between the primary pull-through in relation to bowel function outcome. Children with fecal incontinence report difficulties in areas of family life, social life, school, and work. Yanchar and Soucy [39] have shown a strong association between fecal incontinence and negative effects on social life and social activities, poorer QOL[28], and poor psychosocial function[40]. These effects continue into adulthood where data has revealed that half of the adults who had occasional fecal soiling complained that their work lives were affected [56].

Children 12 years or less have been shown psychosocially to be more distressed (such as embarrassment, distress/discomfort and family difficulties) due to bowel dysfunction, in comparison to children older than 12 years of age [41]. Bowel function concerns included constipation, diarrhea, fecal soiling, abdominal pain and flatulence. Children 12 years or less missed significantly more school due to bowel dysfunction (51%) compared to children over 12 years (4%). Children 12 years or less had to avoid particular foods in their diet more (53%) [in order to improve stooling patterns] compared to children over 12 years (22%). These foods tended to be sweets, dairy products, citrus fruits, yeast, carbohydrates, and soft drinks.

HD had a significant negative impact on family/social functioning with 28% of the families experiencing financial difficulties due to HD, 35% reporting difficulties in public places, 13% reporting a negative impact on their marital relationship due to daily stressors and associated bowel dysfunction, and parents expressed feelings of depression (32%), confusion (46%), anxiety (56%) and difficulty in getting interested in their child's future (11%). Family and extended family was the most important support system when caring for the HD patient[41].

Fifty-percent of the young adults with HD (over 12 years) endorsed feelings of depression, confusion and anxiety, and found it difficult to get interested about their future with HD; however, 63% were hopeful about their future. Overall, 18% of children with HD were clinically depressed, 24% with high state anxiety, 56% with high trait anxiety, 4% with behavioral problems, and 38% with low self-concept. Clinical depression and anxiety was worse in patients older than 12 years [41].

Although the relationship between fecal incontinence and QOL has been a repeated finding and would lead to the impression that children with HD must have a lower QOL than healthy children, this is by no means a universal finding. Impaired QOL has been found in studies using a non-validated QOL instrument [28,146], however, evidence to the contrary has been found using standardized instruments. Diseth showed that teenagers with HD showed no difference in psychiatric morbidity, behavior problems, or global assessment compared with their healthy peers [40] and Goyal [147] noted the same in patients with anorectal malformations.

A quality of life evaluation performed on Dutch patients treated for anorectal malformations or Hirschsprung's disease was conducted and showed that patients with ARM report systematically lower generic quality of life than patients with HD, none of the comparisons achieved statistical significance. Patients with ARM did report more disease-related physical problems (e.g., fecal incontinence) and psychosocial problems (e.g., poor body image) than patients with HD. Patients that had permanent ostomies reported severe dysfunction on all generic quality of life areas[148].

Mills [55] showed an unexpected higher QOL scores across all QOL scales for girls in all age groups. This is a difference not noted in healthy children. The good news is that bowel function and psychosocial distress improves with increasing age [1,46,149,150]' and it is suggested that patients and families learn over time to cope with chronic physical health problems. When Moore [46] evaluated their patient population with 3 separate scoring systems, (Kelly Clinical Score, Wingspread Scoring System, Holschneider Clinical and Electromanometric Score) more than 55% to 70% of patients had excellent anorectal control, with 24% to 35% having a fairly good result. The use of Quality-of-Life Scoring Criteria for children – ages 8 to 16 years [146] is a very reasonable approach to note issues in the patients' diet, daily life, school absence, relationship to peers, and emotional problems. The criteria involves soiling, incontinence, school absence, unhappy or anxious, food restrictions, and peer rejection.

Conclusions

Fecal soiling is common and affects the patient's quality of life. Surgical techniques should be subjected continuously to improvement analysis in an effort to improve this concern. Because children with HD have persistent bowel function problems after surgical correction, it is crucial to inform the parents about this observation after surgery so they have realistic expectations of their child's level of functioning. Counseling should be offered for both the child and their family as studies have shown that children with HD experience distress and anxiety specifically due to bowel dysfunction. They can then be given strategies to cope with the physical problems. Failure to address psychosocial problems from an early age could increase the development of psychiatric morbidity in these children and families with HD. Possible venues for education could include seminars, workshops, and support groups. It should be emphasized that long-term regular follow-up examinations, medication therapy, and toilet training strategies may be required. These follow-ups will allow the physician to monitor the child's bowel function and prevent complications that may worsen into adulthood. It is clear that children with HD will not inevitably develop psychosocial problems, however, when caring for such a patient, physicians need to be aware of the impact HD may have on the psychosocial well-being of the patient and family.

References

[1] Sherman JO, Snyder ME, Weitzman JJ, Jona JZ, Gillis DA, O'Donnell B et al. A 40-year multinational retrospective study of 880 Swenson procedures. *J Pediatr Surg* 1989;4:833-8.

[2] Bourdelat D, Vrsansky P, Pagés R, Duhamel B. Duhamel operation 40 years after: A multicentric study. *Eur J Pediatr Surg* 1997;7:70-6.

[3] Fuchs O, Booss D. Rehbein's procedure for Hirschsprung's disease. An appraisal of 45 years. *Eur J Pediatr Surg* 1999;9:389-91.

[4] Suita S, Taguchi T, Yanai K, Kamimura T, Nakao M, Ikeda K. Long-term outcomes and quality of life after Z-shaped anastomosis for Hirschsprung's disease. *J Am Coll Surg* 1998;187:577-83.

[5] Rescorla FJ, Morrison AM, Engles D, West KW, Grosfeld JL. Hirschsprung's disease. Evaluation of mortality and long-term function in 260 cases. *Arch Surg* 1992;127:934-42.

[6] Duhamel B. Retrorectal and transanal pull through procedures for the treatment of Hirschsprung's disease. *Dis Colon Rectum* 1964;7:455-8.

[7] Soave F. Hirschsprung's disease: a new surgical technique. *Arch Dis Child* 1964;39:116-24.

[8] Swenson O, Bill AH. Resection of rectum and rectosigmoid with preservation of the sphincter for benign spastic lesions producting megacolon: an experimental study. *Surgery* 1948;24:212-20.

[9] Rehbein F. Intraabdominelle resktion oder Rektosigmoidektomie bei der Hirschsprung'schem Krankheit. *Chirurg* 1958;29:336-9.

[10] Langer JC, Fitzgerald PG, Winthrop AL, Srinathan SK, Foglia RP, Skinner MA et al. One-stage versus two-stage Soave Pull-through for Hirschspung's disease in the first year of life. *J Pediatr Surg* 1996;31:33-6.

[11] Shankar KR, Losty PD, Lamont GL,Turnock RR, Jones MO, Lloyd DA et al. Transanal endorectal coloanal surgery for Hirschsprung's disease: experience in two centers. *J Pediatr Surg* 2000;35:1209-13.

[12] De la Torre L, Ortega A. Transanal versus open endorectal pull-through for Hirschsprung's disease. *J Pediatr Surg* 2000;35:1630-2.

[13] Minford JL, Ram A, Turnock RR, Lamont GL, Kenny SE, Rintala RJ et al. Comparison of functional outcomes of Duhamel and transanal endorectal coloanal anastomosis for Hirschsprung's disease. *J Pediatr Surg* 2004;39:161-5.

[14] So HB, Schwartz DL, Becker JM, Daum F, Schneider KM. Endorectal pull-through without preliminary colostomy in neonates with Hirschsprung's disease. *J Pediatr Surg* 1980;15:470-1.

[15] De la Torre-Mondragon L, Ortega-Salgado JA. Transanal endorectal pull-through for Hirschspurng's disease. *J Pediatr Surg* 1998;33:1283-6.

[16] Engum SA, Grosfeld JL. Long-term results of treatment of Hirschsprung's disease. *Semin Pediatr Surg* 2004;13:273-85.

[17] Cilley RE, Statter MB, Hirschl RE, Hirschl RB, Coran AG. Definitive treatment of Hirschsprung's disease in the newborn with a one-stage procedure. *Surgery* 1994;115:551-6.

[18] Carcassonne M, Morisson-Lacombe G, Letourneau JN. Primary corrective operation without decompression in infants less than three months of age with Hirschsprung's disease. *J Pediatr Surg* 1982;17:241-3.

[19] Van der Zee DC, Bax NM. Duhamel-Martin procedure for Hirschsprung's disease in neonates and infants: One-stage operation. *J Pediatr Surg* 1996;31:901-2.

[20] Georgeson KE, Fuenfer MM, Hardin WD. Primary laparoscopic pull-through for Hirschsprung's disease in infants and children. *J Pediatr Surg* 1995;30:1017-22.

[21] Lobe THE, Schropp KP. Duhamel pull-through for Hirschsprung's disease, in Lobe THE, Schropp KP (eds): *Pediatric Laparoscopy and Thoracoscopy*. Philadelphia: PA, Saunders; 1994. p. 207-12.

[22] Curran TJ, Raffensperger JG. The feasibility of laparoscopic Swenson pull-through. *J Pediatr Surg* 1994;29:1273-5.

[23] Smith BM, Steiner RB, Lobe TE. Laparoscopic Duhamel pull-through procedure of Hirschsprung's disease in children. *J Laparoendosc Surg* 1994;4:273-6.

[24] Curran TJ, Raffensperger JG. Laparoscopic Swenson pull-through: A comparison with the open procedure. *J Pediatr Surg* 1996;31:1155-6.

[25] Vieira Travassos D, Bax NMA, Van der Zee DC. Duhamel procedure: a comparative retrospective study between an open and a laparoscopic technique. *Surg Endosc* 2007;21:2163-5.

[26] Conway SJ, Craigie RJ, Cooper LH, Turner K, Turnock RR Lamont GL et al. Early adult outcome of the Duhamel procedure for left-sided Hirschsprung disease: A proscpective serial assessment study. *J Pediatr Surg* 2007;42:1429-32.

[27] Rintala RJ, Lindahl H. Is normal bowel function possible after repair of intermediate and high anorectal malformations. *J Pediatr Surg* 1995;30:491-4.

[28] Bai Y, Chen H, Hao J, Huang Y, Wang W. Long-term outcome and quality of life after the Swenson procedure for Hirschsprung's disease. *J Pediatr Surg* 2002;37:639-42.

[29] Kubota A, Kawahara H, Okuyama H, Oue T, Tazuke Y, Okada A. Clinical outcome of laparoscopically assisted endorectal pull-through in Hirschsprung's disease; comparison of abdominal and perineal approaches. *J Pediatr Surg* 2004;39:1835-7.

[30] El-Sawaf MI, Drongowski RA, Chamberlain JN, Coran AG, Teitelbaum DH. Are the long-term results of the transanal pull-through equal to those of the transabdominal pull-through? A comparison of the 2 approaches for Hirschsprung's disease. *J Pediatr Surg* 2007;42:41-7.

[31] Fujiwara N, Kaneyama K, Okazaki T, Lane GJ, Kato Y, Kobayashi H, et al. A comparative study of laparoscopy-assisted pull-through and open pull-through for Hirschsprung's disease with special reference to postoperative fecal continence. *J Pediatr Surg* 2007;42:2071-4.

[32] Langer JC, Minkes RK, Mazziotti MV,Skinner MA Winthrop AL. Transanal one-stage Soave procedure for infants with Hirschsprung's disease. *J Pediatr Surg* 1999;34:148-51.

[33] Bufo AJ, Chen MK, Shah R,Gross E Cyr B, Lobe TE. Analysis of the costs of surgery for Hirschsprung's disease: One-stage laparoscopic pull-through versus two-stage Duhamel procedure. *Clin Pediatr* 1999;38:593-6.

[34] van Leeuwen K, Geiger JD, Barnett JL, Coran AG, Teitelbaun DH. Stooling and manometric findings after primary pull-throughs in Hirschsprung's disease: Perineal versus abdominal approaches. *J Pediatr Surg* 2002;37:1321-5.

[35] Nasr A, Langer JC. Evolution of the technique in the transanal pull-through for Hirschsprung's disease: Effect on outcome. *J Pediatr Surg* 2007;42:36-40.

[36] Kohno M, Ikawa H, Konuma K, Masuyama H, Fukumoto H, Morimura E et al. Is high amplitude propagated contracton present after transanal endorectal pull-through for Hirschsprung's disease? *Pediatr Surg Int* 2007;23:981-86.

[37] Till H, Heinrich M, Schuster T, Schweinitz D. Is the anorectal sphincter damaged during a transanal endorectal pull-through (TERPT) for Hirschsprung's disease? A 3-dimensional, vector manometric investigation. *Eur J Pediatr Surg* 2006;16:188-91.

[38] Pratap A, Gupta DK, Shakya VC, Adhikary S, Tiwari A, Sherestha P et al. Analysis of problems, complications, avoidance and management with transanal pull-through for Hirschsprung disease. *J Pediatr Surg* 2007;42:1869-76.

[39] Yanchar NL, Soucy P. Long-term outcome after Hirschsprung's disease: Patients' perspectives. *J Pediatr Surg* 1999;34:1152-60.

[40] Diseth TH, Bjornland K, Novik TS, Emblem R. Bowel Function, mental health, and psychosocial function in adolescents with Hirschsprung's disease. *Arch Dis Child* 1997;76:100-6.

[41] Athanasakos E, Starling J, Ross F, Nunn K, Cass D. An example of psychological adjustment in chronic illness: Hirschsprung's disease. *Pediatr Surg Int* 2006;22:319-25.

[42] Catto-Smith AG, Coffey CMM, Nolan TM, Hutson JM. Fecal incontinence after the surgical treatment of Hirschsprung's disease. *J Pediatr* 1995;127:954-7.

[43] Fortuna RS, Weber TR, Tracy Jr FT, Silen ML, Cradock TV. Critical analysis of the operative treatment of Hirschsprung's disease. *Arch Surg* 1996;131:520-4.

[44] Foster P, Cowan G, Wrenn Jr EL. Twenty-five years' experience with Hirschsprung's disease. *J Pediatr Surg* 1990;25:531-4.

[45] Menezes M, Corbally M, Puri P. Long-term results of bowel function after treatment for Hirschsprung's disease: A 29-year review. *Pediatr Surg Int* 2006;22:987-90.

[46] Moore SW, Albertyn R, Cywes S. Clinical outcome and long-term quality of life after surgical correction of Hirschsprung's disease. *J Pediatr Surg* 1996;31:1496-502.

[47] Reding R, de Ville de Goyet J, Gosseye S, et al. Hirschsprung's disease: A 20-year experience. *J Pediatr Surg* 1997;32:1221-5.

[48] Teitelbaum DH, Coran AG. Long-term results and quality of life after treatment of Hirschsprung's diseae and allied disorders, in Holschneider A, Puri P (eds): *Hirschsprung's Disease and Allied Disorders.* Second Edition. Amsterdam, The Netherlands: Harwood Academic Publishers; 2000. p. 457-66.

[49] Teitelbaum DH, Coran AG. Reoperative surgery for Hirschsprung's disease. *Semin Pediatr Surg* 2003;12:124-31.

[50] Drossman D, Sandler R, McKee D. Bowel patterns among subjects not seeking health care. *Gastroentertology* 1982;83:529-34.

[51] Teitelbaum DH, Drongowski RA, Chamberlain JN, Coran AG. Long-term stooling patterns in infants undergoing primary endorectal pull-through for Hirschsprung's disease. *J Pediatr Surg* 1997;32:1049-52.

[52] Shorter NG, Garrow E. Correspondence: Bowel plication in the management of Hirschsprung disease. *J Pediatr Surg* 2007;43:2140-2.

[53] van Kuyk EM, Brugman-Boezeman ATTM, Wissink-Essink M,Severijnen RS, Festen C, Bleijenberg G. Defecation problems in children with Hirschsprung's disease: A biopsychosocial approach. *Pediatr Surg Int* 2000;16:312-6.

[54] Marty TL, Seo T, Matlak ME,Sullivan JJ, Black RE, Johnson DG. Gastrointestinal function after surgical correction of Hirschsprung's disease: Long-term follow-up in 135 patients. *J Pediatr Surg* 1995;30:655-8.

[55] Mills JLA, Konkin DE, Milner R, Penner JG, Langer M, Webber EM. Long-term bowel function and quality of life in children with Hirschsprung's disease. *J Pediatr Surg* 2008;43:899-05.

[56] Iwai N, Deguchi E, Kimura O,Kubota Y, Ono Shimadera S. Social quality of life for adult patients with anorectal malformations. *J Pediatr Surg* 2007;42:313-7.

[57] Holschneider AM, Börner W, Buurman O, Caffarena PF, von Issendorf H, Kaiser G et al. Clinical and electromanometrical investigations of postoperative continence in Hirschsprung's disease – an international workshop. *Z Kinderchir* 1980;29:39-48.

[58] Baxter NN, Rothenberger DA, Lowry AC. Measuring fecal incontinence. *Dis Colon Rectum* 2003;46:1591-605.

[59] Sillen U, Hagberg S, Hedlund H,Rubenson A, Sörsensen SE. Early complications and long-term results of colorectal resection ad modum Rehbein for Hirschsprung's disease. *Z Kinderchir* 1987;42:362-5.

[60] Moore SW, Millar AJW, Cywes S. Long-term clinical, manometric and histological evaluation of obstructive symptoms in the postoperative Hirschsprung's patient. *J Pediatr Surg* 1994;29:106-11.

[61] Nagasaki A, Ikeda K, Suita S. Postoperative sequential anorectal manometric study of children with Hirschsprung's disease. *J Pediatr Surg* 1980;15:615-9.

[62] Heikkinen M, Rintala R, Luukkonen P. Long-term anal sphincter performance after surgery for Hirschsprung's disease. *J Pediatr Surg* 1997;32:1443-6.
[63] Keshtgar AS, Ward HC, Clayden GS, de Sousa NM. Investigations for incontinence and constipation after surgery for Hirschsprung's disease in children. *Pediatr Surg Int* 2003;19:4-8.
[64] Liu DC, Rodriquez J, Hill CB, Loe WA Jr. Transanal mucosectomy in the treatment of Hirschsprung's disease. *J Pediatr Surg* 2000;35:235-8.
[65] Höllwarth ME, Rivosecchi M, Schleef J, Deluggi S, Fasching G, Ceriati E et al. The role of transanal endorectal pull-through in the treatment of Hirschsprung's disease: A multicenter experience. *Pediatr Surg Int* 2002;18:344-8.
[66] Bjornland K, Diseth TH, Emblem R. Long-term functional, manometric, and endosonographic evaluation of patients operated upon with the Duhamel technique. *Pediatr Surg Int* 1998;13:24-8.
[67] Kuwahara M, Iwai N, Yanagihara J, Tokiwa K, Fukata R. Endosonographic study of anal sphincters in patients after surgery for Hirschsprung's disease. *J Pediatr Surg* 1999;34:450-3.
[68] Benninga MA, Wijers OB, van der Hoeven CW, Taminiau JA, Klopper PJ, Tytgat GN et al. Manometry, profilometry and endosonography: Normal physiology anatomy of the anal canal in healthy children. *J Pediatr Gastroenterol Nutr* 1994;18:68-77.
[69] Carneiro PMR, Brereton RJ, Drake DP, Kiely EM, Spitz L, Turnock R. Enterocolitis in Hirschsprung's disease. *Pediatr Surg Int* 1992;7:356-60.
[70] Teitelbaum DH, Qualman SJ, Caniano DA. Hirschsprung's disease. Identification of risk factors for enterocolitis. *Ann Surg* 1998;207:240-4.
[71] Ikeda K, Gota S. Diagnosis and treatment of Hirschsprung's diseae in Japan: An analysis of 1628 patients. *Ann Surg* 1984;199:400-5.
[72] Weitzman JJ. Management of Hirschsprung's disease with the Swenson procedure with emphasis on long-term follow-up. *Pediatr Surg Int* 1986;1:100-4.
[73] Kleinhaus S, Boley SJ, Sheran M, Sieber WK. Hirschsprung's disease: A survey of the members of the Surgical Section of the American Academy of Pediatrics. *J Pediatr Surg* 1979;14:588-97.
[74] Sarioglu A, Tanyel FC, Buyukpamukcu N, Hicsonmez A. Clinical risk factors of Hirschsprung-associated enterocolitis. I: Preoperative enterocolitis. *Turk J Pediatr* 1997;39:81-9.
[75] Vieten D, Spicer R. Enterocolitis complicating Hirschsprung's disease. *Semin Pediatr Surg* 1998;13:263-72.
[76] Surana R, Quinn FMJ, Puri P. Evaluation of risk factors in the development of enterocolitis complicating Hirschsprung's disease. *Pediatr Surg Int* 1994;9:234-6.
[77] Hackam DJ, Filler RM, Pearl RH. Enterocolitis after the surgical treatment of Hirschsprung's disease. Risk factors and financial impact. *J Pediatr Surg* 1998;33:830-3.
[78] Teitelbaum D, Cilley R, Sherman N, Bliss D, Uitylugt ND, Ranaud EJ et al. A decade experience with the primary pull-through for Hirschsprung's disease in the newborn period; A multi-center analysis of outcomes. *Ann Surg* 2000;232:372-80.

[79] Bill AH, Chapman ND. Then enterocolitis of Hirschsprung's disesase: Its natural history and treatment. *Am J Surg* 1962;103:70-4.

[80] Teich S, Schisgall RM, Anderson KD. Ischemic enterocolitis as a complication of Hirschsprung's disease. *J Pediatr Surg* 1998;21:143-5.

[81] Grosfeld JL, Ballantine TVN, Csicsko JF. A critical evaluation of the Duhamel operation for Hirschsprung's disease. *Arch Surg* 1978;113:454-9.

[82] Berry CL, Fraser GC. The experimental production of colitis in the rabbit with particular reference to Hirschsprung's disease. *J Pediatr Surg* 1968;3:36-42.

[83] Menezes M, Puri P. Long-term outcome of patients with enterocolitis complicating Hirschsprung's disease. *Pediatr Surg Int* 2006;22:316-8.

[84] Swenson O. Partial internal sphincterectomy in the treatment of Hirschsprung's disease. *Ann Surg* 1964;160;540-50.

[85] Singh R, Cameron BH, Walton JM, Farrokhyar F, Borenstein SH, Fitzgerald PG. Postoperative Hirschsprung's enterocolitis after minimally invasive Swenson's procedure. *J Pediatr Surg* 2007;42:885-9.

[86] Kobayashi H, Hiradawa H, Surana R, O'Briain DS, Puri P. Intestinal neuronal dysplasia is a possible cause of persistent bowel symptoms after pull-through operation for Hirschsprung's disease. *J Pediatr Surg* 1995;30:253-7.

[87] Polley T, Coran AG, Wesley JR. A ten-year experience with ninety-two cases of Hirschsprung's disease. Including sixty-seven consecutive endorectal pull-through procedures. *Ann Surg* 1985;202:349-55.

[88] van Leeuwen K, Teitelbaum DH, Elhalaby EA, Coran AG. Long-term follow-up of redo pull-through procedures for Hirschsprung's disease: Efficacy of the endorectal pull-through. *J Pediatr Surg* 2000;35:829-33.

[89] Tariq GM, Brereton RJ, Wright VM. Complications of endorectal pull-through for Hirschsprung's disease. *J Pediatr Surg* 1991;26:1202-6.

[90] Agarwala S, Bhatnagar V, Mitra DK. Long-term follow-up of Hirschsprung's disease: Review of early and late complications. *Indian Pediatr* 1996;33:382-6.

[91] Woolside JR, Crawfor ED. Urodynamic feature of pelvic plexus injury. *J Urol* 1980;124:657-8.

[92] Blaivas JG, Barbalias GA. Characteristic of neural injury after abdominoperineal resection. *J Urol* 1983;129:84-7.

[93] Chang PL, Fan HA. Urodynamic studies before and/or after abdominaoperineal resection of the rectum for carcinoma. *J Urol* 1983;130:948-51.

[94] Yalla VS, Andriole GL. Vesicourethral dysfunction following pelvic visceral ablative surgery. *J Urol* 1984;132:503-9.

[95] Leveckis J, Boucher NR, Parys BT, Reed MW, Shorthouse AJ Anderson JB. Bladder and erectile dysfunction before and after rectal surgery for cancer. *Br J Urol* 1995;76:752-6.

[96] Holschneider AM, Kraeft H, Scholtissek C. Urodynamische Untersuchungen von Blasenentleerungsstorungen bei Analatresie und Morbus Hirschsprung. *Z Kinderchir* 1982;35:64-8.

[97] Ates O, Hakguder G, Kart Y,Olguner M, Akgür FM. The effect of dilated ganglionic segment on anorectal and urinary functions during 1-stage transanal endorectal pull through for Hirschsprung's disease. *J Pediatr Surg* 2007;42:1271-5.

[98] Russell MB, Russell CA, Niebuhr E. An epidemiological study of Hirschsprung's disease and additional anomalies. *Acta Paediatr* 1994;83:68-71.

[99] Quinn FM, Surana R, Puri P. The influence of trisomy 21 on outcome in children with Hirschsprung's disease. *J Pediatr Surg* 1994;29:781-3.

[100] Caniano DA, Teitelbaum DH, Qualman SJ. Management of Hirschsprung's disease in children with trisomy 21. *Ann J Surg* 1990;159:402-4.

[101] Hackam DJ, Reblock K, Barksdale EM, Redlingler R Lynch J, Gaines BA. The influence of Down's syndrome on the management and outcome of children with Hirschsprung's disease. *J Pediatr Surg* 2003;38:946-9.

[102] Morabito A, Lall A, Gull S, Mohee A, Bianchi A. The impact of Down's syndrome on the immediate and long-term outcomes of children with Hirschsprung's disease. *Pediatr Surg Int* 2006;22:179-81.

[103] Stephen FD, Durham-Smith E. Classification, identification and assessment of surgical treatment of anorectal anomalies ("Wingspread classification"). *Pediatr Surg Int* 1986;1:200-5.

[104] Catto-Smith AG, Trajanovska M, Taylor RG. Long-term continence in patients Stephen with Hirschsprung's diseases and Down syndrome. J Gastroenterol Hepatol 2006;21:748-753.

[105] Book L, Hart A, Black J, Feolo M, Zone JJ, Neuhausen SL. Prevalence and clinical characteristics of celiac disease in Downs syndrome in a US study. *Am J Med Genet* 2001;98:70-4.

[106] Rogers J. Continence – lessons in control. *Nurs Times* 1998;94:66-8.

[107] Jasonni V, Martucciello G. Total colonic aganglionosis. *Semin Pediatr Surg* 1998;7:174-80.

[108] Yann R, Yves A, Dominique J, Thierry Y, Oliver G, Florence L.Improved quality of life by combined transplantation in Hirschsprung's disease with a very long aganglionic segment. *J Pediatr Surg* 2003;38:422-4.

[109] N-Fekete C, Ricour C, Martelli H, Jacob SL, Pellerin D.Total colonic aganglionosis (with or without ileal involvement): A review of 27 cases. *J Pediatr Surg* 1986;21:251-4.

[110] Bickler SW, Harrison MW, Campbell TJ, Campbell JR. Long-segment Hirschsprung's disease. *Arch Surg* 1992;127:1047-40.

[111] Ikeda K, Goto S. Total colonic aganglionosis with or without small bowel involvement: An analysis of 137 patients. *J Pediatr Surg* 1986;21:319-22.

[112] Martin LW. Surgical management of Hirschsprung's disease involving the small intestine. *Arch Surg* 1968;97:183-7.

[113] Anupama B, Zheng S, Xiao X. Ten-year experience in the management of total colonic aganglionosis. *J Pediatr Surg* 2007;42:1671-6.

[114] Escobar MA, Grosfeld JL, West KW, Scherer LR, Rouse TM, Engum SA et al. Long-term outcomes in total colonic aganglionosis: A 32-year experience. *J Pediatr Surg* 2005;40:955-61.

[115] Hoehner JC, Ein SH, Shandling B, Kim PC. Long-term morbidity in total colonic aganglionosis. *J Pediatr Surg* 1998;33:961-6.

[116] Stockmann PT, Philippart AI. The Duhamel procedure for Hirschsprung's disease. *Sem Pediatr Surg* 1998;7:89-95.

[117] Kimura K, Nishijima E, Muraji T, Tsugawa C, Matsumoto Y. A new surgical approach to extensive aganglionosis. *J Pediatr Surg* 1981;16:840-3.

[118] Lal D, Nichol PF, Harms BA, Go LL Lund DP. Ileo-anal S-pouch reconstruction in patients with total colonic aganglionosis. *J Pediatr Surg* 2004;39:7-9.

[119] Kim HG, Lee PW, Garza J, Duggan C, Fauza D, Jaksic T. Serial transverse enteroplasty for short bowel syndrome: A case report. *J Pediatr Surg* 2003;38:881-5.

[120] Meier-Ruge W. Ueber ein Erkrankungsblid des Colon mit Hirschsprung Symptomatik. *Verh Dtsch Ges Pathol* 1971;55:506-11.

[121] Lassman G, Wurnig P. Lokale ganglienzellhyperplasie in der submucosal am oralen ende des aganglionaren segments bei morbus Hirschsprung. *Z Kinderchir* 1973;12:236-43.

[122] Schmittenbecher PP, Sacher P, Cholewa D, Haberlik A, Menardi G, Moczulski J et al. Hirschsprung's disease and intestinal neuronal dysplasia: A frequent association with implications for the postoperative course. *Pediatr Surg Int* 1999;15:553-8.

[123] Estevão-Costa J, Fragoso AC, Campos M, Carvalho JL. An approach to minimize postoperative enterocolitis in Hirschsprung's disease. *J Pediatr Surg* 2006;41:1704-7.

[124] Fadda B, Pistor G, Meier-Ruge W, Hofmann-von Kap-her S, Müntefering H, Espinoza R. Symptoms, diagnosis, and therapy of neuronal intestinal dysplasia masked by Hirschsprung's disease. *Pediatr Surg Int* 1987;2:76-80.

[125] Hanimann B, Inderitzin D, Briner J, Sacher P. Clinical relevance of Hirschsprung-associated neuronal intestinal dysplasia (HANID). *Eur J Pediatr Surg* 1992;2:147-9.

[126] Meier-Ruge W, Ammann K, Bruder E, Holschneider AM, Schärli AF, Schmittenbecher PP et al. Updated results on intestinal neuronal dysplasia (IND B). *Eur J Pediatr Surg* 2004;14:384-91.

[127] Kobayashi H, Wang Y, Hirakawa H, O'Briain DS, Puri P. Intraoperative evaluation of extent of aganglionosis by a radid acetylcholinesterase histochemical technique. *J Pediatr Surg* 1995;30:248-52.

[128] Meyrat BJ, Lesbros Y, Laurini RN. Assessment of the colon innervation with serial biopsies above the aganglionic zone before the pull-through procedure in Hirschsprung's disease. *Pediatr Surg Int* 2001;17:129-35.

[129] Skába R, Frantlová M, Horák J. Intestinal neuronal dysplasia. *Eur J Gastroenterol Hepatol* 2006;18:699-701.

[130] Poceta JS, Strandjord TP, Badura RJ Jr. Milstein JM. Ondine curse and neurocristopathy. *Pediatr Neurology* 1987;3:370-2.

[131] Rohrer T, Trachsel D, Engelcke G, Hammer J. Congenital central hypoventilation syndrome associated with Hirschsprung's disease and neuroblastoma; case of multiple neurocristopathies. *Pediatr Pulmonol*ogy 2002;33:71-6.

[132] Ghose SI, Squire BR, Stringer MD, et al. Hirschsprung's disease: Problems with transitional zone pull-through. *J Pediatr Surg* 2000;12:1805-9.

[133] Tam PKH, Boyd GP. Origin, course and endings of abnormal enteric nerve fibers in Hirschsprung's disease defined by whole mount immunohistochemistry. *J Pediatr Surg* 1990;25:457-61.

[134] Miura H, Ohi R, Tseng SW, Takahashi T. The structure of the transitional and aganglionic zones of Auerbach's plexus in patients with Hirschsprung's disease: A computer-assisted three-dimensional reconstruction study. *J Pediatr Surg* 1996;31:420-6.

[135] White FV, Langer JC. Circumferential distribution of ganglion cells in the transition zone of children with Hirschsprung's disease. *Pediatr Dev Pathol* 2000;3:216-22.

[136] Farrugia MK, Alexander N, Clarke S, Nash R, Nicholls EA, Holmes K. Does transitional zone pull-through in Hirschsprung's disease imply a poor prognosis? *J Pediatr Surg* 2003;38:1766-9.

[137] Lynn HB. Rectal myectomy in Hirschsprung's disease, a decade of experience. *Arch Surg* 1975;110:991-4.

[138] Abbas BS, Forootan H. Role of anorectal myectomy after failed endorectal pullthrough in Hirschsprung's disease. *J Pediatr Surg* 1994;29:1307-9.

[139] Wilcox DT, Kiely EM. Repeat pull-through for Hirschsprung's disease. *J Pediatr Surg* 1998;33:1507-9.

[140] Weber TR, Tortuna RS, Silen ML, Dillon PA. Reoperation for Hirschsprung's disease. *J Pediatr Surg* 1999;34:154-6.

[141] Sarioglu A, Tanyel CF, Büyükpamukcu N, Hiçsönmez A. Redo operations of Hirschsprung's disease. *Int Surg* 1998;83:333-5.

[142] Langer J. Repeat pull-through surgery for complicated Hirschsprung's disease: Indications, techniques, and results. *J Pediatr Surg* 1999;34:1136-41.

[143] Schweizer P, Berger S, Schweizer M, Holschneider AM, Beck O. Repeated pull-through surgery for complicated Hirschsprung's disease – principles derived from clinical experience. *J Pediatr Surg* 2007;42:536-43.

[144] Gobran TA, Ezzat A, Hassan ME,O'Neill J. Redo transanal endorectal pull-through: A preliminary study. *Pediatr Surg Int* 2007;23:189-93.

[145] Dibley MJ, Goldsby JB, Staehling NW, Trowbridge FL. Development of normalized curves for international growth reference: historical and technical considerations. *Am J Clin Nutr* 1987;46:736-48.

[146] Bai Y, Yuan Z, Wang W, Zhao Y, Wang H, Wang We. Quality of life for children with fecal incontinence after surgically corrected anorectal malformation. *J Pediatr Surg* 2000;35:462-4.

[147] Goyal A, Williams JM, Kenny SE, Lwin R, Baillie CT, Lamont GL et al. Functional outcome and quality of life in anorectal malformations. *J Pediatr Surg* 2006;41:318-22.

[148] Hartman EE, Oort FJ, Aronson DC, Hanneman MJ, van der Zee DC, Rieu PN, Madern GC et al. Critical factors affecting quality of life of adult patients with anorectal malformations or Hirschsprung's disease. *Am J Gastroenterol* 2004;99;907-13.

[149] Hsu WM, Chen CC. Clinical and manometric evaluation of postoperative faecal soiling in paitents with Hirschsprung's disease. *J Formos Med Assoc* 1999;98:410-4.

[150] Sarioglu A, Tanyel CF, Senocak ME. Complications of the two major operations of Hirschsprung's disease: A single centre experience. *Turk J Pediatr* 2001;43:219-22.

In: Hirschsprung's Disease: Diagnosis and Treatment
Ed: Ramón Núñez and Manuel López-Alonso
ISBN: 978-1-60741-349-3

Chapter XXIV

Variant Hirschsprung's Disease

Prem Puri

The typical patient with Hirschsprung's disease is a newborn presenting with delayed passage of meconium and abdominal distension or a young child presenting with severe chronic constipation. The diagnosis is confirmed by the histological and histochemical evaluation of suction rectal biopsies which demonstrate absence of ganglion cells in the submucosa and increased acetylcholinesterase (AChE) activity in the lamina propria. However, there are a number of patients who clinically resemble Hirschsprung's disease despite the presence of ganglion cells in rectal biopsy. Various terms have been used to describe these conditions such as "chronic idiopathic intestinal pseudoobstruction", "pseudo-Hirschsprung's disease", "neonatal intestinal pseudo-obstruction" and "intestinal hypoperistalsis syndrome". There is a growing interest to further investigate these relatively rare functional bowel disorders, since the diagnosis and management of these patients continues to be a challenge for clinicians. Over the past two decades our group has focused its research interest into delineating variant Hirschsprung's disease based on specific histochemical, immunohistochemical and electronmicroscopic studies.

Since 1981, it has been our policy to obtain suction rectal biopsy specimens from patients who have severe chronic constipation or are suspected to have functional intestinal obstruction. The suction rectal biopsy specimens are obtained at 3, 5 and 7 cm from the pectinate line and examined by conventional hematoxylin and eosin (H&E) staining, histochemistry and immunocytochemical staining. If the results of suction rectal biopsy show normal AChE activity in the lamina propria and muscularis mucosae with normally appearing ganglion cells or without ganglion cells, and the patient continues to have signs and symptoms of obstruction or severe constipation, we perform a full-thickness rectal biopsy. Immediately after the biopsy specimen is obtained, the tissue is divided into four parts and processed for H&E staining, AChE histochemistry, NADPH-diaphorase histochemistry, immunohistochemistry (PGP9.5, peripherin, nNOS, NCAM, NGFR and c-kit)and electronmicroscopic studies. If necessary, further full-thickness bowel biopsies or seromuscular bowel biopsies are obtained for additional investigations using whole-mount preparation technique.

Between 1981 and 2003, full-thickness bowel biopsy or resected surgical specimens from 151 patients (61 boys and 90 girls) with clinical symptoms suggesting HD, were examined in our research laboratory. Their ages ranged from 1 day to 9 years. One hundred and three patients had onset of symptoms in the neonatal period. Eighty-three patients were from Ireland and in 68 patients, biopsy material was sent to our laboratory from other countries. Table 1 shows various functional bowel disorders diagnosed using different histological techniques.

Table 1. Variant Hirschsprung's Disease (1981-2007)

Intestinal neuronal dysplasia	73
Hypoganglionosis	17
Immature ganglia	9
Internal sphincter achalasia	41
Smooth muscle disorders	22
Total	**162**

Intestinal Neuronal Dysplasia

Intestinal neuronal dysplasia (IND), a clinical condition that resembles Hirschsprung's disease (HD), was first described by Meier-Ruge [1] in 1971 as a malformation of the enteric plexus. In 1983, Fadda et al [2] subclassified IND into two clinically and histologically distinct subtypes. Type A occurs in less than 5% of cases, is characterized by congenital aplasia or hypoplasia of the sympathetic innervation, and presents acutely in the neonatal period with episodes of intestinal obstruction, diarrhoea and bloody stools. The clinical picture of Type B resembles HD and is characterized by malformation of the parasympathetic submucous and myenteric plexuses and accounts for over 95% of cases of isolated IND. IND occurring in association with HD is of Type B. The characteristic histologic features of IND B include hyperganglionosis of the submucous and myenteric plexuses, giant ganglia, ectopic ganglion cells, and increased acetylcholinesterase (AChE) activity in the lamina propria and around submucosal blood vessels [3,4].

The incidence of isolated IND has varied from 0.3% to 40% of all suction rectal biopsies in different centres [5-8]. IND immediately proximal to a segment of aganglionosis is not uncommon and often presents as persistent obstructive symptoms after a pull-through operation for HD [9]. Some investigators have reported that 25% to 35% of patients with HD have associated IND [2,3,9]. However, others have rarely encountered IND in association with HD [10]. The uncertainty regarding the incidence of IND has resulted from the considerable confusion regarding the essential diagnostic criteria [11]. The diagnostic difficulty is centered on a wide variability encountered in the literature, not only in terms of age of the patient, the type of specimen examined and the stains performed, but also the diagnostic criteria used [11]. Many investigators have raised doubts about the existence of

IND as a distinct histopathologic entity [12-14]. It has been suggested that the pathologic changes seen in IND may be part of normal development or may be a secondary phenomenon induced by congenital obstruction and inflammatory disease [14,15]. One strong piece of evidence that IND is a real entity stems from animal models. Recently, two different *Hox11L1* knockout mouse models have been generated. In both cases, homozygous mutant mice were viable, but megacolon developed at the age of 3 to 5 weeks. Histological and immunohistochemical analyses showed hyperplasia of myenteric ganglia, a phenotype similar to that observed in IND[16-18]. However, the mutation screening of this gene in 48 patients with IND did not show any sequence variant, either causative missense mutation, or neutral substitution [19]. More recently Von Boyen et al [20] reported abnormalities of the enteric nervous system in heterozygous endothelin B receptor (EDNRB)-deficient rats resembling IND in humans. They showed that a heterozygous 301-bp deletion of the EDNRB gene led to abnormalities of the submucous plexus, such as giant ganglia, hyperganglionosis and hypertrophy of the nerve fiber strands. These findings support the concept that IND may be linked to a genetic defect.

Since the first description in 1971, most controversy surrounding IND has been regarding which histologic diagnostic criteria are required for definitive diagnosis. The presently recognized diagnostic criteria, previously reported by our group and supported by others, are hyperganglionosis and giant ganglia, in addition to the presence of at least 1 of the following on suction rectal biopsy: ectopic ganglia in the lamina propria, increased AChE-positive nerve fibers around submucosal blood vessels and in the lamina propria[3,4,11,21,22]. However, Lumb and Moore [23] feel that giant ganglia can be a normal feature in normal bowel having identified them in segments of adult bowel removed during surgery for colorectal carcinoma. To overcome the confusion in diagnostic criteria, Borchard et al [24], produced guidelines for identifying IND in mucosal rectal biopsies. These comprised two obligatory criteria (hyperplasia of the submucous plexus and an increase in AChE-positive nerve fibers around submucosal blood vessels) and 2 additional criteria (neuronal heterotopia and increased AChE activity in the lamina propria). In our experience, hyperganglionosis and giant ganglia are the most important features for the diagnosis of IND in suction rectal biopsies, except in the newborn, where hyperganglionosis is a normal finding [4].

Another controversial area surrounding IND is whether the histologic findings are age-related. The recent description of hyperganglionosis, considered to be one of the most important criteria of IND, as an age-dependent finding, has caused further confusion. Recent studies have found that the enteric nervous system continues to develop in the postnatal period. Wester et al [25,26] investigated the number of ganglion cells per ganglion and ganglion cell density in whole-mount preparations of the submucous plexus of normal distal colon and found a marked decrease of ganglion cells density with increasing age, but the number of ganglion cells per ganglion remained constant. Knowledge of the ganglion cell density of the normal human enteric nervous system is scant, apparent by the huge variation among reports of the normal neuron density in the myenteric plexus. The reported density varies more than 200 times among the different studies [27-30]. This results in difficulties defining conditions such as hyperganglionosis. Schofield and Yunis [31,32] reported that 8.3% of 456 investigated cases had features of IND, using increased AChE activity in the lamina propria and hyperganglionosis (defined as more than 5 ganglia per high-power field in the submucosa) as diagnostic criteria. These patients had a high incidence of prematurity, indicating that some histological features of IND may be related to age and development. Age-related alterations of the enteric ganglia were discussed further by Smith [10], who described a significantly higher number of submucous ganglia in children under 4 weeks of age compared with older children. It would be desirable with better knowledge of the enteric nervous system and also with quantitative diagnostic criteria of IND to distinguish normal variation from pathological conditions. Moore et al [33] introduced a morphological scoring system based on the findings of hyperganglionosis, giant ganglia, maturity of neurons, heterotopic neuronal cells and AChE activity in the lamina propria, muscularis mucosa or adventitia of submucosal blood vessels. Hyperganglionosis and increased AChE activity of nerve fibers in the lamina propria were of major importance in this scoring system.

Suction rectal biopsy is the principal method for the diagnosis of disorders of intestinal innervation. It is necessary to include a sufficient amount of submucosa in the suction biopsy specimens. Traditionally, hematoxylin and eosin staining and AChE histochemistry (Fig 1) in suction rectal biopsy specimens have provided the basis for the diagnostic evaluation of IND.

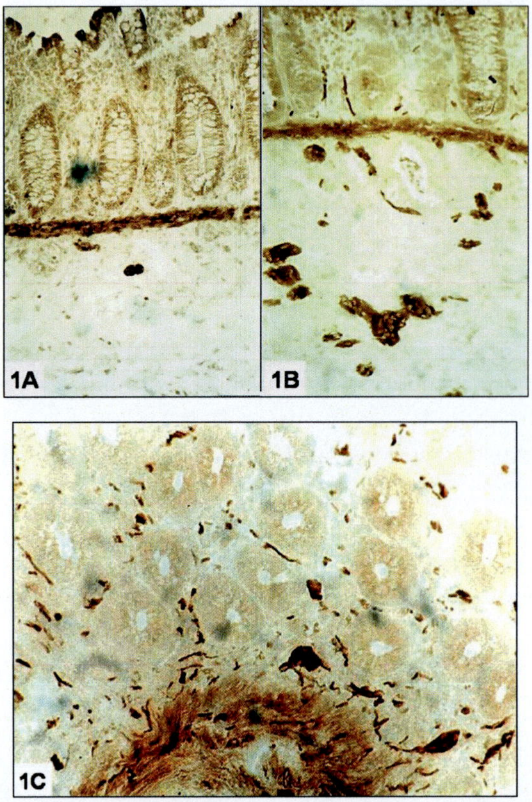

Figure 1.AChE staining (A) Normal rectal suction biopsy (B) Rectal suction biopsy from a patient with IND showing hyperganglionosis, giant ganglia and increased AChE activity in the lamina propria (C) ganglia cells in the lamina propria in IND (original magnification x125).

However, there has been discussion about whether AChE histochemistry is sufficient for the accurate diagnosis of IND and other additional staining techniques have been proposed.

Meier-Ruge et al suggest lactate-dehydrogenase histochemistry [34,35]. In our laboratory, newer neuronal markers currently are being used, such as reduced nicotinamide-adenine dinuleotide phosphate (NADPH) diaphorase histochemistry and immunohistochemistry using antibodies raised against neural cell adhesion molecule, Protein Gene Product 9.5 (PGP9.5), S-100, Peripherin and Synaptophysin. Ganglion-cell counting can be difficult. Standard Immunohistochemical techniques, using antibodies raised against neuron specific enolase or PGP 9.5, which are commonly used to display the enteric nervous system, are less suitable for cell counting because they stain not only the cell bodies but also the axonal processes. Recently, cuprolinic blue staining has been proposed as the method that stains the largest number of ganglion cells [26]. Furthermore, this method stains only the cell bodies and not the axons, which makes it relatively easy to distinguish the individual cells. The whole-mount preparation elegantly shows 3-dimensional morphology of the submucous and myenteric plexuses in IND, demonstrating markedly increased number of ganglion cells compared to controls.

Current treatment of IND Type B is in the first instance conservative, consisting of laxatives and enemas. In the majority of patients the clinical problem resolves or is manageable in this way. If bowel symptoms persist after at least 6 months of treatment, internal sphincter myectomy should be considered. Recently Gillick et al [36] reported results of treatment in 33 patients with IND followed-up for periods ranging from 1 to 8 years (mean, 2.4 years). Twenty-one (64%) patients had a good response to conservative management and currently have normal bowel habits. Twelve patients (36%) underwent internal sphincter myectomy after failed conservative management. Seven of these patients now have normal bowel habits. Two patients were able to stay clean with regular enemas. Three patients who continued to have persistent constipation after myectomy and underwent resection of redundant and dilated sigmoid colon now have normal bowel habits. Scharli reported that 13 of the 22 cases required internal sphincter myectomy, which resulted in satisfactory results in 90% of the patients within 3 months. Resection and pull-through operation is rarely indicated in IND. The indication for surgery should not be determined on the basis of histopathological findings alone: rather the decision must be based on the individual patient's clinical symptoms.

Hypoganglionosis

Isolated hypoganglionosis is rare. Clinically, it resembles HD [5,37,38]. Failure to pass meconium may be the first symptom in the neonatal period, whereas infants and older children present with chronic constipation. The diagnosis of hypoganglionosis by means of suction biopsy is difficult. Rectal suction biopsy results with absent or low level of AChE activity in the lamina propria and absence or reduction of submucosal ganglion cells may raise suspicion of hypoganglionosis. A full-thickness rectal biopsy allows the inspection of the myenteric plexus and is essential for the diagnosis of hypoganglionosis. The characteristic histologic features of hypoganglionosis include sparse and small myenteric ganglia, absent or low AChE activity in the lamina propria, hypertrophy of muscularis mucosae and circular muscle [39]. Meier-Ruge et al [40] performed morphometric measurements in resected bowel specimens from patients with hypoganglionosis and found a dramatic decrease in plexus area and nerve cell number in the myenteric plexus and an increase in distance between ganglia.

Gut innervation has a complex, 3-dimensional structure, which is difficult to appreciate on thin sections. The whole-mount preparation technique produces a 3-dimensional picture to better show the structure of neuronal networks and their relationship of branching and interconnecting nerve fibers to each other and to the neighbouring tissues [21]. This technique therefore is especially useful for the investigation of pathologic changes in the submucosal and myenteric plexuses such as hypoganglionosis [41]. The great advantages for the histologic evaluation become obvious when whole-mount preparations are compared with sections.

Recently, a marked reduction in myenteric and muscular c-kit positive interstitial cells of Cajal (ICCS) in the large bowel of patients with isolated hypoganglionosis has been suggested to contribute to motility dysfunction [42]. Furthermore, abnormality of the neuromuscular junction has been reported in hypoganglionosis which may further contribute to disturbances in gut motility [43].

There is little information regarding the genetic basis of isolated hypoganglionosis. Inoue and coworkers [44] performed mutation screening of RET and GDNF gene in children with hypoganglionosis but found no sequence variants, either causative missense mutation or neutral substitution.

Treatment of hypoganglionosis is similar to Hirschsprung's disease involving resection of the affected segment and pullthrough operation.

Immature Ganglia

Immature ganglia are usually seen in the biopsy results from premature infants presenting with functional intestinal obstruction. Acetylcholinesterase staining of suction rectal biopsy specimens show small ganglia and ganglion cells. However, AChE histochemical technique usually fails to distinguish small ganglia from nerve supporting cells (enteric glia). NCAM and NADPH-diaphorase staining methods can usually clearly show small ganglion cells that are the same size as enteric glial cells. Cathepsin D has been further used to show the maturation of enteric ganglion cells [45]. The histological proof of maturation of ganglion cells in the myenteric plexus of young infants was accompanied by the improvement of the bowel function, ie. peristalsis. The treatment of patients with immature ganglia is conservative consisting of laxative and enemas.

Internal Sphincter Achalasia

The internal anal sphincter (IAS), which is a specialized smooth muscle continuation of the circular muscle layer of the rectum, plays an important role in the maintenance of anorectal continence and in the pathophysiology of incontinence and constipation [46]. The IAS relaxes in response to rectal distension, a phenomenon called the rectosphincteric inhibitory reflex, which is mediated by intramural nerves descending from the rectum to the IAS. The IAS receives adrenergic, cholinergic and nonadrenergic, noncholinergic (NANC) innervation. Several investigators have reported that IAS relaxation is brought about by the activation of intramural NANC nerves. Recently, it has been shown that nitric oxide (NO) is the NANC neurotransmitter mediating neurogenic relaxation of the human internal sphincter.

Internal anal sphincter achalasia (IASA) is a clinical condition with presentation similar to Hirschsprung's disease but with the presence of ganglion cells on suction rectal biopsy. The diagnosis of IASA is made on anorectal manometry, which shows the absence of rectosphincteric reflex on rectal balloon inflation. Previously, IASA has been referred to as ultrashort segment Hirschsprung's disease (HD) [47]. The ultrashort segment Hirschsprung's disease, which is a rare condition, is characterized by an aganglionic segment of 1 to 3 cm long and normal acetylcholinesterase (AChE) activity in the lamina propria and increased AChE activity in the muscularis mucosae [48]. Many patients who are considered to have ultrashort HD on abnormal anorectal manometric findings show presence of ganglion cells and normal acetylcholinesterase (AChE) activity in suction rectal biopsies. Many investigators have therefore suggested that the term IASA is more suitable because it reflects more accurately failure of relaxation of the internal sphincter, which is the causative factor in this condition [47,49]. The exact pathogenesis and pathophysiology of IASA is not understood fully. Altered intramuscular innervation has been reported in IASA and this is believed to be responsible for the motility dysfunction seen in these patients. Hirakawa et al [46] reported absence of nitrergic innervation within the IAS muscle in patients with IASA and suggested that nitrergic nerve depletion may play an important role in the development of IASA. More recently, Oue and Puri [50] reported defective innervation of the neuromuscular junction (NMJ) of the IAS in patients with IASA. If the NMJ is abnormal, the neurotransmitter chemicals synthesizing neurons cannot be transmitted to muscle cells, thereby causing motility dysfunction. Altered distribution of c-kit positive interstitial cells of Cajal (ICCs) has been reported in the internal sphincter of patients with internal sphincter achalasia which may further contribute to motility dysfunction in these patients [51].

Posterior internal sphincter myectomy has been recommended as the treatment of choice for patients with internal sphincter achalasia. De Caluwe et al [52] reported bowel function in 15 consecutive patients with IASA 2 to 6 years after posterior internal sphincter myectomy. At the time of follow-up, 7 patients had regular bowel motions and were not on any laxatives. Six patients had normal bowel habits but were on small doses of laxatives. One patient was able to stay clean with regular enema regimen. One patient required resection of dilated and redundant sigmoid colon and now has normal bowel habits with laxatives.

Recently, intra-anal injection of botulinum toxin has been used to treat patients with IASA [53]. This treatment modality has been found to be safe and effective but only short-term treatment in these children.

Smooth Muscle Cell Disorders

These patients who show no apparent innervation abnormalities in the pathologic specimens demonstrate abnormalities of smooth muscle cells on electron-microscopy. The outcome of smooth muscle disorders is usually poor. There are two main types of smooth muscle cell abnormalities (1) perinuclear vacuolation and (2) "central core" degeneration. All nine patients in the latter group had Megacystis-microcolon intestinal hypoperistalsis syndrome (MMIHS).

Perinuclear Vacuolation

All 10 patients in this group showed identical findings in the smooth muscle cells such as perinuclear vacuolation with well-preserved mitochondria and an increase in collagen, whereas neuronal components appeared quite normal ultrastructurally. Six of the 10 patients had marked lipofuscin deposition in smooth muscle cells. These patients usually have no peristaltic contractions in the bowel. Nine of the 10 patients in our series have died.

Megacystis-Microcolon-Intestinal Hypoperistalsis Syndrome

Megacystis microcolon intestinal hypoperistalsis syndrome (MMIHS) is a rare congenital and generally fatal cause of functional intestinal obstruction in the newborn [54,55]. This syndrome is characterized by abdominal distension caused by a distended non-obstructed urinary bladder, microcolon and decreased or absent intestinal peristalsis (Fig 2).

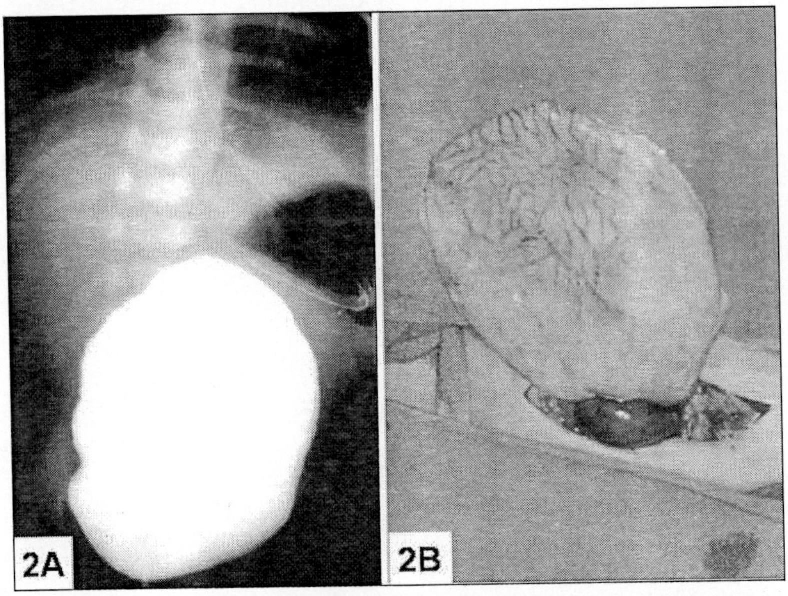

Figure 2. (A) Voiding cystourethrogram showing massively dilated bladder in a newborn with MMIHS. (B). Operative photograph of the large urinary bladder in the same patient.

Usually incomplete intestinal rotation and shortened small bowel are associated. Although more than 100 cases have been reported in the literature, the etiology of this syndrome is not yet fully understood. Puri et al [56] in 1983 reported two newborns with

MMIHS in whom light microscopy of the intestine showed thinning of the longitudinal muscle coat and abundant amounts of connective tissue between the muscle fibers. Electron microscopic evaluation of the smooth muscle cells of the ileum and bladder showed disorganization of myofilaments, cytoplasmic central core "vacuolar type" degeneration and abundant interstitial connective tissue proliferation. These smooth muscle abnormalities are seen in all hollow viscera including urinary bladder and uterus. Since their report, a number of other investigators have confirmed the presence of thinning of the longitudinal muscular coat of the bowel and vacuolation and degeneration in smooth muscle cells of bowel and bladder in this syndrome [57]. More recently, Piotrowska et a [58] reported deficiency of contractile and cystoskeletal proteins in smooth muscle cells in MMIHS bowel and Rolle et al reported markedly increased collagen deposits within the bladder wall [59]. Furthermore, MMIHS has been reported to be associated with loss or deficiency of interstitial cells of Cajal (ICCS) in the bowel of these patients [60]. ICCs are pacemaker cells which are densely distributed throughout the whole gastrointestinal tract. ICCs have important functions in neurotransmission, generation of slow waves and regulation of mechanical activities in the gastrointestinal tract especially for co-ordinated peristalsis.

The management of patients with MMIHS is frustrating. A number of prokinetic drugs and gastrointestinal hormones have been tried without success. Surgical manipulation of the gastrointestinal tract has generally been unsuccessful. The outcome of this condition is generally fatal. The need for surgical intervention should be made carefully and individualized, in that most explorations have not been helpful and probably are not necessary.

References

[1] Meier-Ruge W: Ueber ein Erkrankungsbild des Kolon mit Hirschsprung Symptomatik. *Ver Deutsch Ges Pathol*, 1971; 55: 506-10.

[2] Fadda B, Maier WA, Meier-Ruge W, et al: Neuronale intestinale Dysplasie. Eine kritische 2-Jahresanalyse klinischer und bioptischer Diagnose. *Z Kinderchir*, 1983;138: 284-7.

[3] Schaerli AF: Neuronal intestinal dysplasia. *Pediatr Surg Int*, 1992; 7: 2-7.

[4] Kobayashi H, Hirakawa H, Puri P: What are the diagnostic criteria for intestinal neuronal dysplasia? *Pediatr Surg Int*, 1995;10: 459-64.

[5] Puri P: Variant Hirschsprung's disease. *J Pediatr Surg*, 1997; 32: 149-57.

[6] Meier-Ruge W: Epidemiology of congenital innervation defects of the distal colon. *Virchows Arch* V *Pathol Anat*, 1992:420: 171-7.

[7] Milla PJ, Smith VV: Intestinal neuronal dysplasia. *J Pediatr Gastroenterol Nutr*, 1993: 17: 356-7.

[8] Martuciello G, Caffarena PE, Lerone M, et al: Neuronal intestinal dysplasia: Clinical experience in Italian patients. *Eur J Ped Surg* 1994; 4: 287-92.

[9] Kobayashi H, Hirakawa H, Surana R, et al: Intestinal neuronal dysplasia is a possible cause of persistent bowel symptoms after pull-through operation for Hirschsprung's disease. *J Pediatr Surg*, 1995; 30: 253-9.

[10] Smith VV: Isolated intestinal neuronal dysplasia: A descriptive histological pattern or a distinct clinicopathological entity? In: Hadziselimovic F, Herzog B (eds): *Inflammatory Bowel Disease and Morbus Hirschsprung's Disease*. Dordrecht,The Netherlands: Kluwer Academic; 1992.p. 203-214

[11] Puri P, Wester T: Intestinal neuronal dysplasia. *Semin Pediatr Surg*, 1998; 7:181-6.

[12] Csury L, Pena A: Intestinal neuronal dysplasia: Myth or reality? Literature review. *Pediatr Surg Int*, 1995; 10: 441-6.

[13] Kapur RP: Neuronal dysplasia: a controversial pathological correlate of intestinal pseudoobstruction. *Am J Med Genet*,2003; 122A: 287-93.

[14] Lake BD: Intestinal neuronal dysplasia. Why does it only occur in parts of Europe? *Virchows Arch*, 1995; 426: 537-39.

[15] Oguzkurt P, Senocak ME, Akcoren Z, Buyukpamukcu N: Diagnostic difficulties in neuronal intestinal dysplasia and segmental colitis. *J Pediatr Surg*, 2000; 35: 519-21.

[16] Hatano A, Aoki T, Dezawa M, Yusa S, Iitsuka Y, Koseki H, Taniguchi M, Tokuhisa T: A novel pathogenesis of megacolon in Ncx/Hox11L1 deficient mice. *J Clin Invest*,1997; 100: 795-801.

[17] Shirasawa S, Yunker AMR, Roth KA, Brown GA, Horning S, Korsmeyer SJ: Enx (Hox11L1)-deficient mice develop myenteric neuronal hyperplasia and megacolon. *Nat Med*, 1997;3: 646-50.

[18] Yamataka A, Hatano M, Kobayashi H, Wang K, Miyahara K, Sueyoshi N, Miyano T: Intestinal neuronal dysplasia-like pathology in Ncx/Hox11L.1 gene-deficient mice. *J Pediatr Surg*, 2001; 36: 1293-6.

[19] Costa M, Fava M, Seri M, Cusano R, Sancandi M, Forabosco P et al: Evaluation of the Hox11L1 gene as a candidate for congenital disorders of intestinal innervation. *J Med Genet*, 2000; 37:E9.

[20] von Boyen GB, Krammer HJ, Süss A, Dembowski C, Ehrenreich H, Wedel T: Abnormalities of the enteric nervous system in heterozygous endothelin B receptor deficient (spotting lethal) rats resembling intestinal neuronal dysplasia. *Gut*, 2002;51:414-9.

[21] Rolle U, Nemeth L, Puri P: Nitrergic innervation of the normal gut and in motility disorders of childhood. *J Pediatr Surg* 2002;37: 551-67.

[22] Rolle U, Piotrowska AP, Puri P. Abnormal vasculature in intestinal neuronal dysplasia. *Ped Surg Int*. 2003; 19: 345-8.

[23] Lumb PD, Moore L: Are giant ganglia a reliable marker of intestinal neuronal dysplasia B (IND B). *Virchows Arch*, 1991; 432:103-6.

[24] Borchard F, Meier-Ruge W, Wiebecke B, Briner J, Muntefering H, Fodisch HJ, Holschneider AM, Schmidt A, Enck P, Stolte M: Innervationsstoerungen des Dickdarms – Klassifikation und Diagnostik. *Pathologe*,1991; 12: 171-4.

[25] Wester T, O'Briain S, Puri P. Morphometric aspects of the submucous plexus in whole-mount preparations of normal human distal colon. *J Pediatr Surg*, 1985; 33: 619-22.

[26] Wester T, O'Briain S, Puri P. Notable postnatal alterations in the myenteric plexus of normal human bowel. *GUT*, 1999; 44; 666-74.

[27] Smith VV: Intestinal neuronal density in childhood: a baseline for the objective assessment of hypo- and hyperganglionosis. *Pediatr Pathol*, 1993; 13: 225-37.

[28] Ikeda K, Goto S, Nagasaki A, et al: Hypogenesis of intestinal ganglion cells: a rare cause of intestinal obstruction simulating aganglionosis. *Z Kinderchir* 1988; 43: 52-3.

[29] Meier-Ruge W, Morger R, Rehbein F: Das hypoganglionaere Megakolon als Begleiterkrankung bei Morbus Hirschsprung. *Z Kinderchir*, 1970; 8: 254-64.

[30] Yunis EJ, Schofield DE. Intestinal neuronal dysplasia in a case of sigmoid stenosis. *Pediatr Pathol*, 1992; 12:275-80.

[31] Schofield DE, Yunis EJ. What is intestinal neuronal dysplasia? *Pathol Ann*, 1992; 27:249-62.

[32] Schofield DE, Yunis EJ. Intestinal neuronal dysplasia. *J Pediatr Gastroenterol Nutr*, 1991; 12:182-9.

[33] Moore SW, Laing D, Kaschula ROC, et al. A histological grading system for the evaluation of co-existing NID with Hirschsprung's disease. *Eur J Pediatr Surg*, 1994; 4:293-7.

[34] Meier-Ruge W, Bronnimann PB, Gambazzi F, et al. Histopathological criteria for intestinal neuronal dysplasia of the submucous plexus (type B). *Virchows Arch*, 1995; 426:549-56.

[35] Meier-Ruge W. Is intestinal neuronal dysplasia really a myth or an invented disease? *Pediatr Surg Int*, 1995; 10:439.

[36] Gillick J, Tazawa H, Puri P: Intestinal neuronal dysplasia: Results of treatment in 33 patients. *J Pediatr Surg*,2001; 36: 777-9.

[37] Schaerli AF: Standardization of terminology of dysganglionoses. *Pediatr Surg Int*, 1995; 10: 440.

[38] Kobayashi H, Yamataka A, Lane GJ, Miyano T. Pathophysiology of hypoganglionosis. *J Ped Gastroenterol Nutr*, 2002; 34: 231-5.

[39] Puri P, Fujimoto T: Diagnosis of allied functional bowel disorders using monoclonal antibodies and electronmicroscopy. *J Pediatr Surg*, 1988; 23: 546-54.

[40] Meier-Ruge WA, Brunner LA, Engert J, et al. A correlative morphometric and clinical investigation of hypoganglionosis of the colon in children. *Eur J Pediatr Surg*, 1999: 9:67-74.

[41] Watanabe Y, Ito F, Ando H, Seo T, Kaneko K, Harada T, Iino S. Morphological investigation of the enteric nervous system in Hirschsprung's disease and hypoganglionosis using whole-mount colon preparation. *J Pediatr Surg*, 1999: 34:445-9.

[42] Rolle U, Yoneda A, Solari V, Nemeth L, Puri P. Abnormalities of c-Kit positive cellular network in isolated hypoganglionosis. *J Ped Surg*, 2002; 37: 709-714.

[43] Kobayashi H, Li Z, Yamataka A, Lane GJ, Miyano T. Overexpression of neural cell adhesion molecule (NCAM) antigens on intestinal smooth muscles in hypoganglionosis: is hypoganglionosis a disorder of the neuromuscular junction? *Pediatr Surg Int*, 2003; 19:190-3.

[44] Inoue K, Shimotake T, Tomiyama H, Iwai N. Mutational analysis of the RET and GDNF gene in children with hypoganglionosis.*Eur J Pediatr Surg*, 2001; 11:120-3.

[45] Tatekawa Y, Kanehiro H, Kanokogi H, Nakajima Y, Nishijima E, Muraji T, Imai Y, Tsugawa C, Toyosaka A, Nakano H. The evaluation of meconium disease by distribution of cathepsin D in intestinal ganglion cells. *Pediatr Surg Int*, 2000; 16:53-5

[46] Hirakawa H, Kobayashi H, O'Briain S, et al: Absence of NADPH-diaphorase activity in internal anal sphincter (IAS) achalasia. *J Pediatr Gastroenterol Nutr*, 1995: 20: 54-8.

[47] Neilson IR, Yazbeck S: Ultrashort Hirschsprung's disease: Myth or reality. *J Pediatr Surg*, 1990; 25: 1135-8.

[48] Meier-Ruge W: Ultrashort segment Hirschsprung's disease: An objective picture of the disease substantiated by biopsy. *Z Kinderchir*, 1985; 40: 146-50.

[49] Lake BD, Puri P, Nixon HH, et al: Hirschsprung's disease An appraisal of histochemistry demonstrated acetylcholinesterase activity in suction rectal biopsy specimens as an aid to diagnosis. *Arch Pathol Lab Med*, 1978; 102; 224-47.

[50] Oue T, Puri P: Altered intramuscular innervatio and synapse formation in internal sphincter achalasia. *Pediatr Surg Int*, 1999; 15: 192-4.

[51] Piotrowska AP, Solari V, Puri P. Distribution of interstitial cells of Cajal in the internal anal sphincter of patients with internal anal sphincter achalasia and Hirschsprung's disease. *Arch Pathol Lab Med*, 2003; 127: 1191-5.

[52] De Caluwe D, Yoneda A, Akl U, Puri P. Internal anal sphincter achalasia: outcome after internal sphincter myectomy. *J Ped Surg*, 2001; 36: 736-8.

[53] Ciamarra P, Nurko S, Barksdale E, Fishman S, Di Lorenzo C. Internal anal sphincter achalasia in children: clinical characteristics and treatment with Clostridium botulinum toxin. *J Pediatr Gastroenterol Nutr*, 2003; 37:315-9.

[54] Berdon WE, Baker DH, Blanc WA, et al: Megacystis-microcolon-intestinal hypoperistalsis syndrome: A new cause of intestinal obstruction in the newborn. Report of radiologic findings in five newborn girls. *Am J Roentgenol*, 1976; 126: 957-64.

[55] Granata C, Puri P. Megacystis microcolon intestinal hypoperistalsis syndrome. *J Pediatr Gastr Nutr*, 1997; 25:12-4.

[56] Puri P, Lake BD, Gorman F, et al: Megacystis-microcolon-intestinal hypoperistalsis syndrome: A visceral myopathy. *J Pediatr Surg*, 1983; 18: 64-9.

[57] Rolle U, O'Briain S, Pearl RH, Puri P. Megacystis-microcolon-intestinal hypoperistalsis syndrome: evidence of intestinal myopathy. *Ped Surg Int* 2002: 18: 2-5

[58] Piotrowska AP, Rolle U, Chertin B, De Caluwe D, Bianchi A, Puri P. Alterations in smooth muscle contractile and cytoskeleton proteins and interstitial cells of Cajal in megacystis microcolon intestinal hypoperistalsis syndrome. *J Ped Surg* 2003; 38: 749-55.

[59] Rolle U, Puri P. Structural basis of voiding dysfunction in megacystis microcolon intestinal hypoperistalsis syndrome. *J Pediatr. Urol*. 2006: 2: 277-84.

[60] Rolle U, Piotrwska AP, Puri P. Interstitial cells of Cajal in the normal gut and in interstial motility disorders of childhood. *Pediatr Surg Int*. 2007: 23: 1139-52.

In: Hirschsprung's Disease: Diagnosis and Treatment
Ed: Ramón Núñez and Manuel López-Alonso
ISBN: 978-1-60741-349-3

Chapter XXV

Intestinal Transplant in Hirschsprung's Disease and Intestinal Pseudoobstruction

Manuel López Santamaría and Francisco Hernández Oliveros

Introduction

Gastrointestinal Dysmotility (GD) is a general term applied to a group of disorders characterized by failure to produce normal peristalsis in the otherwise anatomically normal intestine. It covers a series of conditions including Chronic Intestinal Pseudo-Obstruction Syndrome (CIPOS), Hirschsprung´s disease and related neuromuscular disorders (Intestinal Neuronal Dysplasia). Some gastrointestinal structural abnormalities may also be complicated by the development of dysmotility, i.e. patients with a history of malrotation, atresia, enterocolitis or gastroschisis repair, frequently present an abnormal motility that limits tolerance for enteral feeding, even when the length of residual small bowel is apparently sufficient [1]. Moreover, an experimental animal model has recently demonstrated an association between Gastroschisis and delayed maturation of intestinal pace-maker cells [2].

Permanent Intestinal Failure (IF) is defined as the inability of the small bowel to provide sufficient fluid and nutrient digestion and absorption so as to satisfy body nutrient and fluid requirements in adults or growth in children [3]. However, the definition of IF remains a matter of debate and its diagnosis is based primarily on a long-term dependency on total parenteral nutrition (PN). Short Bowel Syndrome is the most frequent cause of IF in both adults and children, but some children with intestinal motility disorders can also develop irreversible IF.

Many patients with IF can maintain good nutritional status with PN, wich has been described as the artifitial gut, by analogy to the artificial kidney of renal dyalisis [4]. However, with time, some patients develop life-threatening complications related to PN, and in those cases, Intestinal Transplantation (IT) is the logical therapeutic option.

Although the intestine was one of the first organs to be experimentally transplanted [5], the initial results of bowel transplantation in humans were disappointing [6], and thus, the intestine was considered a forbidden organ for clinical transplantation for nearly three decades [7]. The introduction of Tacrolimus [8] (FK506) as a new immunosupressor in the late 80´s [9,10], and the steady improvements in immunosuppression over the last 15 years have made IT a feasible procedure for patients with irreversible intestinal failure [11]. Nowadays, IT may be applied with remarkable success in selected cases and IT is no longer considered an "experimental" procedure.

As of March 2005, a total of 1292 transplants had been registered at the International Intestinal Transplantation Registry (children and adults); motility disorders comprises 17% of the indications in children (CIPOS 9%, Hirschsprung disease 7%, other motility disorders 1%). In the same series, Gastroschisis accounted for 22% of the indications for pediatric IT (http://www.intestinaltransplant.org).

The present chapter will therefore analyze the role for IT in motility disorders. Most of the topics such as indications, surgical techniques, post surgical management, etc, are irrespective of the nature of IF (SBS, diarrhea, motility disorders), and as a consequence, they will be disccussed in a general way. However, aspects of IT that are specific to motility disorders will also be commented. According to the purpose of this book, we will focus in motility disorders coursing with an anatomically intact intestine as in Hirschsprung's Disease and CIPOS. Given their special characteristics, we shall not discuss anatomically produced Gastrointestinal Dysmotility like Gastroschysis.

Surgical Techniques for Intestinal Transplantation

Intestinal transplantation is evolving, and this includes the surgical techniques [12,13]. Three types if IT have been described in humans: isolated IT, combined liver and IT and multivisceral IT [14]. The original techniques have recently been adapted to patients' specific needs, resulting in innovative transplant techniques [15]. The original techniques and their modifications will be discussed in this section.

Isolated Intestinal Transplantation

Isolated Intestinal transplantation ITT is the simplest form of intestinal transplantation. It has been used in patients with intestinal failure without liver disease or gastric dysmotility [16]. IIT usually involves transplantation of the jejuno-ileal segment of the bowel; the colon is not routinely transplanted; nevertheless, the inclusion of the colon or part of the colon with the graft can be particularly beneficial for patiens transplanted for Hirschsprung disease or others motility disorders (see later).

Arterial inflow to the intestinal graft can be made through either the superior mesenteric artery (SMA) of the receptor or their infrarenal aorta, if the recipient´s SMA is too short or has small caliber as occurs in most patients with short bowel syndrome. In this case a donor arterial interposition graft (usually the iliac artery) is generally used [17]. Venous outflow is towards the superior mesenteric vein or toward the inferior cava when the former is not accessible or an existing hepatic fibrosis might impair the graft's venous return. When the inferior vena cava is thrombosed a possible alternative is the left renal vein or the inferior mesenteric vein [18].

Hepatointestinal Transplantation

This technique is indicated in cases of IF associated to end-stage liver disease. Other indications are the existence of portal hypertension and porto mesenteric thrombosis, IT may also be indicated due to intestinal ischemia produced by hypercoagulability since the liver transplantation would correct the coagulation disorder [19]. This is the most frequent type of transplantation in children [11], a point that is related with the different etiologies for intestinal failure in the two age groups, but especially with children's greater susceptibility to developing parenteral nutrition associated liver disease (PNALD, see below). Currently the most common technique for a combined liver/intestinal transplant includes the donor's pancreatic-duodenal complex. This procedure simplifies surgery both in the donor and recipient, and avoids the severe and frequent biliary complications that occurred with the original technique [20].

Arterial inflow to the hepatointestinal graft can be obtained either from the recipient's infrarenal or supraceliac aorta [12]. An extension graft from donor thoracic aorta is generally used in order to perform the anastomosis of the graft in a more superficial plane. The receptor's remaining abdominal viscera must be drained, either through the graft's portal system or via a portocava anastomosis [21].

Multivisceral Transplantation

Classically, this term referred to a transplantation of three or more abdominal viscera, usually stomach, duodenum, pancreas, liver and/or intestine (Figure 1), but, since the acceptance of "en bloc" hepatointestinal transplantation, multivisceral transplantation usually refers to cases in which the stomach or part of the stomach is included with the graft [11].

Gastrointestinal Tract Reconstruction

When the recipient retains native foregut, as occurs in an isolated intestine or hepatointestinal transplantation, upper gastrointestinal tract reconstruction is made between the recipient duodenum or jejunum and the proximal jejunum of the donor [17]. In a multivisceral transplantation, reconstruction was initially made with an esophago gastrostomy anastomosis, but this was seen to be associated to severe gastro-esophagic reflux in a significant number of cases so that currently it is preferred to conserve the receptor's gastroesophagic junction, preserving the left gastric artery, and performing a gastro-gastric anastomosis [17]. Pyloroplasty is absolutely necessary_because of the loss of vagal innervation after transplant.

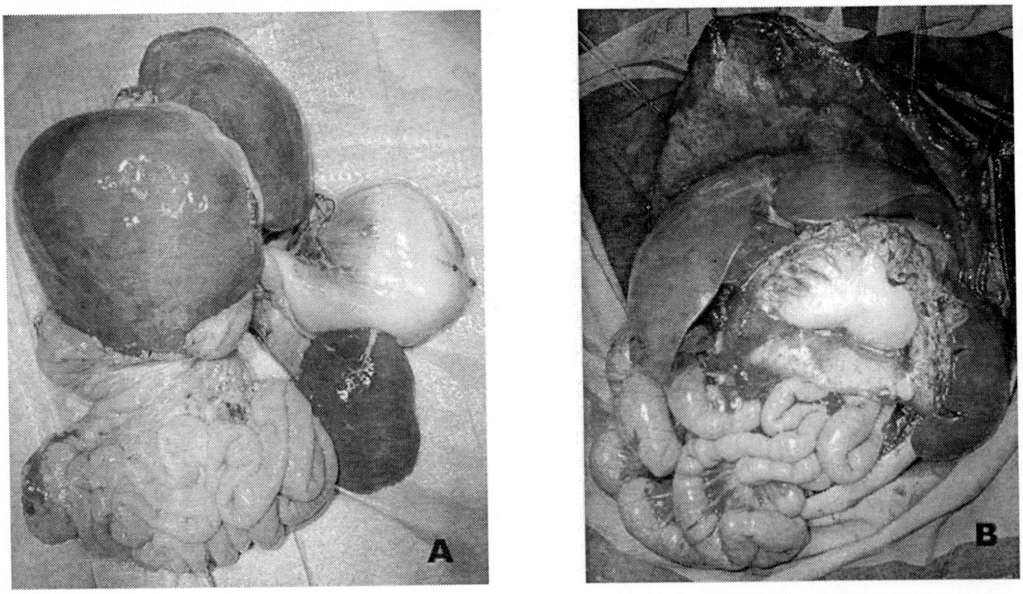

Figure 1.Multivisceral graft. A. graft. B. After revascularization. The graft includes the stomach, duodenum, pancreas, spleen, liver and small bowel.

Distal gastrointestinal reconstruction is usually done exteriorizing the transplanted terminal ileon, either as a terminal, side to end (Bishop-Koop) or double barrel ileostomy (Mikulicz) ileostomy.

Abdominal Wall Closure

Many children subjected to IT have previously undergone multiple abdominal interventions, often with more or less extensive intestinal resections and developed intestinal fistulae, and in these cases wall infections are also frequent problems [17]. All of this can result in shrinkage of the abdominal cavity and loss of abdominal cavity domain. Therefore, closure of the abdominal wall after transplantation can be sometimes extremely difficult or even impossible to perform. The first step towards a comfortable closure is the choice of donor, a small-for-size donor is the best choice; nevertheless, various surgical techniques have been developped in order to accommodate larger grafts, including skin or muscle flaps [22], and inflatable expanders so as to stretch the abdominal cavity before transplantation [23]. Abdominal wall closure can also be done in steps, using a prosthetic mesh /usually Gore-Tex, polyetrafluorethylene, (PTFE). The Miami Group has described an abdominal wall transplantation that includes subcutaneous cell tissue, muscle and aponeurosis, with a vascular pedicle consisting of the iliac arteries and veins, preserving the epigastric vessels, which ensure the viability of the wall graft. They report using this procedure on ten occasions with acceptable results [24], but so far no other group has reported this technique.

Innovative It Techniques

In the last years the original techniques have been modified and important refinements have allowed us to cover different necessities of the IF patients needing transplantation.

Currently, small children represent the majority of candidates for small bowel transplantation. An important limitation in pediatric IT is the scarcity of size-matched donors, particularly when the recipient candidate is a very young child in need of a liver-intestine transplant (LIT). Once enlisted for LIT, the waiting list time may be as high as a year [25], with a very high pretransplantation mortality, being estimated as close to 50% among candidates between 0 and five years of age [26]. As a consequence many of the innovative techniques aim at increasing the donor-pool for thes children.

Reduzed-Sized Orthotopic Composite Liver-Intestinal Transplantation

The technical basis for this procedure has no difference from the liver reduction techniques described in the early 80´s in liver transplantation. The LIT graft is procured en bloc with the duodenum, the head of the pancreas and the small bowel. The liver is reduced on the back table, using an extrahilar approach, thus withouth any dissection in the portal triad. As occurred with the techniques for reducing a graft liver, this technique makes it possible to use grafts from donors up to four or five time greater than the recipient. Some bowel lengh reduction can also be performed after revascularization, in cases when the graft is still too large [27]. The intestinal resection should always involve the mid-jejunum, and the length of intestine to be resected is determined according to availability of abdominal domain. As the graft comes from a larger donor, as much as 60% of intestine can be resected without imparing graft function (Figure 2).

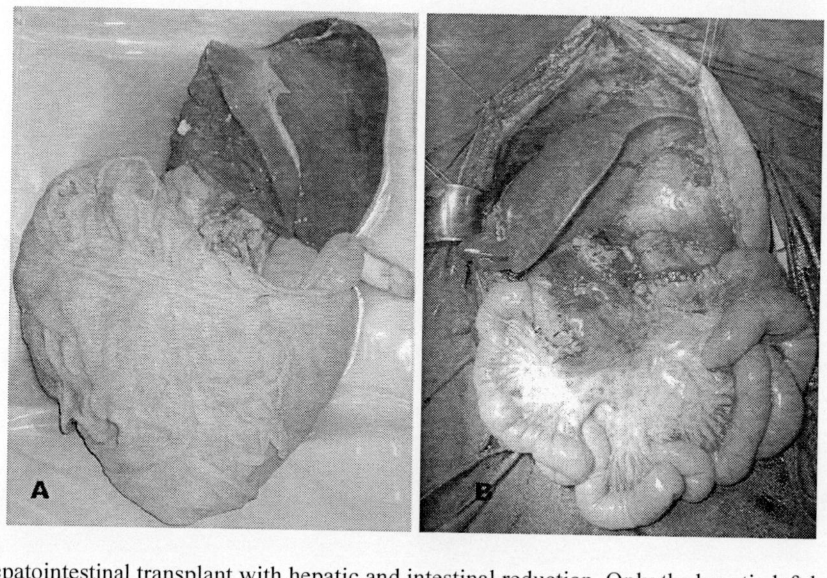

Figure 2. Hepatointestinal transplant with hepatic and intestinal reduction. Only the hepatic left lateral segment (Couinaud´s segments II-III) have been transplanted. 200 cm of mid small bowel were also resected after revascularization, leaving with the graft only 120 cm of small bowel.

Sequential Liver Intestinal Transplantation (Slit)

Hepatointestinal transplantation is usually performed in a composite way (i.e.) including the duodenum and the head of the pancreas of the donor, with the hepatic hilum intact). LIT can salso be performed using a non composite technique, transplanting each organ separately. SLIT can be performed asynchronically or synchronically. In the former, the liver is transplanted first and the intestine is transplanted later, once hepatic function is normalized and the malnutrition secondary to hepatopathy has improved. In the second modality, both organs, liver and intestine are transplanted separately in the same surgical procedure [28]. Compared with the composite LIT, non composite LIT allows the use of larger donors (up to ten times heavier), replacement of the intestinal or liver graft leaving the other component untouched, as well as offering the technical possibility of employing liver intestinal grafts from a living donor.

Isolated Intestinal Transplantation with Grafts from a Living Donor

Although living-donor small bowel transplantation (LSBT) is not routinely performed, the use of living donor grafts has been successfully developed in renal, hepatic, pancreatic and lung transplantation. LSBT can reduce waiting time, thus decreasing pretransplant mortality, and avoiding the progression of the hepatopathy in the children on the intestinal transplant list. The graft consists of a long segment of terminal ileum (approximately 150 cm long), with the arterial inflow given by the ileocolic artery, and the outflow by the ileocolic vein. In all cases, the donor´s ileo-cecal valve, in continuity of a segment of 20 cm of terminal ileum and at least 60% of small bowel should be preserved [29,30]. Up to now, a total of 30 LSBT have been reported, and the results have been similar than those with a cadaveric donor [11].

Liver Transplant Without It

Althouth no applicable to cases with intestinal dysmotility, we will still comment on this option which is useful in children with Short Bowel Syndrome (SBS) in whom, if it were not for the progression towards severe liver disease, the length of the residual intestine might be long enough to achieve complete digestive autonomy. In selected cases, an alternative to combined liver-intestine transplantation could be isolated liver transplantation, wich aims at breaking the vicious circle of malabsortion and stunting related to the hepatopathy. This technique is only aplicable to infants and very young children who have tolerated an enteral intake over 50% before end-stage liver disease develops [31].

Extended use of Multivisceral Transplantation

Recently proposed for use in children with a very low body weight as a substitution of a combined liver-intestine transplant. Small children with end-stage liver disease normally have splenomegaly due to portal hypertension; the stomach and duodenum are usually dilated and some of them have experienced previous episodes of pancreatitis. Resection of the native stomach, duodenum and pancreas can extirpate potentially dysfunctional organs, allow a larger cavity to place the graft, permit direct access to the abdominal aorta and maintain the continuity of the gastrointestinal tract, which is transplanted orthotopically; fewer intestinal and vascular anastomoses are needed (the receptor's abdominal viscera do not need venous drainage), and it makes it possible to use lower weight donors. Another additional advantage is that it allows better control of hemorrhage if there is advanced portal hypertension making it possible to clamp the celiac trunk and the superior mesenteric artery of the receptor early during the procedure [16].

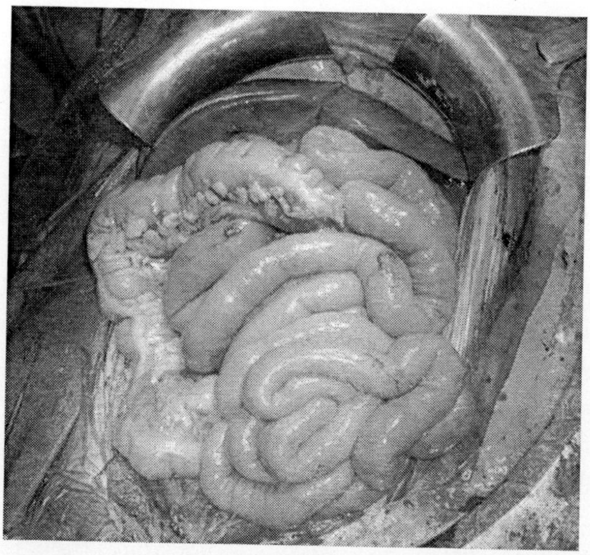

Figure 3.Hepatointestinal transplantation in a 8 year old girl with extensive Hirschsprung disease. The ileocecal valve, cecum, ascending and right colon have been included with the graft. Subsequently the patient underwent a Swenson procedure in order to restore fecal function.

Technical Considerations Regarding IT for Motility Disorders

Although early studies considered the inclusion of the colon a risk factor after IT [32], subsequent studies have shown that allograft colon inclusion has no impact on results [33,34]. Besides, including the ileocecal valve significantly enhances the fluid reabsorption capacity, improving the watery diarrhea without increasing infection. Nowadays, the colon or the part of the colon is included with the graft in cases when the native colon has been lost, either anatomically or functionally. In children with extensive intestinal aganglionosis (EIA) the aim of IT is not only to achieve intestinal autonomy, but also to restore colonic function with normal continence. Currently, the right colon with the ileocecal valve is included with the graft and a colon pull-through procedure is performed once the patient has achieved intestinal autonomy, followed by ileostomy closure several weeks afterwards (Figure 3). Very good results in terms of faecal continence have been reported [35].

For children with CIPO who have undergone IT, the graft to use is also a matter of debate. The dysmotility usually affects the entire gastrointestinal tract, and some groups advocate multivisceral transplants with removal of native stomach, duodenum and colon [36,37]. However, in a report by Sigurdsson that includes 8 cases [38], these large multivisceral grafts did not eliminate the underlying problem of pervasive dysmotility (all the patients who received allograft stomachs continued to have delayed gastric emptying). Similar results have been achieved excluding the stomach and colon from the graft, and, currently, many groups follow the OMAHA philosophy of "less may be better" [39].

Intestinal Transplantation Indications

Intestinal transplantation should only be considered in children with permanent intestinal failure, but in some cases, the irreversibility of the IF can be difficult to confirm [40]. In Children with extreme short bowel syndrome (SBS), or children with congenital intestinal epithelial disorders, it is easy to foresee the irreversibility of the IF. However, cases in which SBS is not extreme, or children with chronic intestinal pseudo obstruction (CIPOS), irreversibility is not as apparent, and it is mandatory that all conventional therapeutic options be exhausted before IT can be indicated [41]. Extensive Hirschsprung disease, involving the entire or almost the entire small bowel is a very rare form of Hirschsprung Disease (HD), accounting for less that 1% of the cases [3]. The severity of the intestinal failure is related to the length of small bowel involved, and the probability of irreversible intestinal failure and subsequent permanent TPN dependency is high if the normal ganglionic bowel is shorter than 50 cm [42]; besides, all of the cases present dysmotility in the remaining normal small bowel and this is more likely to be a congenital defect rather than a consequence of bowel distension as a deficit in Cajal cells has been documented in the remaining normal small bowel in patients with extensive HD. Surgical procedures like reverse loops, Kimura procedure longitudinal myectomy or bowel lengthening do not improve intestinal absorption {Yann, 2003#22}. Extensive intestinal aganglionosis can be considered a severe form of SBS without a functional colon, and thus, these patients represent a specific population of high risk candidates for IT.

Transplantation Criteria

Intestinal Transplantation has been primarily used only as a life-saving therapy for patients who failed TPN therapy and those with life-threatening complications [43,44]. Such limited indications were implemented during the early developing phase of the procedure because of the high mortality associated with the procedure in the early period [43]. Nevertheless, a significant improvement in results over the last 15 years now allows a wider use of IT. According to the Work Group at the International Intestinal Transplantation

Symposium, in Brussels in July 2005 [45], "Intestinal transplantation is indicated for patients with irreversible intestinal failure expected to die prematurely on Parenteral Nutrition". This affirmation implicitly modifies the earlier criterion in referring "as early as possible" for IF patients with a probable poor evolution [46] and recommends that they be "immediately" referred to transplant centers for evaluation as possible candidates, even in the absence of TPN related complications. Recommendations about referral of children for assessment of suitability for IT are made in mind of the fact that early referral is a key factor in improving IT results. The importance of early referral is even more critical when one considers that a better recipient selection is one of the factors that has most contributed to the improved results as reflected in the IT Internal Registry reports for 2003 and 2005 [11.47].

Currently accepted criteria for IT are as follows (Table I)

Table I. Indications for intestinal transplantations

INDICATIONS FOR INTESTINAL TRANSPLANTATION [46]	
Permanent Intestinal failure (PIF) associated to life-threatening complications	Liver disease Impending loss of central venous access Recurring sepsis Frequent episodes of serious dehidratation
PIF that virtually always results in early death despite optimal parenteral nutrition	Ultra-short small bowel Congenital intractable epithelial disorders
PIF with high mortality and poor quality of life	Frequent hospitalizations Chronic Intestinal Pseudoobstruction Syndrome (some cases)

Impending or overt liver failure (increased serum bilirrubin and /or liver enzyme levels, splenomagaly, thrombocytopenia, gastroesophageal varices, coagulopathy, stoma bleeding, hepatic fibrosis or cirrhosis [48]. Hepatic damage (Parenteral Nutrition Associated Liver Disease (PNALD) is the most frequent and most severe complication to develop in IF patients. Some 40% to 60% of children requiring long term PN and about 25% to 40% of adults receiving home PN develop liver damage of variable intensity [46]. The clinical spectrum of lesions includes hepatic steatosis, cholestasis, cholelythiasis and hepatic fibrosis. A progression to biliary cirrhosis, portal hypertension and liver failure is not usual in adult, but more frequent in children and new born [49]. Causes are multifactorial, but the loss of lymphoid tissue associated to the intestine (in SBS), the existence of hepatobiliary sepsis [50-52], as a consequence of alterations in intestinal microflora, as well as the hepatic immaturity in premature baby makes them more vulnerable and is implicated in the progression to hepatic failure [53]. Other important mechanisms include the absence of nutrients in the intestinal lumen resulting gastrointestinal hormone hyposecretion, reduced bile flow and biliary stasis, which lead to the development of cholestasis, biliary sludge and lithiasis, which, in turn, increase liver dysfunction. In Preterm new born, a taurine or cisteine deficit may contribute to liver damage, while in older children and adults, a choline deficit, lipid emulsions and manganese toxicity may be associated factors. Among patients at higher risk of developing this complication are newborns with early jaundice (before the 3rd or 4th month of life), and SBS cases that have undergone multiple laparotomies, have an ultra SBS or cases with absence of intestinal continuity. The development or appearance of signs of portal hypertension in jaundiced patients may indicate a progression of their liver damage. Structurally, the damage is progressive, starting with fibrosis in any or its degrees and continuing to cirrhosis (Figure 4).

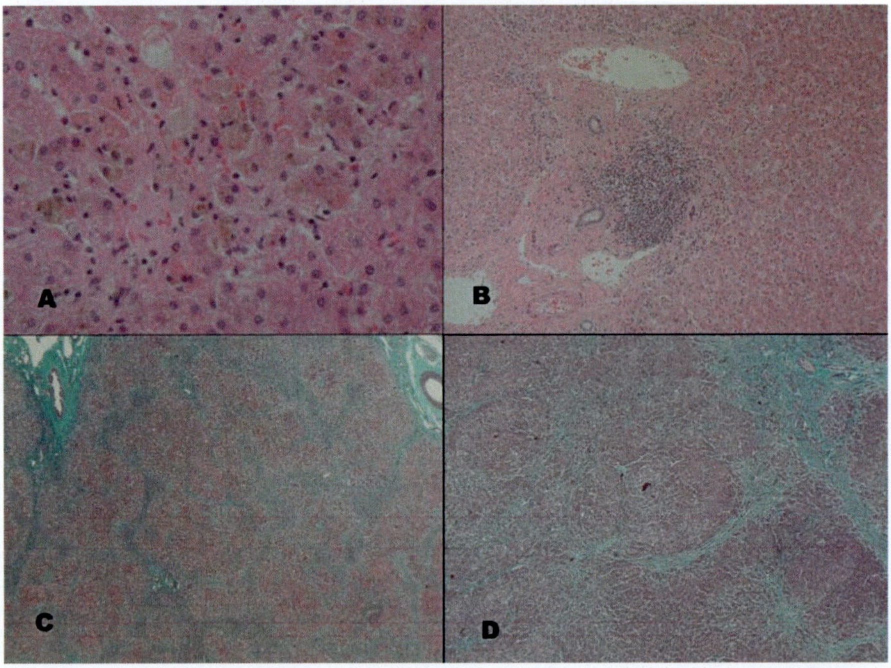

Figure 4. Progression of parenteral nutrition associated liver disease from cholestasis (A) to liver cirrhosis (D). Intermediate steps B and C show periportal inflammatory infiltrate and bridging fibrosis respectively.

It has recently been proposed that PNALD, or parenteral nutrition related liver damage, be replaced by "Intestinal Failure-related liver disease"[3] which is more general that the earlier term and better reflects the multifactorial nature of this syndrome, since, in fact, the most important elements leading to cholestasis are related with the impairment of intestinal function and bacterial overgrowth.

Impending loss of central venous access: children at high-risk for requiring PN indefinitely and who are also in danger of losing all usual vascular access are appropriate candidates for IT [46]. Referral to IT centers must not be delayed until difficult approaches are needed (Figure 5).

Currently, permanent intestinal failure associated to the loss of half of conventional access (jugular and femoral veins in small children, jugular, subclavian and femoral veins in larger children) is an accepted indication for IT [54].

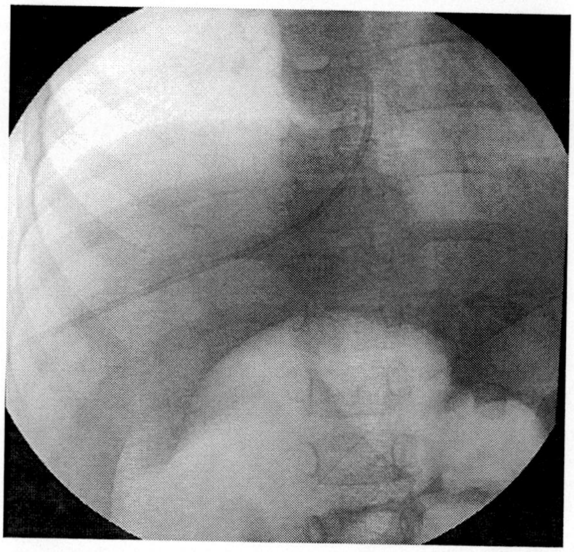

Figure 5. Transhepatic inserction of a Broviac catheter in a patient with thrombosis of superior and inferior vena cava.

Recurring sepsis: Factors such as prolonged requirement for central venous lines, the translocation of micro organisms and the loss of lymphoid tissue associated with the intestine (in SBS cases) are considered responsible for the elevated infectiou complication rate in IF patients. The frequency and mortality rate for these complications has been notably decreased and patients with frequent infections with limited morbidity should not be considered as potential IT candidates. On the contrary, patients who develop metastatic infectious complications, such as a cerebral abscess, endocarditis and/or multiorgan failure should be evaluated as IT candidates. Equally, patients who are multiresistent germ carrriers (e.g. Vancomicin resistant Enterococcus faecium) and who frequently develop catheter infections with these germs, should also be considered IT candidates. The American Gastroenterological Association (AGA) recommends IT in cases of permanent IF associated with 2 episodes or more of systemic sepsis secondary to line infection per year, 1 episode of line-related fungemia, septic shock, or acute respiratory distress syndrome [46,54].

Intestinal failure virtually always results in early death despite optimal PN [46]:

[1] Cases with ultrashort intestinal syndrome, such as duodeno-colic anastomosis, non reconstructible intestine, SBS that is shorter than 10 cm in small children or less than 30 cm in larger children, severe traumas that damage the main branch of the superior mesenteric artery, intraabdominal tumors, (usually desmoids) that require nearly total intestinal resection (Figure 6), etc. As there is no possibility of intestinal adaptation, it is advised to go ahead with the indication for IT before complications related with PN develop [46,54,55].

[2] Congenital intestinal mucosa syndrome that course with untreatable diarrhea such as microvillous inclusion disease, tufting enteropathy etc. As in the section above, it is better to transplant before there is any irreversible hepatic damage that would

necessitate a combined liver-intestinal transplant. Currently, children with fecal loses over 10% of body weight per day are considered candidates for early IT [46,54,55].

[3] Intestinal Failure associated with high morbidity and poor quality of life. In the absence of obvious life-threatening complications IT may still be appropriate. A few children with short bowel syndrome may have sufficiently high and erratic fluid losses to consistently appropriate replacement impossible outside a hospital. These patients may be unable to attend school or participate in other age-appropriate activities. Similarly, children with the most severe form of CIPOS may be effectively disabled because of chronic massive gastrointestinal dilatation refractory to stomal decompression or partial gastrointestinal resection {DiLorenzo, 1999 35, Faure, 1999 #36}. These children should also be considered for IT although they have not yet developed the usual indications [46].

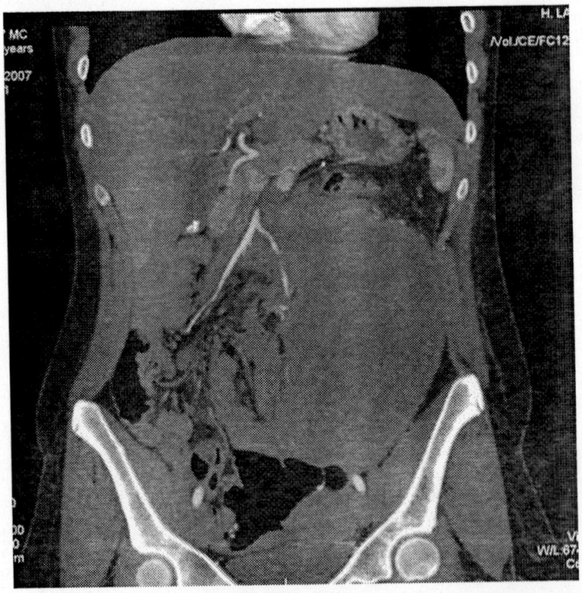

Figure 6. Desmoid tumor in a teenage girl with Gadner disease. The tumor infiltrates small bowel, duodenum and pancreas. The patient underwent a modified multivisceral graft (see text).

Contra-Indications for Intestinal Transplantation

The exclusion criteria are not different from those habitual in other solid organ transplantation and can be grouped as absolute or relative [46,54,55].

Absolute Criteria:

- Deep or progressive neurological deficit.
- Life-threatening extradigestive illnesses.
- Active Sepsis
- Malignancies

- Severe and unsolvable psychosocial problems.

Relative Critera:

- Immunodeficiency
- Drug dependency/Addiction
- Impossibility of ensuring central venous access during the first 6 months post transplantation.
- Benign neoplasias with unclear/doubtful prognosis.

Postoperative Care

Immunosuppresion Treatment

Tacrolimus (Prograf®) is the base immunosuppresion drug [56], in association or not with corticosteroids, azatioprin (Imurel®) or Micofenolate Mofetil (Cell Cept®) [57]. Alternatively, Rapamicine (Sirolimus®) may be used as immunosuppression induction for the first 3 to 6 months in substitution of azatioprin or Micofenoate, or even as the base immunosuppression if there is calcineurinic-induced nephrotoxicity [58] (Tacrolimus). However, its use is controversial given its pernicious effect on healing and the report (plus another of our own personal experience) of three cases of graft thrombosing microangiopathy [48,59,60]. Induction with interleukin-2 antireceptor monoclonal antibodies (humanized like Daclizumab, Zenapaz®, or chimeric like Basiliximab, Simulect®), have made it possible to significantly reduce the rate of rejection and helped improve results.

Immunosuppression strategy has recently changed; the receptor's lymphocyte population is modified by the administration of drugs that produce the complete perioperative depletion of native lymphocytes (tolerogenic immunosuppression) [61]. For this purpose, the following immunosupression inductors are employed: anti-thymocyte rabbit globulin (Timoglobulin), which depletes T lymphocytes, or Campath 1H (anti CD-52 cells), which almost completely depletes the T and B lymphocyte populations, and natural killer cells that last nearly six months [62]. Campath has been only rarely used in children and more experience is needed to evaluate the results. Nevertheless, the use of any of these drugs makes it possible to reduce Tacrolimus levels and avoid the use of corticosteroids.

Immunosuppression is monitored by controlling blood levels of Tacrolimus, which is kept at between 15-20 ngr/ml during the first month post transplant, and then tapered progressively to 5-10 ngr/ml from the sixth month post transplant. The administration of E1 prostaglandin in the initial phase is widely accepted in order to counter act the renal toxicity of tacrolimus, given its beneficial effect on microcirculation. Corticosteroids, if used, are administered as methyl-prednisolone at initial doses of 20 mg/kg, and gradually reduced to 2 mg/kg in the week after transplantation. The maintenance dose is 0.3 mg/kg.

Treatment of Rejection Episodes

If the Tacrolimus levels are maladjusted, the dose is increased or intravenous administration is employed so as to reach the desired levels. Rejection episodes are treated with a methylprednisolone boluses and, if the rejection is cortico-resistent, the treatment options are anti-CD3 monoclonal antibodies, Mofetyl Micophenolate or Rapamicine [56]. Recently, Campath 1H or Thymoglobulin have been proposed as alternative treatments. Some refractory rejections episodes have been successfully treated with anti alfa necrosis factor (Infliximab) monoclonal antibodies [63].

Anti Infection Treatment

The need of central venous lines and the increased bacterial translocation from the transplanted intestine (as a consequence of damage from the preservation, rejection, stasis, etc), necessitates the use of systemic antibiotics, including antifungal medications [41]. The use of antiviral agents over long time periods is also advisable, given the frequency of opportunistic germ infections [32]. All patients receive selective intestinal decontamination for the first few weeks post transplant and prophylaxis for Pneumocystis carinni with trimetroprim-sulfametoxazol twice weekly.

Complications

Many complications in IT are a consequence of the peculiarities of the gastrointestinal tract, and among these one of the most important is its wealth of lymphoid tissue and its physiological colonization by germs; the intestinal lumen is estimated to contain some 10^{14} bacteria of 400 different species [41,64].

Technical Complications

Despite the difficulty of the procedure, particularly in some variants, technical complications are not frequent, except in very small children (under two years of age), in whom technical problems are responsible for half of the instances of graft loss [32]. Billiary complications (fistulae, dehiscences, stenoses, etc.) were frequent in intestinal-liver transplantations in the past. These problems have now disappeared with the acceptance of the "en bloc" technique that does not require billiary reconstruction (hepaticojejunostomy). Necrotizing enterocolitis is a rare and serious complication because it is accompanied by intestinal gangrene [65]. The pathogenesis is unknown, but phenomena of ischemic reperfusion after the cold graft ischemia are suspected, as well as hypovolemia after diarrhea and dehydration. In some cases abdominal wall closure is a real,challenge; particularly in children with a congenital short bowel syndrome, since the volume of their abdominal cavity is reduced; also they have undergone multiple prior intrabdominal surgeries, with intestinal fistulae and/or ostomies, and have frequently lost important amounts of abdominal wall due to intrabdominal infection [63].

Rejection

Rejection is the most frequent complication in IT and the most frequent cause of graft loss [16,21,44]. Diagnosis is frequently difficult, and although biochemical markers like fatty acid adhesion protein [66], Chromo 51 tetra acetic diamine ethylene acid permeability studies [67], and more recently citruline serum levels have been evaluated [68], rejection diagnosis is still based on histological criteria (Table II).

Table II. Histologic criteria for grading intestinal allograft acute cellular rejection (ACR)

Grade	Histologic findings [69]
Indeterminate for ACR	Minimal localized inflammatory infiltrate, minimal crypt ephitelial injury, increased crypt epitelial apoptosis (< 6 apoptotic bodies/10 crypts), no to minimal architectural distortion, no mucosal ulceration, changes insufficient for the diagnosis of mild ACR
Mild ACR	Mild localized inflammatory infiltrate with activated lymphocytes, mild crypt epithelial injury, increased crypt apoptosis (>apoptotic bodies/10 crypts), mild architectural distortion, no mucosal ulceration.
Moderate ACR	Widely dispersed inflammatory infiltrate in lamina propia, diffuse crypt epithelial injury, increased crypt apoptosis with focal confluent apoptosis, more prominent architectural distortion, possible mild to moderate intimal arteritis, no mucosal ulceration.
Severe ACR	Features of moderat ACR plus mucosal ulceration; possible severe intimal arteritis or transmural arteritis may be seen.

For this purpose regular endoscopic sampling, or when the situation warrants it, is the habitual diagnostic procedure [56]. Video-endoscopy with magnification correlates quite well with the histological data, but its use is not very widespread [16]. Histologic criteria to standardize rejection degree have been developed, and are widely accepted [69,70]. Acute rejection is histologically characterized by activated lymphocyte infiltration of the lamina propia, crypt epithelium damage and apoptosis. It is stratified as light, moderate/mild and severe. Chronic rejection as an entity is developing with the increased experience with IT [71]. It courses with diarrhea and hemorrhages, and radiologically demonstrable areas of stenosis and dilation. Histologically it is characterized by plasmocytary infiltrate, ulcerations, and vellosity and crypt loss. Besides of the direct damage from the immune response, the epithelial lesion is also a consequence of the obliterating arteriopathy, as the endothelium is also a target tissue of this type of rejection (Figure 7).

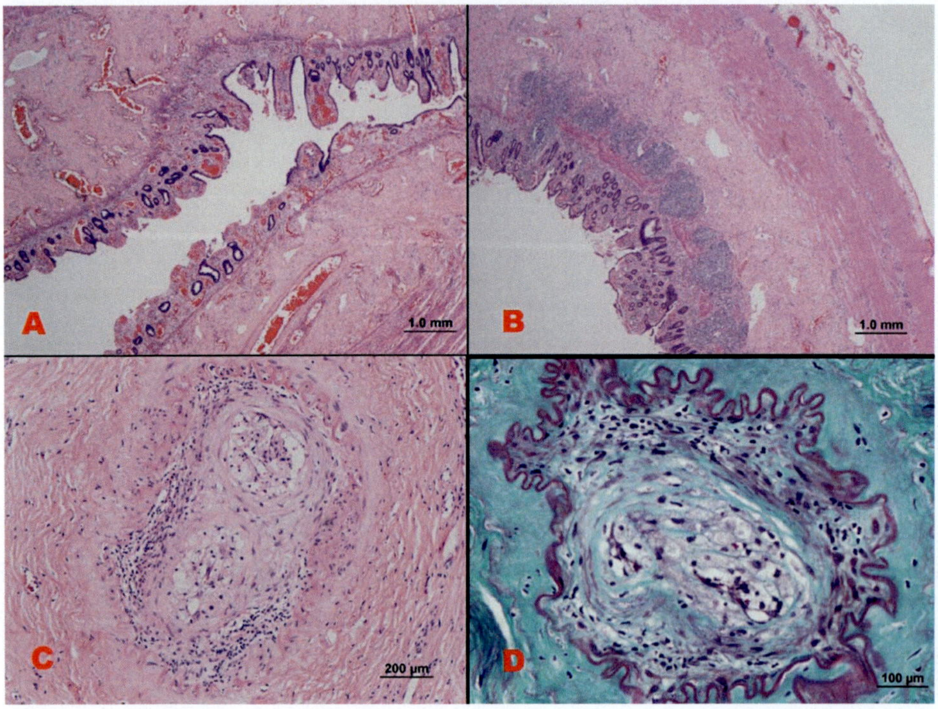

Figure 7. Chronic rejection. A: regenerative surface epithelium, intestinal lumen narrowing with mucosal ulcerations and crypt loss. B: as in A, associated to thickenin and fibrosis afecting all intestinal layers. C and D: obliterative arteriopathy.

Sepsis

Sepsis is the second most common complication and the main cause of death, responsible of 50% of all deaths in IT patients [16,21,44]. The use of central venous catheters, intraperitoneal infections or sepsis due to technical problems (dehiscence, perforation, necrosis, etc.) and intraluminal infections due to the increased intestinal mucosa permeability to microorganisms are all predisposing factors for the development of septic phenomena [72]. Also, there is a close relation between sepsis and rejection that is not common with other solid organ transplants, as consequence of the increased translocation after a rejection episode in the intestine [73,74].

Opportunistic Infections

Immunosuppression received by an IT recipient is higher than in liver, heart or kidney transplants. Consequently, opportunist infections are more frequent with IT than with other solid organ transplants [32]. Cytomegalovirus infection has been an important source of morbidity, although it is now well controlled by the combination of preventive measures [75] and prophylaxis with the systematic peritransplant use of ganciclovir and hyperimmune gamma globulin [76,77]. Adenovirus infections are responsible for many cases of postransplantation diarrhea [78], and infections from organisms not yet described in other solid organ transplants have been related with IT, such as calcivirus infection, which produces a secretory diarrhea [79]. Epstein-Bar infection is also frequent and its implications will be commented in the next paragraph.

Post Transplantation Lymphoproliferative Disorders

These lesions are usually related to Epstein Barr virus (EBV) infection [80,81]. EBV has a special affinity for B lymphocytes, which have a specific surface receptor for this virus. In the context of a cellular immunity deficit secondary to the immunosuppressive medication, infected B lymphocytes proliferate, in some cases becoming malign, generally in the form of a non Hodgkin's B Cell lymphoma. Children are more susceptible than adults to this complication and the incidence in some series is close to 30% of patients [82,83]. Treatment consists in the reduction and/or withdrawal of immunosuppression and the administration of antiviral drugs. An anti CD 20+ (Rituximab) has recently become available and it constitutes a second line treatment [84]. A low dose monochemotherapy is recommended in the absence of response and malignization [85]. An effective method for preventing lymphoproliferation is the determination of the viral load in peripheral blood with DNA amplification techniques so as to adjust immunosuppression levels in infected children [86].

Dysmotility and Diarrhea

Postransplantation secretory diarrhea can on occasion constitute a severe problem, particularly in children [74]. In some cases it is associated with rejection and it responds to an increase in the immunosuppression dose [63], but in other cases etiology is not clear, the action of certain pathogens, usually virus [78,79], motility disorders [87], denervation leading to an altered sympathetic nerve tone, etc., have all been suspected. Inflammatory and immunological mechanisms, the lymphatic dis-connection, intestinal denervation, the increased intraluminal osmotic load brought about by malabsorption of hydroxylated fatty acids, carbohydrates and bile salts, graft vs. host disease [88] and adverse effects of immunosuppression (particularly Micophenolate Mofetyle) have also been implicated in this problem.

Food Adversion

This problem is quite frequent, particularly in children with intestinal failure secondary to neonatal problems who had never received food orally, as well as in patients with chronic intestinal idiopathic pseudo obstruction, who relate oral feeding with earlier disagreeable experience of abdominal pain, gases, etc [89-91]. It does not seem to correct itself with time, and in some cases psychological support is necessary. At 5 years after IT over half of the transplanted children experience this complication [89].

Graft Versus Host Disease

This disease produces diarrhea, skin lesions (Figure 8) and cholestasis. Despite the large lymph tissue load in the transplanted intestine, surprisingly few patients develop this complication [92].

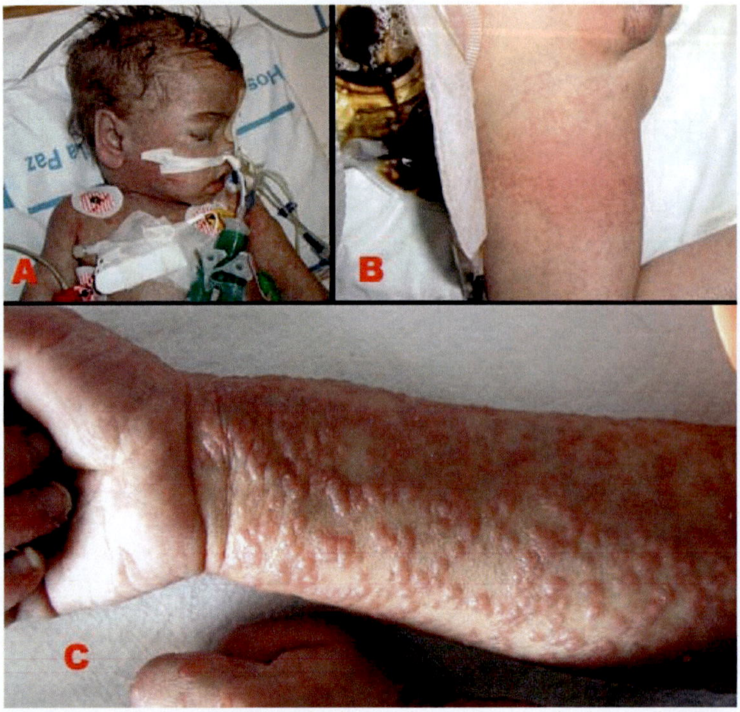

Figure 8. Cutaneous changes in cases of graft versus host disease after IT.

Recurrence of Disease

So far, a recurrence of the underlying disease has only been reported in cases of Crohn's Disease [93,94], or intrabdominal tumors, mainly desmoids [95].

Results of Intestinal Transplantation

The data of the International Intestinal Transplantation Registry provide a reference of the modern reach of this procedure. Between April 1 1985 and March 31 2005, 1,295 intestinal transplants have been done on 1,210 patients, of whom 658 were alive at the end of the study. Broken down by years, only after 2001 do more than 100 transplants per year begin to be performed and only three hospitals in the world had an experience of more than 100 transplants. In the last two years, only 29 hospitals in the world have performed an intestinal transplant.

The most reliable source on the results of intestinal transplantation is also the International Intestinal Transplant Registry, which is updated every two years making it possible to identify difficult to detect tendencies in regard to the results of individual centers. The last report was presented in Brussels, June/July 2005, at the IX International Intestinal Transplantation Symposium, and of the most outstanding results, is the important improvement in terms of graft and patient survival, superior to 80% at one year in the May 2003 – May 2005 period. Factors influencing this improvement were the magnitude of the center's experience (over 10 transplantations); improved recipient selection (characterized by a higher rate of patients who come to transplantation from their homes) and the use of some immunosuppression inductor, whether anti interleukin 2 receptor antibodies, timoglobulin or Campath (Table III).

Table III. Multivariant análisis of factors that influenced in the improvement of results. Period 2000-2005 (Data from Internacional Registry of Intestinal Transplantation)

	Graft		Patient	
	p	*RR*	*p*	*RR*
IT grouped by year	0.0308	0.58	*ns*	
Experience <10 cases	0.0530	2.11	0.00530	2.14
Pretranaplant state (hospitalized/home)	0.0006	0.43	0.0004	0.40
First IT	0.0024	0.29	0.0040	0.30
Induction only with FK506	*ns*	-	0.0098	3.92

Over 75% of the patients who survive the first 6 months post transplant achieve complete digestive autonomy, and are free of parenteral nutrition, with a good quality of life, measured in the registry by the Karnofsky Index. However, this improvement has primarily been achieved in the first year post transplantation, and nevertheless, the log term results have not improved significantly with time. Therefore, the challenge is to increase investigation and develop new strategies to prevent late complications.

In summary, the factor that have contributed the most over the last 15 years to the important improvement in intestinal transplantation results, allowing its clinical acceptance, are the following:

- Refinements of surgical technique [96]
- Advances in the understanding and treatment/management of the most frequent complications [56]
- Standardization of the degrees of rejection [69].
- Identification of the atypical characteristics of rejection [97]
- Better understanding of transplantation immunology [98]
- Improved receipient selection [47]

Intestinal Rehabilitation Units

Intestinal failure is a very complex problem and requires a super specialized treatment by extremely motivated professionals with a great deal of experience. Despite this few centers offer all the possible treatment options and treat all the stages of intestinal failure from the beginning through to transplantation [3]. Although many important advances are occurring in the field of intestinal failure, the activity in this field is very compartmentalized, particularly in regards to treatment and it is still frequent to observe that the different available options are employed in an uncoordinated way with hardly any or no interrelation among the professionals managing the patients.

It nevertheless seems realistic to accept that centralizing cases in centers that can integrate all possible therapeutic options is the best tool to improve results, decrease complication rates and reduce the extraordinarlily elevated cost of any of the treatment modalities for IF.

One of the most interesting aspects of IT is that it has allowed some centers to evolve into Intestinal Rehabilitation Units that integrate a multidisciplinary team for the three basic procedures in treating intestinal failure: nutritional support, pharmacology and surgery, including intestinal transplantation, an evolution like the one that twenty years ago lead to the creation of specialized hepatology units from the programs established to perform liver transplantations [99].

The mission of the Intestinal Rehabilitation Units consists in eliminating or reducing the need for parenteral nutrition in IT patients through an individualized plan including dietary, medical and surgical measures, in an attempt to simultaneously improve the patient's quality of life and longevity, at the same time as it minimizes the cost of treatment and of the complications [100]. The basis is that there is no single optimum procedure and on the contrary, the probability of success is highest with the appropriate evaluation that is carried out by an experienced multidisciplinary team that can pay attention to the smallest details [100].

With this purpose the Intestinal Rehabilitation Units are made up of a multidisciplinary group of professionals interested in intestinal failure. This team is composed of gastroenterologists, surgeons with experience in the autologous reconstruction of the intestine and in transplantation, dietary specialists, coordinators, specialized nursing staff, psychologists/psychiatrists, specialists in the care of ostomies, wounds and fistulas, and social workers [100,101].

The following clinical tasks are relevant for the evaluation unit [100]:

- Physical, biochemical and radiological evaluation of the patient.
- Education and training of the patient and caretakers
- Nutritional support
- Weaning from parenteral nutrition.
- Treatment of intestinal failure complications.
- Psycho-social support.
- Different surgical options, including autologous intestinal reconstruction and intestinal transplantation.

- Pharmacological options in intestinal failure treatment.

The benefits of the Intestinal Rehabilitation Units extend to all areas [3,100-103]: result optimization, decreases in mortality and complication rates, reduced costs, improved interaction among professionals and the different treatment modalities, greater flexibility for fast treatment adjustments, more dynamic communications of the patient and family members with caretakers as well as the patient's perception of a continuum in the treatment they are receiving. Other advantages are the greater possibility of the patient and their families to meet other patients with similar problems (the creation of patient associations is desirable) and the possibility to have a large enough number of cases to be able to develop clinical research programs. Beside, the elevated cost of nutritional support as well as the creation of an ever-larger population of IF patients necessitates the development of a national control and management policy [104]. Centers that can offer all of the therapeutic options improve results and optimize costs [105,106]; so promoting Intestinal Rehabilitation Units should be a priority. In fact, and although it is paradoxical, one of the immediate results of the nutritional rehabilitation units is the decrease in the need for parenteral nutrition and transplantation in a significant number of patients, something we have been able to observe in our own experience.

Finally, early treatment of intestinal failure in reference centers is a key to identifying as soon as possible the eventual irreversibility of the intestinal failure and makes it possible to perform transplantation at the most appropriate time [3]. This objective is particularly interesting if one considers that early referral reduces pretransplantation mortality (close to 50% in children under 2 years of age), and in many cases it is possible to avoid a combined transplantation including the liver, and, as reflected in the results in the International Intestinal Transplantation Registry, the improved receptor selection (impossible to perform if there is no early referral) constitutes one of the questions that has most influenced the improvement in IT results [11].

References

[1] Connor FL, Di Lorenzo C. Chronic intestinal pseudo-obstruction: assessment and management. *Gastroenterology* 2006; 130:S29-36.

[2] Midrio P, Faussone-Pellegrini MS, Vannucchi MG, Flake AW. Gastroschisis in the rat model is associated with a delayed maturation of intestinal pacemaker cells and smooth muscle cells. *J Pediatr Surg* 2004; 39:1541-7.

[3] Goulet O, Ruemmele F. Causes and management of intestinal failure in children. *Gastroenterology* 2006; 130:S16-28.

[4] Scribner BH, Cole JJ, Christopher TG, et al. Long-term total parenteral nutrition. The concept of an artificial gut. *Jama* 1970; 212:457-63.

[5] Lillehei RC, Goott B, Miller FA. The physiological response of the small bowel of the dog to ischemia including prolonged in vitro preservation of the bowel with successful replacement and survival. *Ann Surg* 1959; 150:543-60.

[6] McAlister VC, Grant DR. Clinical small bowel transplantation. In Grant DR, Wood R, eds. *Small bowel transplantation*: A Hodder Arnold Publication, 1994. p. 121 - 132.

[7] Abu-Elmagd K, Todo S, Tzakis A, et al. Three years clinical experience with intestinal transplantation. J *Am Coll Surg* 1994; 179:385-400.

[8] Starzl TE, Todo S, Fung J, et al. FK 506 for liver, kidney, and pancreas transplantation. *Lancet* 1989; 2:1000-4.

[9] Abu-Elmagd K, Fung JJ, Alessiani M, et al. The effect of graft function on FK506 plasma levels, dosages, and renal function, with particular reference to the liver. *Transplantation* 1991; 52:71-7.

[10] Warty V, Diven W, Cadoff E, et al. FK506: a novel immunosuppressive agent. Characteristics of binding and uptake by human lymphocytes. *Transplantation* 1988; 46:453-5.

[11] Grant D, Abu-Elmagd K, Reyes J, et al. 2003 report of the intestine transplant registry: a new era has dawned. *Ann Surg* 2005; 241:607-13.

[12] Starzl TE, Todo S, Tzakis A, et al. The many faces of multivisceral transplantation. *Surg Gynecol Obstet* 1991; 172:335-44.

[13] Todo S, Tzakis AG, Abu-Elmagd K, et al. Intestinal transplantation in composite visceral grafts or alone. *Ann Surg* 1992; 216:223-33.

[14] Todo S, Tzakis A, Abu-Elmagd K, et al. Abdominal multivisceral transplantation. *Transplantation* 1995; 59:234-40.

[15] Kato T, Ruiz P, Thompson JF, et al. Intestinal and multivisceral transplantation. *World J Surg* 2002; 26:226-37.

[16] Kato T, Tzakis AG, Selvaggi G, et al. Intestinal and multivisceral transplantation in children. *Ann Surg* 2006; 243:756-64.

[17] Kato T, Tzakis A, Selvaggi G, Madariaga J. Surgical techniques used in intestinal transplantation. *Curr Opin Organ Transplant* 2004; 9:207-13.

[18] Mueller AR, Pascher A, Platz KP, et al. Modified surgical technique in clinical small bowel transplantation: donor and recipient management. *Transplant Proc* 2002; 34):2265-7.

[19] Grant D, Wall W, Mimeault R, et al. Successful small-bowel/liver transplantation. *Lancet* 1990; 335:181-4.

[20] Sudan DL, Iyer KR, Deroover A, et al. A new technique for combined liver/small intestinal transplantation. *Transplantation* 2001; 72:1846-8.

[21] Abu-Elmagd K, Reyes J, Bond G, et al. Clinical intestinal transplantation: a decade of experience at a single center. *Ann Surg* 2001; 234:404-16.

[22] Carlsen BT, Rudkin GH, Farmer D. Complicated abdominal wall closure in intestinal transplant recipients. *Curr Opin Organ Transplant* 2005; 10:128-31.

[23] Alexandrides IJ, Liu P, Marshall DM, et al. Abdominal wall closure after intestinal transplantation. *Plast Reconstr Surg* 2000; 106:805-12.

[24] Levi DM, Tzakis AG, Kato T, et al. Transplantation of the abdominal wall. *Lancet* 2003; 361:2173-6.

[25] Bueno J, Ohwada S, Kocoshis S, et al. Factors impacting the survival of children with intestinal failure referred for intestinal transplantation. *J Pediatr Surg* 1999; 34:27-32.

[26] Fryer J, Pellar S, Ormond D, et al. Mortality in candidates waiting for combined liver-intestine transplants exceeds that for other candidates waiting for liver transplants. *Liver Transpl* 2003; 9.:748-53.

[27] de Ville de Goyet J, Mitchell A, Mayer AD, et al. En block combined reduced-liver and small bowel transplants: from large donors to small children. *Transplantation* 2000; 69:555-59.

[28] Fishbein T, Florman S, Gondolesi G, Decker R. Noncomposite simultaneous liver and intestinal transplantation. *Transplantation* 2003; 75:564-65.

[29] Gruessner RW, Sharp HL. Living-related intestinal transplantation: first report of a standardized surgical technique. *Transplantation* 1997; 64:1605-07.

[30] Testa G, Panaro F, Schena S, et al. Living related small bowel transplantation: donor surgical technique. *Ann Surg* 2004; 240:779-84.

[31] Horslen SP, Sudan DL, Iyer KR, et al. Isolated liver transplantation in infants with end-stage liver disease associated with short bowel syndrome. *Ann Surg* 2002; 235:435-9.

[32] Todo S, Reyes J, Furukawa H, et al. Outcome analysis of 71 clinical intestinal transplantations. *Ann Surg* 1995; 222:270-80.

[33] Goulet O, Sauvat F, Ruemmele F, et al. Results of the Paris program: ten years of pediatric intestinal transplantation. *Transplant Proc* 2005; 37:1667-70.

[34] Reyes J, Bueno J, Kocoshis S, et al. Current status of intestinal transplantation in children. *J Pediatr Surg* 1998; 33:243-54.

[35] Yann R, Yves A, Dominique J, et al. Improved quality of life by combined transplantation in Hirschsprung's disease with a very long aganglionic segment. *J Pediatr Surg* 2003; 38:422-4.

[36] Masetti M, Rodriguez MM, Thompson JF, et al. Multivisceral transplantation for megacystis microcolon intestinal hypoperistalsis syndrome. *Transplantation* 1999; 68:228-32.

[37] Loinaz C, Mittal N, Kato T, et al. Multivisceral transplantation for pediatric intestinal pseudo-obstruction: single center's experience of 16 cases. *Transplant Proc* 2004; 36:312-3.

[38] Sigurdsson L, Reyes J, Kocoshis SA, et al. Intestinal transplantation in children with chronic intestinal pseudo-obstruction. *Gut* 1999; 45:570-4.

[39] Iyer K, Kaufman S, Sudan D, et al. Long-term results of intestinal transplantation for pseudo-obstruction in children. *J Pediatr Surg* 2001; 36(:174-7.

[40] Goulet O, Sauvat F. Short bowel syndrome and intestinal transplantation in children. *Curr Opin Clin Nutr Metab Care* 2006; 9:304-13.

[41] Goulet O, Jan D, Brousse N, et al. Intestinal transplantation. *J Pediatr Gastroenterol Nutr* 1997; 25:1-11.

[42] Fouquet V, De Lagausie P, Faure C, et al. Do prognostic factors exist for total colonic aganglionosis with ileal involvement? *J Pediatr Surg* 2002; 37:71-5.

[43] Abu-Elmagd KM. Intestinal transplantation for short bowel syndrome and gastrointestinal failure: current consensus, rewarding outcomes, and practical guidelines. *Gastroenterology* 2006; 130:S132-7.

[44] Grant D. Intestinal transplantation: 1997 report of the international registry. Intestinal Transplant Registry. *Transplantation* 1999; 67:1061-4.

[45] Goulet O. Are the needs and indications for bowel transplantation changing? In *Symposium IISBT,* ed. Brussels: IXth International Small Bowel Transplantation Symposium, 2005.

[46] Kaufman SS, Atkinson JB, Bianchi A, et al. Indications for pediatric intestinal transplantation: a position paper of the American Society of Transplantation. *Pediatr Transplant* 2001; 5:80-7.

[47] Grant D. Small bowel transplant registry. In *Symposium IISB*T, ed. Brussels: IXth International Small Bowel Transplantation Symposium, 2005.

[48] Franco A, Hernandez D, Capdevilla L, et al. De novo hemolytic-uremic syndrome/thrombotic microangiopathy in renal transplant patients receiving calcineurin inhibitors: role of sirolimus. *Transplant Proc* 2003; 35:1764-6.

[49] Kelly DA. Intestinal failure-associated liver disease: what do we know today? *Gastroenterology* 2006; 130:S70-7.

[50] Kaufman SS, Loseke CA, Lupo JV, et al. Influence of bacterial overgrowth and intestinal inflammation on duration of parenteral nutrition in children with short bowel syndrome. *J Pediatr* 1997; 131:356-61.

[51] Sondheimer JM, Asturias E, Cadnapaphornchai M. Infection and cholestasis in neonates with intestinal resection and long-term parenteral nutrition. *J Pediatr Gastroenterol Nutr* 1998; 27:131-7.

[52] Wolf A, Pohlandt F. Bacterial infection: the main cause of acute cholestasis in newborn infants receiving short-term parenteral nutrition. *J Pediatr Gastroenterol Nutr* 1989; 8:297-03.

[53] Watkins JB, Szczepanik P, Gould JB, et al. Bile salt metabolism in the human premature infant. Preliminary observations of pool size and synthesis rate following prenatal administration of dexamethasone and phenobarbital. *Gastroenterology* 1975; 69:706-13.

[54] American Gastroenterological Association medical position statement: short bowel syndrome and intestinal transplantation. *Gastroenterology* 2003; 124:1105-10.

[55] Kaufman S. Indications for intestinal transplantation and graft allocation. *Curr Opin Organ Transplantation* 2004; 9:220-24.

[56] Horslen SP. Optimal management of the post-intestinal transplant patient. *Gastroenterology* 2006; 130:S163-9.

[57] Al-Hussaini A, Tredger JM, Dhawan A. Immunosuppression in pediatric liver and intestinal transplantation: a closer look at the arsenal. *J Pediatr Gastroenterol Nutr* 2005; 41:152-65.

[58] Fishbein TM, Florman S, Gondolesi G, et al. Intestinal transplantation before and after the introduction of sirolimus. *Transplantation* 2002; 73:1538-42.

[59] Saikali JA, Truong LD, Suki WN. Sirolimus may promote thrombotic microangiopathy. A*m J Transplant* 2003; 3:229-30.

[60] Paramesh AS, Grosskreutz C, Florman SS, et al. Thrombotic microangiopathy associated with combined sirolimus and tacrolimus immunosuppression after intestinal transplantation. *Transplantation* 2004; 77:129-31.

[61] Reyes J, Mazariegos GV, Abu-Elmagd K, et al. Intestinal transplantation under tacrolimus monotherapy after perioperative lymphoid depletion with rabbit anti-thymocyte globulin (thymoglobulin). *Am J Transplant* 2005; 5:1430-6.

[62] Tzakis AG, Kato T, Nishida S, et al. Preliminary experience with campath 1H (C1H) in intestinal and liver transplantation. *Transplantation* 2003; 75:1227-31.

[63] Fishbein TM. The current state of intestinal transplantation. *Transplantation* 2004; 78:175-8.

[64] Wells CL. Colonization and translocation of intestinal bacterial flora. *Transplant Proc* 1996; 28:2653-6.

[65] Khan FA, Kato T, Berho M, et al. Graft failure secondary to necrotizing enterocolitis in multi-visceral transplantation recipients: two case reports. *Pediatr Transplant* 2000; 4:215-20.

[66] Mittal NK, Tzakis AG, Kato T, Thompson JF. Current status of small bowel transplantation in children: update 2003. *Pediatr Clin North Am* 2003; 50:1419-33.

[67] Watson CJ, Wraight EP, Neale G, et al. Radionuclide studies in intestinal transplantation. Diagnosis of rejection and assessment of permeability. *Transplantation* 1996; 61:155-7.

[68] Pappas PA, A GT, Gaynor JJ, et al. An analysis of the association between serum citrulline and acute rejection among 26 recipients of intestinal transplant. *Am J Transplant* 2004; 4:1124-32.

[69] Wu T, Abu-Elmagd K, Bond G, et al. A schema for histologic grading of small intestine allograft acute rejection. *Transplantation* 2003; 75:1241-8.

[70] Ruiz P, Bagni A, Brown R, et al. Histological criteria for the identification of acute cellular rejection in human small bowel allografts: results of the pathology workshop at the *VIII International Small Bowel Transplant Symposium. Transplant Proc* 2004; 36:335-7.

[71] Noguchi Si S, Reyes J, Mazariegos GV, et al. Pediatric intestinal transplantation: the resected allograft. *Pediatr Dev Pathol* 2002; 5:3-21.

[72] Goulet O. Intestinal failure in children. *Transplant Proc* 1998; 30:2523-5.

[73] Fryer J, Grant D, Jiang J, et al. Influence of macrophage depletion on bacterial translocation and rejection in small bowel transplantation. *Transplantation* 1996; 62:553-9.

[74] Goulet O. Complications after intestinal transplantation: traditional and new. *Pediatr Transplant* 1999; 3:89-91.

[75] Kusne S, Manez R, Frye BL, et al. Use of DNA amplification for diagnosis of cytomegalovirus enteritis after intestinal transplantation. *Gastroenterology* 1997; 112:1121-8.

[76] Burroughs M, Sobanjo A, Florman S, et al. Cytomegalovirus matching does not predict symptomatic disease in intestinal transplantation. *Transplant Proc* 2002; 34:946-7.

[77] Farmer DG, McDiarmid SV, Winston D, et al. Effectiveness of aggressive prophylatic and preemptive therapies targeted against cytomegaloviral and Epstein-Barr viral disease after human intestinal transplantation. *Transplant Proc* 2002; 34:948-9.

[78] Pinchoff RJ, Kaufman SS, Magid MS, et al. Adenovirus infection in pediatric small bowel transplantation recipients. *Transplantation* 2003; 76:183-9.

[79] Kaufman SS, Chatterjee NK, Fuschino ME, et al. Calicivirus enteritis in an intestinal transplant recipient. A*m J Transplant* 2003; 3:764-8.

[80] Collins MH, Montone KT, Leahey AM, et al. Post-transplant lymphoproliferative disease in children. *Pediatr Transplant* 2001; 5:250-7.

[81] Tanner JE, Alfieri C. The Epstein-Barr virus and post-transplant lymphoproliferative disease: interplay of immunosuppression, EBV, and the immune system in disease pathogenesis. *Transpl Infect Dis* 2001; 3:60-9.

[82] Preiksaitis JK. Epstein-Barr virus infection and malignancy in solid organ transplant recipients: strategies for prevention and treatment. *Transpl Infect Dis* 2001; 3:56-9.

[83] Cockfield SM. Identifying the patient at risk for post-transplant lymphoproliferative disorder. *Transpl Infect Dis* 2001; 3:70-8.

[84] Berney T, Delis S, Kato T, et al. Successful treatment of posttransplant lymphoproliferative disease with prolonged rituximab treatment in intestinal transplant recipients. *Transplantation* 2002; 74:1000-6.

[85] Gross TG, Hinrichs SH, Winner J, et al. Treatment of post-transplant lymphoproliferative disease (PTLD) following solid organ transplantation with low-dose chemotherapy. *Ann Oncol* 1998; 9:339-40.

[86] Finn L, Reyes J, Bueno J, Yunis E. Epstein-Barr virus infections in children after transplantation of the small intestine. *Am J Surg Pathol* 1998; 22:299-309.

[87] Sarr MG. Motility and absorption in the transplanted gut. *Transplant Proc* 1996; 28:2535-8.

[88] Yagi M, Masutani H, Iwasa K, et al. Changes of mucosal immunologic function in graft-vs-host reaction after small bowel transplantation. *Transplant Proc* 1992; 24:1503-4.

[89] Kosmach-Park B, Iurlano K, Smith A, et al. Current status of pediatric intestinal transplant recipients: care requirements and patient outcomes. In *Symposium VtISBT,* ed. Stockholm, Sweden: VII th International Small Bowel Transplant Symposium, 2001.

[90] Snell L, Randolph S. Home care management of intestinal transplant recipients. *Prog Transplant* 2004; 14:299-310.

[91] Silver HJ, Castellanos VH. Nutritional complications and management of intestinal transplant. *J Am Diet Assoc* 2000; 100(6):680-4, 687-9; quiz 685-6.

[92] Mazariegos GV, Abu-Elmagd K, Jaffe R, et al. Graft versus host disease in intestinal transplantation. *Am J Transplant* 2004; 4:1459-65.

[93] Kaila B, Grant DR, Pettigrew N, et al. Crohn´s disease recurrence in a small bowel transplant. *Am J Gastroenterol* 2004; 99:158-162.

[94] Sustento-Reodica N, Ruiz P, Rogers A, et al. Recurrent Crohn's disease in transplanted bowel. *Lancet* 1997; 349:688-91.

[95] Moon JI, Selvaggi G, Nishida S, et al. Intestinal transplantation for the treatment of neoplastic disease. *J Surg Oncol* 2005; 92:284-91.

[96] Kato T, Gaynor JJ, Selvaggi G, et al. Intestinal transplantation in children: a summary of clinical outcomes and prognostic factors in 108 patients from a single center. *J Gastrointest Surg* 2005; 9:75-89.

[97] Ishii T, Mazariegos GV, Bueno J, et al. Exfoliative rejection after intestinal transplantation in children. *Pediatr Transplant* 2003; 7:185-91.

[98] Tinckam KJ, Sayegh MH. Transplantation tolerance in pediatric recipients: lessons and challenges. *Pediatr Transplant* 2005; 9:17-27.

[99] Schaffner F. The history of liver disease at The Mount Sinai Hospital. *Mt Sinai J Med* 2000; 67:76-83.

[100] Brown CR, DiBaise JK. Intestinal rehabilitation: a management program for short-bowel syndrome. *Prog Transplant* 2004; 14:290-6.

[101] DiBaise JK, Young RJ, Vanderhoof JA. Intestinal rehabilitation and the short bowel syndrome: part 2. *Am J Gastroenterol* 2004; 99:1823-32.

[102] Sudan D, DiBaise J, Torres C, et al. A multidisciplinary approach to the treatment of intestinal failure. *J Gastrointest Surg* 2005; 9:165-76.

[103] Koehler AN, Yaworski JA, Gardner M, et al. Coordinated interdisciplinary management of pediatric intestinal failure: a 2-year review. *J Pediatr Surg* 2000; 35:380-5.

[104] Howard L. Home parenteral nutrition: survival, cost, and quality of life. *Gastroenterology* 2006; 130:S52-S59.

[105] Goulet O, Baglin-Gobet S, Talbotec C, et al. Outcome and long-term growth after extensive small bowel resection in the neonatal period: a survey of 87 children. *Eur J Pediatr Surg* 2005; 15:95-101.

[106] Beath SV, Booth IW, Murphy MS, et al. Nutritional care and candidates for small bowel transplantation. *Arch Dis Child* 1995; 73:348-50.

In: Hirschsprung's Disease: Diagnosis and Treatment
Ed: Ramón Núñez and Manuel López-Alonso

ISBN: 978-1-60741-349-3

Chapter XXVI

Nutritional Status, Situations of Nutritional Risk, and Nutrition in Hirschsprung's Disease

Emilio Blesa and Luis Lassaletta

Nutritional Status

Maintaining normal nutritional status is necessary in any healthy person, and is equally so in sick patients, or at least we must attempt to approach it as closely as possible. When a sick patient is going to be operated on, sometimes with complex and serious surgery in which there may occur severe infections, or when fragments of the gut will be extirpated or temporarily excluded from transit, it is essential to try to confront these challenges with a good state of nutrition and to maintain it during and after recovery.

In children with Hirschsprung's disease (HD), it is not always easy to achieve an adequate nutritional status. The possible reasons are manifold. Until diagnosis, the child may have suffered crises of intestinal obstruction or subobstruction. He may suffer severe enterocolitis before or after surgical correction. Temporary enterostomies may need to be performed. And resection of part or all of the colon may be performed, sometimes also including portions of variable length of the small intestine. All this changes temporarily or permanently the patients' digestive function.

Nutritional Evaluation

An obligatory part of the comprehensive evaluation of any child due to undergo surgery is the assessment of nutritional status [1]. The overall subjective assessment that we make on the basis of the anamnesis and physical examination, while useful, is far from easy, especially in children. One usually adds therefore an objective evaluation which, in its simplest and most economic and practical form for the present purposes, includes anthropometric measurements that are easy to take – weight, length/height, cranial circumference, and brachial circumference. These can then be used to calculate various indices complementing the basic information, which together are generally enough to know to what extent the patient may present little or unbalanced body growth [2,3].

Measurement of Bodily Growth and Constitution

Measurement of bodily growth and constitution is the most important component of the evaluation of nutritional status. The variables used can be compared with those considered normal for the healthy population of equal age and sex, and expressed as percentiles, percentages, or standardized z-scores [3].

Anthropometric Measurements

Weight

This together with height is the anthropometric variable most widely used to assess nutritional status. It provides data of interest on total body mass and detects nutritional alterations in patients with either acute or chronic pathologies [4,5]. In the newborn and infants, the evaluation of the weight must take the birth weight into account, and the aim must be to attain an average daily weight gain of 25–30 grams until they reach a similar weight to that of term infants with normal weight for the same age [2].

Length/Height

This also reflects total body mass, but by itself is usually only pathological by default in situations of chronic malnutrition [4,5].

Cranial Circumference

This is used primarily in children from birth to age three, and its value is compared against reference tables. Its reduction suggests a prolonged period of malnutrition [5].

Brachial Circumference

This is more used in pre-school and school-age children to obtain information on the protein-calorie nutritional status and lean body mass [3,6]. In infants and young children, it is useful for the calculation of indices of interest that will be commented on in the following paragraphs.

Indices

Relative Weight And Height Percentages

For each variable, these are the measured value divided by the P_{50} for the corresponding sex and age, multiplied by one hundred.

Weight Percentage Relative to the Expected Value for the Height

Similar to the previous case, but with height replacing age in the calculation [3].

Body Mass Index

This reflects a proportion between weight and height, according to the formula: *weight (in kg)/height (in m)*^{2}. This is a measure of under- or over-weight, the latter in children and adolescents usually as a result of adiposity [7].

Acute and Chronic Malnutrition

For Waterlow [8], there exists acute malnutrition when the weight percentage relative to the expected value for the height is less than 90%: *mild* if this index is between 90% and 80%, *moderate* between 80% and 70%, and *severe* less than 70%.

A good alternative in patients under the age of three or where the measurements of weight or height are unreliable is the method of McLaren [3]. This is to use the ratio between the brachial and the cranial circumferences. Values between 0.31 and 0.28 indicate *mild* acute malnutrition; those between 0.28 and 0.25, *moderate*; and less than 0.25, *severe*.

To evaluate chronic malnutrition, Waterlow [8] uses the relative height, regarding chronic malnutrition to be *mild* for values between 95% and 90%, *moderate* if it is between 90% and 85%, and *severe* if it is less than 85%.

In malnourished patients, the recommendations are [3]:

- For mild malnutrition, aggressive oral nutritional rehabilitation.
- For moderate malnutrition, aggressive enteral nutrition, by nasogastric tube or gastrostomy if necessary.
- For severe malnutrition, parenteral nutrition (PN) if enteral nutrition is insufficient.

Situations of Nutritional Risk in Hirschsprung's Disease

As is noted in other chapters of this book which give detailed descriptions of the situations that we shall refer to as causes of nutritional risk, until HD patient's disease is treated or throughout their lives for some of them, they will present situations in which their proper nutrition is going to be threatened and even occasionally made practically impossible.

The key factors that, singly or in association, are causes of malnutrition in these patients are summarized in the following diagram:

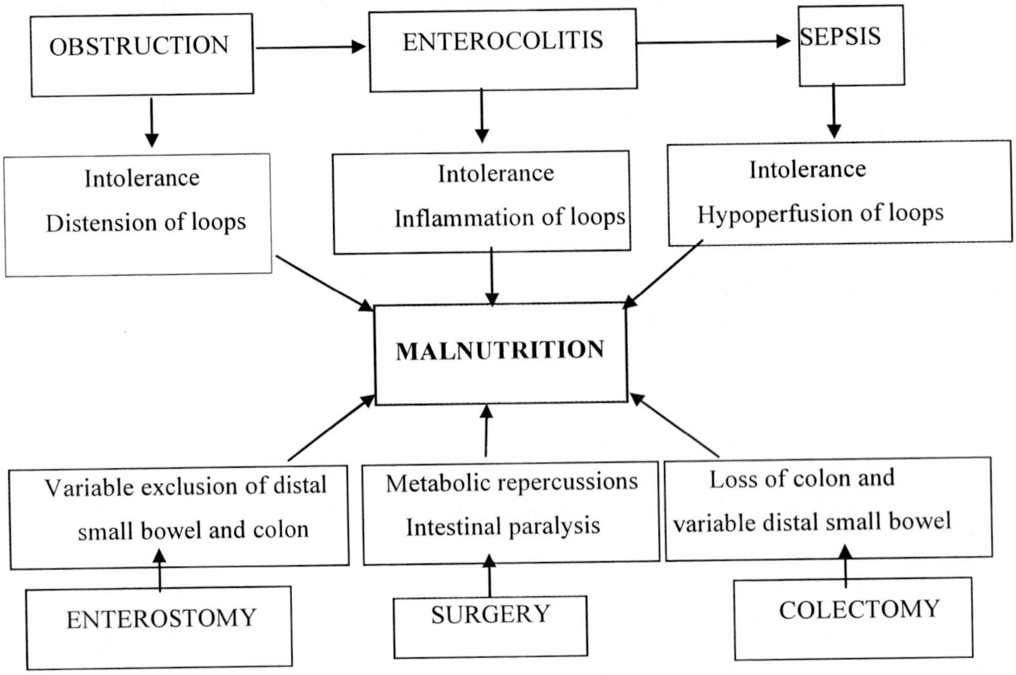

Among the surgical procedures applied to these patients, in addition to the enterostomy and colectomy with more or less distal intestine included, in most of them a partial resection of the colon is performed. This is almost always rectosigmoidal. Together with some colostomies, it suppresses or excludes the distal large bowel, without apparent repercussions on the patient's nutritional status.

Obstruction, Enterocolitis, Sepsis

Three clinical manifestations or complications typical of HD are obstruction, enterocolitis, and sepsis. These are often interrelated, particularly in the newborn and infant. They all lead to gastrointestinal intolerance and, if prolonged or repeated, to acute malnutrition. This is because nutrient contributions can not be made normally for sufficient time, or they have to be interrupted on several occasions without enough time between them to compensate the malnutrition that was secondary to this or previous crises. They act through the distension, inflammation, or hypoperfusion of the loops involved.

Sometimes doubts in the diagnosis, with delay in deciding to introduce parenteral nutrition, in performing a colostomy or enterostomy, or in implementing programmed rectal wash-outs, keep the child in a situation of nutrient deficiency which ends by affecting his weight and the associated indices, with delayed weight gain and acute malnutrition [6,7].

These children, who will eventually require surgery, are converted into critically ill surgical patients, with the concomitant repercussion postoperatively. When in addition there is sepsis, the complexity of their management is even greater. Therefore, when HD is suspected, within a margin of days or a few weeks the diagnosis should be confirmed or ruled out, and the most appropriate therapeutic measures implemented with no unnecessary delay [9,10]. At the same time, all necessary measures must be taken to provide the nutrients required to achieve the patient's adequate nutritional status [1].

Enterostomies

Enterostomies are best avoided by extirpating the aganglionic zone and pulling the well-innervated zone through to the anus. Sometimes however, they are unavoidable. Almost all patients who need them have total colonic aganglionosis (TCA). They are the price to pay to avoid prolonged PN with its concomitant complications, as well as the risk of enterocolitis, intestinal obstruction, and even perforation [10]. Their consequences are also important, and are related to the amount of affected ileum excluded distal to the enterostomy, and to the exclusion of the colon.

The intestine excluded from transit by a proximal enterostomy no longer performs its functions. It becomes a possible cause of malabsorption, the more so the greater its length, and is always a cause of accelerated transit due to the loss of the "ileal brake" represented by the resistance of the ileocæcal junction, with its role as an "ileal pylorus" [11–18].

The ileum's absorption function, for the purposes that interest us here, is exerted primarily on fluids from the jejunum, with the salts they contain, and on the absorption of vitamin B12 and bile salts [11,12].

Losses through abundant liquid stools due to ileostomy may lead to grave electrolyte disorders. Together with the water lost, there is a loss of sodium, potassium, bicarbonate, zinc, and magnesium. Fæcal elimination of more than 45 ml/kg/day through the enterostomy is considered to be dangerously high [1]. These losses have been reported to range from 10 to 58 ml/kg/day. Among other effects, hyponatræmia, metabolic acidosis, and hypochloræmia have especially to be taken into account [19].

The sodium loss in infants with enterostomy has been estimated at 90 mEq/1000 g of fæces, with an average of 3.3 mEq/kg/day [20]. These losses can be monitored by the decreases in blood and urine sodium levels. One very important consequence of sodium deficiency is the failure to thrive, together with malnutrition. Even when they are provided sufficient calories, these patients fail to gain weight normally until they are given sufficient sodium to reverse this situation [19].

Metabolic acidosis is the consequence of bicarbonate loss through the enterostomy, and the kidney's inability to eliminate acidic radicals in the presence of sodium depletion [19].

In all these patients there may occur malabsorption of carbohydrates, fats, and proteins. Among other factors, this is related to the exclusion of the colon, the particularities of which will be discussed below.

Exclusion of the Colon, Colectomy, Colostomy

Neither in patients with enterostomy, even though this preserves the colon, nor in those with colectomy, as is the case after the definitive surgery for TCA, can the colon perform its normal functions. Only in those ileostomies in which the colon has not yet been removed may its endocrine function persist, at least in part. The functions of the colon are, *inter alia*:

Absorption and Secretion of Water and Electrolytes

Of the large volume of chyme that the ileum evacuates daily into the colon, over 90% is absorbed. Together with the water, almost all the ions are absorbed, with very little sodium being lost. Most of this absorption takes place in the proximal colon. But when the colon is affected by irritative processes, such as bacterial colitis, its mucosa not only absorbs less, but can even secrete and hence lose large quantities of water and electrolytes as diarrhœa [21,22]. Without the colon's action, insufficient of these substances are absorbed, and they are eliminated through the enterostomy or through the anus after ileoanal anastomosis.

Caloric Absorption

Following an ileostomy or when the colon is removed, there is a loss of the capacity that corresponded to the colon of caloric absorption from the carbohydrates, fats, and proteins that the ileum, especially if it has been partially resected, would have evacuated into it. In general, the greater the amount of ileum removed, the greater is this loss [23].

Complex carbohydrates (starch and fibre) are fermented by the flora of the colon, especially in the cæcum, and transformed into short-chain fatty acids (SCFA) – acetic, propionic, butyric which, once absorbed, provide a not inconsiderable amount of energy, up to 10% of the total [24,25].

The colon also has capacity to absorb medium chain triglycerides (MCT) and proteins, which may reach it especially after major resections of the small bowel [25–27].

Given the above, it has to be accepted that in cases of extensive aganglionosis, with variable resections of the ileum, with ileostomies, or with ileoanal anastomosis after colectomy, the capacity to make use of enteral nutrients is clearly impaired relative to patients with short bowel but intact colon [28].

Secretion of Peptide YY (PYY)

Peptide YY is released after stimulation of the duodenum by fats and glucose. It is produced in endocrine cells of the distal jejunum, colon, and rectum. It inhibits gastric secretion, delays gastric emptying, reduces intestinal motility with a resulting increase in transit time, and acts to brake transit in the distal ileum [29]. It works by preventing the secretion of secretin and cholecystokinin, and reduces the intestinal secretion stimulated by intestinal vasoactive peptide. It consequently limits water loss in enterostomies or after resections [30–32]. Its levels are raised after partial ileal resection, and lowered after proctocolectomy [33–35].

The consequence of colectomies is the loss of functions that correspond to the colon, with little or no scope for compensation by the unresected small bowel. With a colostomy, however, only the secretory function and absorptive function of the large bowel distal to the stoma is excluded, while the endocrine function is retained. The colon proximal to the stoma, which is usually long, adapts to recuperate at least partially the function of the total colon. The result is that the patient usually adapts well to the colostomy, allowing normal nutrient intake. In sum, the complications of colostomies, whatever their indication, do not usually involve alterations of nutritional status [36,37]. Whenever possible, the ileocæcal junction and the largest available fragment of colon must be preserved [38,39].

Nutrition

The current preoperative management and surgical treatment of HD give good results in most patients. Given all the forms of the disease, their nutritional problems do not seem too important [40,41], and indeed these aspects are not considered in most publications in this regard. This is becoming even more true with the ever earlier application of surgery, often practised in the first few months or even weeks of life, avoiding in most patients the repeated subobstruction, enterocolitis, and sepsis which are frequent causes of acute malnutrition [9,10]. Indeed, there can be no better way of obviating alterations in nutritional status.

Despite this generalization of definitive neonatal surgery in TCA patients, sometimes subobstructive crises, enterocolitis, or the lack of a secure diagnosis of HD and its extension force PN to be initiated with its far from inconsiderable number of concomitant problems [9,10]. This is seldom the case in rectosigmoidal and colonic forms of affectation.

It is in patients with TCA in whom the obstruction and enterocolitis make PN or the performance of enterostomies obligatory that situations of acute and, in the long term, chronic malnutrition arise most frequently. The reported frequency and intensity vary according to the authors, from those who do not even describe it in their series, through others who consider it a minor or very rare problem, to those who stress not only its high frequency but its apparent tendency to persist and even become worse in the long term. This would suggest that chronic malnutrition, left to a standard diet unadapted to the particular nutritional requirements of the affected patient, is not resolved by any sufficient adaptation of the child's residual intestine to its resected situation [42–49].

Acute Malnutrition

States of acute malnutrition usually affect patients who for short periods of time, from days to a few weeks, for the reasons discussed above, do not have adequate nutrient intake. They are in general detected by the defect in weight and acute electrolyte disorders. They mainly affect the newborn and very young infants. The infant without serious nutritional problems tolerates well a lack of caloric intake for 5 to 7 days [1].

Above all, nutrition must at no time be neglected in patients in whom a final diagnosis of HD has yet to be established or obstructive or infectious complications have arisen which have led to postponement of surgery, especially if these complications are repeated. The nutrition of these patients will generally consist of [1,11]:

- Breast milk whenever it is well tolerated.
- Standard formula milk as for healthy patients.
- Diet that is normal for the patient's age.
- Special formulas for patients with poor tolerance to normal foods for their age. These must be isotonic, and preferably with carbohydrates in the form of maltodextrin, hydrolyzed proteins, and about half of the fat intake in the form of medium chain triglycerides (MCT). These diets are easily digested and absorbed. Otherwise, one can try feeding with simple carbohydrates and protein hydrolysates alone.
- Parenteral nutrition, either supplementary or total, if adequate enteral nutrition is impossible, in all cases maintaining some enteral intake.

Overall in infants with HD, a preoperative exclusive diet of breast milk has been possible in almost half of the patients, and standard formulas in more than one third. Only a small fraction have required special diets [41]. The recommended method of feeding is [1,41]:

- Giving the breast or bottle whenever possible.
- If oral tolerance is inadequate, enteral nutrition, preferably by nasogastric tube. At least initially, slow perfusion for 2 to 3 hours is better than a "bolus".
- Greater volumes and concentrations are tolerated by stomach than by jejunum.
- If direct stomach feeding will be for longer than 6 to 8 weeks, it is preferable to perform a gastrostomy.
- With direct gastric intake, there is increased risk of pathological gastrœsophageal reflux, in which case this and gastric emptying must be evaluated so as to feed through a nasojejunal tube or a jejunostomy, despite the complications involved, or even to perform gastrœsophageal antireflux surgery.
- In patients with an absolute diet, oral intakes have to be resumed as soon as possible.
- To increase the oral intake, it must be borne in mind that increases in volume are better tolerated than increased osmolarity.

These recommendations apply both preoperatively and after enterostomies or the definitive surgery. The following diagram is a synthesis of the pathogenicity of these situations:

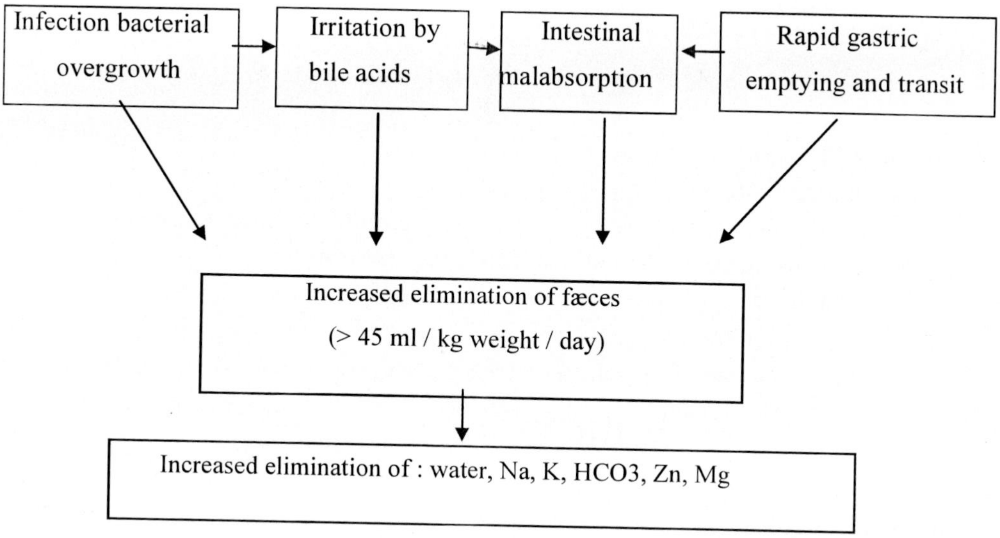

In these patients, infection often leads to abundant liquid fæcal losses. A major cause is bacterial overgrowth, especially in ostomies and pull-throughs performed with aganglionic or obstructed segments. In these cases, as in the enterocolitis typical of unoperated HD, retention of chyme leads to bacterial overgrowth, and this to enteritis, with increased losses through the stoma or anus, and sepsis due to bacterial translocation. The increase of bacteria in the gut can be monitored by the levels of D-lactase, indicanuria, or exhaled hydrogen [1,12].

The effect of pathological flora on bile salts is their deconjugation, with the formation of large amounts of bile acids whose cathartic effect leads to increased fluid loss in the fæces. As they are not reabsorbed normally, the pool of bile salts is diminished, and may become insufficient to emulsify the ingested fats. Consequently, there can appear malabsorption of fats [1,12], as evidenced by their increase in the fæces. Also, malabsorption of carbohydrates will be indicated by the detection in the stools of a $pH<5.5$ or an amount $>0.5\%$ of reducing substances, and malabsorption of proteins by an increase in alpha 1-antitrypsin. In addition, vitamin B12 malabsorption should always be taken into account.

It is therefore necessary in all patients with an enterostomy or ileoanal pull-through to monitor electrolyte metabolism, bile salt deficiency, macronutrient and vitamin B12 malabsorption, the possible onset of bacterial overgrowth, and accelerated gastric emptying and digestive transit. Any alteration in these parameters must be promptly corrected.

In general, nutritional disorders subsequent to enterostomy depend to a great extent on the length of the ileal segment excluded. In patients with TCA and an enterostomy performed at less than 50 centimetres from the ileocæcal junction, prognosis is good, with short-term total or supplementary PN. Enterostomies at more than 100 centimetres, however, are accompanied by high morbidity and mortality, and require total PN for months or years. They are authentic cases of short bowel syndrome [12,50-53].

In cases where the evolution is good, the recommendations regarding the type and form of nutrient intake are the same as were described above. In cases where enteral nutrition is slow to be tolerated, is tolerated only partially, or there is malabsorption, the following considerations may be taken into account [1,11,12,54]:

- Exclusive oral tolerance may not be achieved until months or even years have passed [50].
- Initially, the most urgent and important consideration is to ensure sufficient water and electrolyte intake.
- In patients with ileostomies, the amounts eliminated through them have been reported to be between 10 and 58 ml/kg/day, with an average of 31 ml/kg/day in infants requiring supplementation and 16 ml/kg/day in those who do not.
- The sodium requirements of infants with ileostomy are usually between 6 and 10 mEq/kg/day, although this can vary. In any case, sodium intake should be sufficient to maintain urine levels at values greater than 10 mEq/litre. Potential overload should be monitored [19,20]. Administration is as NaCl.
- It is also necessary to provide HCO3 when there is excessive lose in the fæces. The amount will depend on the serum levels of Na, Cl, and HCO3. Administration is as NaHCO3.
- It should be borne in mind that when the aim is not just that the patient should have an adequate weight gain, but should recover any weight lost, the potassium requirements will rise in proportion to the desired weight to recuperate.
- Oral contributions, even if minimal, should be initiated as soon as they can be tolerated. Hyperosmolarity must be avoided.
- This replacement of PN has to be gradual, starting with 5% of total calorie intake, with small increases every 3 to 7 days, depending on the tolerance.
- Opioids that prolong transit, such as loperamide, may be useful in selected patients and at specific times. They should be avoided in those who have already presented or are at risk of bacterial overgrowth.
- The probable causes of bacterial overgrowth, such as stenosis of an ostomy or their realization in aganglionic intestine, should be corrected surgically.
- If there is malabsorption of carbohydrates, their quantity should be reduced.
- Malabsorption of fats can be improved with greater percentage contributions of MCT, but always contingent on administering sufficient essential fatty acids (>2% of the total calorie intake).
- In the case of malabsorption of fats, there needs to be parenteral administration of water-soluble vitamins.
- Malabsorption of protein hydrolysates can be compensated by presenting them in the form of dipeptides to facilitate absorption.
- In patients with excluded or extirpated colon, bile salt chelants may lessen their reabsorption and lead to their decrease in the enterohepatic circulation, with poorer emulsion of ingested fats.
- In major exclusions or resections of the ileum, parenteral administration of vitamin B12 is necessary, together with any mineral that is not being absorbed normally (Cl, K, Mg, Ca, Zn, Fe).
- The detection of anæmia requires treatment.

- There is currently no evidence for any positive effect on the evolution of these patients of various drug treatments when groups of treated *versus* untreated children are compared. This applies as much to inhibitors of gastric secretion as to glutamine, growth hormone, or other growth factors [12].

When there is so little residual intestine that, despite being treated by specialists in the treatment of intestinal failure in children, sufficient enteral nutrition and the withdrawal of PN can not be attained, the last resort is intestinal transplant [54–56].

Chronic Malnutrition

In HD patients, chronic malnutrition usually occurs in those with TCA where the colon has been extirpated together with varying amounts of distal ileum, and a pull-through has been performed of the normally innervated zone, which is anastomosed to the anal canal. It is generally of protracted evolution, and is a consequence of the loss of function of the resected colon and small bowel which can not be compensated by the residual intestine. The same may occur in patients in whom an enterostomy is maintained for long periods of time.

Among its causes are shortened transit times and the loss of the digestive and absorptive function of the suppressed small and large intestines. As a result, the fæces have a looser consistency and greater volume than in the normal population, and the number of stools per day is from 3 to 5 in most patients [40,42]. This entails a greater loss of water, and possibly also of electrolytes, sugars, fats, and proteins that could have been processed and absorbed by the resected small intestine and the colon. Consequently, the water requirements are usually greater and too much sodium may be lost. Also, the reduced digestibility of the dietary intake may lead to insufficient calorie availability, with its repercussion on growth.

There is reference to deficient bodily growth in most publications that report long-term follow-up of patients operated on for HD [40], especially those with TCA [44–49]. There is a typical lag in height [8], with or without a lag in weight. Therefore, long-term monitoring of variables as simple as weight or height can detect growth retardation, and then to a study of possible malabsorption of nutrients. Their compensation must be adapted to the particularities of each patient, striving always to use normal nutrients that are natural and well-tolerated by most patients. At times a patient may require special dietary supplements to ensure a well-balanced caloric supply with the different macronutrients administered [44]. Other anthropometric indices can detect alterations in the protein or fat compartments, and help design modifications in the diet to optimize the type of nutrients with respect to digestion and absorption [3,7].

One can not fail to note, however, that while publications describing the long-term nutritional evolution of patients who had undergone surgery for HD emphasize that the appearance of chronic malnutrition is very frequent, they restrict themselves to recommending the control and treatment of these patients by specialists in nutrition, making hardly any reference to what type of nutritional or therapeutic measures are recommended [47,48].

In the authors' experience, we obtained data from a comparison of a group of 10 HD patients who underwent a rectosigmoidectomy with another 7 who underwent a colectomy with removal of part of the distal ileum. After a mean follow-up time of 5 years 7 months, they showed significant differences in the variables shown in the Figure 1.

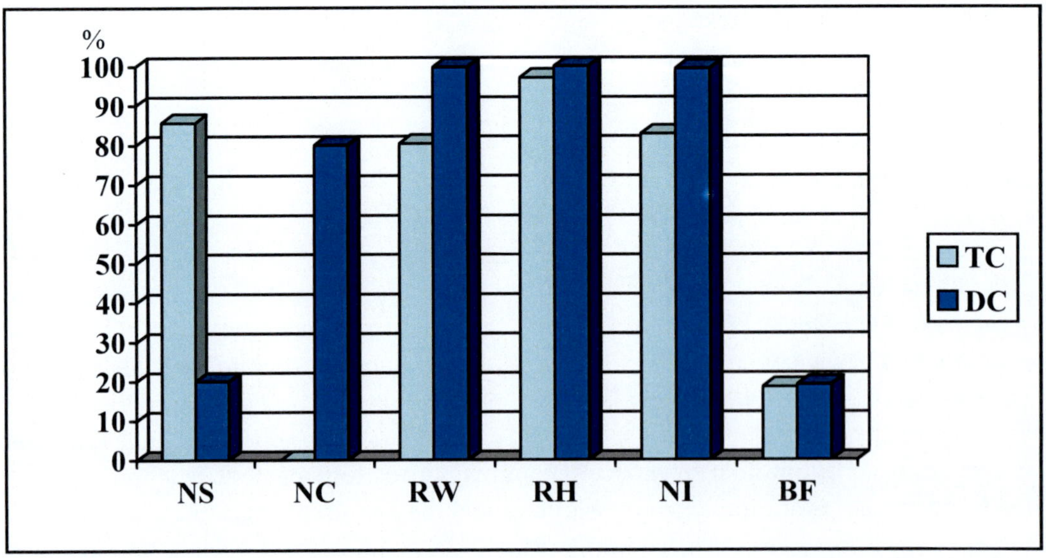

TC: Total colectomy; DC: Distal colectomy (rectosigmoidectomy); NS: number of stools ≥3; NC: normal consistency; RW: relative weight; RH: relative height; NI: nutritional index; BF: total body fat.

Figure 1. Comparison of a group 10 HD patients with distal colectomy and another 7 with total colectomy.

In our experience, the HD patients treated with a total colectomy had looser and more frequent stools than those who had a rectosigmoidectomy, as well as a poorer state as a whole, with significantly lower weight and height and worse nutritional state. Their proportions of total body fat were similar. These observations suggest that colectomy has a negative effect on nutrition, being the cause of mild malnutrition in some patients.

In view of the above, it seems advisable to monitor, at least throughout their pædiatric age, the potential nutritional deficiency in HD patients who have undergone total colectomy. The objective will be to detect and treat the consequences, and avoid correctable complications such as anæmia, and others such as retardation in growth which the patient will be incapable of compensating once past the age of growth. Moreover, the consistency and number of stools may be improved with diets tailored to the patient's ability to digest and absorb them as effectively as possible.

References

[1] Teitelbaum DH, Coran AG. Nutritional support. In Grosfeld JL, O`Neil JA Jr, Fonkalsrud EW, Coran AG (eds) *Pediatric Surgery*. Philadelphia: Mosby Elsevier; 2006. p. 194-220

[2] Cooper A, Jakobowski D, Spiker J, Floyd T, Ziegler MM, Koop CE: Nutrition assessment: An integral part of the preoperative pediatric surgical evaluation. *J Pediatr Surg* 1981; 16: 554-61.

[3] Phillips SM, Motil KJ. Measurement of growth and body composition in children, in *Up To Date*, Rose BD (ed). Up To Date, Wellesley, MA, 2003.

[4] Jelliffe, DB. *The assessment Of the nutritional status of the community*. Monograph series No 53, World Health Organization, Geneva 1966.

[5] Mascarenhas MR, Zemel B, Stallings VA. Nutritional assessment in pediatrics. *Nutrition* 1998; 14: 105-15

[6] Wong WW, Stuff JE, Butte NF, Smith EO, Ellis KJ:. Estimating body fat in African American and white adolescent girls: a comparison of skinfold-thickness equations whith a 4- compartment criterion model. *Am J Clin Nutr* 2000; 72: 348-54

[7] Mei Z, Grummer-Strawn LM, Pietrobelli A, Goulding A, Coran MI, Dietz WH: Validity of body mass index compared with other body composition screening indexes for the assessment of body fatness in children and adolescents. *Am J Clin Nutr* 2002; 75: 978-85.

[8] Waterlow, JC. Cassification and definition of protein-calorie malnutrition. *Br Med J* 1972; 3: 566-9

[9] Carcassonne M, Guys JM, Morisson-Lacombe G, Kreitmann B. Management of Hirschsprung`s disease: Curative surgery before 3 months of age. *J Pediatr Surg* 1989; 24: 1032–4.

[10] Coran AG, Teitelbaum DH. Recent advances in the management of Hirschsprung`s disease. *Am J Surg* 2000; 180: 382–7.

[11] Vanderhoof JA, Young J. Pathophysiology of the short bowel syndrome in children, in *Up To Day*, Rose BD (ed). UP To Day, Welleslley, MA, 2007.

[12] Vanderhoof JA, Young J. Management of the short bowel syndrome in children, in *Up To Day*, Rose BD (ed). UP To Day, Welleslley, MA, 2007.

[13] Ullin AW, Shoemaker WC, Deutsch, J. The ileocecal valve and papilla. *Arch Inter Med* 1956; 97: 409-20

[14] Ullin AW, Deutsch J. Visualization of ileocecal papilla in a living subject. *Gastroenterology* 1950; 16: 444-9

[15] Cummings JH, James WPT,Wiggins HS. Role of the colon in ileal resection diarrhoea. *Lancet* 1973; 1: 344-7

[16] Richardson JD, Griffen WO. Ileocecal valve substitutes as bacteriologic barriers. *Am J Surg*, 1972; 123: 149-53

[17] Singleton AO, Redmond DC, McMurray JE. Ileocecal resection and small bowel transit and absorption. *Ann Surg* 1964; 159: 690-4

[18] Stahlgren LH, Umana G, Roy R, Donnelly J: A study of intestinal absorption in dogs followings massive small intestinal resection and insertion of an antiperstaltic segment. *Ann Surg* 1962; 156: 483-92.

[19] Bower TR, Pringle KC, Soper RT. Sodium deficit causing decreased weight gain and metabolic acidosis in infants with ileostomy. *J Pediatr Surg* 1988; 23: 567-72.

[20] Schwarz KB, Ternberg JL, Bell MJ, Keating JP. Sodium needs of infants and children with ileostomy. *J Pediatr* 1.983; 102: 509–13.

[21] Willis S, Kisielinski K, Klosterhalfen B, Schumpelick V. Morphological and functional adaptation of the small intestine after colectomy and ileal pouch-anal anastomosis in rats. *Int J Colorectal Dis* 2002; 17: 85–91.

[22] Mibu R, Itoh H, Nakayama F. Effect of total colectomy and mucosal proctectomy on intestinal absorptive capacity in dogs. *Dis Colon Rectum* 1987; 30: 47–51.

[23] Nordgaard I, Hansen BS, Mortensen PB. Importance of colonic support for energy absorption as small-bowel failure proceeds. *Am J Clin Nutr* 1966; 64: 222–31.

[24] LaMont JT. Why fibre is good for you. *The Lancet* 1994; 343: 372.

[25] Jeppesen PB, Mortensen PB. Colonic digestion and absorption of energy from carbohydrates and medium-chain fat in small bowel failure. *JPEN* 1999; 23: S 101–S105.

[26] Jeppesen PB, Mortensen PB. The influence of a preserved colon on the absorption of medium- chain fat in patients with small bowel resection. *Gut* 1998; 43: 478–83.

[27] Heine W, Wutzke KD, Richter I, Walther F, Plath C. Evidence of colonic absorption of protein nitrogen in infants. *Acta Paediatr Scand* 1987; 76: 741-4.

[28] Nordgaard I, Hansen BS, Mortensen PB. Colon as a digestive organ in patiens with short bowel. *The Lancet* 1994; 343: 373–6.

[29] Carvajal SH, Mulvihill SJ. Intestinal peptides and their relevance in pediatric disease. *Sem Pediatr Surg* 1995; 4: 9–21.

[30] Sharman-Koendjbiharie M, Piena-Spoel M, Hopman WPM, Albers MJIJ, Jansen J*BMJ*, Tibboel D. Gastrointestinal hormone secretion after surgery in neonates with congenital intestinal anomalies during starvation and introduction of enteral nutrition. *J Pediatr Surg* 2003; 38: 1.602–6.

[31] Nightingale JMD, Kamm MA, van der Sijp jr. M, Ghatei MA, Bloom SR, Lennard-Jones JE. Gastrointestinal hormones in short bowel syndrome. Peptide YY may be the "colonic brake" to gastric emptying. *Gut* 1996; 39: 267–72.

[32] Ternent CA, Staab P, Thorson AG, Blatchford GJ, Christensen MA, Thompson JS et al. Ileoanal pouch function and release of peptide YY. *Dis Colon Rectum* 1998; 41: 868–74.

[33] Adrian TE, Path MRC, Savage AP, Fuessl HS, Wolfe K, Besterman HS, Bloom SR. Release of peptide YY (PYY) after resection of small bowel, colon or pancreas in man. *Surgery* 1987; 101: 715–9.

[34] van Battum PLH, Hopman WPM, Salemans JMJI, Kuijpers JHC, Nagengast FM, Jansen *BMJ*. Impaired release of peptide YY in patients with proctocolectomy and ileal pouch-anal anastomosis. *Scand J Gastroenterol* 1999; 34: 404–8.

[35] Adrian TE, Ferri G-L, Bcarese-Hamilton AJ, Fuessl HS, Polak JM, Bloom SR. Human distribution and release of a putative new gut hormone, peptide YY (PYY). *Gastroenterology* 1985; 89: 1070-7.

[36] Nour S, Stringer MD, Beck J. Colostomy complications in infants and children. *Ann R Coll Surg Engl* 1.996; 78: 526-30.

[37] Chirdan LB, Uba FA, Ameh EA, Mshelbwala PM. Colostomy for high anorectal malformation: an evaluation of morbidity and mortality in a developing country. *Pediatr Surg Int* 2008;24:407-10.

[38] Davidoff AM, Hebra A, Balmer D, Templeton JM, Schnaufer L. Management of the gastrointestinal tract and nutrition in patients with cloacal exstrophy. *J Pediatr Surg* 1996; 31: 771-3.

[39] Levitt MA, Mak GZ, Falcone Jr RA, Peña A. Cloacal exstrophy—pull-through or permanet stoma? A review of 53 patients. *J Pediatr Surg* 2008; 43: 164-70.

[40] Marty TL, Seo T, Matlak ME, Sullivan JJ, Black RE, Johnson DG. Gastrointestinal function after surgical correction of Hirschsprung`s disease: Long-term follow-up in 135 patients. *J Pediatr Surg* 1995; 30: 655-8.

[41] Langer JC, Durrant AC, de la Torre L, Teitelbaum DH, Minkes RK, Caty MG, et al. One-stage transanal Soave pullthrough for Hirschsprung`s disease. *Ann Surg* 2.003; 238: 569-76.

[42] N-Fékété C, Ricour C, Martelli H, Lortat-Jacob S, Pellerin D. Total colonic aganglionosis (with o without ileal involvement): A reviw of 27 cases. *J Pediatr Surg* 1986; 21: 251-4.

[43] Kimura K, Nishijima E, Muraji T, Tsugawa C, Matsutmo Y. Extensive aganglionosis: Further experience with the colonic patch graft procedure and long-term results. *J Pediatr Surg* 1988; 23: 52-6.

[44] Endo M, Watanabe K, Fuchimoto Y, Ikawa H, Yokoyama J. Long-term results of surgical treatment in infants with total colonic aganglionosis. *J Pediatr Surg* 1994; 29: 1310-14.

[45] Hoehner JC, Ein SH, Shandling B, Kim CW. Long-term morbidity in total colonic aganglionosis. *J Pediatr Surg* 1.998; 33: 961-8.

[46] Núñez R, Cabrera R, Agulla E, Moreno C, Serrano A, Ortiz C, Blesa E. Aganglionismo cólico con afectación ileal. Plastia ileocólica. *Cir Pediatr* 2001; 14: 76-8.

[47] Tsuji H, Kiely EM, Drake DP, Pierro A. Management and long-term follow-up of infants with total colonic aganglionosis. *J Pediatr Surg* 1999; 34: 158-62.

[48] Hernández F, Rivas S, Ávila LF, Leal N, Martínez L, Murcia J, et al. Aganglionismos extensos. Tratamiento y resultados a largo plazo. *Cir Pediatr* 2003; 16: 54-7.

[49] Anupama B, Zheng S, Xiao X. Ten-year experience in the management of total colonic aganglionosis. *J Pediatr Surg* 2007; 42: 1.671-6.

[50] Levy M, Reynolds M. Morbidity associated with total colon Hirschsprung`s disease. *J Pediatr Surg* 1992; 27: 364-7.

[51] Suita S, Taguchi T, Kamimura T Yanai K. Total colonic aganglionosis with or without small bowel involvement: a changing profile. *J Pediatr Surg* 1.997; 32: 1537-41.

[52] Fouquet V, De Lagausie P, Faure C, Bloch J, Malbezin S, bauman C, aigrain Y. Do prognostic factors exist for total colonic aganglionosis with ileal involvement?. *J Pediatr Surg* 2002; 37: 71-5.

[53] Wildhaber BE, Teitelbaum DH, Coran AG. Total colonic Hirschsprung`s disease: 28-year experience. *J Pediatr Surg* 2005: 203-7.

[54] Booth IW. Enteral nutrition as primary therapy in short bowel síndrome. *Gut* 1994; Supl. 1: S69-S72.

[55] Goulet O, Ruemmele F. Causes and management of intestinal failure in children. *Gastroenterology* 2006; 130: S16-S28.

[56] Bond GJ, Reyes JD. Intestinal transplantation for total/near total aganglionosis and intestinal pseudo-obstruction. Sem *Pediatr Surg* 2004; 13: 286-92.

Annex: Hirschsprung's Disease: The Parents' Experience and Informed Consent for Hirschsprung's Disease

Chapter XXVII

Hirschsprung's Disease: The Parents' Experience

Sheyla Leal, Mª Carmen Vicente and Ángela Del Hoyo

Introduction

The authors of this chapter are parents whose children have undergone operative repair for Hirschsprung's disease (HD). We want to contribute to this book our experience with this disease, namely, what we have learnt about it with our children, so that it can be made use of by other families. Parental care, especially nursing (irrigating the colon with serum, washing out its content) and digital rectal manipulation (dilation of the anus and rectum with the finger), is essential for successful treatment of this disease. Family members must therefore know these techniques in detail.

Our first contact with HD came after the birth of our babies. At that time we wanted to obtain information about this disease that we could understand easily. We found, however, that there was little documentation oriented to parents about HD, including when we looked for it on the Web.

The chapter consists of two parts: "*Hirschsprung's Disease in our Children*", which is a detailed account of the clinical histories of three patients our children with this disease, and "*Observations and Advice for Parents*", based on our experience with this disease.

Hirschsprung's Disease in our Children

In the following, each of the three families will describe the case of their child. It is the experience lived through with this disease during diagnosis, and before and after the operation.

Because of the different extent of intestine affected, these cases represent three forms of HD. In one child, the HD involved the rectum and sigmoid colon (the commonest form of this disease). In another, it reached the splenic flexure (long segment Hirschsprung's disease).And the third had a rare form of the disease called total colonic aganglionosis with the entire colonand a segment of terminal ileum affected.

Case 1: Patient with Rectosigmoid Hirschsprung's Disease

Our child is now 5 years old, and was operated on at 5 months of age for rectosigmoid HD. The pregnancy was with standard prenatal care, to term, and without incident. The prenatal ultrasound scans were normal. There is no family history of this disease. Delivery was in hospital, with the aid of a vacuum extractor. When the child was born, he was well. Weight: 2.800 kg.

He was under observation for 12 hours for premature rupture of the amniotic sac. When feeding was begun, he did not want to take the breast or the bottle, and neither did he pass the meconium. He vomited frequently, and the abdomen became distended.

At 2 days old (still without passing the meconium), we were referred to another hospital for suspected intestinal pathology, where he was hospitalized for 8 days. On the 2nd day after admission, anorectal manometry was performed, and was suggestive of HD. We had never heard this word, so that the doctor had to explain what this condition consisted of. He told us that this disease was due to a lack of nerve cells of the intestinal plexuses. This caused an alteration of the peristalsis or intestinal transit in the affected segment. He also informed us that to confirm that diagnosis they had also to do a rectal biopsy and a contrast enema, but that with the suspicion of HD they must start special care (nursing and digital rectal manipulation) to help the baby defæcate. With this nursing care, the baby passed the meconium and flatus. The abdominal distension disappeared, and he began to tolerate oral feeding.

Prior to discharge from the hospital, we were taught how to perform the nursing care and the rectal manipulation because, for a few months, we would have to help him at home to defæcate. We did not find it easy to learn how to do the nursing care, so that initially we went to the hospital frequently. They explained to us that, at this stage, the greatest complication our child could have was enterocolitis (infection of the mucus of the colon, characterized by anorexia, vomiting, abdominal distension, diarrhœa or absence of stools, and fever).

One day we decided that we had to overcome this situation, since, after all, "who better than the parents to look after him". So we really set about learning to do the nursing care, and soon were doing it superbly. At every visit to the surgeon, he encouraged us by telling us how well we were doing everything.

At 2 months, the contrast enema showed a narrow rectosigmoidal segment followed by a dilated zone, suggestive of the disease. The rectal biopsy confirmed the aganglionosis. With our nursing care, the child evolved very well. We were immensely reassured seeing our child grow like other normal children. At 5 months, he was operated on. The day before, he was prepared with total intestinal irrigation. Everything in the operation went well, and the attention of the hospital was extraordinary. The operation was transanal. The correctness of the pull-through was visualized laparoscopically.

The child passed a very bad time immediately after the operation. His abdomen swelled, and he was vomiting to "expel the anæsthesia". He was discharged at 7 days, by when he was again passing stools. The surgeon recommended that in the postoperative period we continue with the nursing cares for at least 1 or 2 months. We were to start at 12 days after surgery, but at 10 days, before starting the nursing, he presented severe enterocolitis. Fortunately, we realized it soon because he had high fever, swollen abdomen, did not want to eat, and did no stools. We recall that the digital rectal manipulation caused him to expel very liquid and fetid stools. He was admitted again at the hospital. He needed intravenous antibiotics, and fasting for a few days. Then everything went fine.

For a few months, he took a special milk (casein hydrolysate) and medication (metronidazol). We did regular rectal wash-outs (one a day) for about 2 months, and anal stimulation with Hegar's dilators for 4 months. We always had a water-based paste (zinc oxide, talc, glycerine, and distilled water) to use to prevent perianal dermatitis.

The child evolved wonderfully. His height and weight were always above the normal percentile for his age. In the visits to both the surgeon and the pædiatrician we always got good news. Our son is now four years old, and is very well. He is a lovely child, full of vitality, and has no problems with food. He likes almost everything to eat, and has a very good appetite. Sometimes he does stools every day (normal consistency), and at other times he finds it more difficult and it takes two days. He no longer wears nappies, and his fæcal and urinary continence is normal. Reeducation for sphincter control was very simple.

Very infrequently, we have performed some specific nursing care. He is almost never sick, and is very cheerful. When we look at him, it takes all our cares away. It gives us great joy to see that he is so strong, and had it not been for the advances in medicine, the story would have been very different.

Case 2: Patient with Long Segment Hirschsprung's Disease

Our child at present is 4 years old, and underwent surgery at 6 months of life for long segment HD.

The pregnancy was with standard prenatal care, and to term. There occurred some incidents: sciatica at 6 months, hypoglycæmia, arterial hypotension, and mild losses of consciousness. Delivery was in hospital, and normal (eutocic). Birth weight: 3.585 kg. It was more than 3 days before the meconium was passed, which was with the aid of a saline serum enema administered with a bulb syringe. There is a family history of Hirschsprung's disease, because my husband had had an operation for total colonic aganglionosis. But when our child was born, I was not well acquainted with my husband's disease nor did I know that it could be hereditary.

The child was discharged at 3 days, and for nearly a month we were going from doctor to doctor without knowing what he had. He was constipated and had colic caused by gases. We went several times to the emergency department of our hospital because of chronic constipation and distended abdomen. He was prescribed Micralax to facilitate evacuation of stools, but it did not solve the problem.

At 26 days old, his pædiatrician decided to move him to another hospital suspecting that he could have some intestinal pathology. At this hospital, he was evaluated by the pædiatric surgeon who decided to transfer him to another referral hospital for anorectal manometry. Following this test, the doctor informed us that our child probably had Hirschsprung's disease, and that for its confirmation a rectal biopsy and a contrast enema were necessary.

The contrast enema at 1 month old showed that the transition zone was at the splenic flexure, and the full thickness rectal biopsy confirmed the aganglionosis. They informed me that if the nursing cares and rectal manipulation with the finger did not resolve the intestinal obstruction a colostomy would have to be performed. We were also informed that the greatest complication that could arise before the definitive surgery was enterocolitis. They explained to us in detail the clinical manifestations of this complication.

In the hospital, they taught us how to perform the nursing cares and the rectal manipulation. Both were indispensable for the child's fæcal evacuation. It was not easy because this was a long segment aganglionosis. But I (the mother) decided to avoid the intestinal derivation. The child was 1 month old, and the surgeon wanted to wait a few months before doing the definitive surgery. I used a Levin tube (16 Fr) and a rectal tube (22 Fr), and physiological saline serum. I did the nursing cares 2 or 3 times a day, and the rectal manipulation once a day. My child was saved from the need for a colostomy, so avoiding the discomfort of an intestinal derivation and the complications of this surgery.

At 4 months, a follow-up contrast enema re-confirmed that the transition zone was at the splenic flexure. They commented on something that was very important to me, and that was that the nursing cares were effective because the colon was not dilated, and this meant that I was doing it very well. The cleansing of the contrast enema is very important. I took three hours with the nursing cares until the intestine was clean. There can not be any remnant left over. Our son had gone these months without suffering any complications.

At 6 months old and weighing 8 kg, he had the operation. He was admitted the day before, and on that afternoon he underwent the intestinal cleansing (total intestinal irrigation and rectal enemas). Before the surgery, he was administered prophylactic antibiotics. The operation was performed without complications. Ligature of the left mesocolon was performed by laparoscopy (Ligasure). This was followed by the transanal endorectal pull-through. 50 cm of the colon was resected. The coloanal anastomosis was completed without tension and without other complications.

Following the operation, from not having to open the abdomen as was the case in my husband's time, our son recovered very quickly. He was 48 hours in the intensive care unit. In the ward, oral tolerance was begun, gradually increasing the enteral contribution with casein hydrolysate. On day 5 after the operation, the rectal probe was withdrawn, and he passed liquid and lumpy stools. He was discharged on day 7.

The food at home for 2 months was a special milk (casein hydrolysate). This milk suited him very well. For 2 months, we did 2 sessions of nursing cares a day, and for 4 months anal stimulation with Hegar's dilators (12–15). There were no complications.

My son is now 4 years old. He has urinary and anal sphincter control. He does 2 stools a day. With vaccines he has had no problem, but with antibiotics yes. Some antibiotics cause him constipation and others diarrhœa. When he gets a cold, I usually give him one or two sessions of the nursing care to wash out medications and avoid "bugs" growing in his intestine.

Sometimes his stools are quite acidic, and can burn the skin of his bottom. The surgeon recommended us creams with zinc oxide (Lassar's paste) to prevent perianal dermatitis. Our child's bottom is now always impeccable.

Finally we can say with joy that my son is a healthy child, that as the operation was with a laparoscopic approach he has not been left with any scar and he can be proud of a perfect body.

Case 3: Patient with Total Colonic Aganglionosis with Ileal Involvement

Our son is 24 months old, and has had surgery for total colonic aganglionosis with ileal involvement. At 1 month old, he had an ileostomy, and at 4 months old the definitive operation.

Pregnancy

The pregnancy was twins, with standard prenatal care by the gynæcologist. In the third trimester, I had slight bleeding, so I rested for 2 weeks. After that, all check-ups (monthly) were normal – the babies were in perfect condition.

At 30 weeks, I was recommended relative rest. The children were born at 36 weeks in hospital. Delivery was normal (eutocic). The first twin weighed 2.360 kg and the second 2.380 kg. Length: 47 cm each.

First Hours of Life

The first hours passed without incident for both twins. After the first 24 hours, my second twin passed meconium and my first had not. To begin with, we saw everything as normal, but as the hours passed and there was still no stool, we began to worry. The problem began when the child began to vomit. We put this down to the epidural. He vomited everything that he took in. When the pædiatrician examined him, he introduced a probe into the anus but no meconium was passed. At 48 hours old, he was moved to the newborn ward.

Admission to the Newborn Ward

On admission to the newborn ward, normal feeding was stopped, and parenteral feeding was initiated. The child continued to vomit, no meconium was passed, and the abdomen was distended. One could even appreciate some intestinal loop through the abdominal wall. The pædiatrician explained to us that there were various diseases that could cause the our child's symptoms. One was Hirschsprung's disease. He recommended that we should look for information on the Web.

The first test that was performed was a simple abdominal Rx. We were informed that it showed dilated loops of the small intestine, but that there was no complete intestinal obstruction. The next study was an enema with gastrografin. It shows stiffened edges of the colon wall, and œdema of the right colon mucus (enterocolitis). No transition zones were observed. With this study, he evacuated meconium, but not sufficient. Rectal irrigation (nursing) was therefore begun to be repeated various times a day, and rectal manipulation to stimulate defæcation. At 10 days following admission, an anorectal manometry study showed absence of the recto-anal inhibitory reflex (RAIR, a reflex of defæcation), a typical finding in HD. But the surgeon told us that confirmation of the diagnosis required a rectal suction biopsy, which was advisable to delay until about the child was about 1 month old. The biopsy was performed at 29 days of life, and was compatible with Hirschsprung's disease.

First Operation: Ileostomy

Given the impossibility of decompressing the intestine effectively with the nursing care and rectal manipulation, at 1 month old it was decided to perform a laparotomy. In the course of this procedure, a narrowed segment of the terminal ileum could be appreciated, with a clear transition zone, followed by a dilated zone. The intraoperative biopsies confirmed Hirschsprung's disease and total colonic aganglionosis. The aganglionic segment was about 10 cm long, and the dilated segment of ileum about 25 cm. An ileostomy with a loop stoma was made in healthy (normal calibre) intestine at about 35 cm from the ileocæcal junction.

In the operation everything went fine. He left the operating room awake, and stayed only two days in the intensive care unit, after which he returned to the newborn ward. At 48 hours, bile was already being passed through the ileostomy. The doctors recommended that we should learn how to place the enterostomy collecting bags. We had to take very good care of the stoma and the skin around it which could easily become irritated. This zone had to be dry and very clean. A bag had to be found that did not irritate the skin, etc. The bag is used until the child has the definitive operation. He had parenteral feeding for a few days. This was then progressively reduced according to his tolerance of continuous enteral and oral feeding. We went home when he was tolerating food by mouth well, his fæces were more or less lumpy instead of liquid, and we knew how to change the stoma bags.

Care at Home

After three months in the hospital, we were scared to go home. We thought that we would not be able to look after him properly without the help of the doctors and nurses, but really being at home is not like being anywhere else. The care that the child required was feeding with a formula milk that his digestion did not have to process too much, and changing the bag and hygiene of the stoma. For a month everything went well until the ileostomy began to prolapse more and more. Also, the fæces were sometimes fairly liquid. The surgeon told us he had either to redo the ileostomy or to do the definitive operation, and that, given the child's overall state and his weight (6 kg), he considered the second option most advisable.

Second Operation: The Definitive Surgery

They explained to us that they had two possible surgical alternatives. They could exclusively join the healthy ileum to the anus, or they could join about 10 cm of the right colon to the healthy ileum (ileocolonic pouch) and anastomose the healthy ileum to the anus by transanal pull-through. During the operation, the surgeons opted for the second. They removed about 35 cm of non-functional ileum and the rest of the colon.

The operation went without complications, and he was awake when he was taken to the intensive care unit, where he remained for 3 days. He was then switched to the normal ward. Recovery was painful for the child, because the pain-killers did not have much effect. He began to pass stools through the rectal probe at a few hours. Healing of the ileostomy was perfect; it did not get infected. On day 2 postoperatively, he began with parenteral feeding.On day 8, he was started on mixed feeding (parenteral and enteral) which was maintained for some 3 weeks. When on day 10 the rectal probe was withdrawn, the stools were very frequent and liquid, and, despite all the care, caused perianal excoriation. With the introduction of cholestyramine resin and loperamide, the stools became more pasty.

To treat the perianal excoriation, we tried all sorts of protective and cicatrizing creams, but nothing really worked. The best was thorough cleansing with soap and water after each stool, drying, and applying Mercurochrome. At 2 weeks, we started with anal dilation and again the nursing cares. Initially, we just watched how the doctors and nurses did it, and then we did it together. It was difficult, but the surgeon explained to us that it was the only way that the child would not present complications such as enterocolitis and stenosis at the site of the anastomosis. Little by little, our fear gave way to practice. Three weeks afterwards, the parenteral feeding was withdrawn, and feeding was entirely enteral and oral. The perianal excoriation improved, and the stools had greater consistency. At last, the child was discharged.

Recovery at Home

The arrival home was incredible. The hardest part was done. Now we had to deal with the perianal lesions and prevent diarrhœa. The child had a delay in vaccinations. Following the administration of one vaccine, he developed severe gastroenteritis, with dehydration that required hospitalization. The endoscopy of the ileocolonic pouch showed major hyperplasia of Peyer's patches in the ileal mucus. The lining of the colon was normal. A couple of months passed, and our only problem was the anal irritation, because the child ate very well (the special formula milk casein hydrolysate). His introduction to ordinary foods was the contrary of other babies he began with purées and cereals, and progressed to fruit at the end because they are more acidic and help to pass more stools. His feeding depended on the consistency of the fæces. Usually his diet was normal, but if the fæces were liquid he was given a more astringent diet. His weight and height are within the normal percentiles. He has no anæmia, since part of the terminal ileum was conserved. He was recently hospitalized again with severe viral gastroenteritis. Once this was controlled, he went back to his usual diet. Currently he is well. We continue doing some nursing cares as well as the perianal care since the slightest neglect to do so leads to the skin becoming irritated again.

Observations and Advice for Parents

Our intention with the observations and advice in this second part of the chapter is that they will be useful for other parents of children with HD. First of all, we wish to de-dramatize the severity of this disease, since, after surgery, most children have a good quality of life.

We also want to stress something that is essential in the parents' context. This is that both of them should know about any diseases they suffer from, especially if they are hereditary. HD can pass from parent to child as in Case 2. Therefore, if either parent has it, they must understand that if their child exhibits the same symptoms it might have the disease. This would help the early suspicion of the disease, and hence contribute to preventing its complications (enterocolitis, bowel obstruction, malnutrition, etc.) and make it possible to carry out the surgical repair at an earlier age.

The early suspicion of the disease is also greatly aided by the clinical datum of the first passing of meconium [1-3]. Our 3 children all presented delays of more than 48 hours in evacuating meconium. But in one of them, this was insufficiently valued by the pædiatricians. Probably this was because this disease is the great unknown at a popular level, and even for some pædiatricians.

We would like to emphasize here that, as we saw during the diagnostic phase of our children, anorectal manometry is extremely useful for the early suspicion of this disease. It should be performed for every newborn with a delay of over 24 hours in passing meconium so as to screen for those with absence of the recto-anal inhibitory reflex (RAIR), *i.e.*, with suspected HD [4]. In these neonates, nursing care should be initiated already until a rectal biopsy has confirmed or ruled out the disease. If aganglionosis is confirmed, these cares will continue of course until the operation [5-7].

From our experience, we can say that the *nursing* and *digital rectal manipulation* are the two most beneficial things that parents can do to care for a child with HD. They facilitate fæcal evacuation, ensure adequate nutrition, prevent enterocolitis, and obviate the need for a colostomy (see chapter XIII).

The irrigation nursing is done with rectal tubes of sizes 12–18 Fr, depending on the patient's age. We advise using thicker rather than thinner tubes as they do less damage. The tube is lubricated with vaseline and gently introduced into the anus until it reaches the dilated zone or until it drains the fæcal content (Figure 1A).

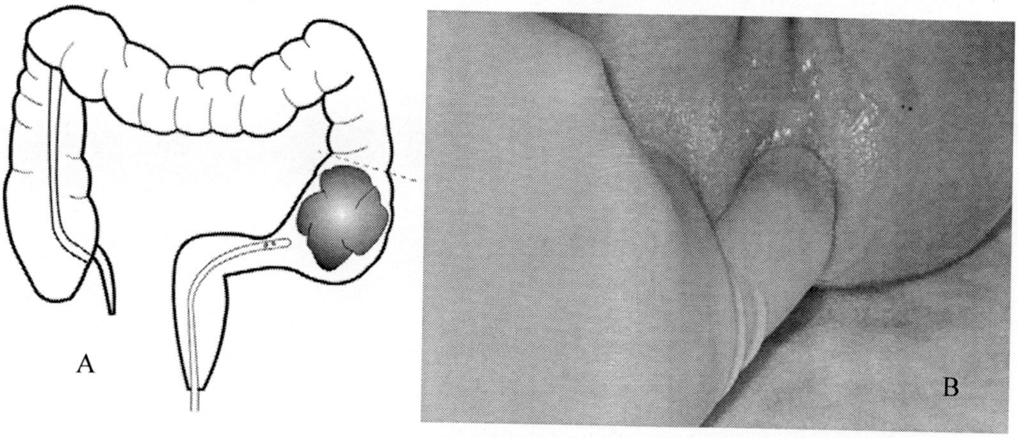

Figure 1. A: For the nursing care to be effective, the irrigation tube must reach the dilated zone. The fæcal content can then be washed out correctly. B. Rectal manipulation must be done with the little finger so as not to harm the anorectum.

When the tube is in the colon, irrigations are performed with physiological saline solution (a 25 ml bolus in the neonate, and up to 50–100 ml in older infants) to wash the fæcal content out through the tube. Irrigation is continued until the fluid coming out is clear. To avoid electrolyte disturbance, all the infused solution should be removed. The frequency of these nursing cares have to be adapted to the clinical situation. One a day may be sufficient, but it is the doctor who must establish the frequency [6]. Rectal perforation is rare, but may occur while carrying out these nursing procedures.

The rectal manipulation in the newborn is done with the little finger so as not to harm the anorectum (Figure 1B). The finger should be introduced gently but completely. Rectal stimulation stimulates decompression of the colon because it distends the rectum and the internal anal sphincter, thereby facilitating the evacuation of fæces. Again, the frequency with which it should be done will be set by the doctor. We saw (Case 1) that a simple digital rectal manipulation can help evacuate the flatus and fæces from the colon.Currently the aim is for the nursing care procedures and the digital rectal manipulation to replace intestinal derivations whenever possible (Cases 1 and 2). With extensive aganglionosis (Case 3), however, these cares are insufficient to overcome the intestinal obstruction. Effective intestinal decompression then requires the surgeon to create a stoma which opens out to the skin a healthy segment of the intestine (colostomy or ileostomy [8-10].

The stoma requires special care involving the active participation of the parents, nurse, surgeon, and, if possible, a specialist in enterostomy [8]. The parents should have learnt before leaving the hospital how to handle the collecting bags to avoid the fæcal content contacting the peristomal skin. Ileostomies, especially the highest, usually excrete a more liquid content (which is more corrosive for the skin), so that these patients must be monitored periodically to prevent cutaneous lesions. A great variety of collecting bags are marketed for all ages. They can be one-piece bags with bag and seal forming a single unit, or two-piece bags with a baseplate that adheres to the skin and a bag that fits into the plate (Figure 2 A, B, C and D). The two-piece devices are more comfortable for the child.

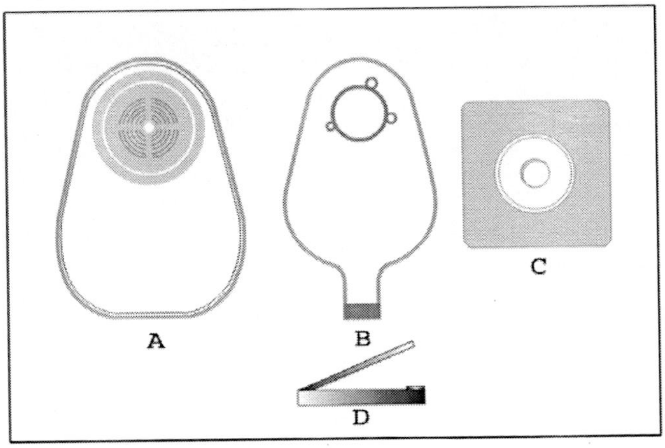

Figure 2. Bags for enterostomy. A. Closed one-piece bag with skin barrier. B. Two-piece system drainable bag. C. Baseplate with rim for two-piece system. D. System for closing drainable bags.

The bag may be closed or open at the bottom, and with or without filter. The central disc of the plate will be cut out according to the size of the stoma so that the peristomal skin does not come into contact with the fæcal content. The bag will be changed as required by the rate of intestinal evacuation, and the baseplate every 4-5 days, or if it comes unstuck. Information can be found on the Web of commercial providers (*e.g.*, Coloplast, Convatec, Cases, and Hollister) of products related to stoma care. It is also important that parents have good communication with the doctors, and that they are well informed about the disease. They must understand how to recognize the first symptoms of enterocolitis (rejection of food, vomiting, abdominal distension, fever, and diarrhœa). They should take the child to the hospital when these arise.

In recent years, there have been great advances in the surgical treatment of HD [11]. The aim of this treatment is to remove the pathological (aganglionic) segment, and join the healthy intestine to the anus or rectum. At present, in over 75% of patients (rectosigmoidal aganglionosis), this treatment is performed at a very young age, transanally, in a single surgical step, and without leaving visible scars [11,12]. The results are very satisfactory. In extensive aganglionosis, however, especially total colonic aganglionosis with ileal involvement, the diagnosis, treatment, and postoperative management are very complex. The incidence of complications (dehydration, enterocolitis, anæmia, and short-bowel malnutrition) is high [9,13,14]. Hydration is essential in this type of aganglionosis because these patients tend to lose fluids quickly. They require periodic check-ups, and long-term monitoring of their weight and height development.

To prevent postoperative stenosis of the anastomosis, anal dilation is necessary [15]. We advise rubbing the dilator with a cloth to warm it up a bit and then lubricating it well. It is introduced gently into the anus. These dilations are usually performed for 4–6 months. In the first month they are done daily; in the second every 3 days; in the third twice a week; and then, for 2 or 3 months, once a month.

One of the biggest problems of extensive aganglionosis, especially total colonic aganglionosis, is the care of the perianal area. In this type of aganglionosis, there tend to occur periods of diarrhœa producing anal excoriation. In addition to treating the diarrhœa, the perianal zone should be kept very clean and dry (washing with neutral soap and water after each stool). In many cases, the association of zinc oxide and talc is very effective at preventing and curing dermatitis. Many protective and regenerative creams are marketed (Zincospray, Lutsine Eryplast, Lasser's paste, A-Dermin Epitheliale). To prevent the perianal skin from chafing with the nappies, it is useful to place a gauze impregnated with one of these creams between the buttocks.

Training for anal sphincter control with patients who have undergone surgery for HD should be done as with any other child. It will begin when the child expresses its readiness to follow its parents' teachings. It is usually said that the child is able to start anal sphincter control when it can climb a stair without support (at about 24 months). The child should be accustomed to defæcate at a certain time, preferably in the morning at waking or after meals. Some HD patients may require more time in anal sphincter training to achieve control, and in others fæcal incontinence secondary to the surgery may impede their control of the anal sphincter.

Finally we would advise parents of children with this disease to have a lot of patience and perseverance with the care and treatment of their children. We must never lower our guard, since even if our child is doing very well we must not discontinue the care and medication until the doctor says it is advisable.

Acknowledgments

We are grateful to Dr Ramón Núñez and to Dr J. Luis Cordero, for their collaboration and advice in this chapter. Also, we want to thank all the staff of the Hospital Materno-Infantil (Complejo Hospitalario Universitario) of Badajoz for their excellent professionalism.

References

[1] Coran AG, Teitelbaum DH. Recent advances in the management of Hirschsprung's disease. *Am J Surg*, 2000; 180:382-7.

[2] Loening-Bauke V, Kimura K. Failure to pass meconium: diagnosing neonatal intestinal bstruction.*Am Fam Physician* 1999;60:2043-50.

[3] Kessmann J. Hirschsprung's disease: diagnosis and management. *Am Fam Physician*, 2006; 74:1319-22.

[4] Núñez R, Cabrera R, Moreno C, Agulla E, Vargas I, Blesa E. Utilidad de la manometría anorrectal en el diagnóstico neonatal de la enfermedad de Hirschsprung. *Cir Pediatr*, 2000; 13:16-9.

[5] Herek Ö: A new colonic lavage method for infants with Hirschsprung' disease. *Pediatr Surg Int*, 2001; 17:671.

[6] Ghinelli C, Del Rosi C: Treatment of Hirschsprung`disease without colostomy. *Peadtr Surg Int.* 1993;8:27-30.

[7] Cabrera García R, De Agustí JC. *Manual para padres de niños y niñas con Enfermedad de Hirschsprung*. Sevilla: Hospitales Universitarios Virgen del Rocío; 2007. pp.1-14.

[8] Casasa JM, Broto J, Jimenez AI, Boix-Ochoa J. Derivaciones intestinales en el tratamiento de la enfermedad de Hirschsprung. *An Esp Pediatr*, 1987; 281-3.

[9] Núñez R, Cabrera R, Agulla E, Moreno C, Serrano A, Ortiz C, Blesa E. Aganglionismo cólico con afectación ileal. Plastia ileocolica. *Cir Pediatr*, 2001; 14:76-81.

[10] Somme S, Langer JC. Primary versus staged pull-through for the treatment of Hirschsprung disease. *Semin Pediatr Surg*, 2004; 13:249-55.

[11] De La Torre-Mondragón L, Ortega-Salgado JA. Transanal endorectal pull-through for Hirschsprung's disease. *J Pediatr Surg*, 1998; 33:1283-86.

[12] De La Torre-Mondragón L. Enfermedad de Hirschsprung. Mitos y realidades a 120 años de su descripción. *Acta Pediatr* Mex, 2008:29:139-46.

[13] Wildhaber BE, Teitelbaum DH, Coran AG. Total colonic Hirschsprung's disease: A 28-year experience. *J Pediatr Surg*, 2005; 40:203-7.

[14] Vieten D, Spicer R. Enterocolitis complicating Hirschsprung's disease. *Semin Pediatr Surg*, 2004; 13:263-72.

[15] Hackam DJ, Filler RM, Pear RH. Enterocolitis after the surgical treatment of Hirschsprung's disease: Risk factors and financial impact. *J Pediatr Surg*, 1998; 33:83.

In: Hirschsprung's Disease: Diagnosis and Treatment
Ed: Ramón Núñez and Manuel López-Alonso
ISBN: 978-1-60741-349-3

Chapter XXVIII

Informed Consent and Hirschsprung's Disease

Mª Ángeles López De La Torre

Nowadays, the concept of informed consent is undeniable; however, this concept evolved slowly before it was incorporated into the different legal systems. The classic clinical relationship model, known as "*paternalism*", is now part of the past. This involved the doctor making decisions on the patients' behalf based on the principle of welfare and has now been replaced by a new model based on *"patient autonomy"* with patients free and able to make decisions regarding their own health.

In Spain, the most recent regulatory background can be found in Article 43 of the Spanish Constitution, which speaks of the "*right to health*" in the widest sense [1]. This principle was the subject of a basic state regulation development via Law 14/1986, 25 April, on General Healthcare, articles 10 and 11 of which set out the charter of rights and duties of users of the health system, among which are patients' rights with regard to informed consent [2].

Later on, Royal Decree 63/1995, of 20 January, on Healthcare Services Regulation within the National Health Service (Spanish Official Gazette No. 35 of 10 February, 1995) was an important step forward, as it included informed consent as an additional provision (as well as surgical interventions, laboratory tests, healthcare transport, etc.) in terms of clinical documentation. This regulation was revoked by Royal Decree 1030/2006, of 15 September, establishing the Common Service Portfolio of the National Health Service and its updating procedure (Spanish Official Gazette No. 222, of 16 September, 2006), although the right to informed consent was also set out in article 10.1.

The Council of Europe's Convention for the Protection of Human Rights and Human Dignity is specifically relevant with regard to the application of Biology and Medicine as part of the Spanish legal system [3]. This Convention deals explicitly, in detail and at great length, with the need to acknowledge patients' rights, including the right to information, informed consent and the privacy of information about people's health, seeking to harmonise the law governing these matters in different countries.

Basic Law 41/2002, dated 14 November, governing Patient Autonomy and the Rights and Obligations regarding Clinical Information and Documentation, completes the provisions that the General Healthcare Law sets out as general principles. As this is a Basic Law (according to the provisions of article 149.1.1.ª and 16.ª of the Constitution), it has precedence over all possible regional laws governing the same aspects since it came into force [4]. The Autonomous Communities or regions are also obliged to take the necessary measures to adapt to it [5].

However, although it is basic Law, the provisions regarding healthcare information, information for exercising freedom of choice of doctor and healthcare centre, the informed consent of the patient and clinical documentation will be additionally applicable to medical research projects, organ harvesting and transplant procedures, the application of assisted human reproduction procedures and others which lack specific regulations [6].

Law 41/2002 strengthens and gives special treatment to the patient's right to autonomy and specifically establishes as a basic principle that *"Generally, the prior informed consent of patients and users is required for all actions in the healthcare area. This consent, which must be obtained once the patient has received appropriate information, shall be given in writing in the circumstances foreseen in the Law"*.

The Supreme Court has held that *"It is an essential element of the lex artis ad hoc standard" and has even stressed "The relevance of lacked informed consent, considering this is a violation of lex artis ad hoc standard, is evidence of the abnormal operation of the healthcare service" [7]. Furthermore, the Contentious-Administrative Court classifies the patient's informed consent as a "Clinical Act" [8].*

It must be noted that the Jurisprudence has progressively shaped the concept of *"lex artis ad hoc" in numerous judgements, defining it as "The criteria for assessing the suitability of the specific medical act performed by the medical professional, whether scientist or clinician, taking into account the specific characteristics of its author, the profession, the complexity of the act and the essential importance to the patient and, where appropriate, the influence of endogenous factors, the condition and intervention of the patients, their family members or the healthcare organisation itself to classify this act compliant or noncompliant with the normal procedure used" [9].*

There are two essential concepts developing the above, these being the legal right of the patient/parents/legal representative to the healthcare information and informed consent, which are not considered as two separate items but which form part of one another. These aspects are analysed below.

I Healthcare Information

Law 41/2002 defines medical information as *"All data, whatever its form, class or type, giving knowledge of a person's physical or mental state of health, or ways to conserve, care for, improve or recover it"*.

It is a right.- Patients have the right to know, in the event of any action within the healthcare service, all the information available on it, with the exception of the circumstances set out in the Law.

It also establishes the patient's duty to provide truthful and accurate information about his physical condition or health, and to collaborate in obtaining this, especially when this is in the public interest or for healthcare reasons.

a) Right holder.- The patient holds the right to his own healthcare information.

Others linked to the patient by family or *de facto* relationships may also be informed:

- When so permitted by the tacit or express consent of the patient.
- When, in the judgement of the attending physician, the patient is not capable of understanding the information because of his physical or mental condition.

In the event of this incapacity, the patient has a right to be informed in a manner suitable to his ability to understand. The healthcare professional must inform the patient's legal representative.

Taking into consideration that, at present, most patients are diagnosed in the neonatal period or when they are being breastfed [10] the recipients of the information will be their parents or legal representatives. In other words, here we are entering the area of consent granted by a representative as foreseen in Law 41/2002.

b) Guarantor of compliance with the right to the information.- The person who must guarantee the information is the patient's attending physician. The professionals caring for him during the healthcare process or applying a technique or a specific procedure to him, are also bound to inform him.

In any case, all professionals acting in healthcare activities are bound not only to use the techniques correctly, but also to comply with their duties to provide information and clinical documentation.

So far we can conclude that informed consent is a coin with two faces. One the one hand, it is the patient's right, and on the other it is the doctor's duty.

c) The time at which the information must be provided.- The information must be provided before the consent is obtained. There is no legally established period during which the information must be provided, but it must be given sufficiently in advance to allow the patient to calmly reflect and then to make a free, responsible decision.

It must be remembered that, without information, or with incomplete or defective information, consent cannot be properly given. Furthermore, it is also true to say that the consent cannot be ratified subsequent to the medical act.

d) Manner of providing the information.- As a general rule, this is given verbally, a record of this being entered on the medical history.

It is to be noted that the Supreme Court quashes and revokes a Judgement by the Central Court with regard to the entries made on medical histories, stating the following:

"The Central Court's error was to consider the content of the medical history as untouchable, as facts proven, without realising that the medical history is no more than the story of a medical process, which may or may not be true, when compared with the other evidence. Not doing so, or if it has been done, not showing how it has been done, gives the medical history the nature of indisputable truth, which shall not be allowed" [11].

It is important to emphasise that the burden of proof that the information has been given falls on the healthcare professional, meaning that if it is given in written form it will be much easier to prove that the information has been given.

This theory has undergone a clear evolution since an initial favourable moment by placing the burden of proving the lack of information or informed consent on the plaintiff. The reason for this reversal of the burden of proof lies both in the doctrine of ease of proof [12] and therefore the more advantageous situation of professionals for providing proof, and the impossibility of being able to prove negative facts, which puts the party with the burden in a defenceless situation, which is against the principle of effective legal protection. Thus, the judgement by the Civil Division of the Supreme Court of 16 October, 1998 stated that

"The obligation to inform corresponds to the professionals performing the intervention and to the hospital". Other, more recent judgements have concurred in this [13].

e) Extent and content of the information.- On the one hand, we have Law 41/2002 establishing that "When faced with submitting to any healthcare act, the patient has the right to know <u>all</u> the information available on it, with the exceptions set out by the Law" and on the other, states that "The informed consent must be obtained after the patient has received appropriate information and the patient or user has the right to make a free choice, after receiving the appropriate information, among the available clinical options".

In spite of the foregoing, the Law still fails to define the concepts of *"all"* and *"appropriate"*, only stating that the minimum information shall consist of:

- The purpose and nature of the intervention (Law 41/2002 defines what is understood by intervention within the healthcare field: *"All actions taken for preventative purposes, diagnoses, therapies, rehabilitation or research").*
- The risks relating to the patient's personal or professional circumstances.
- The consequences.

Other principle of the aforementioned Law regulating the "*Conditions of the information and written consent*" tells us that "*The healthcare professional shall provide the patient with the following basic information before obtaining his informed consent*":

- The relevant or important consequences that the intervention is to certainly cause.
- The contraindications.
- The risks relating to the patient's personal or professional circumstances.
- The likely risks under normal circumstances, according to the experience and the state-of-the-science or directly related to this type of intervention.

Risks considered very serious, which are rare but exceptional, should also be included. There is a judgement by the Supreme Court which ordered a surgeon to pay compensation for not having informed the patient of the high risk of an injury which only presented in 2% of cases; in other words, that every 100 interventions, a negative result was obtained in two [14].

The judgement by the Supreme Court (1st Civil Division) of 12 January 2001, sheds a great deal of light on the concepts of typical and preventable risks, ruling "*That typical risks cannot be confused with foreseeable risks, as foreseeability has no relationship with the statistical likelihood or frequency of the event. If the risk is typical (and therefore foreseeable) it must be notified, although the statistical percentage of such an event occurring may be minor. Its typical nature makes it necessary and obligatory to provide information about it*".

In the aforementioned judgement of 31 July 1996, an odd comparison is made to differentiate foreseeability from likelihood. The court ruled:

> "The foreseeability is evident. It can be said to be very slight, and will be unforeseeable at the moment it is going to happen, but if there is evidence it happens in two of every one hundred cases, it has already been foreseen. Something similar happens in a lottery game. The prizes are not won very often, but it is foreseen that they will be won" [15].

This theory on the obligation to inform of the typical risks is upheld by the prestigious jurists Julio Cesar Galán Cortés [16], Ricardo de Lorenzo y Montero and Javier Sánchez Caro [17], among others.

Taking the foregoing into consideration with regard to,

> "The patient or user has the right to choose freely, after the receiving appropriate information, from among the medical options available" and "The patient or user's power to choose, freely and voluntarily, from two or more healthcare alternatives"

another point to add to the information content would be the following:

- The treatment alternatives and their risks, discomfort and side effects, as well as the explanation of the criteria that have led the doctor to his decision to recommend one procedure over the others. The possibility of doing nothing should also be included.

On this point, the lack of information based on the fact that there is no alternative treatment, it is to be noted that this argument was rebutted by the Civil Division of the Supreme Court, which stated:

> "The theory of the first instance judgement, which does not attribute consequences to the lack of information based on the grounds that there is no alternative to the treatment, does not affect the obligation to do so and to obtain the informed consent prior to the intervention, as the right to decide belongs to the patient and it affects his health and therefore, it is not who informs him but the person from whom he receives the information, adopting the most advantageous solution in his interests. To find otherwise would be tantamount to finding that diseases or interventions that have only one treatment, according to the state-of-the-science, do not require informed consent."[18]

f) Information requirements. The medical information forms part of all the healthcare actions. Law 41/2002 states that it shall be:

- True. If the healthcare professional has doubts, these must be expressed.
- The patient shall be told in a comprehensible, appropriate manner of his needs and will be helped to make decisions in accordance with his own free will.

Jurisprudence holds that the information given to the patient must be

> "Specific, correct, true, honest, continuous, precise and comprehensive; to enable it to be completely understood by its recipient, it must include all the facts within their reach, and must also be sufficient to provide clear, accurate data to enable a decision to be made regarding whether or not to undergo the intervention recommended or proposed by the medical services" [19].

Patients/parents/legal representatives are entitled to ask questions, as the communication between them and their doctor must be bi-directional.

It is true that the information is not limited to a single act, but must be provided on a continuous basis. It must be taken into consideration that any subsequent incidents may influence the willingness of the patients/parents/legal representatives to give their consent.

Acronyms, abbreviations, formulas and technical words must be avoided, and the information must be specifically adapted to the level of understanding of the person for whom it is intended.

g) Limits to the information. The patients' right to healthcare information may be limited by the certified existence of a therapeutic need state (empowering the doctor to act professionally without first informing the patient, when for objective reasons, knowledge of his own condition could be seriously injurious to his health). In such a case, the doctor will provide a reasoned explanation of the circumstances in the medical history and will inform the persons connected to the patient by family or *de facto* relationship of their decision.

There must be sufficient proof of the aforementioned "*objective reasons*" which, in any case, will be applied arbitrarily.

In this respect, if we consider the systematic context of the principle, that is, within the right to information, we can conclude that this therapeutic privilege cannot operate as such when this information is basic and prior to a medical intervention involving a serious risk to the patient's health [20].

h) The right not to be informed.- All persons have the right not to be informed if that is their wish. However, this right is limited by the following:

- The health interests of the patient himself, of third parties or the group.
- The therapeutic demands of the case.

When the patient expressly waives his or her right to be informed, this wish is to be respected and the waiver shall be put down in writing, without prejudice to obtaining his informed consent prior to the corresponding intervention.

II Consent

Law 41/2002 defines this as "*The free, voluntary and conscious agreement of the patient, while being of sound mind after receiving appropriate information, to an action that will affect his health*".

Acting individuals.

Who must give consent? In the case of paediatric patients, consent is given by a representative pursuant to Law 41/2002. One of the circumstances when consent is given by a representative is:

- When a minor patient is not intellectually or emotionally able to understand the implications of the intervention, the consent will be given by the minor's legal representative after having listened to the patient's opinion if he is over 12 years of age. In the case of minors who are neither incapable nor incapacitated, but emancipated or aged over sixteen years, the representative's consent is not required. However, in interventions presenting a serious risk, according to the health professional's judgement, the parents will be informed and their opinion will be taken into account when making the corresponding decision.

The representative giving consent will be sufficient for the circumstances and proportional to the needs that must be met, always in favour of the patient and respecting their personal dignity. The patient will participate to the greatest degree possible in the decision-making throughout the healthcare process.

Who must obtain the consent? The jurisprudence is unanimous in considering that it is the doctor who is responsible for obtaining the patients' prior informed consent [21].

b) Form of consent.- Generally speaking, this will be verbal. However, it must be given in writing in the following cases: Surgical intervention, diagnostic procedures and invasive therapies and, generally, the administration of procedures that involve known risks or drawbacks with foreseeable negative repercussions on the health of the patient.

The written consent of the patient/parents/legal representative will be necessary for each of the actions specified in the above paragraph, reserving the right to incorporate annexes and other general-type data and will include sufficient information about the procedure being administered and the risks involved.

In any case, the doctor in charge must weigh up each case, and the more doubtful the result of the intervention the more important it is to obtained the prior written, informed consent of the patient/parents/legal representative.

Consent requirements

- *Informed*: Consent given without full knowledge of the facts is tainted and therefore invalid. This is what is known as *"uninformed consent"* [22].
- *Free and voluntary*: The informed consent given by a person who is not acting voluntarily is neither ethically nor legally acceptable. There should therefore be no *"coercion"* (pressure exerted by another to force their agreement or behaviour), *"manipulation"* (intervention using skilful methods and, on occasions, tricks, which distort the truth or justice, or to serve private interests) or *"persuasion"* (moving, obliging someone with reasons to believe or do something).
- *Specific*: With regard to the generic documents, the Supreme Court has stated that "*Those are ethically and legally invalid documents that merely obtain the patient's signature because, although they may provide the patient with some information, this is not in their interest nor does it meet the standard of what is reasonable for them to understand the seriousness and scope of their disease, the purpose of the therapy proposed, with the typical risks of the procedure, originating from their condition and other possible therapeutic alternatives. It is, in short, basic, personalised information, in which the patient plays an active role to consent or reject an intervention based on it*" [23].

- *Prior to the intervention*: It is important that this document be dated.

A judgement by the Fourth Division of the Provincial Balearic Island Court of 13 February 2001, ordered a healthcare professional to pay compensation to a patient for not respecting his right to information, as the patient had signed the informed consent document practically at the doors of the operating theatre. The healthcare professional alleged that the information given to the patient was correct, and that the latter signed the informed consent sheet. Nevertheless, the sentence established that

> "*What cannot be disputed is that the complete information must be provided before the decision to consent to the corrective surgical operation is made, and that this is not given by the mere fact of having a document signed minutes before the operation and in circumstances in which, for obvious sociological and personal or individual reasons, it cannot be expected that the patient signing the document may give a though-out response or freely given consent, especially when the party proffering the document for signature is not the doctor or surgeon who should perform the operation. In fact, we are now at this stage of evidence production because, in spite of the fact that the burden of proof corresponded in this case to the defendant, it has not been possible to certify that the information on the risk of hypercorrection and consequential loss of visual acuity was offered sufficiently in advance for the consent to be given freely nor that it was provided by the appropriate, professionally qualified person*".

The Fourth Division of the Santa Cruz de Tenerife Provincial Court stated in a ruling issued on 17 January 2007 that

> "Consent given in this manner (in the anteroom to the operating theatre, or later, once anaesthetised, in the operating theatre itself, for a surgical intervention about which the patient has not been informed and for which they have not been prepared) cannot be considered valid or effective for the purposes intended here, since it is against medical practice and informed consent requirements which, as set out widely in the provisions of the fifth legal ground of the judgement appealed, demand that a patient who is to undergo a surgical intervention gives his or her express consent for this intervention once precise information has been provided on the scope and consequences of the intervention to be performed. This did not occur in this case, since the aforementioned information was not even provided, nor was it enough to give it in the anteroom to the operating theatre or in the operating theatre itself, when the patient had already been anaesthetised, as an oral response under those circumstances would not be sufficient. Informed consent, regardless of whether it may be verbal or written, demands otherwise: peace, reflection, consultation with other specialists and if required, with the couple, which is incompatible with the stress suffered by the patient in the operating theatre or the anteroom".

- *Written*: The jurisprudence has unified its criteria and the doctrine of "*ease of proof*", currently set out in article 217 of the Law 1/2000 of Civil Proceedings, of 7 January, is also applicable in these cases. In this way, the reversal of the burden of proof is applied, *"meaning that the burden of proof with regards to the existence of appropriate informed consent falls on the healthcare professional, who is in the most advantageous situation for certifying this" [2].*

The judgement by the 1st Civil Division of the Supreme Court, of 12 January 2001, goes on about this stating that

> "The superior position of doctors in the legal process for the purposes of demonstrating that consent does exist, and the fact that the patient can be asked to prove the positive

facts on which they are basing their assertion, but not the preventative or extinctive facts, for which the burden of proof corresponds to the doctor accused".

Likewise, it must be remembered that the informed consent document forms part of the minimum content to include in the medical history and that the professionals involved are bound to complete the aspects relating to direct patient care.

c) What to do in cases where the patient/parents/legal representatives waive the right to receive information.- As discussed above, it is possible to waive the right to the information but in spite of this, it will be necessary to obtain prior consent before the intervention proposed.
d) Exceptions to informed consent.- Healthcare professionals may perform vital medical interventions for the sake of the patient's health, without need for their consent, in the following cases:

- When there is a risk to public health based on the health grounds established by law. In any event, once the pertinent measures have been taken, pursuant to the provisions of Spanish Organic Law 3/1986, of 14 April, on special public health measures (Spanish Official Gazette number 102, of 29 April, 1986), whenever these measures involve the patients' admission to the hospital against their will, legal authorities must be notified within 24 hours.

This Organic Law empowers the responsible healthcare authorities to protect public health and prevent its loss or deterioration, adopting measures for examination, treatment, hospitalisation and control. These measures may be adopted provided that [25]:

There is a healthcare emergency or need.

- There are rational indications leading to the assumption that the health of the general population is at risk due to the specific state of health of a person or a group of persons or because of the health conditions in which an activity is carried out.
- When there is an immediate serious risk to the physical or psychical integrity of the patient and it is not possible to obtain their authorisation, consulting, circumstances permitting, their family members or persons related *de facto* to them.

In any case, the facts of the situation must be recorded on the medical history, as must the healthcare professionals' decision to intervene without obtaining the patient's consent.

The doctor must not venture beyond the boundaries in such exceptional circumstances. A gynaecologist who performed a tubal ligation after an emergency caesarean section without the patient's consent was given a criminal sentence.

"The hysterectomy would have been obligatory if the haemorrhage had not been controlled, as it had been, and the ligation required the patient's consent. The correctness of the action did not give the doctor the right to do this without consent, unless it had been necessary to make an urgent decision in this respect, because of the imminent danger to the life or integrity of people" [26].

e) Revocation.- The patient or his legal representative are free to revoke their consent in writing, at any time, without giving reasons and without being prejudiced as a result.

f) Teaching or research projects.- All patients or users have the right to be informed of the possibility of undergoing procedures for prognosis, diagnosis and therapies being used in a teaching or research projects, which must not, under any circumstances, involve an additional risk to health.

g) Drug research in patients suffering from Hirschsprung's Disease.-

- Clinical trials: Clinical trials of drugs for human use shall be conducted according to the provisions of the specific regulations [27].

For this purpose, the administration of an investigational drug to a single patient shall not be considered a clinical trial when this is done in the scope of usual medical practice and with the sole purpose of obtaining a therapeutic benefit for the patient, which shall be governed by the regulations on compassionate use set out in article 28 of Royal Decree 223/2004, of 6 February, governing Clinical Trials of Drugs.

The aforementioned regulations define informed consent as

"The decision, which must be set out in writing and be dated and signed, to participate in a clinical trial, adopted voluntarily by persons capable of giving their consent having been duly informed and documented regarding its nature, importance, implications and risks."

When the person subject to the trial is not capable of giving his or her consent, the decision must be made by their legal representative as follows:

- If the person subject of the trial is a minor: The minor's parents' or legal representative's informed consent shall be obtained. The consent must set out the minor's presumed consent and can be revoked at any time, at no prejudice to the patient. When the minor is aged 12 or over, their consent to participate in the trial must also be obtained.
- Minors shall receive information about the trial, its risks and benefits according to their ability to understand, from staff experienced in dealing with minors.
- The researcher shall accept the explicit wishes of the minor to refuse to participate in the trial or to withdraw at any time, when he or she is capable of forming an opinion based on the information received.
- The sponsor of the clinical trial shall inform the Public Prosecutor of the authorisations for clinical trials whose population includes minors.

Persons subject to a trial must give their consent once the objectives, risks and drawbacks of the trial, as well as the conditions under which it is conducted, have been understood, based on a prior interview with the researcher or a member of the research team, and once having been informed of their right to withdraw from the study at any time at no prejudice to them.

The consent shall be documented through an information sheet given to the person in question and the consent document itself. The information sheet shall contain only relevant information, expressed in clear terms, understandable by the persons in question, and shall be drafted in these persons' own language.

The persons participating in a clinical trial, or their legal representative, may revoke their consent at any time, without giving a reason and without being prejudiced as a result.

When the clinical trial is of specific interest to the population in which the research is conducted and there are reasons justifying the need for the investigational drug to be administered, a person may be included in a clinical trial without obtaining prior consent in the following cases:

- If there is an immediate serious danger to the physical or psychical integrity of the individual, there is no appropriate treatment alternative in clinical practice and it is not possible to obtain their legal representative's consent. In this instance, circumstances permitting, family members or other persons related *de facto* to these individuals shall be consulted in advance.
- If the individuals in question are not capable of making decisions because of their physical or psychical condition and have no legal representative. In this instance, consent will be given by family members or other persons related *de facto* to them.

In both cases, these circumstances and the manner in which one should proceed must be foreseen in the trial documentation approved by the Ethical Committee of Clinical Research, and the person in question or their legal representative should be informed as soon as possible and must give consent to continue in the trial, if appropriate.

- Post-authorisation studies of an observational nature with drugs for human use affecting patients with Hirschsprung's Disease: These shall be governed by specific regulations [28].

h) Clinical research with healthcare products in patients affected by Hirschsprung's Disease. This shall be governed by specific regulations [29].

i) Refusal of treatment.- All patients and users have the right to refuse treatment, except when otherwise established by the Law. Their refusal of treatment shall be set out in writing. Furthermore, all healthcare professionals involved in healthcare activities are bound to abide by the patient's free and voluntary decisions.

In the event that the treatment prescribed is rejected, the patient or user will be invited to sign a voluntary discharge. If the patient declines to sign, the management of the healthcare centre, at the request of the doctor in charge, may issue a compulsory discharge under the conditions foreseen by the Law.

The fact of not accepting the treatment prescribed will not lead to a compulsory discharge when alternative treatments are available, even when these are palliative in nature, provided that these are provided by the healthcare centre and accepted by the patient. These circumstances must be duly documented.

When the patient refuses to be discharged, the centre management, after having examined the corresponding medical report, shall listen to the patient and, if the patient still refuses, will refer the matter to the Court, for the decision to be confirmed or revoked.

In addition to the above, in the Autonomous Community of Andalusia, regulations have been passed specifically for cases involving paediatric patients in which, when there is a conflict of interests, and in the case of a rejection of treatment by the parents or guardians, the child's interest shall prevail [30]. In these cases, those responsible for the healthcare services and the healthcare personnel themselves are specifically bound to inform the relevant bodies of the Regional Government of Andalusia responsible for the protection of minors, the legal authorities or public prosecutor, of any facts that may indicate the existence of situations where minors may be vulnerable or at risk, and to collaborate with them to prevent and resolve such situations in the interests of the minor.

In this sense, Organic Law 1/1996, of 15 January, on legal protection for minors (Spanish Official Gazette no. 15, of 17 January 1996) establishes that

> "Minors shall have the right to receive the care they need with full respect for ethical, religious and cultural beliefs of the minor and their parents, provided that these do not endanger the life of the minor or public health, in which case the dispositions of the authorities and law in force shall be observed".

The Supreme Court has determined with absolute certainty that,

> "The minor's right to life and health cannot give in to the declaration of freedom of choice and objection by the parents"

a clear reference to the cases involving Jehovah's Witnesses [31].

j) Does obtaining informed consent exonerate the doctor from liability? Within the scope of the Law, correctly obtaining the consent document does not exonerate the doctor from possible liability incurred from professional malpractice.

Jurisprudence dictates that informed consent requires the patient's acceptance of the inherent or associated risks and consequences of the authorised intervention, although it does not exonerate the doctor from medical liability based on injury attributable to negligent acts by the healthcare professional or the poor operation of the centre or medical service. In this latter sense, the 3rd Contentious Administrative Division of the Supreme Court insists that

"The existence of informed consent does not oblige the patient to accept any risks deriving from inappropriate healthcare service" [32].

k) Legal consequences of the lack of or defective informed consent.- Healthcare professionals and public and private healthcare centres that fail to comply with the duty to inform and the informed consent of the patient may lead to, depending on the case, public liability, pecuniary liability and even criminal liability; without prejudice to any disciplinary measures that may be taken by the work centre itself [33].

A doctrine sector holds that the doctor's failure to comply with the duty to inform and, consequentially, the omission of or poor informed consent, is not immediately and automatically related to the payment of compensation, which requires the identification of damage deriving from the materialisation of a risk of which the patient was not informed prior to the medical intervention, correctly performed from a technical standpoint, to be able to establish public liability on the grounds of this infringement, as public liability can exist without blame but not without damage.

Therefore, even when the lack of informed consent constitutes medical malpractice and a violation of the *lex artis,* this being a prerequisite and essential element of the same, its absence cannot give rise to public liability *per se* if the medical action did not cause any harm to the patient [34].

This legal reasoning is supported by the statement that

"Although informed consent is the axis of medical activity, its absence only generates liability when the patient has suffered some kind of harm" [35].

Furthermore, the Provincial Court of Palma de Mallorca has found the lack of informed consent on its own, without the need for the patient to make a complaint [36].

The widely-commented decision of the 1st Civil Division of the Supreme Court dated 12 January 2001 holds that,

"The sentence is possible in cases of lack of or defective information; although the medical procedure may be correct"

precisely because the court itself long held that information forms part of the *lex artis*.

Jurisprudence insists that in cases where there is a lack of or deficient healthcare information, the patient is deprived of the right to obtain clarification before giving consent and making decisions deriving from this, the right to new consultations, the right to choose or the right to delay the performance of the medical act. In these cases, the healthcare professional and health centre where health care has been provided shall incur public or pecuniary liability, according to whether the centre is public or private. Therefore, according to the 1st Division of the Supreme Court.

"Although the doctor's action had been performed in accordance with the rules of lex artis, the healthcare centre and the doctor are jointly and severally liable to pay the compensation in question for denying the patient the right to information and the possible choices with regard to the intervention which he or she was to undergo" [37].

In criminal law, and with regard to the crime of injury or malpractice, the existence of the informed consent document does not exonerate the doctor from incurring criminal liability, with the exception of the three circumstances set out in article 156 of the Criminal Code, (i.e. in organ transplants performed in accordance with the Law, sterilisations and sex reassignment surgery carried out by healthcare professionals, except when the consent has been obtained incorrectly, or for a price or compensation, or the party giving consent is minor or incapable; in which case neither the patient's nor their legal representatives' consent shall be valid [38].

Failure to obtain informed consent has occasionally been ruled to constitute serious mental distress, different and separate from the bodily injury deriving from the intervention and, therefore compensable.

An interesting legal and jurisprudential study [39] concludes

"That on the grounds that it is indisputably set out in the regulations establishing the patient's rights to healthcare information and informed consent, relating to rights such as freedom, autonomy and human dignity, it is logical to relate the behaviours threatening these regulations with prejudice to these rights; prejudice or damage which, thus formed, is intrinsically impossible to assess from a merely pecuniary standpoint, as are the rights damaged." The author believes that from this approach, the next step could be "The acknowledgement of the right to compensation for this specific injury, which would imply including it as an independent item among all compensable damages, compatible, where appropriate, with others that could apply to compensation for damages of a different nature and origin. Finally, and based on this, it would be difficult to deny this compensation when, although no other type of injury is alleged or acknowledged by the court, the lack of information and informed consent has been proven".

The distinguished senior judge from the 3rd Contentious-Administrative Division of the Supreme Court, Mr Juan Antonio Xiol Ríos, already stated at the 7th Healthcare Law Conference that the lack of informed consent generates compensable mental distress different from the bodily harm that may be caused.

Examples of judgements deeming the omission of informed consent leads to the existence of compensable mental distress include, among others:

- Judgement by the 3rd Contentious-Administrative Division of the Supreme Court, of 4 April 2000, holds that "There is no doubt, however, that by omitting the informed consent, the minor's representatives were deprived of the opportunity to consider the advisability of rejecting the operation, avoiding its risks and of ensuring and confirming the need for the surgical intervention, making it impossible for the patient and his family members to have due knowledge of the risks involved when he underwent the operation. This situation cannot be irrelevant from the point of view of the principle of personal autonomy, essential to our Law, which demands that all persons be aware, as far as possible and to the extent to which they desire, of the situation in which they find themselves, that decisions they are entitled to make should not unjustifiably be taken on their behalf and that people whose health is in serious danger should be permitted to take preventative measures of all kinds. This situation of unconsciousness caused by the lack of information attributable to the Healthcare Authority of the risk existing, absolutely independently from the unfortunate crystallisation in the results of the operation, which is not causally linked to this lack of information or that this may have been successful, is in itself serious mental distress, different and separate from the bodily harm deriving from the intervention".

- Judgement by the 1st Civil Division of the Supreme Court, 23 November 2007:"The damage caused by this lack of information exclusively affects the parents-plaintiffs, who have suffered mental distress from being denied the necessary information to make their decisions in an appropriate manner... It is certainly difficult to quantify the mental distress in such a case, although it may result from the parents' need to adapt to a new personal, family and economic situation and, as stated in the judgement of 21 December 2005 (Law report 2005, 10149) to the special care required from an unforeseen or extraordinary circumstance for them, as is the case with the birth of a child with Down's Syndrome".
- Judgement by the 1st Civil Division of the Supreme Court, of 29 May 2003: The Court considers that failure to provide the appropriate prior information "Not practicing this correctly is an omission constituting guilt on the part of the healthcare service under articles 1902 and 1903 of the Civil Code and Constitutional Regulations (articles 43 and 51-1 and 2)". It also establishes compensation "including the pecuniary damages and mental distress caused".

l) Privacy/Confidentiality.- A citizen's right to privacy derives from the provisions of article 18 of the Spanish Constitution of 1978, and is implemented, among others, by the Organic Law on Civil Protection of Honour, Intimacy and one's Own Image, of 5 May 1982 (Spanish Official Gazette number 115, of 14 May 1982).

Law 41/2002 establishes as a *basic principle:*

"That human dignity, the upholding of free will and intimacy shall guide all activities aimed at obtaining, using, filing, keeping and disclosing medical information and documentation".

This regulation forms intimacy as a right, thus
"All people are entitled to the confidentiality of their medical information, and that nobody may access this without the prior authorisation set out by Law".

In turn, Organic Law No 15/1999, of 26th December, for the Protection of Personal Data (Spanish Official Gazette no. 298, of 14 December 1999) qualifies data relating to the health of citizens as "*specially protected data",* establishing a uniquely strict regimen for obtaining, keeping and transferring such information [40].

The Deontological and Medical Ethics Code of 31 March, 1999, also includes the duty for medical secrecy (articles 14 to 17).

Article 72.c) of Law 55/2003, of 26 December, of the Framework Statute for statutory personnel in health services, classes as a very serious offence

> "Breaking the required confidentially of data relating to the centre or institution or personal intimacy of users and the information relating to the process and stay in the institutions or healthcare centres" and also establishes that "very serious violations shall be corrected with one of the following penalties: a) Dismissal from the service, b) Mandatory transfer to a different location, c) Suspension of functions (no longer than six years and no less than two years)".

For its part, article 199.2 of Organic Law 10/1995, of 23 November of the Criminal Code, punishes the professionals who breach their professional duty of confidentiality and disclose another's secrets. This behaviour is punishable with prison of between one and four years, a fine of twelve to twenty-four months and a ban from practising the profession for between two and six years.

The typical action punished is reflected in the verb "disclose" which includes all communication to third parties for which consent or authorization has not been given by the patient/parents/legal representative.

With regard to obtaining photographs of paediatric patients to be published either in scientific journals or other media, prior, written and signed consent is required. The Supreme Court has stressed that

> "images of minors are specially protected by our legal system" [41].

III Conclusions

This paper is intended to shed light on the main questions relating to informed consent and to help and encourage Healthcare Professionals to carry out their documentary work to excellent standards. There is no doubt that with your medical skills and experience as clinician, and with an understanding of the subject, the introduction (effective and efficient) of informed consent may become, not only a gratifying task, but also a safety task, and at the same time will be of help in facing possible claims or complaints, and especially, their success.

I am based on the principle that no human activity can ever be expected to be ineffable neither can this be demanded in the area of doctors' liability. In addition, there must be considered that the nature of the doctor's liability is the obligation of activity (or means) not results. The idea held is that the obligation is not to obtain a result (the patient's health) but to provide the most appropriate service in order to achieve such a result [42].

Within the scope of the Autonomy of Will, Informed Consent is therefore not only an ethical demand [43] but also a legal requirement. It constitutes a Fundamental Human Right acknowledged in international texts on Human Rights and Spanish Law. It is one of the most recent incorporations made in the theory of Human Rights, a necessary consequence or explanation of the traditional rights to life, physical integrity and freedom of thought. The right to personal freedom, to make one's own decisions with regard to one's own person and life itself and consequential to self-determination over one's own body [44] and, therefore, can be demanded not only from the point of view of the doctrine, but also from the legal standpoint.

References

[1] Art. 43 of the Spanish Constitution of 27 December 1978 (*Spanish Official Gazette* No. 311, of 29 December, 1978).

[2] Law 14/1986, 25 April, on General Healthcare (*Spanish Official Gazette* 102, dated 29 April 1986. Sections 5, 6, 8, 9 and 11 of article 10 and section 4 of article 11 have been revoked).

[3] Also known as the Oviedo Convention, the city where it was signed on 4 April 1997. It was ratified by Spain on 5 October 1999 and came into effect on 1 January 2000 (*Spanish Official Gazette* No. 251, of 20 October, 1999).

[4] 1st Additional Provision of Basic Law 41/2002, dated 14 November, governing Patient Autonomy and the Rights and Obligation regarding Information and Clinical Documentation (*Spanish official gazette*. No. 274, of 15 November 2002).

[5] There are Regional Laws subsequent to Law 41/2002 regulating these aspects: Law 1/2003 of 28 January, on Patient Rights and Information in the Autonomous Community of Valencia; Law 5/2003 of 4 April, on health (Balearic Islands); Law 8/2003 of 8 April (Castile-León) on Rights and Duties of Health Persons; Law 5/2003 of 9 October, Essential Prior Statement of Agreement (Andalusia); Law 3/2005 of 7 March, amending Law 3/2001, of 28 May Regulation on Informed Consent and the Medical History of Patients (Galicia); *Law 3/2005*, of 8 July, on Health Information and Autonomy of the Patient (Extremadura); Law 6/2005 of 7 July, on The Prior Statement of Agreement Regarding Own Health (Castile-La Mancha); *Law 1/2006*, on 3 March, on Prior Agreement (Balearic Islands).

[6] 2nd Additional Provision of Basic Law 41/2002, dated 14 November, governing Patient Autonomy and Rights and Obligations regarding Information and Clinical Documentation (Spanish official gazette. No. 274, of 15 November 2002).

[7] Judgements by the 1st Civil Division of the Supreme Court, of 2 October 1997, 3 October 2000 and 17 April 2007 as well as Judgements by the 3rd Contentious-Administrative Division of the Supreme Court of 30 March 2004, 20 September 2005 and 16 January 2007.

[8] Judgements by the 1st Civil Division of the Supreme Court, of 29 May 2003, 21 December 2005 and 21 December 2006.

[9] Judgements by the 1st Civil Division of the Supreme Court, of 2 March 1991, 2 March 1990, 20 October 1997 and 23 May 2006.

[10] López- Alonso, M. Chapter 9.

[11] Judgement by the 1st Civil Division of the Supreme Court, of 17 June 1998.

[12] Doctrine which is nowadays included in art. 217 of Law 1/2000, of 7 January, on Civil Proceedings (Spanish Official Gazette, number 7, of 8 January 2000)
[13] Judgements by the 1st Civil Division of the Supreme Court of 28 December 1998, 2 March 2000, 25 September 2003, 21 December 2005 and 18 May 2006.
[14] Judgement by the 1st Civil Division of the Supreme Court, of 31 July 1996.
[15] Comment on the judgement of 12 January 2001 of the Civil Division of the Supreme Court. Santiago Pelayo Pardos, Social Security Administration Lawyer, Member of the Management Board of the Spanish Healthcare Association, Actualidad de Derecho Sanitario, Opinion piece.
[16] El consentimiento informado del usuario de los servicios sanitarios [The healthcare service user's informed consent] Julio César Galán Cortés, Lawyer and Doctor of Medicine, Ed. Colex, Madrid 1997.
[17] Responsabilidad legal del profesional sanitario [The healthcare professional's legal liability] Ricardo de Lorenzo y Montero and Javier Sánchez Caro, Spanish Healthcare Law Association Training Plan. Madrid 2000.
[18] Judgements by the 1st Civil Division of the Supreme Court, of 8 September 2003 and 10 May 2006.
[19] Judgement by the 1st Civil Division of the Supreme Court, of 29 May 2003.
[20] Tratamiento legal y jurisprudencial del consentimiento informado [Legal treatment of informed consent] Ignacio Sancho Gargallo, Senior Judge, Working Paper no.: 209. Barcelona, April 2004.
[21] Judgements by the 1st Civil Division of the Supreme Court, 23 November 2007, which makes reference to the judgements of 25 April 1994, 31 July 1996, 16 October 1998, 10 November 1998, 28 December 1998, 19 April 1999, 26 September 2000, 12 January and 27 April 2001, 29 May and 8 September 2003, 7 April and 29 October 2004, 20 September 2005, 15 May and 26 June 2006, 6, 19 and 29 June 2007, 19 July 2007, etc.
[22] Judgement by the 1st Civil Division of the Supreme Court, of 26 September 2000.
[23] Judgement by the 1st Civil Division of the Supreme Court, of 15 November 2006, and by the 3rd Contentious Administrative Division of the same Court, of 21 March 2007.
[24] Judgements by the 1st Civil Division of the Supreme Court, on 16 October 1998, 28 December 1998, 19 April 1999, 2 March 2000, 12 January 2001 and 8 September 2003.
[25] Tratamiento legal y jurisprudencial del consentimiento informado [Legal treatment of informed consent] Ignacio Sancho Gargallo. Senior Judge, Working Paper no.: 209. Barcelona, April 2004.
[26] Judgement by the 2nd Criminal Division of the Supreme Court, of 26 October 1995.
[27] Royal Decree 223/2004, of 6 February, regulating Clinical Trials of Drugs (Spanish Official Gazette Number. 33, of 7 February 2004).
[28] Royal Decree 1344/2007, of 11 October, governing the reporting of adverse drug events related to drugs for human use (Spanish Official Gazette number 262 of 1 November, 2007).
[29] Royal Decree 1143/2007, of 31 August (Spanish Official Gazette number 210 of 1 September 2007) which has been amended Royal Decree 634/1993, of 3 May (Spanish Official Gazette number 126 of 27 May 1993), on healthcare active implantable products; Royal Decree 414/1996, of 1 March, governing healthcare products (Spanish

Official Gazette number 99 of 24 April 1996) and Royal Decree 1662/2000, of 29 September (Spanish Official Gazette number 235 of 30 September 2000).

[30] Law 1/1998, of 20 April, on Rights and Care of Minors in Andalusia (Official Gazette of the Government of Andalusia No. 53, of 12 May 1998).

[31] Judgement by the 2nd Criminal Division of the Supreme Court, of 17 June 1997.

[32] Judgements by the 3rd Contentious-Administrative Division of the Supreme Court, of 10 October 2000 and 7 June 2001.

[33] Arts. 70 to 75 Law 55/2003, of 26 December, of the Framework Statute of statutory personnel in healthcare services (Spanish Official Gazette No 301, of 17 December 2003)

[34] Consentimiento informado y nexo causal en la responsabilidad médica [Informed consent and causation in medical liability] Julio César Galán Cortés, Actualidad Jurídica Aranzadi no. 716/2006.

[35] Judgement by the 1st Civil Division of the Supreme Court, of 23 July 2003.

[36] Judgement by the 4th Division of the Provincial Court of Palma de Mallorca, of 4 October 1996.

[37] Judgement by the 1st Civil Division of the Supreme Court, of 8 September 2003.

[38] Organic Law 10/1995, of 23 November of the Criminal Code (Spanish Official Gazette no. 281, of 24 November 1995).

[39] Responsabilidad sanitaria por incumplimiento del deber de información al paciente [Healthcare liability due to failure to comply with the duty to inform the patient] Mª Luisa Arcos Vieira, Universidad Pública de Navarra, Cuadernos de Aranzadi Civil no. 27/2006 (Studies).

[40] This Organic Law has been implemented by Royal Decree 1720/2007 of 21 December (Spanish Official Gazette No 17, of 19 January 2008).

[41] Judgement by the 1st Civil Division of the Supreme Court, of 18 October 2004.

[42] Judgement by the 1st Civil Division of the Supreme Court, of 21 December de 2005, which refers to the decisions of 8 May 1991, 20 February 1992, 13 October 1992, 2 February 1993, 20 September 1994, 16 February 1995, 15 October 1996, 13 December 1997, 9 December 1998, etc.

[43] Judgement by the 1st Civil Division of the Supreme Court, of 16 October 1998, which reminds that it is a deontological duty prior to the General Healthcare Law.

[44] Judgements by the 1st Civil Division of the Supreme Court, of 12 January 2001 and 11 May 2001.

Index

A

AAP, 306, 358
abdomen, 132, 188, 204, 223, 225, 232, 234, 235, 244, 263, 333, 431, 432, 433, 434
ablations, 16
abnormalities, 26, 33, 38, 62, 65, 78, 80, 81, 83, 84, 98, 126, 163, 186, 272, 292, 293, 324, 326, 329, 330, 332, 338, 340, 358, 375, 379, 381, 385
absorption, 55, 160, 206, 209, 210, 217, 294, 295, 358, 385, 392, 410, 417, 418, 422, 423, 425, 426
absorption coefficient, 160
abstinence, 186, 195
ACC, 97, 98
accidental, 210, 217
accounting, 27, 52, 192, 392
accuracy, 119, 157
ACE, 350
acetylcholine, 47, 58, 63
acetylcholinesterase, 63, 70, 77, 107, 108, 118, 119, 120, 121, 180, 181, 183, 193, 274, 359, 370, 373, 374, 379, 384
achalasia, 121, 151, 169, 258, 309, 315, 374, 379, 384
acid, 23, 28, 32, 43, 71, 90, 92, 181, 185, 186, 194, 195, 211, 298, 330, 399
acidic, 329, 417, 434, 437
acidosis, 417
ACR, 399
actin, 58
action potential, 46, 47, 49
activation, 30, 40, 45, 46, 47, 49, 91, 102, 332, 379
active site, 92
acute, 186, 336, 337, 395, 399, 408, 409, 414, 415, 416, 419
acute rejection, 409
acute respiratory distress syndrome, 395
adaptation, 298, 395, 419, 426
adenine, 62, 359, 377
adenosine triphosphate, 47
adhesion, 20, 31, 33, 42, 43, 69, 206, 271, 284, 325, 330, 377, 383, 399
adhesions, 227, 258, 278, 283, 284, 298, 328, 355
adiposity, 415
adjustment, 299, 365
administration, 161, 208, 210, 211, 327, 328, 336, 337, 338, 397, 398, 401, 408, 422, 436, 450, 453
adolescents, 131, 136, 284, 365, 415, 425
adult, 20, 43, 121, 132, 207, 208, 210, 255, 314, 349, 353, 354, 364, 366, 371, 375, 393
adulthood, 290, 361, 363
adults, 21, 23, 32, 45, 131, 136, 207, 307, 350, 354, 361, 362, 385, 386, 393, 401
adventitia, 376
aerobic, 207, 210
aetiology, 117, 119
Africa, 134, 306
African American, 425
afternoon, 210, 211, 433
age, 63, 65, 73, 75, 76, 77, 88, 94, 100, 108, 117, 120, 130, 131, 135, 141, 150, 151, 154, 155, 156, 170, 176, 177, 178, 180, 185, 189, 190, 191, 208, 210, 222, 230, 249, 251, 259, 263, 267, 269, 271, 272, 273, 283, 284, 291, 294, 298, 299, 308, 310, 321, 323, 325, 328, 330, 337, 338, 343, 350, 351, 352, 353, 354, 355, 357, 358, 360, 361, 362, 363, 364, 374, 375, 387, 389, 396, 398, 405, 414, 415, 420, 424, 425, 431, 432, 437, 439, 449
agents, 76, 332, 338, 398
aggregates, 19, 32
aggregation, 32

aging, 354
aid, 159, 207, 384, 431, 432
air, 138, 141, 143, 161, 162, 170, 183, 185, 188, 193, 226, 335
alanine, 40
albinism, 85, 105
alcohol, 184, 186, 194, 195
algorithm, 133, 333
allele, 41, 102
allergy, 196
allograft, 391, 392, 399, 409
allosteric, 44
alpha, 102, 103, 421
alpha5 chains, 43
alternative, 203, 213, 263, 273, 285, 387, 390, 398, 415, 448, 454, 455
alternatives, 296, 311, 436, 447, 450
American Academy of Pediatrics, 69, 82, 100, 135, 158, 312, 320, 341, 355, 367
amino acid, 28, 57, 90, 92
amniotic, 431
amorphous, 118
amplitude, 50, 51, 143, 148, 351, 365
ampulla, 131, 132, 146, 200
AMR, 382
Amsterdam, 83, 260, 308, 366
anaerobes, 210, 211, 336
anaerobic, 207, 209, 210, 336
anaerobic bacteria, 336
anaesthesia, 118, 221
anal fissures, 132
anal inhibitory reflex, 128, 193, 435, 437
analgesia, 236
anastomoses, 251, 305, 391
anastomosis, 115, 116, 189, 203, 206, 207, 211, 217, 225, 226, 227, 229, 230, 231, 232, 233, 234, 235, 236, 238, 239, 247, 248, 249, 250, 251, 253, 256, 258, 259, 260, 262, 264, 265, 275, 282, 283, 284, 286, 294, 295, 302, 306, 307, 308, 309, 313, 314, 325, 338, 339, 344, 353, 356, 363, 364, 387, 395, 418, 426, 433, 436, 439
anatomy, 68, 185, 221, 367
anemia, 300
anencephaly, 79
Anglo-Saxon, 197
animal models, 15, 27, 52, 63, 67, 87, 375
animals, 28, 29, 48, 49, 331, 333
ankles, 245
anorexia, 431
ANS, 56, 60, 65
antecedents, 73, 75, 77, 275
antibiotic, 211, 212, 216, 218, 222, 248, 251, 337, 340, 344
antibiotics, 128, 202, 207, 208, 210, 211, 212, 216, 218, 248, 278, 283, 327, 336, 337, 338, 347, 355, 398, 432, 433
antibody, 48
antigen, 336
antiviral agents, 398
antiviral drugs, 401
anus, 45, 50, 83, 126, 127, 134, 143, 164, 174, 196, 198, 213, 223, 225, 229, 232, 233, 234, 245, 246, 256, 261, 263, 265, 282, 283, 307, 308, 309, 310, 311, 337, 352, 353, 417, 418, 421, 430, 434, 436, 437, 439
anxiety, 362, 363
aorta, 386, 387, 391
aplasia, 374
apnea, 185
apoptosis, 25, 27, 29, 399
apoptotic, 399
appendix, 130, 135, 202, 290, 293, 294, 302
appetite, 432
application, 146, 181, 210, 239, 257, 261, 275, 313, 358, 359, 419, 443, 444
arginine, 62
argument, 448
Ariel, 181
arrest, 32, 61, 88
arterial hypertension, 92
arterial hypotension, 432
arteries, 224, 264, 388
arteritis, 399
artery, 157, 180, 223, 224, 225, 244, 264, 386, 387, 390, 391, 395
ascending colon, 109, 118, 119, 130, 163, 203
Asian, 134
aspiration, 170, 210
assessment, 52, 64, 71, 88, 268, 271, 296, 310, 311, 314, 350, 353, 356, 359, 362, 364, 369, 382, 393, 405, 409, 413, 425
astringent, 437
asymptomatic, 153
Atlantic, 307
atopic dermatitis, 192
atresia, 79, 83, 129, 184, 188, 191, 193, 196, 275, 276, 291, 293, 301, 385
atrial septal defect, 84, 101
atrophy, 112, 117
attacks, 321

Aurora, 84
autonomic nervous system, 56, 95, 97, 105, 330
autonomy, 390, 391, 403, 443, 444, 457
autosomal dominant, 89, 90, 93, 94, 95
autosomal recessive, 28, 89, 96, 98
availability, 26, 37, 353, 389, 423
avoidance, 229, 286, 343, 365
awareness, 290
axon, 42, 43, 49, 59
axon terminals, 49
axonal, 21, 23, 50, 377
axons, 21, 42, 58, 377

B

B lymphocytes, 401
babies, 272, 276, 284, 430, 434, 436
bacteria, 60, 185, 210, 328, 329, 330, 331, 332, 336, 340, 398, 421
bacterial, 60, 68, 211, 294, 327, 328, 330, 332, 333, 336, 337, 338, 339, 340, 345, 346, 355, 358, 394, 398, 408, 409, 418, 421, 422
bacterial infection, 336, 337
Balearic Islands, 460
barium, 159, 160, 161, 163, 164, 170, 203, 204, 223, 277, 291, 335
barium enema, 159, 160, 161, 163, 170, 203, 204, 223, 291, 335
barium sulphate, 160
barrier, 185, 328, 329, 330, 331, 340, 345, 439
barriers, 425
basal lamina, 32, 39, 71
Bax, 116, 121, 240, 287, 313, 364
BBG, 338
behavior, 36, 189, 362
behavioral problems, 362
behaviours, 47, 457
Belgium, 306
beliefs, 455
beneficial effect, 397
benefits, 165, 207, 212, 306, 310, 360, 405, 453
benign, 128, 192, 193, 363
betadine, 232
bias, 271
bicarbonate, 209, 217, 417
bile, 129, 393, 401, 417, 421, 422, 435
bile acids, 421
biliary cirrhosis, 393
binding, 23, 24, 30, 31, 32, 40, 103, 329, 406
biomarker, 195
biomarkers, 186, 195
biopsies, 107, 109, 110, 114, 115, 118, 119, 120, 128, 131, 160, 165, 167, 171, 172, 174, 176, 180, 181, 189, 191, 202, 203, 204, 223, 224, 226, 244, 255, 256, 261, 276, 285, 292, 293, 339, 351, 359, 360, 370, 373, 374, 375, 379, 435
biopsy, 76, 107, 109, 110, 116, 118, 119, 120, 128, 131, 134, 137, 150, 151, 152, 153, 155, 156, 157, 158, 159, 160, 164, 165, 166, 167, 170, 171, 172, 173, 174, 175, 176, 177, 178, 179, 180, 181, 183, 186, 187, 188, 189, 190, 191, 193, 195, 197, 212, 224, 225, 244, 245, 246, 252, 261, 262, 263, 274, 276, 277, 282, 301, 309, 326, 335, 336, 338, 339, 340, 348, 352, 356, 373, 374, 375, 376, 377, 378, 379, 384, 431, 433, 435, 437
bipolar, 223
birth, 21, 23, 28, 74, 75, 76, 81, 88, 104, 127, 129, 151, 156, 183, 185, 186, 188, 189, 194, 197, 299, 350, 414, 430, 458
birth weight, 75, 127, 129, 185, 194, 299, 414
births, 55, 73, 74, 88, 127, 289, 357
bladder, 80, 192, 196, 222, 231, 232, 234, 235, 244, 263, 380, 381
blame, 456
bleeding, 118, 171, 236, 244, 258, 280, 393, 434
blood, 46, 57, 210, 211, 232, 238, 246, 269, 270, 296, 297, 319, 329, 331, 332, 345, 356, 374, 375, 376, 397, 401, 417
blood flow, 46
blood pressure, 210
blood supply, 238, 296, 297, 356
blood vessels, 57, 374, 375, 376
bodily injury, 457
body composition, 425
body fat, 424, 425
body image, 362
body mass index, 415, 425
body weight, 391, 396
bolus, 60, 337, 420, 438
Boston, 63, 70, 138, 156, 221
botulinum, 338, 352, 379
bowel obstruction, 76, 125, 130, 236, 270, 291, 292, 297, 298, 325, 437
bowel perforation, 130
boys, 55, 269, 272, 374
bradycardia, 185
brain, 23, 46, 56, 57, 69, 84
branching, 378
Brazil, 311
breast milk, 420

broad spectrum, 211, 329
Brussels, 393, 403, 408
burn, 434
butyric, 418
bypass, 353

C

cadherin, 31, 43, 90
cadherins, 33
caecum, 16, 18, 19, 25, 28, 29, 31, 32, 35, 38, 61, 163, 165, 166
caesarean section, 452
calcium, 23, 127
caliber, 226, 258, 261, 262, 264, 292, 386
calibration, 255, 257
caloric intake, 420
calorie, 414, 422, 423, 425
CAM, 31, 43, 378
canals, 151
cancer, 52, 91, 94, 100, 368
candidates, 236, 290, 389, 392, 393, 394, 395, 396, 407, 411
capillary, 291, 301
capsule, 34, 69, 170
carbohydrates, 329, 361, 401, 417, 418, 420, 421, 422, 426
carbon, 48, 59, 263
carbon dioxide, 263
carbon monoxide, 48, 59
carcinoma, 81, 87, 94, 102, 104, 291, 301, 359, 368, 375
cardiovascular system, 79
cartilage, 15, 85, 291, 301
case study, 303
casein, 432, 433, 436
cast, 310
category a, 80
catheter, 138, 139, 140, 142, 156, 198, 199, 208, 210, 231, 235, 259, 263, 278, 290, 320, 337, 358, 395
catheters, 138, 199, 200, 400
causation, 462
cDNA, 61, 103
cecum, 34, 68, 187, 391
Celiac disease, 357
cell, 15, 17, 21, 23, 24, 25, 26, 27, 30, 31, 32, 33, 35, 36, 37, 38, 39, 41, 42, 43, 46, 47, 48, 49, 50, 52, 57, 58, 59, 60, 61, 65, 68, 69, 85, 91, 102, 105, 111, 115, 117, 270, 291, 302, 329, 345, 346, 359, 375, 377, 378, 379, 383, 388
cell adhesion, 42, 43, 69, 377, 383
cell body, 25
cell division, 17
cell growth, 291
cell invasion, 37
cell line, 24, 30, 60, 65, 102
cell surface, 32, 58, 65, 91
cellular immunity, 331, 401
central nervous system, 25, 32, 56, 59, 79, 80, 90, 99, 186, 324
cereals, 436
CFA, 418
channels, 48
check-ups, 434, 439
chemicals, 379
chemoattractant, 21
chemotaxis, 24
chemotherapy, 216, 410
chicken, 37
childhood, 69, 95, 119, 133, 181, 290, 299, 354, 382, 384
China, 306, 311
Chi-square, 155
chloral, 170
chloride, 188, 209, 217
cholecystokinin, 34, 418
cholestasis, 358, 393, 394, 402, 408
cholesterol, 98
cholinergic, 23, 36, 56, 57, 58, 63, 69, 378
cholinergic neurons, 23
cholinesterase, 119
chondrodysplasia, 291
chromaffin cells, 81
chromosomal abnormalities, 78, 272, 338
chromosome, 87, 90, 93, 98, 101, 103, 104, 330
chromosomes, 23
chronic illness, 365
chyme, 418, 421
circulation, 422
cirrhosis, 393
citizens, 458
citrus, 361
classes, 93, 205, 459
classical, xi, 56, 116, 118, 119, 335
classification, 68, 76, 77, 78, 79, 88, 89, 326, 369
cleaning, 141, 151, 153, 156, 189, 232
cleavage, 245
cleft lip, 96

cleft palate, 80, 96, 98
clinical presentation, 73, 77, 126, 127, 128, 131, 185, 186, 187, 188, 290, 333
clinical symptoms, 77, 125, 202, 374, 377
clinical trial, 453, 454
clinician, 444, 459
Clostridium botulinum, 384
closure, 15, 207, 215, 299, 306, 307, 358, 388, 392, 398, 406
clusters, 56, 57, 359
CNS, 56, 57, 89, 186
coagulation, 387
coagulopathy, 331, 393
coccyx, 246
codes, 41
coding, 59, 65, 68, 91
coercion, 450
co-existence, 357
cohort, 81, 104, 340, 351
colectomy, 203, 275, 282, 294, 302, 337, 416, 418, 424, 426
colic, 192, 209, 210, 225, 395, 432
colitis, 210, 218, 326, 327, 344, 346, 368, 382, 418
collaboration, xi, xii, 440
collagen, 32, 39, 44, 57, 65, 71, 380, 381
colon cancer, 21
colonisation, 16, 17, 19, 20, 22, 24, 25, 26, 27, 28, 29, 30, 32, 61, 109
colonization, 30, 34, 35, 37, 69, 328, 330, 398
colorectal surgeon, 210, 216
colostomy, 79, 128, 129, 198, 201, 203, 204, 205, 206, 213, 214, 215, 222, 226, 227, 230, 231, 232, 236, 240, 241, 243, 258, 259, 262, 268, 275, 283, 285, 306, 308, 320, 322, 327, 336, 347, 348, 355, 356, 364, 416, 419, 433, 437, 438, 440
communication, 140, 232, 285, 439, 448, 459
community, 425
compensation, 419, 423, 447, 450, 456, 457, 458
complement, 331
complexity, 58, 310, 354, 417, 444
compliance, 445
complications, xi, 76, 150, 153, 156, 165, 169, 171, 172, 188, 201, 202, 206, 210, 214, 215, 216, 221, 226, 230, 236, 237, 238, 245, 250, 251, 252, 258, 259, 260, 261, 270, 283, 284, 286, 290, 294, 295, 297, 298, 299, 305, 310, 311, 321, 336, 341, 352, 357, 358, 360, 363, 365, 366, 368, 385, 387, 392, 393, 395, 396, 398, 403, 404, 410, 416, 417, 419, 420, 424, 426, 433, 436, 437, 439
components, 32, 39, 44, 65, 71, 331, 380
composition, 33, 127, 187, 209
concentration, 25, 29, 65, 211
conceptualization, 78
concordance, 165, 167, 168, 292, 295
condensation, 42
confidentiality, 458, 459
configuration, 131, 255
conflict of interest, 455
confusion, 233, 310, 362, 374, 375
congenital heart disease, 96
congenital megacolon, 82, 87, 100, 135, 168, 212, 239, 341
connective tissue, 58, 192, 381
connectivity, 52
consanguineous, 84
conscious perception, 46
consciousness, 432
consensus, 407
consent, xi, 443, 444, 445, 446, 447, 448, 449, 450, 451, 452, 453, 454, 455, 456, 457, 459, 461, 462
constipation, xi, 46, 53, 55, 64, 76, 77, 87, 93, 115, 120, 121, 125, 131, 132, 136, 165, 167, 169, 181, 184, 190, 192, 193, 198, 200, 236, 238, 259, 267, 273, 283, 287, 291, 305, 307, 308, 324, 349, 350, 352, 353, 354, 360, 361, 367, 373, 377, 378, 433, 434
Constitution, 414, 444
consulting, 452
contamination, 222, 225, 238, 249, 271, 284
contingency, 176, 177
continuity, 60, 245, 259, 305, 350, 390, 391, 394
contractions, 47, 60, 291, 351, 380
control, 19, 29, 30, 32, 33, 42, 45, 56, 57, 58, 60, 65, 67, 68, 95, 170, 191, 201, 205, 206, 215, 223, 238, 272, 273, 278, 279, 283, 301, 308, 314, 325, 326, 330, 331, 332, 338, 340, 352, 357, 362, 369, 391, 405, 423, 432, 433, 440, 452
control group, 272, 273, 325, 326, 330, 331, 357
conversion, 28
copper, 127
corpus callosum, 79, 96, 98
correlation, 21, 27, 92, 95, 99, 104, 125, 295, 297, 361
correlations, 354
corrosive, 205, 438
corticosteroids, 397
cost-effective, 215
costs, 230, 365, 405
Council of Europe, 443
counseling, 93, 99, 134

covariate, 355
covering, xi, 74, 268, 351
cow milk, 193
craniofacial, 79, 80, 92, 94
C-reactive protein, 269, 270
credibility, 137
crest syndrome, 85, 105
crime, 457
critically ill, 417
crystallisation, 458
cues, 31
cultural beliefs, 455
culture, 29, 34, 38, 48, 69
curing, 440
cyst, 84
cysteine, 90
cystic fibrosis, 127, 185, 187, 188, 195
cystourethrogram, 380
cysts, 96
cytomegalovirus, 409
cytoskeleton, 23, 58, 384
cytosolic, 62
cytotoxic, 324, 332
cytotoxicity, 346

D

dairy, 361
dairy products, 361
danger, 202, 394, 453, 454, 458
de novo, 92, 95
deafness, 26, 80, 81, 85, 95, 97, 105, 133
death, 40, 222, 237, 320, 322, 343, 346, 393, 395, 400
deaths, 129, 322, 340, 400
decay, 51
decisions, 443, 448, 454, 456, 458, 460, 462
decompression, 128, 197, 198, 200, 201, 202, 210, 230, 262, 275, 320, 336, 337, 339, 355, 364, 396, 438
decontamination, 207, 210, 211, 398
defecation, 45, 193, 259, 270, 298, 314, 351, 352
defects, 26, 27, 28, 29, 30, 33, 36, 41, 65, 74, 76, 77, 78, 79, 80, 81, 88, 89, 92, 100, 103, 133, 192, 195, 278, 327, 381
defense, 343, 345
deficiency, 52, 62, 298, 300, 324, 332, 381, 416, 417, 421, 424
deficit, 215, 330, 392, 393, 396, 401, 425
deficits, 36, 38
definition, 165, 285, 355, 385, 425
degradation, 330, 345
dehiscence, 203, 206, 207, 211, 237, 247, 248, 283, 356, 400
dehydration, 200, 210, 290, 337, 398, 436, 439
dehydrogenasa, 114
dehydrogenase, 110, 112, 115, 117, 189, 377
dehydrogenases, 117, 173, 176, 178, 179
delayed gastric emptying, 392
delivery, 51
demography, 81
dendrites, 59
denervation, 60, 356, 401
density, 26, 37, 108, 109, 115, 174, 375
depolarization, 52
deposition, 33, 380
deposits, 381
depressants, 186
depressed, 362
depression, 362
derivatives, 16, 19, 21, 26, 30, 40, 44, 48
dermatitis, 283, 432, 434, 440
dermis, 15
descending colon, 20, 32, 110, 160, 163, 165, 248, 261, 264, 268, 272, 284, 294
detection, 75, 81, 283, 421, 422
developing brain, 104
deviation, 117
dexamethasone, 408
diabetes, 185, 187
diabetes mellitus, 185
diagnostic criteria, 189, 192, 374, 375, 376, 381
diamond, 168, 286
diaphragm, 80
diarrhea, 185, 283, 334, 361, 374, 386, 391, 395, 398, 399, 401, 402, 425
diet, 193, 208, 226, 338, 352, 361, 362, 419, 420, 423, 437
dietary, 210, 298, 349, 404, 423
dietary intake, 423
diets, 420, 424
differential diagnosis, xi, 69, 119, 121, 185, 186, 187, 190, 336
differentiation, 19, 21, 22, 23, 24, 27, 28, 29, 30, 32, 34, 36, 39, 40, 44, 65, 66, 291, 330
digestibility, 423
digestion, 55, 186, 385, 423, 426, 435
digestive process, 47
digestive tract, 19, 34, 35, 47, 50, 68, 160, 202, 320, 322

dignity, 449
dilation, 160, 193, 326, 329, 352, 355, 356, 360, 399, 430, 436, 439
dimerization, 91
dipeptides, 422
disabled, 396
discharges, 283
discomfort, 210, 361, 433, 447
discordance, 165, 258
disease gene, 42
diseases, 23, 87, 184, 194, 369, 435, 437, 448
disequilibrium, 91
disorder, 55, 85, 93, 95, 96, 105, 169, 186, 292, 360, 383, 387, 410
displacement, 118
distilled water, 139, 432
distress, 186, 361, 362, 363, 457, 458
distribution, 43, 44, 61, 62, 63, 64, 65, 67, 69, 70, 71, 74, 75, 359, 371, 379, 383, 426
diversity, 44, 58, 329
division, 17, 57, 232, 280, 307, 309
DNA, 30, 31, 40, 101, 188, 401, 409
DNA testing, 188
doctors, 435, 436, 439, 451, 459
dogs, 247, 327, 425, 426
donor, 26, 386, 387, 388, 389, 390, 406, 407
donors, 389, 390, 391, 407
doors, 451
dopamine, 30
dosage, 141, 186
Down syndrome, 80, 203, 211, 321, 322, 323, 324, 325, 335, 338, 355, 357, 369
drainage, 199, 222, 249, 337, 391
drug addiction, 184
drug treatment, 423
drug-induced, 193
drugs, 381, 397, 453, 454, 461
drying, 107, 117, 119, 205, 436
duodenum, 21, 387, 388, 389, 390, 391, 392, 396, 418
duplication, 95, 184
duration, 51, 62, 141, 143, 148, 149, 186, 212, 268, 269, 270, 271, 299, 338, 408
duties, 443, 445
dwarfism, 98
dysplasia, 64, 97, 98, 121, 125, 127, 133, 169, 176, 181, 184, 189, 191, 195, 197, 239, 241, 251, 291, 301, 314, 325, 327, 332, 338, 339, 346, 355, 356, 358, 360, 368, 370, 374, 381, 382, 383, 385

E

E. coli, 330, 331
eclampsia, 185
ECM, 31, 32, 33
ectoderm, 15
edema, 247, 248, 335
education, 404
effluent, 199
Egypt, 311
elderly, 354
electrocautery, 264, 278, 279, 280, 281, 282
electrolyte, 128, 200, 215, 217, 290, 295, 336, 358, 417, 419, 421, 422, 438
electrolyte imbalance, 290, 336
electrolytes, 206, 208, 210, 215, 337, 418, 423
electron, 379
elongation, 19
embryo, 15, 16, 24, 34, 37, 61, 68, 69
embryogenesis, 36, 37
embryonic development, 15, 29, 60
embryos, 18, 20, 27, 35, 36, 40, 43
emotional, 289, 353, 361, 362
emulsions, 393
encephalopathy, 98
encoding, 19, 27, 30, 31, 41, 61, 104
encopresis, 76, 132, 307
endocarditis, 395
endocrine, 43, 57, 81, 94, 101, 104, 418, 419
endoderm, 19
endoplasmic reticulum, 47
endoscopy, 336, 399, 436
endothelin, 39, 91
endothelium, 399
end-to-end, 115
enemas, 141, 151, 153, 156, 160, 168, 170, 172, 185, 192, 193, 200, 203, 207, 208, 211, 213, 217, 222, 243, 259, 308, 337, 351, 377, 378, 433
energy, 418, 426
enolase, 377
enteritis, 327, 332, 337, 338, 346, 409, 410, 421
enterocolitis, ix, xi, 125, 128, 130, 131, 132, 133, 135, 137, 151, 152, 153, 156, 169, 183, 184, 185, 192, 194, 197, 198, 199, 200, 201, 202, 203, 207, 211, 212, 214, 217, 222, 227, 236, 238, 248, 251, 252, 258, 270, 273, 275, 276, 283, 289, 290, 297, 298, 303, 306, 307, 308, 309, 315, 319, 320, 321, 322, 323, 324, 326, 327, 329, 330, 331, 332, 333, 335, 336, 337, 338, 339, 340, 341, 342, 343, 344, 345, 346, 347, 349, 350, 351, 352, 355, 357, 358,

360, 367, 368, 370, 385, 398, 409, 413, 416, 417, 419, 421, 431, 432, 433, 435, 436, 437, 439
enthusiasm, 338
enuresis, 356
environment, 19, 31, 33
environmental factors, 27, 93
enzymatic, 172, 180, 187
enzymatic activity, 187
enzymes, 55, 179
epidemiology, 121, 320
epilepsy, 94, 96, 97
epithelial cells, 329, 330
epithelium, 19, 21, 46, 331, 399, 400
Epstein-Barr virus, 410
erectile dysfunction, 368
erythrocytes, 63, 70
Escherichia coli, 328, 345, 346
esophagus, 58
essential fatty acids, 422
esterase, 345
esterases, 117
esters, 186, 195
ethanol, 195
ethnic groups, 74
ethylene, 399
etiologic factor, 268, 272
etiology, 33, 41, 100, 168, 185, 344, 352, 356, 359, 380, 401
Europe, 73, 382
evacuation, 125, 127, 183, 190, 197, 200, 205, 206, 222, 226, 339, 352, 433, 437, 438, 439
evening, 211
evolution, 79, 155, 159, 191, 193, 200, 203, 326, 333, 336, 337, 359, 393, 404, 421, 423, 446
examinations, 360, 363
exchange transfusion, 180
excision, 268, 350, 355
excitability, 52
excitation, 47
exclusion, 108, 126, 152, 157, 396, 417
excretion, 55
exons, 90, 99
expertise, ix, 99, 311
exposure, 184, 186, 195, 231, 273
expulsion, 155
exstrophy, 427
extracellular matrix, 28, 31, 43, 44, 65, 71

F

faecal, 45, 55, 248, 345, 371, 392
failure, 39, 46, 61, 71, 76, 91, 95, 107, 125, 127, 187, 258, 290, 291, 301, 335, 350, 356, 379, 385, 386, 387, 392, 393, 394, 395, 401, 404, 405, 406, 407, 408, 409, 411, 417, 423, 426, 427, 456, 458, 462
failure to thrive, 76, 125, 290, 291, 336, 417
false negative, 151, 173, 178
false positive, 115, 150, 165, 172, 176, 178
familial, 65, 74, 75, 77, 87, 89, 91, 93, 94, 95, 96, 101, 104, 126, 134
familial dysautonomia, 96
family, 19, 21, 23, 28, 30, 42, 73, 75, 84, 88, 91, 95, 96, 100, 101, 126, 132, 200, 324, 337, 355, 357, 358, 360, 361, 363, 405, 431, 432, 444, 445, 448, 452, 454, 457, 458
family history, 95, 126, 132, 324, 355, 357, 431, 432
family life, 361
family members, 100, 405, 444, 452, 454, 457
family support, 361
fasciculation, 43
fasting, 60, 170, 210, 243, 432
fat, 420, 423, 426
fats, 417, 418, 421, 422, 423
fatty acids, 57, 401, 418
fear, 436
February, 443, 450, 453, 461, 462
feces, 225, 226, 252
feedback, 47
feeding, 185, 192, 236, 271, 335, 337, 385, 401, 420, 431, 434, 435, 436, 437
feelings, 362
feet, 96, 262, 264
females, 90, 92, 192, 223
fetal, 35, 38, 43, 44, 71, 186, 195, 345
fetal alcohol syndrome, 186
fever, 128, 201, 269, 270, 333, 431, 432, 439
fibers, 67, 70, 170, 172, 173, 174, 175, 178, 183, 280, 293, 359, 371, 375, 376, 378, 381
fibroblast growth factor, 43
fibroblasts, 47, 49
fibronectin, 32, 37, 65, 71
fibrosis, 127, 171, 185, 187, 188, 195, 226, 387, 393, 394, 400
filament, 23
film, 163, 276, 291, 335
fistulas, 283, 284, 404
fixation, 83, 196, 291

flatulence, 361
flexibility, 405
flora, 60, 210, 328, 330, 409, 418, 421
flow, 46, 68, 138, 139, 393
flow rate, 139
fluctuations, 141, 143, 150, 151, 152, 156
fluid, 161, 183, 185, 188, 193, 210, 243, 251, 290, 294, 335, 385, 391, 396, 421, 438
fluorescence, 18
Foley catheter, 138, 199, 208, 244
folic acid, 298
follicles, 176, 331
follicular, 118
food, 55, 60, 192, 201, 357, 362, 401, 432, 433, 435, 439
forceps, 116, 152, 170, 225, 245
frameshift mutation, 40
France, xv, 91, 101, 299, 308
free choice, 446
free will, 448, 458
freedom, 444, 455, 457, 460
freedom of choice, 444, 455
Freud, 82
fruits, 361
functional analysis, 42
fusion, 237

G

G protein, 38
gamma globulin, 400
ganglia, 15, 16, 20, 21, 26, 30, 32, 34, 37, 40, 55, 57, 59, 60, 61, 62, 64, 65, 69, 88, 92, 110, 115, 116, 117, 175, 178, 179, 189, 332, 359, 374, 375, 376, 377, 378, 382
ganglion, 20, 23, 31, 35, 37, 42, 57, 59, 61, 65, 67, 111, 114, 115, 120, 127, 169, 170, 172, 173, 174, 175, 178, 180, 183, 189, 192, 193, 262, 263, 276, 277, 283, 293, 294, 335, 355, 359, 371, 373, 374, 375, 377, 378, 379, 383
ganglioneuroblastoma, 85, 301
ganglioneuroma, 95, 105
gangrene, 180, 398
gas, 45, 185, 335
gases, 59, 225, 401, 432
gastric, 60, 185, 194, 210, 276, 386, 387, 392, 418, 420, 421, 423, 426
gastroenteritis, 333, 336, 436
gastrointestinal, xvi, 35, 55, 56, 57, 58, 67, 68, 79, 169, 185, 186, 229, 235, 301, 324, 328, 343, 345, 381, 385, 387, 388, 391, 392, 393, 396, 398, 407, 416, 427
gastrointestinal tract, 35, 55, 56, 57, 58, 67, 79, 169, 328, 381, 387, 391, 392, 398, 427
gastroparesis, 53
gastroschisis, 385
gauge, 296
GDNF, 24, 25, 26, 27, 28, 29, 36, 37, 38, 65, 90, 91, 102, 103, 300, 378, 383
gel, 329
gender, 325
gene, 19, 27, 28, 30, 31, 32, 35, 39, 40, 41, 42, 43, 61, 65, 70, 85, 87, 89, 90, 91, 92, 93, 94, 95, 98, 99, 100, 101, 102, 103, 104, 105, 290, 291, 300, 330, 345, 375, 378, 382, 383
gene expression, 19, 42, 345
gene mapping, 93
general anesthesia, 255, 259
generalization, 419
generation, 39, 44, 381
generators, 47
genes, 19, 26, 27, 30, 32, 33, 35, 42, 65, 66, 74, 87, 88, 89, 90, 92, 93, 96, 99, 100, 102, 105, 300, 330
genetic defect, 81, 375
genetic disease, 87
genetic mutations, 65, 290
genetics, ix, xi, 15, 37, 82, 87, 89, 100, 101, 102, 104, 105, 319, 344
Geneva, 425
genomics, 34
genotype, 27, 92, 95, 99, 104
gentamicin, 211, 231
geographical variations, 74
Germany, 135, 255
germline mutations, 102
gestalt, 90, 92, 96, 97
gestation, 32, 79, 88, 127, 185
gestational age, 150, 151, 154, 155, 156, 185, 299
GFAP, 23
GFP, 17, 25
Gibbs, 168, 301
girls, 196, 269, 272, 355, 362, 374, 384, 425
glass, 188
glia, 34, 35, 36, 38, 43, 57, 60, 68, 117, 378
glial, 15, 16, 22, 23, 24, 27, 32, 35, 38, 40, 44, 57, 65, 102, 378
glial cells, 15, 16, 22, 23, 24, 27, 57, 378
glial fibrillary acidic protein, 23
glial lineage, 23
globulin, 397, 400, 409

gloves, 232, 235
glucagon, 187, 195
glucose, 57, 70, 418
glutamine, 423
glycerin, 193, 276
glycerine, 432
glycol, 208, 209, 215, 216, 217
glycoprotein, 127
glycoproteins, 329, 330, 342, 345
glycosaminoglycans, 65
glycosyl, 27, 91
goals, 137, 358
goiter, 192
gold, 107, 118, 276, 306, 310, 311
gold standard, 107, 118, 276, 306
goodness of fit, 155
Gore, 388
GPI, 27
G-protein, 28, 92
grading, 326, 333, 334, 349, 383, 399, 409
grafting, 16, 21
grafts, 388, 389, 390, 392, 406
grains, 357
Gram-negative, 211, 336
green fluorescent protein, 17, 61
grouping, 349
groups, 28, 58, 61, 74, 75, 78, 134, 138, 155, 174, 230, 236, 237, 249, 250, 251, 269, 271, 272, 273, 299, 354, 357, 362, 363, 387, 392, 423
growth, 19, 26, 27, 32, 35, 36, 43, 91, 94, 98, 131, 186, 192, 236, 291, 296, 298, 300, 328, 358, 371, 385, 411, 414, 423, 424, 425
growth factor, 26, 43, 91, 423
growth factors, 91, 423
growth hormone, 423
guidance, 21, 35, 42, 43
guidelines, 82, 181, 194, 196, 211, 218, 375, 407
guilt, 458
gut, 16, 17, 18, 20, 22, 23, 25, 26, 27, 28, 30, 31, 32, 34, 35, 36, 37, 38, 39, 43, 44, 46, 47, 48, 49, 50, 52, 55, 56, 57, 58, 60, 61, 62, 65, 68, 69, 70, 78, 85, 105, 120, 143, 215, 217, 340, 346, 378, 382, 384, 385, 405, 410, 413, 421, 426

H

handling, 141, 200
hands, 96, 311
haploinsufficiency, 38, 91, 92, 96
haplotype, 91, 102
harm, 244, 438, 456, 457, 458
harvesting, 444
healing, 397
health, 345, 366, 443, 444, 445, 448, 449, 450, 452, 453, 455, 456, 458, 459, 460
health care, 366, 456
health services, 459
healthcare, 443, 444, 445, 446, 447, 448, 449, 450, 451, 452, 454, 455, 456, 457, 458, 459, 461, 462
hearing, 80, 95
heart, 42, 84, 92, 94, 96, 141, 210, 227, 400
heart rate, 141, 210
heavy metal, 160
height, 198, 245, 248, 414, 415, 423, 424, 432, 437, 439
helix, 23
hematoxylin-eosin, 359
hematuria, 222
heme oxygenase, 70
hemorrhage, 171, 178, 184, 391
hemorrhages, 399
hemorrhoidectomy, 354
hemostasis, 247, 249
hepatic failure, 393
hepatic fibrosis, 387, 393
hernia, 80, 184
heroin, 186
heterogeneity, 93, 96
heterogeneous, 19, 92, 95, 99, 100, 169, 344
heterozygotes, 92
high pressure, 50, 278
high risk, 203, 262, 332, 335, 392, 447
high temperature, 172, 174
high-risk, 394
hips, 231
Hispanics, 88
histochemical, 107, 115, 117, 118, 119, 121, 170, 172, 173, 176, 178, 180, 257, 339, 342, 345, 360, 370, 373, 378
histochemistry, 49, 62, 76, 117, 119, 120, 180, 181, 373, 376, 384
histocompatibility antigens, 239
histological, ix, 63, 67, 189, 191, 276, 277, 278, 285, 326, 331, 366, 373, 374, 376, 378, 382, 383, 399
histology, 120, 191, 328
histopathology, xi, 262, 263, 293
Holland, 91
home-care, 209
homology, 92
Hong Kong, 91

hormone, 49, 393, 423, 426
hormones, 49, 381, 426
hospital, 159, 165, 200, 203, 205, 221, 227, 252, 337, 338, 351, 396, 431, 432, 433, 434, 435, 438, 439, 446, 452
hospitalization, 129, 201, 208, 299, 321, 350, 351, 436
hospitalizations, 393
hospitalized, 210, 337, 403, 431, 437
hospitals, 200, 222, 236, 402
host, 26, 36, 328, 401, 402, 410
HSCR, 15, 23, 26, 28, 30, 31, 32, 33, 55, 61, 62, 63, 64, 65, 87, 88, 89, 90, 91, 92, 93, 94, 95, 96, 97, 98, 99, 100
human, 15, 30, 40, 43, 44, 48, 57, 60, 61, 69, 70, 92, 101, 103, 195, 284, 330, 337, 345, 346, 347, 375, 379, 382, 406, 408, 409, 444, 453, 454, 457, 458, 459, 461
human activity, 459
human dignity, 457, 458
humans, 29, 30, 60, 375, 386
husband, 432, 433
hydrate, 170
hydration, 215, 355, 439
hydrocephaly, 79, 98, 99
hydrogen, 421
hydrolysates, 420, 422
hydrolyzed, 420
hydronephrosis, 80, 192
hydrostatic pressure, 58
hygiene, 435
hygienic, 200
hyperalimentation, 358
hypercapnia, 95
hyperparathyroidism, 100
hyperplasia, 41, 63, 94, 118, 175, 176, 178, 183, 189, 375, 382, 436
hypersensitive, 333
hypersensitivity, 210
hypertelorism, 97
hypertension, 185, 391, 394
hyperthermia, 76
hyperthyroidism, 196
hypertrophy, 49, 375, 377
hypoglycemia, 185, 187
hypoperfusion, 416
hypopigmentation, 81, 92, 95, 97, 104
hypoplasia, 80, 81, 85, 96, 97, 98, 105, 118, 291, 301, 374
hypospadias, 80, 96, 97, 98
hypotension, 432
hypothesis, 26, 28, 327
hypothyroidism, 196, 324
hypotonia, 324
hypoventilation, 30, 40, 84, 90, 95, 97, 98, 104, 105, 133, 291, 370
hypoventilation syndrome, 30, 40, 84, 90, 104, 105, 291, 370
hypovolemia, 398
hypovolemic shock, 172
hypoxia, 95, 117, 151
hysterectomy, 452

I

IASA, 379
iatrogenic, 356
ICC, 46, 47, 48, 49, 50, 52, 67, 71
ice, 23, 172
identification, 16, 34, 92, 104, 105, 120, 180, 261, 369, 409, 456
idiopathic, 53, 164, 167, 287, 373, 401
ileostomy, 128, 129, 130, 201, 202, 203, 204, 205, 206, 210, 215, 227, 294, 296, 298, 336, 388, 392, 417, 418, 422, 425, 434, 435, 436, 438
ileum, 17, 25, 61, 62, 68, 78, 130, 134, 163, 166, 167, 185, 186, 189, 194, 203, 215, 225, 275, 276, 289, 291, 293, 295, 296, 298, 303, 332, 358, 381, 390, 417, 418, 422, 423, 424, 431, 435, 436, 437
images, 160, 459
imaging, 61, 84
immune function, 330
immune response, 324, 340, 399
immune system, 329, 332, 410
immunity, 191, 291, 331, 332, 346
immunocytes, 355
immunodeficiency, 98
immunoglobulin, 43, 329
immunoglobulin superfamily, 43
immunoglobulins, 331, 342, 347
immunohistochemical, 69, 71, 373, 375
immunohistochemistry, 62, 64, 70, 371, 373, 377
immunological, 16, 183, 327, 328, 331, 401
immunology, 403
immunoreactivity, 63, 103, 293
immunosuppression, 386, 397, 401, 403, 408, 410
immunosuppressive, 401, 406
immunosuppressive agent, 406
imperforate anus, 83, 134, 184, 193, 196
implementation, 128

impotence, 226
imprinting, 104
in situ, 25, 48, 61, 230, 239, 414
in vitro, 21, 23, 25, 27, 28, 29, 32, 36, 37, 38, 41, 405
in vivo, 21, 27, 28, 29, 32, 37, 38, 44
inactivation, 23, 91
inbreeding, 74
incidence, 26, 67, 73, 74, 75, 76, 77, 78, 79, 80, 81, 82, 87, 88, 89, 95, 100, 126, 127, 128, 132, 135, 136, 137, 152, 153, 156, 166, 178, 185, 202, 207, 211, 216, 238, 248, 252, 262, 269, 273, 289, 291, 297, 320, 321, 323, 324, 325, 328, 339, 351, 352, 355, 356, 357, 358, 359, 374, 376, 401, 439
inclusion, 386, 391, 395
incubation, 117, 121, 359
incubation time, 359
incurable, 116
India, 311
Indian, 82, 83, 134, 368
Indiana, xv
indication, 115, 132, 164, 202, 203, 271, 276, 342, 377, 394, 395, 419
indicators, 332
indices, 159, 164, 165, 166, 414, 416, 423
induction, 15, 211, 231, 262, 397
inductor, 403
inert, 160
infancy, 76, 131, 133, 196, 299, 309, 341
infants, 126, 127, 128, 134, 156, 157, 185, 188, 192, 193, 194, 198, 199, 200, 201, 202, 208, 209, 212, 213, 214, 215, 217, 230, 234, 238, 240, 256, 262, 271, 274, 275, 276, 282, 285, 289, 290, 297, 299, 301, 303, 307, 315, 316, 319, 323, 326, 328, 331, 335, 344, 346, 355, 358, 364, 365, 366, 377, 378, 390, 407, 408, 414, 417, 420, 422, 425, 426, 427, 438, 440
infection, 206, 207, 211, 218, 226, 236, 237, 238, 247, 249, 298, 328, 329, 336, 340, 351, 355, 358, 391, 395, 399, 400, 401, 408, 409, 410, 421, 431
infections, 184, 207, 211, 218, 226, 328, 331, 337, 388, 395, 398, 400, 410, 413
infectious, 210, 216, 290, 324, 327, 395, 420
inferior vena cava, 387, 395
inflammation, 117, 327, 332, 346, 408, 416
inflammatory, 185, 327, 328, 330, 332, 348, 355, 356, 375, 394, 399
inflammatory bowel disease, 348
inflammatory disease, 375
inflammatory response, 328, 355
inflation, 138, 141, 145, 147, 148, 149, 150, 152, 156, 379
informed consent, xi, 443, 444, 445, 446, 447, 448, 449, 450, 451, 452, 453, 455, 456, 457, 459, 461
infringement, 456
ingestion, 60, 193, 209
inheritance, 87, 88, 89, 90, 94, 96, 99, 103
inherited, 27
inhibition, 32, 45, 46, 49, 117
inhibitor, 21
inhibitors, 47, 408, 423
inhibitory, 29, 31, 47, 50, 58, 60, 62, 69, 151, 156, 157, 190, 191, 194, 197, 354, 378
inhibitory effect, 29, 31
initiation, 290, 331, 351
injection, 338, 379
injuries, 188
injury, 32, 185, 236, 354, 368, 399, 447, 455, 457
innervation, 15, 43, 46, 49, 53, 56, 57, 69, 70, 108, 109, 110, 115, 116, 117, 120, 169, 192, 195, 204, 293, 302, 306, 309, 345, 360, 370, 374, 376, 378, 379, 381, 382, 388
innovation, 310, 311, 349
innovative procedures, 311
inositol, 27
insertion, 425
insight, 50
inspection, 377
instability, 185
institutions, 171, 459
instruments, 221, 225, 226, 232, 255, 307, 362
insulin, 187
integration, 65
integrin, 29, 32
integrins, 32, 33, 43
integrity, 330, 354, 452, 453, 454, 460
intensive care unit, 433, 435, 436
interaction, 39, 55, 61, 65, 101, 405
interactions, 19, 27, 29
intercellular adhesion molecule, 32
interdisciplinary, 411
interface, 67
interference, 234
interferon, 324, 346
interleukin, 397, 403
interleukin-2, 397
interneuron, 46, 52
interneurons, 46, 47, 50, 59

interstitial, 34, 46, 47, 48, 50, 52, 53, 55, 58, 67, 70, 90, 92, 93, 101, 127, 133, 134, 293, 332, 346, 378, 379, 381, 384
interval, 177, 351
intervention, 150, 151, 153, 165, 166, 198, 200, 201, 202, 203, 211, 230, 243, 247, 248, 249, 250, 251, 252, 256, 258, 259, 320, 321, 326, 330, 351, 381, 444, 446, 447, 448, 449, 450, 451, 452, 455, 456, 457, 458
interview, 454
intestinal flora, 328, 330
intestinal obstruction, xi, 38, 55, 67, 125, 127, 129, 131, 132, 134, 137, 151, 153, 156, 161, 183, 186, 193, 196, 198, 200, 202, 203, 204, 210, 212, 227, 275, 276, 290, 291, 301, 325, 327, 328, 343, 355, 373, 374, 378, 380, 383, 384, 413, 417, 433, 435, 438
intestinal perforation, 130, 169, 188, 214
intestinal tract, 30, 119, 222, 229, 329
intestine, 15, 16, 17, 18, 19, 20, 21, 22, 23, 24, 25, 26, 27, 28, 29, 30, 31, 32, 33, 34, 35, 37, 43, 45, 46, 47, 49, 55, 60, 61, 62, 69, 75, 88, 125, 159, 163, 188, 193, 197, 198, 199, 200, 202, 203, 204, 206, 209, 213, 226, 229, 232, 245, 256, 289, 295, 297, 326, 327, 329, 330, 331, 332, 336, 345, 346, 357, 358, 381, 385, 386, 387, 389, 390, 391, 393, 395, 398, 400, 402, 404, 406, 407, 416, 417, 419, 422, 423, 431, 433, 434, 435, 438, 439
intimacy, 458, 459
intra-abdominal abscess, 336
intramuscular, 49, 58, 379, 384
intraoperative, 114, 115, 120, 121, 202, 203, 204, 214, 238, 239, 274, 315, 359, 435
intraperitoneal, 185, 400
intravenous, 141, 202, 207, 211, 212, 236, 278, 336, 337, 338, 355, 358, 398, 432
intravenous antibiotics, 211, 278, 336, 337, 432
intravenous fluids, 337
intravenously, 243
intrinsic, 26, 34, 44, 49, 52, 88, 169, 332
intussusception, 184, 215, 278
invaginate, 265
invasive, 24, 25, 32, 33, 138, 201, 230, 270, 271, 311, 328, 368, 450
Investigations, 120, 367
ions, 418
Ireland, xvii, 374
iris, 80, 84, 96, 97
iron, 127, 298, 300
iron deficiency, 300
irrigation, 128, 129, 188, 192, 197, 198, 199, 200, 201, 205, 207, 208, 210, 213, 215, 217, 223, 224, 225, 235, 236, 262, 277, 278, 282, 320, 337, 339, 340, 342, 431, 433, 435, 437, 438
irritation, 436
ischemia, 185, 356, 387, 398, 405
ischemic, 356, 398
Islam, 83, 301
isoforms, 32, 44
isolation, 75, 78, 88, 99
Italy, 91
ITT, 386

J

Japan, xviii, xix, 73, 81, 82, 100, 136, 212, 309, 322, 328, 343, 367
Japanese, 291
jaundice, 394
jejunum, 109, 195, 289, 387, 389, 417, 418, 420
Jordan, 40, 300
judge, 457
judgment, 284
Jung, 314
justice, 450
justification, 155

K

kidney, 34, 38, 44, 69, 80, 96, 385, 400, 406, 417
kidney transplant, 400
killer cells, 332
kinase, 27, 36, 37, 38, 65, 90, 100, 101, 102, 105, 290
knees, 231
knockout, 41, 375
Korean, 120, 181

L

L1, 31, 43, 145
L2, 145
lactase, 421
Lactobacillus, 338, 340
lactose, 338
lamellar, 59
lamina, 21, 63, 77, 107, 108, 112, 113, 116, 118, 119, 172, 173, 174, 175, 179, 293, 331, 332, 373, 374, 375, 376, 377, 379, 399

laminin, 28, 32, 39, 43, 44, 65, 71
language, 454
laparoscope, 263
laparoscopic, 115, 118, 206, 230, 240, 252, 261, 262, 263, 264, 271, 274, 306, 308, 309, 310, 311, 313, 315, 339, 349, 350, 351, 364, 365, 434
laparoscopy, ix, xi, 159, 160, 165, 227, 257, 261, 262, 264, 268, 269, 270, 271, 272, 274, 284, 285, 293, 339, 365, 433
laparotomy, 128, 165, 203, 204, 223, 227, 230, 244, 247, 252, 255, 276, 284, 285, 292, 293, 294, 336, 339, 350, 351, 435
large intestine, 31, 35, 60, 68, 214, 423
larynx, 97
latency, 51, 144, 145, 146, 147, 148, 152
late-onset, 105
latex, 138, 141
law, 444, 452, 455, 457
laxatives, 352, 377, 379
leakage, 262, 325, 356
leaks, 226, 229, 259, 306
lean body mass, 414
learning, 311, 431
legal protection, 446, 455
legal systems, 443
lesions, 92, 205, 327, 363, 393, 401, 402, 436, 438
lethargy, 185, 201, 319
leukocytes, 332
levator, 264
liberation, 223
lifestyle, 349
life-threatening, 385, 392, 393, 396
ligament, 297
ligand, 24, 27, 65, 91, 103
ligands, 27, 42, 91
likelihood, 356, 447
limitation, 389
limitations, 307, 354
linear, 17, 18
linkage, 91, 92, 93
links, 205
lipid, 393
lipofuscin, 380
liquids, 202, 206
liver, 297, 358, 386, 387, 388, 389, 390, 391, 393, 394, 396, 398, 400, 404, 405, 406, 407, 408, 409, 411
liver cirrhosis, 297, 394
liver damage, 393, 394
liver disease, 386, 387, 390, 391, 394, 407, 408, 411
liver failure, 358, 393
liver transplant, 387, 389, 390, 398, 404, 406, 407, 409
liver transplantation, 387, 389, 390, 398, 404, 406, 407, 409
localised, 25, 58, 59
localization, 69
location, 16, 36, 49, 145, 146, 167, 223, 227, 264, 276, 277, 279, 287, 325, 351, 459
locus, 30, 39, 87, 90, 91, 96, 102, 103, 104
London, xiii, 228, 308, 313
long period, 45, 74, 306, 423
longevity, 404
losses, 396, 417, 421, 432
lumbar, 243
lumen, 45, 50, 55, 58, 60, 206, 207, 211, 232, 265, 331, 332, 337, 393, 398, 400
luminal, 57, 144, 187, 329
lung, 217, 390
lying, 25
lymph, 118, 178, 331, 402
lymph node, 118, 178, 331
lymphatic, 176, 401
lymphocyte, 193, 332, 397, 399
lymphocytes, 331, 332, 397, 399, 401, 406
lymphoid, 331, 393, 395, 398, 409
lymphoid follicles, 331
lymphoid tissue, 393, 395, 398
lymphoma, 401
lysis, 325

M

machines, 44
macroglossia, 192
macronutrients, 423
macrophage, 346, 409
macrophages, 332
magnesium, 185, 417
maintenance, 27, 29, 30, 35, 36, 40, 91, 378, 397
malabsorption, 401, 417, 421, 422, 423
males, 74, 90, 92, 154, 223, 236, 283
malignancy, 410
malnutrition, 131, 132, 230, 236, 390, 414, 415, 416, 417, 419, 423, 424, 425, 437, 439
malpractice, 455, 456, 457
maltodextrin, 420
mammals, 28
management, ix, 53, 64, 71, 120, 135, 183, 194, 203, 213, 214, 229, 236, 239, 240, 270, 271, 272, 275,

283, 286, 287, 294, 297, 299, 300, 302, 310, 320, 336, 341, 343, 344, 349, 357, 365, 366, 369, 373, 377, 381, 386, 403, 405, 406, 408, 410, 411, 417, 419, 425, 427, 439, 440, 454, 455
mandates, 128
manganese, 393
manifold, 413
manipulation, 48, 197, 200, 207, 320, 334, 381, 430, 431, 432, 433, 435, 437, 438, 450
mapping, 93, 103, 339
mask, 174
maternal, 76, 185
matrix, 28, 31, 43, 44, 65, 71
matrix protein, 43, 44, 71
maturation, 127, 134, 155, 178, 378, 385, 405
MBP, 208
MCA, 90, 94
meals, 440
measurement, 114, 168, 181
measures, 128, 172, 174, 202, 206, 208, 338, 400, 404, 417, 423, 444, 452, 456, 458
meconium, 76, 107, 125, 126, 127, 128, 129, 131, 132, 134, 135, 137, 153, 154, 155, 161, 166, 169, 183, 184, 185, 186, 187, 188, 189, 190, 191, 194, 195, 197, 212, 290, 291, 301, 333, 334, 373, 377, 383, 431, 432, 434, 435, 437, 440
media, 121, 459
median, 143, 146, 148, 236, 237, 308, 321, 338, 351, 354
mediation, 36
mediators, 31
medical care, 125, 197, 198, 201
medical services, 448
medication, 283, 298, 351, 352, 363, 401, 432, 440
medications, 268, 398, 434
medicine, 432
medulla, 15, 95
melanocytes, 16
men, 74, 88
mental health, 365
mental retardation, 31, 41, 84, 90, 92, 93, 96, 98, 104, 133, 186, 203, 238, 268
mental state, 444
mercury, 170
mesenchyme, 16, 19, 20, 25, 27, 31, 32, 47
mesenteric vessels, 278, 279, 281, 282, 285
mesentery, 295
mesoderm, 19
messengers, 65
meta-analysis, 216, 217
metabolic, 187, 215, 330, 417, 425
metabolic acidosis, 215, 417, 425
metabolism, 98, 408, 421
metastatic, 395
methylprednisolone, 398
Mexico, xvii, 311
Mexico City, xvii
Miami, 388
mice, 15, 16, 19, 20, 21, 23, 24, 28, 29, 30, 31, 32, 34, 36, 38, 39, 41, 44, 61, 71, 103, 133, 331, 345, 346, 347, 375, 382
microarray, 31, 33
microbial, 217, 345
microcephaly, 79, 84, 94, 96, 97, 98, 104
microcirculation, 397
microcornea, 97
microflora, 211, 340, 393
microorganisms, 328, 329, 331, 400
microscopy, 379, 381
migration, 16, 17, 18, 19, 21, 22, 23, 24, 25, 26, 27, 28, 29, 31, 32, 33, 34, 35, 36, 37, 38, 39, 41, 42, 43, 44, 61, 65, 66, 68, 69, 85, 88, 105, 291
migratory properties, 24
milk, 184, 193, 196, 420, 432, 433, 435, 436
mimicking, 196
minority, 75
minors, 449, 453, 455, 459
misfolding, 91
misleading, 115, 117, 359
Missouri, 196
misunderstanding, 285
mitochondria, 380
mitotic, 24, 32
mixing, 60
MMCs, 60
modalities, 404, 405
modality, 309, 379, 390
models, 15, 27, 28, 37, 39, 52, 63, 67, 87, 101, 284, 375
modifier gene, 87, 91, 99
Mofetil, 397
molecular mechanisms, 15, 19, 42
molecular oxygen, 62
molecules, 21, 28, 32, 33, 43, 55, 58, 59, 65
monoclonal antibodies, 383, 397, 398
monogenic, 88, 93
monotherapy, 409
Moon, 410

morbidity, xi, 73, 75, 125, 201, 202, 206, 207, 289, 290, 294, 296, 299, 319, 321, 334, 337, 357, 362, 363, 370, 395, 396, 400, 421, 426, 427
morning, 210, 440
morphogenesis, 19, 27, 35
morphological, 19, 49, 376
morphology, 23, 58, 59, 64, 70, 71, 377
morphometric, 109, 178, 377, 383
mortality, 73, 75, 125, 169, 202, 206, 215, 238, 287, 289, 290, 291, 296, 299, 306, 314, 319, 321, 322, 327, 334, 337, 339, 340, 341, 342, 348, 349, 355, 357, 363, 389, 390, 392, 393, 395, 405, 421, 426
mortality rate, 169, 238, 289, 290, 296, 355, 395
mosaic, 95
mothers, 75, 76, 185, 186
moths, 237
motivation, 357
motor activity, 60
motor function, 127, 267, 268
motor neurons, 46, 47, 50, 58, 59
mouse, 15, 23, 31, 35, 36, 37, 38, 39, 40, 41, 43, 44, 61, 65, 68, 69, 70, 92, 101, 103, 346, 375
mouse model, 15, 39, 40, 101, 103, 346, 375
mouth, 435
movement, 61, 141, 152, 156, 170, 188, 236
MPS, 128
mRNA, 24, 28, 33, 62, 70
MTC, 94
mucin, 326, 330, 338, 342, 345, 346
mucoid, 185
mucosa, 21, 46, 50, 57, 77, 107, 108, 109, 116, 118, 119, 170, 172, 173, 174, 179, 183, 185, 189, 243, 244, 245, 246, 248, 249, 251, 252, 261, 264, 265, 273, 278, 279, 280, 282, 284, 309, 326, 327, 328, 330, 331, 337, 340, 346, 347, 376, 395, 400, 418
mucosal barrier, 327, 330
mucus, 326, 329, 330, 332, 340, 345, 431, 435, 436
multidimensional, 361
multidisciplinary, 352, 404, 411
multipotent, 94
multivariate, 350, 352
murine model, 35, 92
muscarinic receptor, 56
muscle, 20, 28, 31, 32, 39, 44, 45, 46, 47, 48, 49, 50, 52, 53, 55, 57, 58, 60, 62, 63, 65, 68, 69, 77, 187, 204, 223, 262, 264, 265, 280, 281, 293, 306, 307, 354, 374, 377, 378, 379, 380, 381, 384, 388, 405
muscle cells, 20, 28, 31, 32, 49, 50, 55, 57, 58, 379, 380, 381, 405
muscle contraction, 47
muscle relaxation, 62
muscles, 15, 45, 46, 47, 52, 108, 109, 110, 112, 115, 120, 192, 244
muscular dystrophy, 80, 98
muscular tissue, 52
musculoskeletal system, 79
mutant, 23, 27, 30, 39, 44, 70, 71, 375
mutants, 21, 29
mutation, 27, 28, 30, 39, 40, 41, 43, 84, 85, 91, 92, 93, 95, 96, 98, 100, 102, 103, 104, 105, 134, 359, 375, 378
mutations, 27, 28, 30, 39, 40, 41, 43, 65, 71, 89, 90, 91, 92, 94, 95, 96, 98, 99, 100, 101, 102, 103, 104, 105, 290, 300
myelomeningocele, 79, 96
myopathies, 99, 184
myopathy, 192, 196, 384
myosin, 58

N

NA, 81, 102, 213, 378
N-acety, 185, 189
NaCl, 422
NADH, 175, 179
narcotic, 186
NAS, 186
Nash, 120, 371
nasogastric tube, 210, 231, 235, 337, 415, 420
National Health Service, 443
natural, 39, 145, 146, 332, 333, 340, 341, 346, 368, 397, 423
natural killer, 332, 397
natural killer cell, 332, 397
nausea, 209, 335
NEC, 185, 186, 335
neck, 15, 109
necrosis, 172, 251, 326, 398, 400
neglect, 437
Neomycin, 243
neonatal, xi, 62, 75, 119, 125, 126, 127, 130, 131, 133, 134, 137, 138, 150, 151, 153, 154, 155, 156, 157, 158, 159, 160, 166, 169, 171, 172, 178, 181, 186, 187, 192, 194, 195, 197, 200, 201, 202, 212, 213, 227, 230, 236, 240, 251, 257, 260, 276, 284, 285, 286, 290, 292, 293, 294, 297, 312, 316, 320, 322, 340, 348, 373, 374, 377, 401, 411, 419, 440, 445

neonate, 32, 83, 85, 108, 113, 116, 118, 125, 127, 128, 129, 130, 131, 135, 184, 199, 200, 202, 209, 213, 290, 291, 292, 333, 346, 438
neonates, 76, 107, 108, 120, 127, 128, 157, 166, 167, 169, 171, 172, 178, 186, 191, 192, 193, 194, 196, 200, 201, 202, 208, 209, 210, 213, 214, 238, 240, 241, 275, 278, 282, 284, 285, 291, 293, 320, 323, 347, 364, 408, 426, 437
neoplasia, 81, 94, 101, 104
neoplasias, 397
neoplastic, 410
nephrotoxicity, 397
nerve, 32, 36, 44, 57, 58, 61, 62, 63, 70, 75, 77, 107, 108, 109, 110, 111, 112, 113, 115, 116, 117, 118, 119, 172, 173, 183, 293, 356, 359, 371, 375, 376, 378, 379, 401, 431
nerve cells, 36, 61, 107, 108, 110, 112, 115, 116, 117, 359, 431
nerve fibers, 70, 172, 173, 183, 293, 359, 371, 375, 376, 378
nerve structure, 119
nerve trunk, 62, 63, 293
nerves, 39, 56, 57, 60, 63, 69, 70, 108, 291, 356, 378
nervous system, xi, 15, 30, 32, 34, 35, 36, 37, 38, 39, 40, 42, 43, 44, 46, 47, 48, 49, 52, 55, 58, 59, 67, 68, 82, 83, 84, 87, 88, 114, 115, 120, 169, 176, 178, 181, 187, 196, 330, 375, 377, 382, 383
Netherlands, 295, 296, 308, 366, 382
network, 17, 19, 20, 32, 45, 46, 50, 52, 55, 57, 61, 63, 70, 359, 383
neural crest, 15, 16, 34, 35, 36, 37, 38, 39, 40, 41, 42, 43, 44, 60, 61, 65, 66, 68, 69, 71, 80, 83, 84, 85, 87, 88, 94, 95, 100, 103, 105, 291, 359
neural development, 31, 42
neural network, 45, 46, 55
neuroblastoma, 81, 85, 95, 97, 104, 105, 291, 359, 370
neuroblasts, 37, 108, 117
neuroendocrine, 15, 291, 293, 302, 330, 346
neuroendocrine cells, 15, 293, 330
neurofilament, 20, 22
neurogenesis, 38, 40, 65
neurogenic, 169, 192, 196, 379
neurogenic bladder, 192, 196
neurological deficit, 396
neuronal cells, 376
neuronal density, 382
neuronal markers, 22, 24, 377
neuronal migration, 43
neurons, 15, 16, 21, 22, 23, 24, 28, 30, 32, 34, 35, 36, 38, 39, 41, 43, 44, 46, 47, 48, 49, 50, 56, 57, 58, 59, 60, 64, 66, 67, 68, 91, 94, 133, 189, 376, 379
neuropathies, 189
neuropathy, 64, 190
neuropeptides, 58
neurotransmission, 47, 52, 58, 59, 381
neurotransmitter, 23, 47, 49, 59, 62, 63, 69, 133, 379
neurotransmitters, 47, 49, 58, 59
neurotrophic, 24, 65, 102
neurturin, 23, 36, 91, 103
neutrophils, 326
New York, 67, 68, 133, 311, 313
Newton, 40
nicotinamide, 359, 377
nicotine, 62
nitric oxide (NO), 22, 47, 49, 50, 58, 59, 62, 69, 70, 189, 293, 315, 338, 379
nitric oxide synthase, 22, 62, 69, 70, 189, 293
nitrogen, 426
Nixon, 133, 157, 195, 218, 313, 322, 341, 343, 345, 384
nodes, 17, 18, 20, 61, 174
non-adrenergic non-cholinergic, 69
non-invasive, 338
normal children, 208, 345, 353, 431
normal development, 375
norms, 361
North America, 210, 216
Norway, 308
NOS, 22, 62
nuclear, 30
nurse, 205, 438
nurses, 435, 436
nursing, 198, 199, 200, 201, 203, 209, 257, 258, 259, 339, 404, 430, 431, 432, 433, 434, 435, 436, 437, 438
nursing care, 199, 201, 339, 431, 432, 433, 434, 435, 436, 437, 438
nutrient, 385, 416, 419, 421
nutrients, 206, 393, 417, 418, 423
nutrition, xi, 198, 201, 227, 247, 296, 297, 299, 321, 385, 387, 393, 394, 403, 404, 405, 408, 411, 413, 415, 416, 420, 421, 423, 424, 426, 427, 437
nutritional disorders, 421
nystagmus, 80, 97

O

obesity, 96, 98
objectivity, 306
obligation, 446, 447, 448, 459
observations, 25, 28, 29, 92, 228, 310, 312, 354, 408, 424, 437
obstruction, 49, 55, 67, 116, 126, 127, 128, 129, 130, 131, 135, 183, 184, 185, 186, 188, 193, 194, 195, 197, 198, 200, 206, 230, 239, 247, 249, 275, 276, 281, 302, 305, 307, 319, 320, 323, 327, 333, 336, 353, 355, 356, 373, 375, 392, 401, 405, 407, 416, 419, 428
occlusion, 169, 170, 190, 191, 258
odds ratio, 155, 250, 251
oil, 199
old-fashioned, 310, 311
Oman, 74, 82, 136
omission, 207, 456, 457, 458
oncogen, 104
oncogene, 37, 41, 90, 100, 101, 102, 104, 105, 291, 300, 359
opiates, 186
opportunist, 400
opposition, 27
optimization, 405
oral, 49, 50, 60, 94, 170, 185, 189, 207, 208, 209, 210, 211, 212, 216, 217, 218, 283, 328, 338, 401, 415, 420, 422, 431, 433, 435, 436, 451
oral antibiotic, 207, 210, 212, 216, 218
oral antibiotics, 207, 210, 211, 212, 216, 218
organ, 19, 34, 38, 69, 280, 386, 390, 396, 400, 410, 426, 444, 457
organic, 192, 193
organism, 328, 330
orientation, 112, 116, 232, 233, 234
oscillation, 145
oscillations, 50, 141, 144
osmotic, 209, 401
outpatient, 270, 272, 351
ovaries, 234
overload, 200, 422
oxide, 22, 47, 50, 59, 62, 69, 70, 189, 283, 293, 315, 332, 338, 346, 432, 434, 440
oxygen, 62

P

pacemaker, 47, 48, 49, 52, 53, 67, 70, 143, 293, 381, 405
pacemakers, 58
packaging, 346
pain, 131, 132, 209, 210, 319, 351, 361, 401, 436
palliative, 455
palpation, 132, 223, 360
palpebral, 80
pancreas, 35, 387, 388, 389, 390, 391, 396, 406, 426
pancreas transplant, 406
pancreatic, 387, 390
pancreatitis, 391
paracrine, 33, 50
paradox, 99
paradoxical, 405
parameter, 75, 117, 144
parasympathetic, 15, 36, 56, 60, 63, 107, 108, 109, 111, 112, 113, 115, 116, 118, 119, 120, 173, 374
parasympathetic nervous system, 36, 56
parathyroid, 94
parathyroid glands, 94
parenteral, 211, 227, 247, 296, 297, 299, 321, 337, 385, 387, 393, 394, 403, 404, 405, 408, 411, 415, 416, 422, 434, 435, 436
parents, xi, xii, 75, 95, 200, 203, 205, 215, 236, 259, 298, 310, 337, 362, 363, 430, 431, 437, 438, 439, 440, 444, 445, 448, 449, 450, 452, 453, 455, 458, 459
Paris, xv, 52, 53, 253, 312, 314, 407
paternalism, 443
pathogenesis, 43, 46, 63, 65, 66, 119, 187, 320, 327, 328, 333, 341, 343, 345, 379, 382, 398, 410
pathogenic, 185, 330, 340
pathogens, 328, 329, 401
pathologic diagnosis, 230
pathologist, 70, 115, 203, 223, 262, 284, 285, 293, 294, 310, 360
pathologists, 286, 316
pathology, 79, 88, 132, 167, 168, 186, 197, 202, 227, 320, 326, 382, 409, 431, 433
pathophysiology, xi, 52, 55, 65, 119, 120, 133, 221, 319, 344, 346, 378, 379
pathways, 15, 27, 29, 30, 31, 37, 39, 56, 61, 65, 92, 101, 102, 157
patient care, 452
patient management, 71
patterning, 19, 21, 35, 43

pediatric, ix, xi, 71, 85, 121, 215, 216, 217, 218, 230, 289, 292, 294, 306, 308, 309, 310, 311, 341, 354, 355, 386, 389, 407, 408, 409, 410, 411, 425, 426
pediatric patients, 215, 217, 341
peer, 362
peer rejection, 362
peers, 362
pelvic, 16, 45, 171, 222, 229, 232, 235, 247, 248, 255, 275, 280, 281, 284, 291, 295, 306, 308, 309, 311, 335, 356, 360, 368
pelvis, 223, 234, 235, 243, 244, 256, 264, 278, 279, 280, 281, 284, 291, 335
penalties, 459
penetrance, 88, 89, 90, 91, 92, 93, 95, 99, 100
peptide, 47, 418, 419, 426
peptides, 28, 55, 59, 329, 426
percentile, 146, 148, 358, 361, 432
perception, 46, 405
perforated bowel, 130, 202, 326, 333
perforation, 130, 135, 171, 172, 185, 186, 187, 188, 200, 202, 213, 214, 258, 261, 262, 290, 300, 326, 335, 337, 400, 417, 438
perfusion, 138, 185, 296, 420
pericentromeric, 101
perinatal, 194
perineum, 232, 244, 263, 264
periodic, 193, 257, 439
peripheral blood, 401
peripheral nerve, 44, 57
peripheral nervous system, 16, 25, 30, 44, 91, 103
peristalsis, 55, 60, 62, 116, 120, 187, 252, 297, 332, 340, 378, 380, 381, 385, 431
peritoneal, 77, 171, 223, 232, 235, 244, 248, 264, 266, 278, 280, 281, 282, 307, 309, 350
peritoneal cavity, 278, 280, 281
peritoneum, 204, 206, 223, 244, 247
peritonitis, 185, 188, 236
permeability, 399, 400, 409
permit, 49, 107, 244, 359, 391
perseverance, 440
personal autonomy, 457
personal communication, 285
persuasion, 450
perturbation, 31
PGE, 210
pH, 117, 210, 421
phagocytic, 347
phalanx, 97
pharmacology, 404
phenotype, 24, 27, 28, 30, 32, 36, 43, 49, 65, 92, 95, 99, 103, 104, 375
phenotypes, 44
phenotypic, 58, 93, 105
pheochromocytoma, 81
Philadelphia, 134, 194, 364, 424
philosophy, 392
phosphate, 62, 208, 209, 217, 337, 377
phosphorus, 127
photographs, 459
physical health, 362
physicians, 179, 363
physiological, 45, 48, 141, 153, 160, 170, 174, 183, 200, 205, 221, 259, 307, 398, 405, 433, 438
physiology, ix, xi, 52, 157, 341, 367
physiopathology, xi, 306
pig, 36, 68
pilot study, 207, 217
pituitary, 47, 105
placebo, 347
placenta, 185
plasma cells, 331
plasma levels, 406
plastic, 49, 138
plasticity, 32, 68
play, 19, 23, 31, 32, 42, 65, 91, 293, 328, 332, 340, 379
pleasure, ix
plexus, 15, 16, 20, 21, 35, 48, 49, 50, 57, 64, 68, 92, 107, 108, 110, 111, 112, 113, 114, 115, 116, 117, 118, 147, 170, 172, 174, 179, 189, 283, 285, 356, 358, 359, 368, 371, 374, 375, 377, 378, 382, 383
point mutation, 28
point of origin, 60
poisoning, 200
polarity, 21
polydactyly, 80, 84, 96, 97, 98, 101
polyethylene, 208, 209, 215, 216, 217
polymorphisms, 91
polypeptide, 57, 69
polysialic acid, 43
poor, 64, 71, 85, 92, 99, 120, 151, 167, 237, 298, 301, 335, 353, 356, 361, 362, 371, 379, 393, 396, 420, 455, 456
population, 19, 24, 25, 27, 29, 61, 74, 75, 76, 77, 79, 83, 87, 88, 92, 93, 101, 302, 358, 361, 362, 392, 397, 405, 414, 423, 452, 453, 454
population size, 27
portal hypertension, 387, 391, 393
portal vein, 185

ports, 263
positive correlation, 353
postoperative, xi, 79, 115, 116, 120, 128, 133, 135, 191, 205, 207, 211, 216, 222, 223, 226, 227, 235, 238, 258, 267, 268, 270, 271, 272, 281, 282, 283, 284, 297, 305, 307, 308, 309, 311, 320, 321, 322, 323, 324, 325, 327, 332, 336, 337, 338, 339, 340, 341, 342, 343, 351, 352, 353, 354, 355, 356, 357, 358, 359, 365, 366, 370, 371, 432, 439
postoperative outcome, 267, 268, 270, 271, 283
postponement, 420
potassium, 216, 217, 417, 422
powders, 205
power, 326, 375, 447
prebiotics, 340, 348
preclinical, 359
precursor cells, 15, 16, 65
predictors, 168, 286, 352
predisposing factors, 400
preeclampsia, 185
preference, 165, 204, 236
pregnancy, 76, 431, 432, 434
prejudice, 449, 453, 454, 456, 457
premature babies, 155
premature infant, 156, 157, 173, 194, 335, 378, 408
prematurity, 185, 376
prenatal care, 431, 432, 434
preschool, 352
preschool children, 352
pressure, 25, 50, 51, 58, 130, 138, 139, 140, 141, 142, 143, 144, 145, 146, 147, 148, 149, 150, 151, 152, 156, 157, 160, 166, 170, 199, 210, 217, 263, 278, 281, 351, 353, 354, 450
presynaptic, 57
preterm infants, 194
prevention, 55, 211, 218, 283, 320, 340, 342, 410
prevention of infection, 211
preventive, 172, 174, 400
privacy, 444, 458
private, 450, 456
probability, 132, 155, 156, 392, 404
probable cause, 340, 422
proband, 93, 99
probe, 138, 139, 141, 142, 143, 149, 152, 156, 160, 166, 433, 434, 436
probiotic, 337, 340, 348
production, 22, 23, 25, 28, 32, 62, 91, 324, 330, 332, 337, 340, 346, 347, 368, 451
professionalism, 440
progenitor cells, 22, 36
progenitors, 22, 23, 24, 27, 28, 29, 30, 35, 36, 38, 40
progeny, 22
prognosis, 76, 78, 85, 93, 100, 120, 129, 299, 301, 371, 397, 421, 453
prognostic factors, 303, 407, 410, 427
program, 47, 140, 283, 355, 356, 407, 411
prolapse, 204, 206, 215, 225, 436
proliferation, 17, 19, 21, 24, 25, 26, 27, 29, 30, 37, 38, 39, 61, 65, 174, 330, 381
promoter, 30, 102, 345
propagation, 45, 47
property, 328
prophylactic, 100, 211, 248, 340, 433
prophylaxis, 207, 211, 212, 216, 218, 222, 231, 340, 347, 398, 400
propulsion, 308
prosecutor, 455
prostaglandin, 327, 337, 397
prostaglandins, 347
protection, 230, 248, 330, 446, 455
protein, 17, 21, 23, 24, 27, 30, 31, 32, 33, 40, 41, 43, 44, 58, 65, 71, 91, 102, 104, 184, 187, 193, 196, 270, 330, 399, 414, 420, 422, 423, 425, 426
protein hydrolysates, 420, 422
proteins, 21, 24, 27, 31, 381, 384, 417, 418, 420, 421, 423
proteoglycans, 32, 65
protocol, 64, 71, 359
proto-oncogene, 37, 41, 90, 100, 101, 102, 104, 105, 291, 300, 359
PSA, 31
pseudo, 186, 194, 373, 392, 401, 405, 407, 428
pseudocyst, 188
pseudomembranous colitis, 326
Pseudomonas aeruginosa, 329
psychiatric morbidity, 362, 363
psychiatrists, 404
psychosocial development, 361
psychosocial functioning, 361
PTFE, 388
ptosis, 80, 84, 98
public, 362, 445, 452, 455, 456
public health, 452, 455
public interest, 445
pulmonary hypertension, 291
pulse, 141
pus, 319, 326
pylorus, 417
pyramidal, 244

Q

QOL, 361, 362
quail, 16
quality assurance, 215
quality of life, 203, 226, 228, 303, 312, 342, 344, 349, 361, 362, 363, 364, 366, 369, 371, 393, 396, 403, 404, 407, 411, 437
question mark, 292
questionnaire, 268, 269, 272, 298, 350

R

race, 73, 88, 284
racial groups, 78
radio, 160
radiography, 162, 167, 190, 191
radiological, 163, 164, 166, 168, 183, 185, 186, 192, 193, 241, 277, 278, 285, 290, 291, 292, 300, 320, 326, 335, 341, 404
radiologists, 165, 292
random, 23
range, 41, 93, 94, 154, 155, 164, 227, 237, 283, 350, 417
rat, 32, 35, 36, 38, 39, 43, 67, 70, 346, 405
rats, 28, 29, 39, 43, 70, 332, 347, 375, 382, 426
reading, 165, 245
real time, 139
reality, 121, 382, 384
reasoning, 456
recall, 432
reception, 172, 174
receptors, 21, 27, 28, 31, 32, 33, 36, 38, 42, 49, 50, 56, 65, 92, 229
recognition, 43, 92, 93, 290, 355
reconstruction, 202, 206, 238, 370, 387, 388, 398, 404
recovery, 51, 143, 146, 148, 152, 310, 413
rectal examination, 235, 236, 248
rectocele, 354
rectosigmoid, 56, 57, 62, 159, 160, 163, 164, 165, 167, 168, 169, 190, 198, 199, 201, 202, 203, 231, 232, 240, 243, 252, 263, 265, 287, 300, 307, 309, 324, 334, 336, 363, 431
rectum, 45, 50, 51, 55, 56, 63, 76, 77, 78, 108, 110, 116, 117, 118, 119, 126, 127, 129, 130, 131, 132, 134, 141, 142, 143, 147, 156, 163, 164, 168, 173, 180, 187, 188, 196, 200, 202, 203, 207, 221, 222, 223, 224, 225, 229, 230, 231, 232, 234, 235, 238, 243, 247, 248, 255, 256, 257, 264, 265, 268, 271, 278, 280, 282, 291, 307, 308, 309, 310, 336, 350, 358, 363, 368, 378, 418, 430, 431, 438, 439
recurrence, 87, 88, 93, 99, 115, 324, 338, 402, 410
redundancy, 291
reflection, 77, 171, 223, 232, 235, 244, 248, 264, 266, 278, 281, 291, 307, 309, 350, 451
reflexes, 46, 49, 60, 137, 141
refractoriness, 51, 52
refractory, 52, 146, 149, 396, 398
regeneration, 32
regional, 19, 63, 92, 221, 444
registry, 386, 393, 402, 403, 405, 407
regression analysis, 355
regular, 143, 198, 201, 310, 352, 363, 377, 379, 399, 432
regulation, 20, 30, 31, 33, 40, 41, 42, 43, 52, 68, 102, 381, 443, 458
regulations, 444, 453, 454, 455, 457
rehabilitation, 405, 411, 415, 446
rejection, 201, 362, 397, 398, 399, 400, 401, 403, 409, 411, 439, 455
relationship, 75, 76, 87, 146, 151, 195, 324, 325, 362, 378, 443, 447, 448
relationships, 84, 445
relatives, 75, 88, 359
relaxation, 50, 51, 55, 60, 62, 125, 141, 143, 144, 145, 146, 147, 148, 149, 152, 156, 170, 257, 354, 379
relevance, 32, 159, 370, 426, 444
reliability, 107, 120, 138, 157, 159, 163, 164, 165, 166, 176, 177, 214, 239
remission, 226
remodelling, 20, 32
renal, 27, 96, 97, 208, 210, 385, 387, 390, 397, 406, 408
renal function, 406
repair, 294, 325, 354, 355, 358, 364, 385, 430, 437
reparation, 258
reperfusion, 398
repetitions, 47
reproduction, 444
resection, 64, 111, 114, 115, 116, 135, 192, 197, 221, 223, 224, 226, 247, 252, 256, 259, 260, 284, 287, 306, 307, 310, 325, 327, 339, 343, 359, 360, 366, 368, 377, 378, 379, 389, 395, 396, 408, 411, 413, 416, 419, 425, 426
reservation, 405
reservoir, 45, 358
resin, 337, 436

resistance, 50, 199, 211, 280, 337, 417
resolution, 138, 157
resources, 205, 284
respiratory, 95, 186, 210, 217, 395
respiratory failure, 217
retardation, 79, 94, 96, 98, 186, 298, 300, 423, 424
retention, 27, 45, 50, 131, 132, 185, 200, 229, 252, 259, 291, 326, 329, 421
reticulum, 47
retina, 97
retinoblastoma, 81
retinopathy, 96
returns, 235
revascularization, 388, 389
Reynolds, 299, 427
rhythm, 47, 146
right to life, 455
rings, 57
risk, 74, 87, 88, 93, 94, 95, 99, 102, 115, 118, 128, 135, 151, 172, 183, 186, 202, 203, 204, 207, 210, 211, 212, 214, 218, 238, 248, 249, 252, 262, 294, 296, 301, 303, 309, 320, 321, 322, 323, 324, 325, 327, 332, 335, 337, 338, 339, 340, 341, 342, 343, 344, 352, 355, 357, 358, 359, 367, 391, 392, 393, 394, 410, 415, 417, 420, 422, 447, 449, 451, 452, 453, 455, 456, 458
risk factors, 214, 218, 303, 320, 323, 325, 327, 340, 341, 342, 344, 352, 355, 367
risks, 236, 271, 284, 295, 306, 311, 446, 447, 450, 453, 454, 455, 456, 457
rituximab, 401, 410
rodent, 34, 69
rodents, 28
room temperature, 118
rotavirus, 351
rubber, 166, 244

S

safety, 132, 156, 199, 209, 215, 218, 238, 459
saline, 128, 129, 160, 185, 197, 199, 200, 205, 208, 209, 210, 216, 245, 262, 275, 337, 432, 433, 438
salt, 160, 408, 421, 422
salts, 401, 417, 421
sample, 75, 152, 155, 172, 173, 174, 178, 276, 357
sampling, 261, 359, 399
satisfaction, xi, 352
saturation, 141
scaffold, 18
scar tissue, 354
scarcity, 389
schema, 409
school, 361, 362, 396, 414
Schwann cells, 15, 57
sciatica, 432
scores, 269, 353, 354, 362, 414
search, 93, 347, 359
secrete, 328, 418
secretin, 418
secretion, 21, 47, 55, 209, 217, 329, 330, 338, 340, 346, 418, 423, 426
secrets, 459
security, 238, 256
sedation, 138, 140, 155, 157, 170, 351
segregation, 93
seizures, 98
selecting, 197, 271
self-concept, 362
self-control, 259
seminal vesicle, 232
sensation, 67, 350
sense organs, 79
sensing, 45
sensitivity, 48, 126, 146, 155, 156, 165, 172, 179, 183
sensorineural hearing loss, 95
sensors, 45
separation, 280
sepsis, 151, 171, 184, 227, 230, 258, 290, 294, 331, 333, 358, 393, 395, 400, 416, 417, 419, 421
septic shock, 326, 395
septum, 234, 235, 238, 307, 308
sequelae, 289, 329
series, 75, 77, 78, 79, 88, 89, 96, 115, 132, 141, 155, 172, 176, 177, 189, 201, 202, 203, 238, 258, 259, 271, 283, 289, 290, 291, 295, 297, 299, 305, 307, 308, 309, 310, 320, 321, 322, 323, 324, 325, 326, 350, 353, 358, 380, 385, 386, 401, 419, 425
serotonergic, 30
serotonin, 47
serum, 63, 141, 153, 170, 172, 174, 200, 205, 208, 210, 211, 215, 225, 269, 331, 337, 393, 399, 409, 422, 430, 432, 433
services, iv, 159, 203, 455, 459, 462
SES, xii
severity, 125, 268, 270, 299, 320, 339, 351, 352, 392, 437
sex, 65, 73, 74, 87, 88, 92, 93, 99, 102, 299, 355, 414, 415, 457
sex ratio, 93

shape, 165, 268, 272, 273, 292, 351
shock, 172, 185, 326, 333, 334, 337, 395
short period, 419
short-term, 379, 408, 421
sialic acid, 330
sibling, 75, 93, 99
siblings, 75, 82, 87, 93, 104
side effects, 447
Siemens, 139
sigmoid, 46, 47, 62, 64, 77, 88, 119, 161, 164, 168, 207, 224, 232, 249, 253, 258, 259, 261, 263, 264, 268, 269, 271, 277, 278, 291, 292, 293, 299, 302, 309, 310, 350, 377, 379, 383, 431
sigmoid colon, 64, 77, 88, 249, 261, 263, 264, 377, 379, 431
sign, 126, 129, 160, 187, 234, 235, 236, 292, 335, 454
signal transduction, 31
signaling, 30, 40, 41, 42, 43, 44, 91, 95, 102, 290
signaling pathway, 91, 95, 290
signalling, 27, 28, 29, 30, 31, 33, 35, 36, 37, 39, 42, 43, 65
signals, 19, 35, 42, 45, 46, 92, 140
signs, 171, 185, 188, 190, 191, 192, 204, 210, 236, 352, 356, 373, 394
silicon, 264, 265
silk, 223, 232, 278, 279, 282
sites, 20, 44, 58, 103
skeleton, 15
skills, 284, 459
skin, 28, 79, 81, 95, 97, 192, 204, 205, 283, 388, 402, 434, 435, 437, 438, 439, 440
sludge, 393
SMA, 386
small intestine, 16, 19, 23, 25, 28, 29, 36, 53, 57, 68, 88, 166, 192, 193, 199, 234, 289, 295, 296, 297, 347, 357, 358, 369, 409, 410, 413, 423, 426, 435
smooth muscle, 15, 20, 28, 31, 32, 39, 44, 46, 47, 48, 49, 50, 52, 53, 55, 57, 58, 62, 65, 67, 187, 293, 307, 378, 379, 380, 381, 383, 384, 405
smooth muscle cells, 20, 28, 31, 32, 49, 50, 55, 58, 379, 380, 381, 405
SNAP, 62
SNPs, 102
social activities, 361
social group, 75
social life, 354, 361
Social Security, xvii, 461
social support, 404
social work, 404
social workers, 404
sociological, 451
sodium, 209, 217, 338, 417, 418, 422, 423
soft drinks, 361
software, 139, 140
Sonic hedgehog, 19
South Africa, 134, 306
Spain, xiii, xiv, xv, xvi, xvii, xviii, xix, 91, 213, 228, 308, 443, 460
Spanish Constitution, 443, 458, 460
spastic, 129, 159, 363
spasticity, 97
spatial, 16
spatiotemporal, 27, 31, 34, 68
species, 398
specific surface, 401
specificity, 126, 155, 156, 157, 165, 172, 177, 179, 290, 335
spectrum, ix, 99, 104, 105, 211, 292, 329, 333, 393
speculation, 335
speed, 140, 156
sphincter, 45, 47, 50, 52, 58, 77, 88, 117, 121, 125, 141, 147, 150, 156, 157, 169, 170, 200, 225, 229, 245, 248, 256, 257, 258, 259, 264, 267, 271, 287, 305, 307, 308, 309, 316, 320, 327, 333, 338, 351, 352, 353, 354, 355, 363, 365, 367, 374, 377, 378, 379, 384, 432, 433, 438, 440
spinal cord, 57
spindle, 58
spine, 98
spiritual, 361
spleen, 388
splenomegaly, 391
sponges, 225
sponsor, 453
sporadic, 27, 65, 89, 91, 101, 102, 104
S-shaped, 358
SSI, 211
stabilization, 236
stages, 20, 22, 23, 28, 29, 32, 60, 68, 197, 204, 325, 326, 329, 350, 404
standard deviation, 269, 272
standardization, 257
standards, 459
Staphylococcus, 329
starch, 418
starvation, 426
stasis, 199, 327, 328, 332, 339, 355, 393, 398
statistical analysis, 139
statistics, 126

statutory, 459, 462
steady state, 50, 51
stem cells, 23, 27, 30, 39, 40, 44
stenosis, 97, 116, 184, 186, 204, 206, 226, 227, 248, 249, 257, 258, 268, 273, 283, 284, 309, 325, 327, 336, 338, 339, 340, 352, 360, 383, 399, 422, 436, 439
stent, 265
stereotypical, 49
sterile, 172, 174, 244, 262
stimuli, 51, 150
stimulus, 51, 141, 143, 144, 145, 146, 147, 149, 150
stock, 262
stoma, 128, 201, 202, 203, 204, 205, 206, 208, 210, 230, 232, 296, 297, 306, 320, 321, 322, 328, 336, 337, 339, 357, 360, 393, 419, 421, 427, 435, 438, 439
stomach, 16, 19, 27, 30, 47, 53, 57, 109, 387, 388, 391, 392, 420
strain, 331, 346
strategies, 210, 363, 403, 410
stress, 49, 164, 269, 271, 419, 437, 451
stressors, 362
stretching, 50, 271
strictures, 229, 294, 297, 298, 306, 356, 360
stroma, 58
stromal, 53
students, 307
subgroups, 59
subjective, 267, 273, 413
submucosa, 49, 50, 63, 92, 108, 113, 116, 118, 152, 170, 172, 173, 174, 175, 176, 178, 183, 189, 248, 261, 265, 276, 277, 293, 297, 319, 326, 332, 373, 376
substances, 55, 187, 340, 418, 421
substitutes, 425
substitution, 375, 378, 391, 397
substrates, 62
success rate, 295, 360
Sudan, 406, 407, 411
suffering, 100, 156, 323, 433, 453
sugar, 338
sugars, 55, 423
sulfate, 71, 209, 330
sulphate, 32, 160, 185
Sun, 36
supervision, 261, 262, 268
supplements, 423
supply, 246, 264, 296, 423
suppository, 276
suppression, 46
Supreme Court, 444, 446, 447, 448, 450, 451, 455, 456, 457, 458, 459, 460, 461, 462
surgeons, ix, xi, 159, 160, 165, 166, 207, 208, 209, 210, 211, 216, 221, 222, 223, 225, 251, 252, 271, 289, 305, 306, 307, 308, 309, 311, 351, 353, 355, 360, 404, 436
Surgeons, 207, 280, 310
surgeries, 398
surgical intervention, 150, 151, 153, 230, 381, 443, 451, 457
surprise, xi, 311
surveillance, 218, 355
survival, 19, 27, 30, 36, 38, 65, 91, 117, 290, 303, 358, 403, 405, 406, 411
survival rate, 358
surviving, 290
susceptibility, 87, 89, 90, 92, 93, 96, 99, 328, 330, 340, 387
susceptibility genes, 92, 99
suture, 206, 215, 233, 234, 235, 244, 245, 248, 253, 256, 257, 258, 282, 295, 296, 314, 335
swallowing, 60
sweat, 187, 188
sweat chloride test, 188
sweat test, 187
Sweden, 307, 410
sweets, 361
swelling, 87
Switzerland, xiv, xvii, xix
symbiotic, 338
sympathetic, 15, 37, 56, 57, 60, 95, 374, 401
symptom, 131, 187, 188, 377
symptoms, 62, 63, 67, 77, 81, 95, 125, 126, 129, 131, 132, 133, 153, 186, 187, 192, 193, 196, 198, 201, 202, 203, 251, 252, 297, 313, 333, 334, 337, 338, 346, 352, 356, 360, 361, 366, 368, 373, 374, 377, 381, 435, 437, 439
synapse, 50, 384
synapses, 46, 49, 70
synaptic plasticity, 32
synaptic transmission, 59
synbiotics, 347
syndrome, 26, 30, 31, 40, 41, 65, 81, 83, 84, 85, 90, 92, 93, 95, 96, 100, 103, 104, 105, 110, 117, 127, 128, 129, 135, 164, 184, 185, 186, 187, 192, 194, 195, 196, 200, 203, 214, 227, 241, 275, 276, 291, 296, 299, 301, 321, 323, 324, 333, 346, 357, 358, 369, 370, 373, 380, 384, 386, 392, 394, 395, 396, 398, 407, 408, 411, 421, 425, 426

synthesis, 25, 62, 408, 420
systems, 29, 60, 65, 94, 137, 349, 362, 443

T

T lymphocytes, 397
tacrolimus, 397, 408, 409
talc, 432, 440
target population, 29
targets, 21, 57
tau, 61
T-cell, 324, 346
teaching, 453
technology, 230
teenagers, 353, 362
temperature, 160, 185, 210
temporal, 16, 39, 52
tenascin, 44, 65, 71
tension, 46, 62, 204, 232, 238, 249, 264, 265, 282, 283, 433
terminals, 50, 58
territory, 15
testes, 80
TGF, 31, 91
Thai, 196
thawing, 107, 117, 119
therapeutics, 102
therapy, 100, 136, 169, 195, 210, 211, 228, 229, 230, 243, 251, 312, 338, 343, 347, 349, 355, 363, 370, 392, 427, 450
Thomson, 52
thoracic, 84, 97, 387
threat, 328
threatened, 415
threatening, 217, 396, 457
three-dimensional, 64, 371
three-dimensional reconstruction, 371
threshold, 26, 27, 146, 149
thresholds, 57
thrombocytopenia, 393
thrombosis, 387, 395
thrombotic, 408
thyroid, 81, 87, 94, 97, 102, 104, 196, 291, 301, 359
thyroid cancer, 94, 97
thyroid carcinoma, 81, 87, 94, 102, 104, 291, 301, 359
thyroid gland, 196
time consuming, 262
time periods, 257, 398
timetable, 16
timing, 47, 326
tissue, 15, 18, 24, 25, 26, 39, 42, 44, 47, 52, 58, 120, 180, 192, 261, 276, 280, 332, 342, 354, 373, 381, 388, 393, 395, 398, 399, 402
tissue plasminogen activator, 44
T-lymphocytes, 331, 332
tobacco, 256
toddlers, 352, 353
toilet training, 357, 363
Tokyo, xviii, xix
tolerance, 193, 210, 385, 411, 420, 422, 433, 435
tonic, 47, 63
tonometry, 157, 158
total parenteral nutrition, 299, 385, 405
toxic, 76
toxicity, 210, 337, 393, 397
toxin, 328, 337, 338, 344, 352, 379, 384
toxins, 329, 330, 331, 337, 340, 347
traction, 232, 244, 245, 255, 256, 263, 264, 278, 279, 280, 281, 282
trade, 209
tradition, 311
training, 311, 357, 363, 404, 440
trait anxiety, 362
trans, 58, 277, 282, 284
transcription, 19, 23, 29, 30, 40, 65, 92, 102
transcription factor, 19, 23, 29, 30, 40, 65, 92
transcriptional, 33, 41
transducer, 138, 140
transduction, 346
transection, 224
transfer, 433, 459
transformation, 91
transfusion, 171
transgenic, 16, 18, 20, 24, 34, 61
transgenic mice, 16
transgenic mouse, 61
transition, 62, 64, 79, 108, 127, 128, 129, 130, 159, 160, 163, 164, 165, 167, 168, 170, 183, 187, 188, 190, 191, 193, 203, 204, 223, 232, 291, 292, 293, 294, 297, 301, 325, 336, 351, 356, 359, 360, 371, 433, 435
translocation, 327, 332, 338, 340, 395, 398, 400, 409, 421
transmembrane, 27, 28, 42
transmission, 46, 49, 59, 74, 87
transplant, xi, 297, 386, 387, 388, 389, 390, 391, 393, 395, 397, 398, 402, 403, 406, 408, 409, 410, 423, 444
transplant recipients, 406, 410

transplantation, 297, 303, 358, 369, 386, 387, 388, 389, 390, 391, 392, 393, 396, 397, 403, 404, 405, 406, 407, 408, 409, 410, 411, 428
transport, 46, 55, 60, 91, 443
transport processes, 46
transportation, 172
transverse colon, 62, 163, 169, 293
transverse section, 18
trauma, 271, 329, 339
trial, 212, 216, 217, 218, 347, 453, 454
trigeminal, 42
triggers, 45
triglycerides, 418, 420
trisomy, 83, 91, 93, 133, 214, 238, 323, 332, 343, 355, 357, 369
trisomy 21, 83, 91, 93, 133, 214, 323, 332, 343, 355, 357, 369
tubal ligation, 452
tumor, 48, 396
tumors, 53, 291, 307, 395, 402
tumour, 95, 200
tumours, 30, 79, 81, 94, 95
twins, 434
tyrosine, 21, 27, 36, 37, 38, 58, 65, 90, 100, 102, 105, 290
tyrosine hydroxylase, 21

U

Ukraine, 253, 315
ulceration, 319, 326, 327, 335, 399
ulcerative colitis, 326, 342
ultrasound, 126, 431
umbilical hernia, 192
uncertainty, 285, 374
underreported, 353
undifferentiated cells, 23
unfolded, 281
uniform, 19, 26, 138, 165
United Kingdom, xiii, 357
updating, 443
ureter, 264
ureters, 232, 234
urethra, 223, 244, 245, 280
urinary, 84, 101, 231, 235, 259, 263, 286, 313, 356, 369, 380, 381, 432, 433
urinary bladder, 231, 380, 381
urinary dysfunction, 356
urinary tract, 84, 101, 313, 356, 357
urine, 417, 422
Uruguay, 218
uterus, 381

V

vaccinations, 436
vaccine, 436
vacuum, 431
vagal nerve, 57
vagal preganglionic neurons, 56
vagina, 223, 280
vagus, 56, 109
vagus nerve, 56
Valencia, 460
validity, 174
values, 111, 145, 155, 177, 415, 422
vancomycin, 328, 336, 337, 347
variability, 79, 84, 104, 374
variable expressivity, 88
variables, 73, 75, 77, 163, 414, 423, 424
variation, 39, 74, 147, 181, 189, 195, 307, 309, 355, 375
vas deferens, 245, 280
vascularization, 295
vasculature, 382
vasoactive intestinal peptide, 47
vasoactive intestinal polypeptide (VIP), 57, 58, 69
vector, 287, 316, 365
vein, 172, 223, 387, 390
velocity, 45
ventilation, 301
versatility, 287
vertebrates, 15, 21, 60
very low birth weight, 194
vessels, 92, 223, 225, 244, 245, 255, 256, 264, 271, 278, 280, 309, 310, 375, 388
videotape, 139
viral gastroenteritis, 437
virus, 401, 410
virus infection, 410
viruses, 329, 336
viscera, 34, 381, 387, 391
viscoelastic properties, 329
viscosity, 188
visible, 141, 439
vision, 80
visual acuity, 451
visualization, 127, 129
vitamin B1, 298, 417, 421, 422
vitamin B12, 298, 417, 421, 422

vitamins, 422
voiding, 306, 384
volvulus, 79, 83
vomiting, 125, 126, 128, 129, 131, 132, 161, 185, 186, 187, 188, 201, 209, 210, 290, 333, 334, 335, 431, 432, 439
VSD, 97
women, 74, 75, 88, 186
workers, 76, 80, 207, 209, 211, 320, 323, 324, 332, 333, 335, 339
World Health Organization, 425
worry, 434
wound infection, 211, 218, 238, 358
writing, 444, 449, 450, 453, 454

W

waking, 440
Wales, 82, 136, 168, 286, 287
warrants, 358, 399
waste products, 55, 60
water, 139, 157, 187, 200, 209, 217, 295, 329, 337, 358, 417, 418, 419, 422, 423, 432, 436, 440
water-soluble, 187, 422
weakness, 98
wealth, 398
weight gain, 215, 414, 416, 422, 425
Weinberg, 70, 85
welfare, 443
well-being, 363
western countries, 311
Western countries, 73
wetting, 356
white blood cell count, 269, 270, 331
withdrawal, 401, 423

X

X chromosome, 23
X-linked, 99
X-rays, 160

Y

yeast, 340, 361
yield, 172
young adults, 350, 361, 362

Z

zebrafish, 42
zinc, 31, 283, 417, 432, 434, 440
zinc oxide, 283, 432, 434, 440